# Chinese Natural Cures

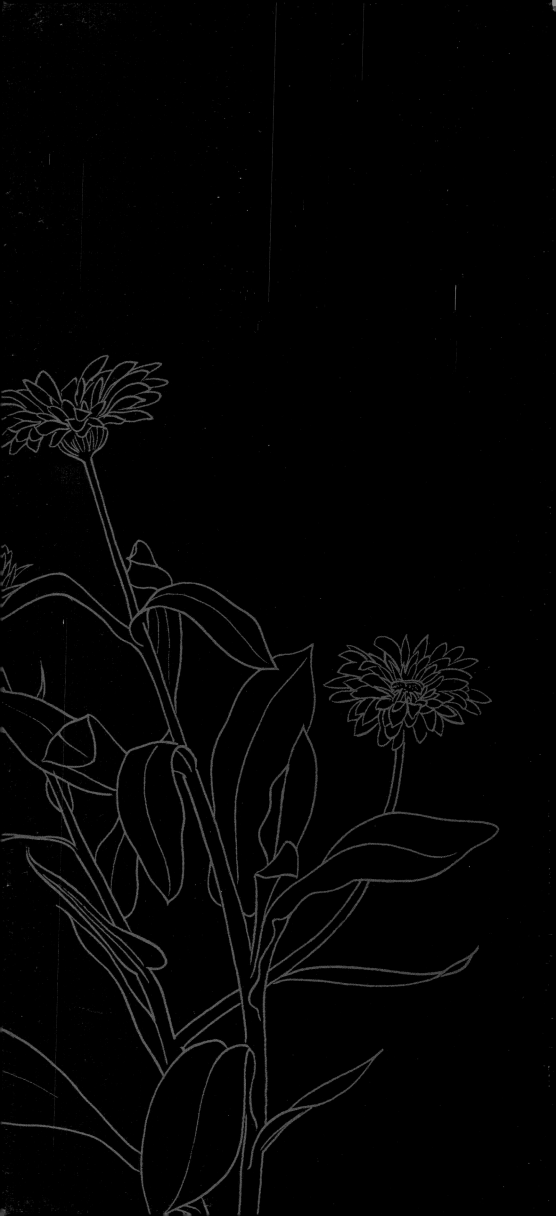

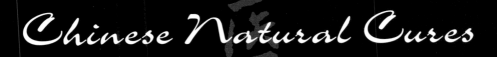

# Chinese Natural Cures

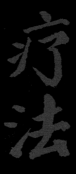

Henry C. Lu

BLACK DOG
& LEVENTHAL
PUBLISHERS
NEW YORK

Published by
Black Dog & Leventhal Publishers, Inc.
151 West 19th Street
New York, NY 10011

Distributed by
Workman Publishing Company
708 Broadway
New York, NY 10003

Text design by Alleycat Design, Inc.
Cover design by 27.12 Design Ltd.

Book manufactured in Hong Kong

ISBN: 1-57912-056-3

h g f e d c b

Library of Congress Cataloging-in-Publication Data

Lu, Henry C.
    Chinese natural cures / Henry C. Lu.
        p.   cm.
    Includes bibliographical references and index.
    ISBN 1-57912-056-3
    1. Medicine, Chinese.        I. Title.
R601.L8748            1999
610'.951--dc21                                98-50126
                                             CIP

*H*enry C. Lu received his Ph.D. degree from the University of Alberta, Edmonton, Canada. He taught at the University of Alberta and the University of Calgary between 1968 and 1971 and has practiced Chinese medicine since 1972. Dr. Lu now teaches Chinese medicine by correspondence. His students live in many countries, including the United States, Canada, England, Australia, Sweden, Italy, Germany, France, New Zealand, Switzerland, Mexico and Japan.

The author is best known for his translation of *Yellow Emperor's Classic of Internal Medicine* from Chinese into English. This translation and Dr. Lu's seven other books are recommended by the Board of Acupuncture Examiners in the United States and used widely in preparation for acupuncture licensing examinations.

Dr. Lu lectures extensively in the United States and maintains close contacts with the developments of Chinese medicine in China, Japan, Taiwan and Hong Kong. He has taken groups of Western doctors to study Chinese medicine in China and Taiwan and has helped many distinguished Western physicians establish themselves as outstanding practitioners of herbalism, acupuncture and manipulative therapy. In March 1982, while leading a group of Western acupuncturists, Dr. Lu was honored for his knowledge of Chinese medical philosophy by Professor Zhao at the Canton College of Traditional Chinese Medicine.

He has received many awards from acupuncture organizations in the United States and Europe. Dr. Lu is a patron of Brisbane College of Traditional Acupuncture and Oriental Medicine in Queensland, Australia, an honorary professor of the Academy of Science for Traditional Chinese Medicine in Victoria, British Columbia and an honorary member of the Acupuncture Association of British Columbia.

Dr. Lu lives in British Columbia with his wife, Janet, their son, Albert and daughter, Magnus. Correspondence with Dr. Lu should be addressed to: International College of Traditional Chinese Medicine of Vancouver, Suite 201, 1508 West Broadway, Vancouver, B.C., Canada, V6J 1W8. The web site for the International College can be found at http://www.tcmcollege.com.

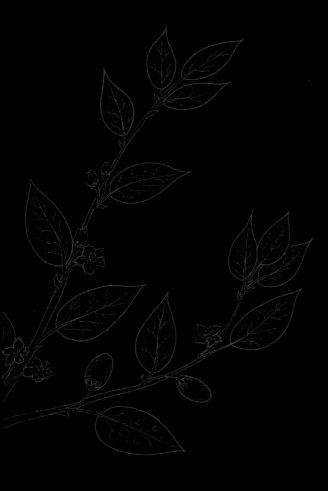

# Table of Contents

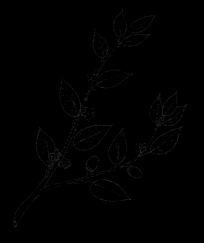

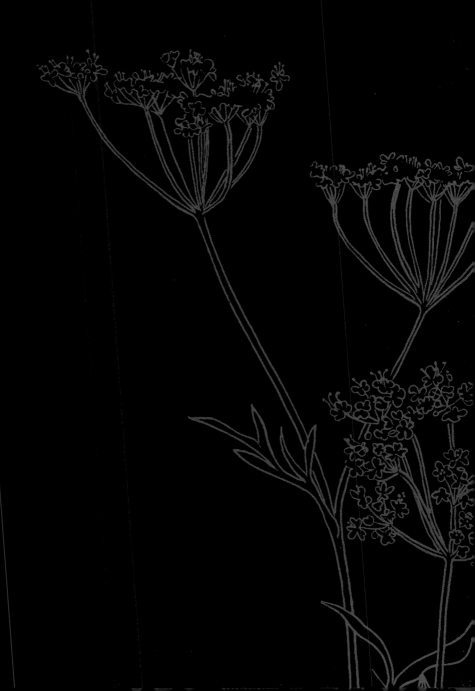

# Philosophy & Methods

Although traditional Chinese medicine is as old as Chinese history itself, if it is new to you, you will likely have many questions about this type of medicine and what it can offer you for your good health. This brief overview of its philosophy and components will help you understand it quickly.

Traditional Chinese medicine includes four distinct methods of treatment: herbology, acupuncture, manipulative therapy and food cures. In addition, it encompasses the remedial exercises *qi-gong* and *tai-ji*.

In China, virtually all kinds of disorders are treated by traditional Chinese medicine. Some disorders may be more effectively treated by acupuncture, others by herbs; still others may be best treated by food cures. In general, pain and muscular symptoms are more effectively treated by acupuncture, skin diseases and diseases of internal organs by herbs. However, it is necessary for a doctor of traditional Chinese medicine to make a diagnosis before deciding what type of treatment would be most effective for a particular patient. When a Western doctor tells a patient that

# The System of Traditional Chinese Medicine

Traditional Chinese medicine goes back over 3,000 years. It was not developed by any particular individual; rather, it grew out of the necessity of maintaining good health among the Chinese people. The ancient Chinese, like all of us, had to struggle against diseases in order to stay in good health. In the process, they came to see the benefits of consuming herbs (known as Chinese herbology today), inserting needles in the body (known as Chinese acupuncture today), eating the right foods (known as Chinese food cures today), massaging the body (known as Chinese manipulative therapy today) and exercising the body (known as *qi-gong* and *tai-ji*).

Today, traditional Chinese medicine is practiced in China side by side with modern Western medicine. There are as many hospitals of traditional Chinese medicine as modern hospitals of Western medicine. From the Chinese point of view, traditional Chinese medicine is on an equal footing with Western medicine; in fact, many Chinese value traditional Chinese medicine over Western medicine.

You may ask why we need traditional Chinese medicine when modern, scientific medicine is available to all of us. The reason is that many diseases and ailments that cannot be cured by Western medicine can be treated by traditional Chinese medicine successfully. It is a fact that many patients experience instant relief of pain when treated with Chinese acupuncture, which cannot be achieved by Western medicine. In addition, traditional Chinese medicine has proven superior to Western medicine in the treatment of skin, liver and kidneys diseases, as well as many other diseases.

When you go to see a doctor of traditional Chinese medicine, the doctor will observe your complexion and look at your tongue, take your pulse and ask you many questions about your symptoms, your eating habits and your food preferences. Then the doctor will come up with a diagnosis of what is wrong with your body and tell you whether you need acupuncture or herbs and what foods are good for you.

there is no cure for a certain disease, it does not necessarily mean that the disease in question cannot be cured by treatments in traditional Chinese medicine either; it only means that there is no cure for the disease by methods of Western medicine.

There are a number of basic differences between the two distinct types of medicine. First of all, Western medicine focuses more on the treatment of symptoms, whereas traditional Chinese medicine focuses more on causes. Western medicine is more useful for first aid and surgery, while traditional Chinese medicine is more useful in treating skin and internal diseases and chronic cases in particular. Many remedies in Western medicine are based upon the results of experiments with animals which may not be effective with the human body. But remedies in traditional Chinese medicine are based upon successful experiences in clinical practice, which are more reliable. Most Western chemical drugs are strong and tend to produce serious side effects. On the other hand, Chinese herbs, acupuncture and food cures are less drastic, can be longer-lasting in effects and, when used the right way, generally do not produce side effects.

Although traditional Chinese medicine and Western medicine operate very differently, it is wise to consult a Western medical doctor in order to get a diagnosis, which may be of some use to a doctor of traditional Chinese medicine and to get the best possible medical care available in modern society.

Traditional Chinese medicine is based, first and foremost, on a classic published in the third century B.C., entitled *Nei-Jing*, or *The Yellow Emperor's Classics of Internal Medicine*. Western medical books often become obsolete in the course of time (most likely within a few years), but many books on traditional Chinese medicine written by Chinese physicians in the past have become timeless classics. The following passage from the above-mentioned celebrated classic may shed some light on the nature of Chinese medicine: "The disease of the five viscera may be compared to a sharp needle in the skin, a stained chair, a knot, or a deposit of mud and sand in a river. One can still remove a needle from the skin, no matter how long ago it was used to prick the body. One can still wash off a stain, no matter how long it has been on the chair. One can still untie a knot, no matter how long ago it was tied. One can still remove a deposit of mud and sand in a river, no matter how long it has been there. Some people assume that a disease cannot be cured, simply because it has a long history, but the truth of the matter is that an outstanding physician can cure a disease for the same reason that one can pull a needle from the skin, wash off a stain from the chair, untie a knot, or clear the blockage from a river. A chronic disease with a very long history can still be cured and those who think otherwise have not really mastered the art of acupuncture."

*It is a fact that many patients experience instant relief of pain when treated with Chinese acupuncture, which cannot be achieved by Western medicine.*

## Philosophy

### YIN AND YANG

Yin and yang are the two most fundamental concepts in Chinese medical philosophy. Rooted in ancient Chinese philosophy, these two opposing concepts are used to account for changes in the universe in a comprehensive manner.

In anatomy, the human body is divided into yin and yang as follows: The internal region is yin, while the external region is yang; the five viscera are yin, while the six bowels are yang; and the tendons and bones are yin, while the skin is yang. In physiology, yin stands for storage of energy, while yang stands for human activities, because yin stays within like a traditional housewife while yang stays in the superficial region to guard against foreign invasion.

In pathology, yin and yang are used to describe two basic patterns of change. When yin wins a victory, yang will be diseased; when yang wins a victory, yin will be diseased. When yang wins a victory, there will be fever; when yin wins a victory, there will be chill. When yang is in deficiency, it will cause chill sensations in the superficial region; when yin is in deficiency, there will be internal heat. In diagnosis, yin and yang symptoms are used to describe the nature of a disease. According to *The Yellow Emperor's Classics of Internal Medicine*," a good physician who has mastered the technique of diagnosis will examine the patient's color and take his pulse and he will classify all symptoms into yin and yang as the first step in making a diagnosis."

In terms of treatment, striking a balance between yin and yang is the most fundamental principle of clinical practice. Among the treatments based on this principle are sedating the excess and toning up the deficiency. *The Yellow Emperor's Classics of Internal Medicine* states, "A hot disease should be treated by cold herbs; a cold disease should be treated by hot herbs….Yin should be treated in a yang disease, yang should be treated in a yin disease."

### THE FIVE ELEMENTS

The five elements are a concept in ancient Chinese philosophy referring to the nature of materials as well as their interrelationships. The concept was later introduced into Chinese medical philosophy for clinical applications. The five elements refer to wood, fire, earth, metal and water. In Chinese medical philosophy, the five-elements theory consists of four laws governing the relationships among the five materials.

According to this theory, the five viscera are viewed as the key organs and the four laws are applied to them. The four laws are the laws of production, control, attack and resisting control. The correspondence between the five elements and the five viscera is as follows: Wood corresponds to the liver, tendons and eyes. Fire corresponds to the heart, blood vessels and tongue. Earth corresponds to the spleen, flesh and mouth. Metal corresponds to the lungs, skin, hair and nose. And water corresponds to the kidneys, bones and ears.

The laws of production and control are used to illustrate the interrelationships among the viscera. For instance, the liver controls the spleen (which is called wood controlling earth), the spleen produces the lungs (which is called earth producing metal) and the lungs control the liver (which is called metal controlling wood). Thus, there are patterns of relationship among the five viscera according the laws.

The laws of attack and resisting control are used to describe pathological changes as well as methods of treatment. For example, since liver disease will affect the spleen, it is called wood attacking earth and should be treated by inhibiting wood and supporting earth. And in treating lungs energy deficiency syndrome, it is necessary to strengthen the spleen and tone up the lungs, which is called developing earth in order to produce metal.

The five-elements theory is based upon clinical experiences and very useful in clinical practice. The four laws of the theory can be summarized as follows:

The first law, the law of production, states that one organ can produce another organ, which indicates a mother-child relationship between the two organs. The mother organ is capable of assisting the child organ in its capacity for growth and nourishment. According to this law, wood produces fire, fire produces earth, earth produces metal, metal produces water and water produces wood.

*When yin wins a victory, yang will be diseased; when yang wins a victory, yin will be diseased.*

*When yang wins a victory, there will be fever; when yin wins a victory, there will be chill.*

The law of control states that one organ can control another organ. According to this law, wood controls earth, earth controls water, water controls fire, fire controls metal and metal controls wood.

The law of attack states that one organ can attack another organ, which means that one organ may abuse its power of control and attack another organ. Thus, an abuse of the second law will lead to the application of this third law. As an example, when the energy of wood is in excess and, at the same time, metal fails to control wood properly, wood will manage to attack earth, which may cause liver-wood in excess with spleen-earth in deficiency. The law of attack falls within the context of pathology.

The fourth law, the law of resisting control, which can also be called the law of rebellion, states that one organ may resist control by another organ, which means that the employee may resist control by the boss, so to speak. This law is a reversal of the law of control and, thus, it falls within the context of abnormal relationships among the internal organs. As an example, under normal circumstances, metal should control wood; but if the energy of metal is in short supply, or if the energy of wood is in excess, wood may resist control by metal, which gives rise to lungs-metal in deficiency with liver-wood in excess.

## ENERGY, BLOOD AND BODY FLUIDS

ENERGY  Energy is the motor of all human activities; all human activities are a function of energy. When energy is disordered, it can cause various types of organ disorders, conversely, organ disorders can cause energy disorders. The disorders of energy are generally divided into two categories: deficiency and excess. Deficiency means shortage, with symptoms of low functioning and decline; excess means too much, with symptoms of congestion and blockage.

With an energy deficiency, there is a functional decline of the internal organs and a low resistance of the organism against the attack of diseases. It can be seen in chronic diseases, aging, or during the recuperating stage of acute diseases. The general symptoms of energy deficiency include white or pale complexion, fatigue, weakness, poor spirits, shortness of breath, too tired to talk, low and feeble voice, excessive perspiration, tongue in light color and weak pulse. In order to treat it, it is necessary to tone up the energy.

An excess of energy manifests itself in energy sluggishness or stagnation. Energy should travel throughout the body without difficulty. However, various factors, including emotional stress, irregular eating, attack of external energies and external injuries, can impact energy circulation negatively and cause energy sluggishness in the chest. They can also cause swelling of the stomach and abdomen with pain if they involve the stomach and intestine, with wandering pain occurring most frequently and swelling more severe than pain. Other symptoms include intestinal rumbling, pain getting better on belching and pain and swelling of breasts in women. In order to treat it, it is necessary to promote the flow of energy and break up energy congestion.

Another type of energy disorder is called energy upsurging, or energy rebellion, which may be seen in cough and asthma due to lungs energy upsurging and in nausea and vomiting as a result of stomach energy upsurging.

BLOOD  Blood is a product of water and grains undergoing energy transformation and it is closely related to the heart, spleen and kidneys. There are three basic types of blood disorders: blood deficiency, blood coagulation and "hot blood."

Blood deficiency means a shortage of blood due to loss of blood or insufficient production of blood. Blood deficiency can be seen in anemia, chronic waste disease, neurosis, parasites and irregular menstruation, with the following symptoms: pale complexion, light color of nails, light color of tongue and fine pulse (there may be an empty pulse after massive bleeding). In order to treat it, it is necessary to tone up the blood or strengthen the energy and tone up the blood at the same time.

Blood coagulation, or blood stasis, can be seen in coronary disease, menstrual pain, suppression of menses, extra-uterine pregnancy, external injuries and carbuncles, with such symptoms as acute pain in the affected region, mostly prickling pain in a fixed region and pain getting worse on pressure or local swelling with lumps, pain in the lower abdomen before menstruation, scant menstrual flow in purple-black color and in lumps and dark purple color of tongue with ecchymosis on the tongue. In order to treat it, it is necessary to activate the blood and transform coagulations.

"Hot blood" is mostly seen in "hot" diseases of external causes, such as measles, scarlet fever and encephalomyelitis; sometimes it can also be seen in such diseases as allergic purpura, aplastic anemia and leukemia, as well as various diseases of bleeding. The following symptoms may be present: red swelling, bleeding, skin eruptions, premature menstruation, excessive menstrual flow in fresh-red color, mental depression, thirst, reddish urine and constipation or fever, red tongue with a yellowish coating and rapid pulse. In order to treat hot blood, it is necessary to cool the blood, clear up heat and counteract toxic effects.

BODY FLUIDS  Body fluids refer to the water in the body under normal circumstances. The functions of body fluids are to water and lubricate internal organs, muscles, skin, hair, membranes and cavities; lubricate the joints; and moisten and nourish the brain, marrow and bones.

Body fluids can be divided into clear fluids and turbid fluids. Clear fluids are spread in the muscles and membranes to moisten the muscles, skin and hair, as well as the cavities of the senses, namely, the eyes, ears, mouth and nose. Perspiration and urine are products of clear fluids. Turbid fluids are spread in the internal organs to nourish such organs as the brain, marrow and bones and to lubricate the joints, but, at the same time, they also have the function of nourishing the muscles.

The production, distribution and excretion of body fluids go through a relatively complicated process in close relationship with the lungs, spleen, kidneys, stomach, small intestine, large intestine and bladder. *The Yellow Emperor's Classics of Internal Medicine* states: "After food enters the stomach, its pure energy is transmitted upward to the spleen; the spleen, in turn, spreads the pure energy to flow upward to the lungs; the lungs reopen and regulate the passage of waterways in order to transmit the energy of water to the bladder below; the pure energy of water then spreads in four directions and travels to irrigate the meridians of the five viscera." This means that the source of water comes from the stomach, which transmits the pure energy to the spleen; through the transporting and transforming functions of the spleen, the fluids from the stomach are sent to the lungs, which spread the fluids to various internal organs.

When foods pass through the small intestine and the large intestine, body fluids will be absorbed through the function of the small intestine in separating the clear fluids from the turbid and the function of the large intestine in transporting and transforming waste matter. This accounts for the assertions in the classic that "the small intestine takes charge of clear body fluids" and "the large intestine takes charge of turbid body fluids." These assertions point to the connection between body fluids and the small and large intestines.

In short, the production, absorption and transportation of body fluids are inseparable from the receiving function of the stomach and the transporting and transforming functions of the spleen. The distribution of body fluids throughout the whole body to moisten the skin and hair and the transformation of body fluids into perspiration and urine are inseparable from the expanding, dispersing, cleaning-up and pushing-downward functions of the lungs, which is why the lungs are considered the upper source of water.

Among the internal organs, the kidneys play a very important role in the production and metabolism of body fluids. This is because all the organs involved in body fluids depend on the warming and pushing power of the kidneys, including the stomach (which receives water), the spleen (which transports and transforms water) and the lungs (which spread and clean up water); in addition, the production and excretion of urine and the metabolism of water throughout the whole body

*Wood corresponds to the liver, tendons and eyes. Fire corresponds to the heart, blood vessels and tongue. Earth corresponds to the spleen, flesh and mouth. Metal corresponds to the lungs, skin, hair and nose. Water corresponds to the kidneys, bones and ears.*

are inseparable from the transforming function of the kidneys. This is why it is said that the kidneys are water organs and they take charge of the water throughout the entire body. Insufficient body fluids and failure of water to transform into body fluids with water retention are the two basic pathological changes in metabolism of body fluids. Insufficient sources and excessive loss and consumption are the two basic causes of insufficient body fluids. The first cause may be due to insufficient intake of water and failure of water to transform into body fluids; the second may be due to the attack of a "hot" pathogen, excessive perspiration, vomiting and diarrhea.

## Causes of Diseases

### THE SIX EXTERNAL PATHOGENS

The six external energies are wind, cold, summer heat, dampness, dryness and fire, which stand for changes in climate during the four seasons. When these six external energies attack the human body through the mouth, nose, or skin to cause superficial disease, they are called the six external pathogenic energies, or the six external pathogens.

WIND  As one of the six external pathogens, wind can cause disease along with another external pathogen; so, a given disease may be caused by a combination of two pathogenic energies, such as wind-cold, wind-heat, wind-dampness, or wind-dryness. Wind is a yang pathogenic energy and, when it causes disease, it will give rise to wandering symptoms and symptoms that change a great deal.

Wind can refer to external wind and internal wind. As one of the six external pathogenic energies, external wind attacks the human body from the outside. Internal wind, on the other hand, causes disease from within. When heat and fire reach their peaks, they may be transformed into internal wind; blood deficiency with yin exhaustion and energy and blood disturbances may also generate internal wind. The symptoms caused by internal wind include vertigo, fainting, twitching, trembling, numbness and dry mouth and eyes.

Injurious wind refers to the disease caused by wind, normally called the common cold. In clinical practice, there are two types: common cold due to wind and cold and common cold due to wind and heat. The two types are treated differently.

COLD  Cold is one of the yin external pathogenic energies that can easily cause harm to yang energy. When a person's yang energy is in deficiency, defense energy will fail to guard the body against foreign invasion; so, cold energy will attack, giving rise to such symptoms as dislike of cold, fever, headache, pain in the body, pain in bones and joints and abdominal pain with diarrhea.

Like wind, cold can be divided into external and internal types. External cold refers to the cold energy that attacks the body from the outside. External cold causes a blockage of yang energy, with such symptoms as dislike of cold, fever, absence of perspiration, headache, pain in the body and superficial and tight pulse. External cold can also refer to a weakening of yang energy in the body, with such symptoms as fear of cold and being very susceptible to an attack of the common cold. Internal cold refers to a weakening of yang energy, with a decline in organ functions that may give rise to disturbances of water transformation, retention of urine and the like.

There can also be a direct attack of cold. Referred to as cold stroke, this is when the cold pathogenic energy attacks while the person is suffering from yang deficiency. The symptoms may include cold limbs and deep and fine or slow and tight pulse.

*The six external energies are wind, cold, summer heat, dampness, dryness and fire, which stand for changes in climate during the four seasons.*

SUMMER HEAT   Summer heat is one of the yang external pathogenic energies. When summer heat attacks the body, it will give rise to such symptoms as headache, fever, thirst, mental depression, excessive perspiration and forceful and rapid pulse. Summer heat can also cause great harm to body fluids, which in turn leads to such symptoms as fatigue, weak limbs and dry mouth. In certain regions, when a great deal of dampness or humidity accompanies a prolonged summer, summer heat can attack the body along with dampness to cause such symptoms as congested chest, nausea, vomiting and diarrhea.

DAMPNESS   Dampness is one of the yin external pathogenic energies. It has a turbid, heavy and sticky nature and it can obstruct the activities of energy transformation performed by the spleen.

There are internal dampness and external dampness and they cause different symptoms. External dampness refers to the dampness outside the human body, such as on the ground, in the air, or of rain and dew. It may give rise to such symptoms as heavy sensations in the head as if being wrapped up by a wet towel, soreness in the back of the neck, congested chest, sore loins, tired limbs and sore joints. Internal dampness refers to a stoppage of dampness within the body normally due to an inability of the spleen to transform dampness because of spleen yang in deficiency. When this occurs, the patient will display such symptoms as poor appetite, diarrhea, abdominal swelling, scant urine, yellowish complexion, edema in the lower limbs, light color of the tongue relaxed pulse.

DRYNESS   Dryness can be divided into internal dryness and external dryness. Both internal dryness and external dryness (one of the six external pathogens) can cause exhaustion to yin fluids. Symptoms of external dryness include pink eyes, dry sensations in the mouth and nose, dry lips, pain in the ribs, dry cough and constipation. With internal dryness, the exhaustion of internal yin fluids is mostly due to a later stage of hot diseases or the result of vomiting and diarrhea, excessive perspiration, excessive bleeding, or improper use of drugs. The symptoms of internal dryness consist of hot sensations as if heat were coming from the bones, mental depression, dry lips, dry tongue, dry skin and dry and withered nails, which are symptoms of yin being harmed by heat.

FIRE   Fire, the sixth external pathogen, can cause the diseases called warm heat and summer heat. Fire is also one of the life forces transformed by yang energy into what is called physiological fire. There are different types of physiological fire, including monarch fire, minister fire and lesser fire. Fire can also refer to a manifestation due to pathological change, which means that all kinds of external pathogenic energies, including the seven emotions (see below) and internal injuries, can transform into fire and turn into pathological fire.

In addition, fire can be differentiated into excess fire and deficiency fire. Excess fire is due to an excess of external pathogenic energies, which are mostly seen in acute hot diseases, with such symptoms as high fever, excessive perspiration, thirst, insanity, pink eyes, red complexion, discharge of blood from the mouth, nosebleed, red tongue, yellowish and dry coating of the tongue and rapid and forceful pulse. Deficiency fire is due to an exhaustion of yin fluids, which is mostly seen in chronic wasting diseases, with such symptoms as being hasty, insomnia, seminal emission with erotic dreams, night sweats, cough with sputum containing blood, red tongue with scant coating and fine-rapid or deficiency-rapid pulse.

## THE SEVEN EMOTIONS

The seven emotions are joy, anger, worry, contemplation, sorrow, fear and shock. The seven emotions can cause disease and, conversely, disorders of the internal organs can cause the seven emotions. *The Yellow Emperor's Classics of Internal Medicine* states: "Anger will force energy to move upward; joy will cause energy to relax; grief will cause energy to disperse; fear will cause energy to move downward; cold will cause energy to constrict; heat will cause a reduction of energy; shock will cause a disorder of energy; labor will consume energy; contemplation will cause energy to coagulate; anger will cause upsurging energy and in severe cases, the patient will display the symptoms of vomiting blood and diarrhea containing undigested foods. Thus, anger will cause energy to move upward. When one is joyful, the energy will remain in harmony and the will is fulfilled so that nutritive and defense energies will flow smoothly.

"Thus, joy will cause energy to relax. When one is in grief, the heart connectives will become cramped, the lungs will be expanded with lobes lifted up, the upper burning space will be blocked up and the nutritive and defense energies will be unable to disperse; as the hot energy is in the internal region, it will extinguish energy. Fear will cause a decline of pure energy; when pure energy is in decline, it will cause a blockage of the upper burning space; when the upper burning space is blocked up, the energy will move downward; when the energy moves downward, the lower burning space will be distended; thus, the energy stream stops. In contemplation, the heart focuses on something, the spirits have a place to return to and the righteous energy stays put; thus, the energy becomes coagulated."

## FOODS AND FATIGUE

When foods cause disease, it is called a food injury. Intoxication, overeating and eating foods with cold or cool energies are common causes. In addition, a prolonged consumption of greasy foods will cause a disorder of the digestive functions and produce internal heat and skin eruptions.

Fatigue is one of the factors that cause deficiency disease. The fatigue may be of an internal organ or due to excessive sex. Also called a bedroom injury, excessive sexual intercourse can harm the kidneys and become a chronic disorder.

*The seven emotions are joy, anger, worry, contemplation, sorrow, fear and shock. The seven emotions can cause disease and, conversely, disorders of the internal organs can cause the seven emotions.*

# The Internal Organs

The internal organs include the five viscera and the six bowels. The five viscera are the liver, heart, spleen, lungs and kidneys. *The Yellow Emperor's Classics of Internal Medicine* states: "The heart is in tune with the blood vessels; its prosperity is manifest in the complexion; its master is the kidneys. The lungs are in tune with the skin; their prosperity is manifest in the hair; their master is the heart. The liver is in tune with the tendons; its prosperity is manifest in the nails; its master is in the lungs. The spleen is in tune with the muscles; its prosperity is manifest in the lips; its master is in the liver. The kidneys are in tune with the bones, their prosperity is manifest in the hair on the head; their master is the spleen." The word "master" refers to the controlling status in the five-elements theory and the word "prosperity" means that when the internal organs are in good health, it will show on body surfaces, such as the hair or the ears or nose.

The six bowels refer to the gallbladder, small intestine, stomach, large intestine, bladder and triple burning space. The following passage is from *The Yellow Emperor's Classics of Internal Medicine*. "The stomach, large intestine, small intestine, triple burning space and bladder are the five organs generated by the energy of the Heaven and their energies bear a resemblance to the energy of the Heaven. Thus, they drain off things without storing them up, they receive turbid energies from the five viscera and they are called transmitting bowels. As they cannot store things up for long, they have to drain things off in due course. The door of physical strength (anus) also acts as the messenger for the five viscera and drains off water and grains without storing them up for long. The so-called five viscera are such that they store up pure energy without draining off and, for that reason, they can be filled to capacity but cannot be oversupplied. The six bowels are such that they transmit things without storing them up and, for that reason, they may be oversupplied but cannot be filled to capacity. The reason is that after foods enter through the mouth, the stomach will be full and the intestines will still be empty. Therefore, it is said that the bowels may be oversupplied but cannot be filled to capacity and that the viscera may be filled to capacity but cannot be oversupplied."

## THE HEART

The heart is the master of the human body and in control of human activities; it is in charge of various parts of the body and coordinates the functions of other internal organs, which is why the Chinese have a saying to the effect that "The heart is the master of the five viscera and the six bowels." The pericardium forms the external defense of the heart and, for this reason, whenever a pathogenic energy tries to attack the heart, it must pass through the pericardium first. When the pericardium is under attack, it may give rise to such symptoms as high fever, coma and delirium, which are considered the symptoms of a diseased pericardium.

The heart is the master of the spirits, which include mental conditions, consciousness and thought. This accounts for the Chinese expression, "The heart is the grand master of the five viscera and the six bowels and it is the residence of the spirits." When the heart is diseased, all related activities will be disordered, giving rise to such symptoms as insomnia, many dreams, forgetfulness and even mental confusion, manifested in incoherent speech and thoughts.

The heart is the master of the blood vessels and its glory is manifest in the face. The blood vessels are the channels through which the blood circulates. The reason that the blood can circulate through the blood vessels is due to the pushing power of the heart. Therefore, the Chinese believe that when energy circulates smoothly, blood will also circulate smoothly; on the other hand, when energy becomes sluggish, blood coagulations may result. The glory of the heart is expressed through a person's complexion, because when the heart is in good condition, the person's complexion will be shiny and reddish and manifest high spirits as well; conversely, when the heart is suffering from blood deficiency, the complexion will be pale and reveal low spirits.

*The Chinese believe that when energy circulates smoothly, blood will also circulate smoothly; on the other hand, when energy becomes sluggish, blood coagulations may result.*

The tongue is the outlet of the heart. The ancient Chinese believed that the heart extends its energy to the tongue; so, when the heart is in harmony, the tongue will be able to differentiate different flavors, which shows the close relationship between the heart and the tongue. The tongue is the external cavity of the heart, so a disease of the heart will be manifested in the tongue. For instance, when the heart is suffering from a deficiency of blood, the tongue will look pale; when the heart is suffering from blood coagulations, the tongue will be decomposed and have ulcers on it; and when the heart cavity is obstructed by sputum, stiffness of the tongue will occur. Therefore, two Chinese phrases are often mentioned in relation to the heart: "the heart with its cavity in the tongue" and "the tongue as the seedling of the heart."

## THE SMALL INTESTINE

The primary function of the small intestine is that of receiving water and grains from the stomach; it is in charge of transformation of foods and differentiating clear energy from turbid energy. When water and grains enter the small intestine from the stomach, they are further digested by the small intestine and the clear energy is absorbed; then they pass through the spleen to be transmitted to various parts of the body to become the material base of human activities. On the other hand, the turbid energy will be passed on to the large intestine and to the bladder for excretion.

The heart and the small intestine are connected to each other through meridians and they form a yin-yang relationship with each other. The small intestine meridian is in the superficial region, whereas the heart meridian is in the deep region. When the heart meridian is suffering from excess fire, it will pass it on downward to the small intestine, causing such symptoms as short streams of reddish urine, burning sensations in

the urethra and pain or discharge of blood on urination, which should be treated by clearing the heart and promoting urination.

Two major syndromes of the heart are blood deficiency of the heart and yin deficiency of the heart. These two syndromes can be seen in general weakness, neurosis and anemia, with the following symptoms: palpitations, depression, insomnia, many dreams, forgetfulness and easily in shock. However, in cases of blood deficiency of the heart, the patient will more likely display pale complexion, pale tongue and a deep and fine pulse and, in cases of yin deficiency of the heart, low fever, night sweats, red zygoma, feeling depressed, hot and dry mouth, red tongue and a fine and rapid pulse. Yin deficiency of the heart should be treated by toning up the yin of the heart, while blood deficiency of the heart should be treated by toning up the blood of the heart and, for both, it is necessary to secure the spirits of the heart.

Energy deficiency of the heart and yang deficiency of the heart are also common syndromes of the heart. They can be seen in heart disease, heart failure, irregular heartbeats, neurosis and shock. In cases of heart energy deficiency, there will be such symptoms as palpitations, shortness of breath, excessive perspiration becoming worse with labor or movements, fatigue, weakness, whitish complexion, congestion in the region before the heart, pale tongue with thin and white coating and a fine and weak or clotting and slowing pulse. In cases of heart yang deficiency, there will be such additional symptoms as cold sensations and cold limbs; in cases of heart yang deficiency prolapse, there will be severe perspiration, coma, extremely cold limbs and disappearing pulse about to exhaust. Heart energy deficiency should be treated by toning up heart energy, heart yang deficiency should be treated by warming up heart yang and heart yang deficiency prolapse should be treated by restoring yang and fixing the prolapse.

## THE LIVER

The liver is one of the most important internal organs in the human body, as it takes charge of storing and regulating the blood throughout the whole body and is also in control of flexing and extending joints and muscles. The liver loves to disperse and grow; it hates to be inhibited and oppressed. Therefore, when the liver is inhibited by the emotion of anger, it will be harmed as a result. For this reason, when the liver is diseased, the patient will display many emotional problems and disturbances. The liver has its outlets in the eyes and forms a yin-yang relationship with the gallbladder. The liver meridian travels around the yin organs (namely, the external genitals), passes through the lower abdomen and spreads around the ribs, with the two branches meeting at the vertex. Thus, when disease occurs in the regions through which the liver meridian passes, the liver should be treated accordingly.

There is a well-known saying in Chinese medicine that goes like this: "The liver is in charge of storing the blood and when a person lies down, the blood will return to the liver for storage. When the person becomes active again, the blood in the liver will flow to all parts of the body once again to meet the needs of various parts of the body."

The liver controls the activities of the tendons, ranging from extension and flexing of joints to nourishment of the tendons. When blood deficiency of the liver occurs, the tendons will suffer from malnutrition, which gives rise to difficulty in extension and flexing of joints, numbness, spasms and the like. In addition, the nails will also change color and appear withered, because the nails are an extension of the tendons.

The eyes and the liver are very closely related to each other. When blood deficiency of the liver occurs, the eyes will suffer from malnutrition, giving rise to such symptoms as dry eyes, blurred vision, or night blindness. When liver-fire burning upward occurs, there will be the symptom of pink eyes. Many eye diseases are related to the liver and should be treated by reference to the liver.

The liver and the gallbladder form a yin-yang relationship with each other, as the liver is a viscus while the gallbladder is a bowel and they are related to each other like brother and sister.

## THE GALLBLADDER

The gallbladder is attached to the liver and situated below the ribs. Although it is one of the six bowels, it differs from other bowels in that its bile is pure as opposed to other bowels that contain turbid substances. When the gallbladder is diseased, the following symptoms will occur: pain in the ribs, bitter taste in the mouth, vomiting of bitter water and jaundice. As the gallbladder and the liver form a yin-yang relationship with each other, the diseases of the gallbladder are often treated by reference to the liver.

Liver and gallbladder dampness-heat is a well-established syndrome that can be seen in acute hepatitis with jaundice, acute cholecystitis and gallstones, with the following symptoms: yellowish appearance of eyeball sclera, apparent pain in ribs, scant urine in reddish-yellow color, fever, thirst, nausea, vomiting, poor appetite, abdominal swelling, yellowish and greasy coating of tongue and wiry and rapid pulse. To treat this syndrome, it is necessary to clear the heat, benefit the dampness, benefit the gallbladder and reduce yellowish appearance.

## THE SPLEEN

The stomach receives foods and digests them and then the spleen digests them for a second time, before sending them to the lungs to be transmitted to all parts of the body.

The most important energy of the human body is what is called "true energy," which is in close relationship with the spleen and the lungs. The spleen sends digested foods to the lungs to be mixed with the energy of the air inhaled by the lungs and the two energies form the important ingredients of true energy. This is why the spleen is capable of producing energy. Therefore, when a person is suffering from energy deficiency accompanied by spleen deficiency, the function of the spleen in producing energy may have already been impaired and should be treated first.

The spleen governs the blood circulating throughout the entire body to prevent the blood from overflowing outside the blood vessels. Energy deficiency of the spleen may impair its function of governing the blood, resulting in various types of bleeding.

As spleen energy is capable of elevating, it can transport pure energy and pure substances of water and grains upward to the lungs and then to other internal organs to be transformed into energy and blood. If spleen energy fails to elevate and caves in instead, then symptoms such as shortness of breath, too tired to talk, chronic diarrhea, prolapse of the anus, prolapse of the uterus and falling of other organs will occur, which are due to middle energy falling.

The spleen likes dryness and dislikes dampness. When the spleen fails to perform its functions of transformation and digestion due to its deficiency, it will generate dampness; conversely, excessive dampness will contribute to the difficulty of the spleen in performing its functions. When the spleen is being troubled by dampness, such symptoms as these will occur: heavy sensations of the head, feeling as if the whole body is sinking down, discharge of watery stools and white and greasy coating of the tongue. For this condition, it is necessary to dry up the dampness and strengthen the spleen and the herbs used should be relatively warm and dry.

## THE STOMACH

The stomach performs the functions of receiving and digesting foods. It is also in charge of pushing down turbid substances. When stomach energy moves downward, water and grains will also move downward, which contributes to digestion, absorption and excretion. If, instead of moving downward, stomach energy moves upward, then it will cause such symptoms as belching, hiccups, nausea and vomiting.

The stomach likes dampness and dislikes dryness. It is very susceptible to the attack of heat, which is called the hot stomach syndrome. When heat attacks the stomach, it will cause harm to stomach fluids and cause such symptoms as dry tongue and mouth and thirst with craving for drink. To treat the hot stomach syndrome, it is necessary to nourish the yin of the stomach and produce fluids.

The spleen and the stomach form a yin-yang relationship, in that the spleen is a yin viscus while the stomach is a yang bowel. The spleen is in charge of elevation, whereas the stomach is in charge of downward movements; the spleen likes dryness, while the stomach likes dampness. They rely on each other in order to exercise control over each other in performing their respective functions of digestion and absorption.

Energy deficiency of both the spleen and the stomach is a distinct syndrome in Chinese medicine. This syndrome may be seen in ulcers, chronic gastritis, chronic enteritis, chronic dysentery, functional disorders of the stomach and intestine, tuberculosis of the intestine, chronic hepatitis and cirrhosis of the liver, with such symptom as poor appetite, belching, swallowing of acid, nausea, vomiting, stomachache with desire for massage, pain getting better after a meal, fullness of stomach, abdominal swelling with discharge of watery stools and edema. Should the disease become chronic, these symptoms will occur: withered and yellowish complexion, fatigue, weakness, loss of weight, light color of the tongue with white coating, fat and tender tongue with tooth marks appearing and soft and weak pulse. To treat this syndrome, it is necessary to strengthen the spleen and harmonize the stomach.

Deficiency coldness of the spleen and the stomach is another common syndrome, called yang deficiency of both the spleen and stomach. It may be seen in ulcers, chronic gastritis, chronic enteritis, chronic dysentery, functional disorder of the stomach and intestine, edema, chronic hepatitis and cirrhosis of the liver, with the following symptoms: abdominal pain, love of heat and warmth, full of clear saliva, hiccups, vomiting, poor appetite, abdominal swelling after meals, fatigue, weakness, cold limbs or scant urine, puffiness, whitish vaginal discharge, light color of the tongue with white-sliding or white-greasy coating and a deep, fine, weak pulse. In treating this syndrome, it is necessary to warm and tone up both the spleen and the stomach.

Another common syndrome, called stomach-fire, may be seen in high-fever stages of various contagious diseases, diabetes, periodontitis and mouth ulcers, with the following symptoms: thirst with craving for cold drink, periodic stomachache with burning sensations, red tongue, yellowish and thick coating of the tongue, dry tongue and big and forceful pulse or sliding and rapid pulse. In order to treat this syndrome, it is necessary to clear and sedate stomach-fire.

Stomach yin deficiency also occurs and may be seen in chronic gastritis, gastric neurosis, indigestion and diabetes, with the following symptoms: dry lips and mouth, lack of appetite, abdominal swelling after meals, discharge of dry stools, dry vomiting, hiccups and dry tongue or burning pain in the stomach, red tongue with scant coating and fine and rapid pulse. To treat this syndrome, it is necessary to nourish the yin of the stomach and clear the heat in the stomach.

## THE LUNGS

The lungs are situated in the thoracic cavity and have the throat as their door and the nose as their outlet. They are a yin viscus, forming a yin-yang relationship with the large intestine, which is a yang bowel. The lungs are in charge of the respiratory energy, or the energy of air. When the lungs fail to control respiratory energy properly, they will give rise to cough, asthma, or difficult breathing.

After foods have passed through the stomach and spleen and been digested properly, they are mixed up with the clear energy of the lungs to become important ingredients of true energy for distribution throughout the entire body. When the lungs fail to distribute true energy properly, such symptoms as fatigue, weakness, shortness of breath, too tired to talk and excessive perspiration will occur, These are all symptoms of the syndrome called energy deficiency of the lungs.

The lungs should be able to expand so that air can go through the nose and the mouth easily. When the lungs fail to expand, congested chest, cough, or asthma may occur. The lungs should also be able to push energy downward and when they fail to do so, cough, asthma, scant urine, or edema may occur.

The lungs are in charge of opening and regulating waterways. Circulation of body fluids is a function of many organs working together as a team, including the lungs. Under normal circumstances, the lungs are capable of sending fluids downward to the kidneys, which pass the fluids to the bladder for excretion. When a pathogenic energy attacks the lungs to impair their normal functions, it will give rise to such symptoms as diminished urination and edema, which is why it is often said that "the lungs are the upper source of water."

The lungs are in charge of the voice, because the production of the voice and the functions of the lungs are closely related to each other. When the lungs are full of energy, the voice will be loud, when the lungs are suffering from energy deficiency, the voice will be feeble. Cold and wind may attack the lungs to cause energy congestion of the lungs, which will give rise to hoarseness or loss of voice. The lungs use the nose as an outlet. The nose is the passage through which air comes and goes, so it is directly related to the lungs. When the lungs are functioning normally, air will go through the nose very smoothly and there will be a normal sense of smell. When the lungs are diseased, it will give rise to nasal congestion, nasal discharge and an impaired sense of smell and, in severe cases, there may be a flickering of the nostrils and difficult breathing.

The lungs are in charge of the skin and the hair. The skin and hair are the outermost regions of the human body and the lungs can send defense energy and body fluids to them for nourishment. When the energy of the lungs is normal, the skin and hair will be moist and smooth and the pores will be well guarded. But as soon as the energy of the lungs becomes deficient, there will be a shortage of defense energy and the outermost regions will not be guarded properly, which will give rise to excessive perspiration and the common cold.

Both the lungs and the heart are situated above the diaphragm, with the lungs in charge of energy and the heart in charge of blood. When energy flows, the blood will circulate and when energy congestion occurs, blood circulation will be impaired. Thus, the lungs and the heart can be seen to work together in control of energy flow and blood circulation.

The lungs are in charge of energy and the spleen can produce energy. Thus, lungs diseases can, in many cases, be treated by toning up spleen energy. For example, a chronic cough with a great deal of white sputum can be treated this way.

The lungs and the large intestine form a yin-yang relationship with each other. Therefore, a cough and asthma due to excessive heat in the lungs can be treated by sedating the large intestine to clear up sputum heat, so the energy of the lungs will move downward, producing relief of the cough and asthma. And constipation, which is a symptom of the large intestine, may be due to energy deficiency of the lungs, in which case, the energy of the lungs should be strengthened to relieve the constipation.

## THE LARGE INTESTINE

The function of the large intestine is to excrete waste matter. When the large intestine is suffering from deficiency, it will cause constipation; when it is suffering from excess, it will cause diarrhea. Dampness-heat of the large intestine is a common syndrome often observed in acute bacillary dysentery, acute onset of chronic dysentery and amebic dysentery, with the following symptoms: abdominal pain, tenesmus, diarrhea with discharge of pus and blood, burning sensations in the anus, short streams of reddish urine, fever, yellowish and greasy coating of the tongue and sliding and rapid pulse. In severe cases, there may be fainting and coma. In order to treat this syndrome, it is necessary to clear up heat and transform dampness in the large intestine.

## THE KIDNEYS

The kidneys are important organs in charge of growth, reproduction and maintenance of the metabolic balance of water. Also, the kidneys are in charge of storing pure substances inherited from one's parents. Thus, the kidneys are innate roots of life. It is also believed that the formation of the fetus begins in the kidneys and that the two kidneys are formed prior to the body itself, so the kidneys can be seen as the roots of the viscera and the bowels as well as the 12 meridians. In clinical practice, some cases of slow growth of an innate nature are dealt with by treating the kidneys. Moreover, the kidneys are situated in the lumbar region and, for this reason, it is said that the loins are the residence of the kidneys; so, when the kidneys are diseased, symptoms may occur across the loins. The kidneys include kidneys yin (true yin, or kidney water) and kidney yang (true yang, or life door-fire).

As already mentioned, the kidneys are in charge of storing pure substances, but "pure substances" refer to two different things. First of all, they refer to the pure substances of the five viscera and the six bowels derived from water and grains that have been digested and transformed by the spleen for distribution throughout the whole body, with extra-pure substances stored in the kidneys for future consumption. The pure substances also refer to those of the kidneys themselves, derived from the innate sources and mixed with the acquired energy of water and grains, which are closely related to the reproduction, growth and aging of the human body. For this reason, when the pure substances of the kidneys are in short supply, a man may suffer from shortage of semen and infertility while a woman may suffer from suppression of menses and infertility, slow growth and premature aging. All of these symptoms should be treated by toning up the kidneys.

The kidneys take charge of water. The regulation of body fluids is closely related to the following three organs: the lungs, spleen and kidneys. This is called energy transformation of the triple burning space and was originally initiated by kidneys yang.

The kidneys are closely related to the growth and the softness or hardness of bones. For instance, in children, a fontanelle not closed after a long period of time can be dealt with by treating the kidneys; the same applies to soft bones in children and to the inability of an adult to stand up for very long due to weak legs. Teeth are extensions of bones and loose teeth or teeth falling out are due to deficiency of kidney energy. The kidneys are in charge of storing pure substances, which generate marrow; marrow nourishes the bones and gathers in the brain. This is why it is said that the brain is the "sea of marrow." Kidneys energy deficiency, which is a common syndrome, may give rise to low intelligence, slow movements and soft bones. In recent years, Chinese acupuncturists have applied the kidney point in auricular acupuncture to treat incomplete growth of the cerebrum in children and aftereffects of brain concussion and the Chinese herbs that tone up the kidneys have been applied to treat aplastic anemia.

Under normal circumstances, the heart and the kidneys remain in balance, depending on each other as well as controlling each other, which is called mutual adjustment of yin and yang or communication between the upper organ and the lower organ. The heart yang is in the upper region, whereas the kidneys yin is in the lower region. The heart yang must rely on the kidneys yin for its supply of yin energy, while the kidneys yin must rely on the heart yang for its supply of yang energy. This interdependence is necessary in order to maintain normal functions of the human body and is called communication between the heart and the kidneys in Chinese medicine. When the heart or the kidneys are disordered, which disrupts the normal relationship between the two organs, insomnia, palpitations, forgetfulness, lumbago and seminal emission can occur, which are the symptoms of the heart and the kidneys being incapable of communicating with each other.

The kidneys are also closely related to the liver. The liver is in charge of storing the blood and the kidneys are in charge of storing pure substances. Pure substances and blood can generate and transform each other, which is why it is said that the liver and the kidneys originate from the same source. Under normal circumstances, kidneys yin will nourish and water liver yin. But when the kidneys are suffering from yin deficiency, the kidneys will be incapable of doing so, which will cause such syndromes as liver yin deficiency and liver yang upsurging. This is called water incapable of nourishing wood in the five-elements theory. On the other hand, yin deficiency of the liver will also cause yin deficiency of the kidneys. When both the liver and the kidneys are suffering from yin deficiency simultaneously, it is called yin deficiency of both the liver and the kidneys, which will cause such symptoms as lumbago, dizziness and being hasty and jumpy.

The kidneys and the bladder are connected with each other through meridians. The condition of the energy of the kidneys has direct bearing on the capacity of the bladder in urination. This is why the kidneys and the bladder are said to form a yin-yang relationship with each other.

## THE BLADDER

The bladder is in charge of storing urine and controlling urination. When the bladder is disordered, it will cause urination disorders and difficult urination. The reason that the bladder is capable of urinating is due to the energy transformation of the kidneys. When the energy transformation of the kidneys breaks down, difficult urination and retention of urine occur. And when the kidneys are suffering from deficiency, dribbling of urine and incontinence take place.

Bladder dampness-heat is a common syndrome observed in urinary infections, urinary calculus and prostatitis, with the following symptoms: frequent urination, pain on urination or difficulty in urination, sudden interruption during urination, reddish-yellow and greasy coating on the tongue and sliding and rapid pulse. To treat this syndrome, it is necessary to clear up heat and remove dampness.

## THE PERICARDIUM

The pericardium is the protector of the heart; it is also its messenger. The pericardium is partially responsible for the symptoms of the heart, such as dizziness and delirium, which are normally considered symptoms of the pericardium as well. The heart is in control of the spirits and it is the great master of the five viscera and the six bowels. When the heart is under attack, the patient will die due to its impact on the spirits; but, according to Chinese medicine, this doesn't happen very often, simply because before the pathogenic energy gets a chance to attack the heart itself, it must attack the pericardium.

## THE TRIPLE BURNING SPACE

The triple burning space refers to the three cavities in the human body, namely, the thoracic cavity (the upper burning space), the abdominal cavity (the middle burning space) and the pelvic cavity (the lower burning space). Why is it called the triple burning space? The reason is that this organ contains three parts, heats up the body and is not really an organ but rather a cavity-like space.

According to *The Yellow Emperor's Classics of Internal Medicine*, "the triple burning space is the irrigation official who builds waterways." However, in performing this duty as the irrigation official, the triple burning space must cooperate with other internal organs, notably, the kidneys, bladder and lungs. The kidneys and the bladder form a yin-yang relationship with each other and the kidneys are connected with the lungs in the upper region. Thus, the triple burning space performs the irrigation duty in cooperation with the kidneys, lungs and bladder and particularly the lower burning space that excretes water into the bladder.

Disorders in the triple burning space may give rise to many urinary symptoms, including suppression of urination, dripping of urine and edema. *The Yellow Emperor's Classics* states, "When the triple burning space suffers from an excess disease, it will cause anuria; when it suffers from a deficiency disease, it will give rise to enuresis." The same classic says, "The symptoms of the diseases of the triple burning space are as follows: congested abdomen, especially hardness in the lower abdomen; anuria that creates a desperate desire to discharge urine; and retention of urine that leads to an accumulation of water in the body and causes swelling."

According to another Chinese medical classic, when heat is present in the upper burning space, it will give rise to cough and pulmonary tuberculosis. According to still another classic, excessive heat in the upper burning space will cause perspiration on the forehead, abdominal swelling, pain in the rib region, dry tongue, scorching mouth and blocked throat; coldness in the upper burning space will cause inability to eat, vomiting of acid, pain in the chest and back, affecting each other and dry and sore throat.

When heat is present in the middle burning space, it will give rise to various types of dry and hard symptoms, such as constipation, abdominal swelling and cough. When the middle burning space suffers from deficiency and cold, it will give rise to incessant diarrhea, indigestion, fullness in the middle and intestinal swelling and rumbling.

When the lower burning space is deficient and cold, it will give rise to enuresis, incontinence of urination and diarrhea. When the lower burning space suffers from excessive heat, it will give rise to discharge of urine containing blood, urination difficulty, suppression of urination and difficult bowel movements

## THE BRAIN, MARROW AND WOMB

In addition to the viscera and the bowels, there are other organs, such as the brain, marrow and womb, which are called the odd and constant organs, in distinction from the viscera and the bowels. Each type of organ performs a different function and, at the same time, is connected with the others and influences the others.

In addition to the brain, marrow and womb, the odd and constant organs include bone, vessels and the gallbladder. It seems that the gallbladder alone occupies a special status in the human body, as it is regarded both as a bowel (as mentioned earlier) and as an odd and constant organ.

The brain is the uppermost organ among the six odd and constant organs and it is the material base of all mental activities. Therefore, the brain is also called "the organ of original spirit." The pathways in which the marrow travels upward and downward extend to the brain on the top and to the coccyx and sacrum at the bottom. This bears a resemblance to the conception of the central nervous system in modern Western medicine.

The brain and marrow are closely connected to the kidneys. The kidneys are in control of bones, bones generate marrow and marrow travels through the brain, which is the "sea of marrow." Hence, when the pure energy of the kidneys is in abundance, the marrow in the brain will be in full supply and, consequently, one will be energetic and in high spirits. The womb in women is a synonym for the uterus, which exists for menstruation and nourishing the embryo and fetus. The function of the uterus is to some extent dependent upon the fullness of the pure energy of the kidneys.

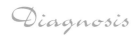

*Diagnosis*

## THE FOUR METHODS OF DIAGNOSIS

The four methods of diagnosis refer to diagnosis by observations, questioning the patient, hearing and smell and taking the pulse. In clinical practice, the four methods are used in combination.

Detecting internal conditions through external manifestations is the key to diagnosis in Chinese medicine. This is based upon the theory that any internal conditions will be manifest externally. Thus, a physician is able to know about the internal conditions of a patient through such external manifestations as complexion, skin conditions and the spirits.

DIAGNOSIS BY OBSERVATIONS  In making a diagnosis through observations, the physician uses the power of his or her eyes to evaluate the patient's spirits, general physical condition (as manifest in muscles, bones and skin), eyes, "outlets," complexion and tongue. In the case of very young patients, fingerprint observation is also included.

Observations of the spirits are intended to determine whether the spirits are there, lost, or prolapsed. A person's spirits are present, or a person is in good spirits, when his or her eyes are active, speech is clear, complexion is moist and shiny and breath is in balance. When a person is in good spirits, a disease can be more easily treated with better results. A person's spirits are lost when his or her eyes are passive, speech is incoherent, complexion is dull and dry and breath is in imbalance. When a person is lacking spirits, a disease may prove more difficult to treat. Prolapse of the spirits refers to a deterioration of the loss of the spirits, which indicates a critical stage of a disease that should be treated as an emergency.

By observing physical conditions, such as of muscles, bones and skin, a physician is able to know about the conditions of a patient's energy and blood. Observations of the spirits as expressed through the eyes can prove useful in understanding the conditions of energy and blood in the internal regions.

Observation of "outlets" is also important. "Outlets" refer to the outlets of the five viscera, namely, the tongue as the outlet of the heart, the nose as the outlet of the lungs, the eyes as the outlets of the liver, the lips as the outlets of the spleen and the ears as the outlets of the kidneys. Observations of these outlets will enable a physician to understand the conditions of the corresponding viscus. For instance, a crimson tongue will indicate burning of heart-fire, blisters on the tongue will indicate dampness-heat in the spleen and ringing in the ears will indicate an exhaustion of the kidneys. However, in making diagnosis, the whole body should be taken into consideration and, for this reason, other aspects of diagnosis should also be taken into account.

Observing a patient's complexion includes evaluating whether the color is deep or superficial and dispersing or gathering and whether the skin is moist or dry. Brightness is seen as a superficial color that indicates a superficial disease; darkness is viewed as a deep color that indicates a deep disease. A light and falling color is one that is dispersing, which generally indicates a new disorder involving the superficial region; a deep and accumulating color is one that is gathering, which usually indicates a chronic and severe disease. A moist appearance of the skin indicates the presence of stomach energy; a withered appearance indicates the decline of stomach energy.

The complexion of a normal person should be shiny and moist, with a mixture of yellow and red. The color of a normal complexion can also be seen in terms of host color and guest color. Host color refers to the base color that varies with individuals, while guest color refers to the color of the face that varies with the climate and other environmental or physical conditions. A normal complexion indicates normal conditions of the five viscera. Likewise, when a person has a very good complexion, it means that the energy conditions of the five viscera are excellent.

The complexion of a person can also be evaluated in terms of "good outlook" or "bad outlook." A moist and bright complexion indicates a good outlook, whereas a withering and dry complexion indicates a bad outlook. As fingerprints are more visible in children than adults, a diagnosis by fingerprint can be used with children under three years old. Diagnosis by fingerprint focuses on the color and density of the print.

*A person's spirits are present, or a person is in good spirits, when his or her eyes are active, speech is clear, complexion is moist and shiny and breath is in balance.*

In making a diagnosis, a physician should use the thumb and forefinger of his or her left hand to hold the tip of the patient's forefinger, while using the thumb of his or her right hand to lightly push the patient's forefinger from the tip towards the base. This way, the print will become more visible.

The physician should observe the print very carefully. A normal fingerprint will appear reddish yellow with a degree of brightness. When the print appears to be floating, it normally points to a superficial disease; when it appears deep, it normally points to a deep disease. A light color of a fingerprint generally points to a deficiency or cold disease; a purple-red color to a hot disease; a blue-purple color to convulsions, wind-cold, pain, indigestion and wind-sputum; and a black color to blood coagulations.

Observation of the tongue, commonly called tongue diagnosis, is an important aspect of diagnosis by observations. It primarily focuses on the coating of the tongue and the quality of the tongue with reference to shape, colors, movement and degree of moisture. There is a Chinese saying that goes like this: "Differentiation of the quality of the tongue enables us to differentiate the five viscera regarding excess and deficiency; observations of the tongue coating enable us to determine how deep the six external pathogenic energies have penetrated into the human body."

The quality of the tongue is also called the body of the tongue. In evaluating the tongue, it is generally believed that the tip of the tongue is symptomatic of the heart and lungs, the sides of the tongue are symptomatic of the liver and gallbladder and the root of the tongue is symptomatic of the kidneys. But these are only broad associations that should be applied with flexibility.

A moist tongue often indicates the presence of sufficient body fluids; a withered tongue often indicates an exhaustion of body fluids. An "old" tongue often indicates an excess disease; a tender tongue often indicates a deficiency disease. When the body of the tongue appears light red, fat and tender, it may

point to a yang deficiency; when the body of the tongue appears thin and bright red, it often indicates a yin deficiency. When the tongue is as shiny as a mirror with a coating, it points to yin deficiency of the liver and kidneys. When the tongue is swollen and painful, it points to excessive fire in the liver.

In terms of the tongue coating, a normal coating is white, but the tongue will have only a thin layer of white and clear coating, which is produced by stomach energy. A pathological white coating of the tongue is primarily due to wind, cold and dampness and it indicates a superficial disease. If the coating appears thin and glossy, it is mostly due to internal cold and dampness or external wind and cold. If the white layer of coating appears dry, it is due to a shortage of fluids. If the white coating occurs in a disease due to an attack of external pathogenic energies, then it generally indicates that these energies are beginning to transform into heat that may cause harm to fluids. A thick layer of white and glossy coating generally points to an excess of internal dampness; if the patient is also suffering from a superficial disease at the same time, it is due to external cold producing internal dampness. A thick layer of white and dry coating is due to heat-harming fluids with an inability of dampness to undergo transformation. A tongue with a white, glossy, sticky, greasy coating is mostly the result of internal sputum and dampness.

A yellow coating of the tongue indicates a hot disease, namely, the presence of the hot pathogenic energy in the internal region. A thin layer of yellow and glossy coating points to a dampness-heat disease and, in a disease of external pathogenic energy, this coating points to the external pathogen transforming into heat in the internal region with fluids remaining unharmed. A thin layer of yellow and dry coating points to the hot pathogen harming yin fluids. A thick layer of yellow and glossy coating points to dampness-heat in the stomach and intestine. A thick layer of yellow and dry coating points to an accumulation of heat-harming fluids. And a yellow and greasy coating of the tongue indicates dampness-heat in the spleen and stomach, dampness-sputum, or indigestion.

DIAGNOSIS BY QUESTIONING THE PATIENT This consists of questioning the patient regarding pain, time of onset, history, habits and so on. Chinese physicians from the past developed 10 essential questions for this purpose, concerning

1  cold and hot sensations,
2  perspiration,
3  head and body,
4  urination and bowel movements,
5  eating,
6  chest,

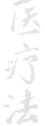

7  hearing,
8  thirst,
9  pulse and color and
10 the spirits.

Subsequently, the ninth and tenth questions have been changed. The ninth question now concerns old diseases and the tenth question the causes of diseases.

DIAGNOSIS BY HEARING AND SMELL    This includes hearing the patient's voice and the sounds of coughing, respiration and so on and smelling the patient's mouth and body. Some diseases may give rise to offensive smells, such as ulcers, tumors, or carbuncles. In some acute contagious diseases or in failure of the liver and kidney functions, there may be special smells to be detected. In addition, when a patient is suffering from heat in the lungs and stomach, he or she may have bad breath; this may also be the case when a patient is suffering from indigestion.

PULSE DIAGNOSIS    Pulse diagnosis involves the use of three fingers to press the radial artery of the wrist, with the throbbing segment of the radial artery divided into three sections, namely, the distal section, middle section and proximal section. To take the pulse is to determine the pulse rate, force, wave and so on. Numerous pulses were discovered in ancient China and about 28 pulses are in frequent use in clinical practice today.

The pulse can tell us about the nature of diseases. For instance, a superficial pulse is symptomatic of a superficial disease, a rapid pulse is symptomatic of a hot disease and a slippery or sliding pulse is symptomatic of a sputum disease, indigestion, excess-heat disease, or pregnancy.

A normal pulse is also called a constant pulse, which is indicative of stomach energy and it appears harmonious, slow, but forceful, neither too fast nor too slow and at about four beats per act of respiration or 70 to 75 beats per minute. Children may display a faster pulse. Pulse rate may also be influenced by physical activities, climate and other environmental conditions.

Abnormal pulse refers to any pulse other than a normal one. For example, a big pulse is an abnormal pulse, unless it is taken when a person is engaged in energetic activities.

The 28 pulses most frequently used in diagnosis include the following: depth-related pulses (1. superficial pulse and 2. deep pulse), frequency-related pulses (3. slow pulse and 4. rapid pulse) strength-related pulses (5. deficiency pulse, 6. excess pulse, 7. big pulse and 8. small pulse), length-related pulses (9. long pulse and 10. short pulse), movement-related pulses (11. slippery pulse, 12. retarded pulse and 13. wiry pulse), change-related pulses (14. abrupt pulse, 15. clotting pulse and 16. intermittent pulse) and combination pulses (17. relaxed pulse, 18. full pulse, 19. disappearing pulse, 20. tight pulse, 21. soft pulse, 22. weak pulse, 23. drumming pulse, 24. persisting pulse, 25. shaking pulse, 26. hidden pulse, 27. dispersing pulse and 28. empty pulse).

## THE EIGHT SYNDROME CLASSIFICATIONS

The eight syndrome classifications are yang syndrome, yin syndrome, superficial syndrome, deep syndrome, cold syndrome, hot syndrome, deficiency syndrome and excess syndrome. Yin and yang are opposed to each other and indicate the different types of disease; superficial and deep are opposed to each other and indicate the regions of a disease; cold and hot are opposed to each other and indicate the nature of a disease; and deficiency and excess are opposed to each other and indicate the conditions of a disease. The superficial, hot and excess syndromes are all yang syndromes; the deep, cold and deficiency syndromes are all yin syndromes.

YANG SYNDROME    A disease that is acute, active, forceful and progressive belongs to the yang syndrome, with such symptoms as red complexion, fever, love of cold, nervousness, dry and cracked lips, love of drinking, loud voice, love of talking, rough breath and constipation. When a symptom belongs to the yang syndrome, the pulse is normally superficial, big, rapid, slippery, excessive and forceful and the tongue is normally red in color with a yellowish and dry coating or even prickles.

YIN SYNDROME    A disease that is chronic, weak, quiet and inhibitive belongs to the yin syndrome, with such symptoms as pale complexion, fatigue, heavy sensations in the body, cold limbs, low voice, quiet with dislike of talking, feeble breath, shortness of breath, decreased appetite, love of heat, long and clear streams of urine and abdominal pain with desire for massage. In the yin syndrome, the pulse is normally deep, fine, slow and weak and the tongue is normally light in color and fat and tender, with a moist and sliding coating.

SUPERFICIAL SYNDROME    A disease that occurs in the skin and hair or in the external regions of the meridians belongs to the superficial syndrome.

DEEP SYNDROME    A disease that occurs in the internal organs belongs to the deep syndrome. For instance, a warm or hot disease due to external causes with the pathogenic energy residing at the superficial region of the body belongs to the superficial syndrome; but when the pathogenic energy enters into the deep region to affect the energy and blood or the internal organs, it belongs to the deep syndrome.

COLD SYNDROME    This syndrome includes all diseases caused by cold pathogenic energy or by a decline in yang energy with yin excess. The symptoms may include low body temperature, pale complexion, withered spirits, fatigue, sleeping with legs curled up, love of warmth, fear of cold, cold abdominal pain that lessens with warmth, absence of thirst or thirst with a craving for hot drink, discharge of watery stools, clear and long streams of urine, pale tongue with a white and sliding coating and deep and slow pulse, which are mostly seen in chronic and weak diseases.

HOT SYNDROME   This syndrome includes all diseases caused by hot pathogenic energy or an excess of yang energy. The symptoms may include fever, depressed feeling, red complexion, dislike of heat, dry lips and mouth, love of cold drink, red and dry lips, constipation, short streams of reddish urine, red tongue with a yellowish and dry or black and dry coating and rapid pulse, which are usually seen in contagious and excess diseases.

DEFICIENCY SYNDROME   This syndrome encompasses all diseases caused by a decline in body energy. The symptoms of this syndrome include pale complexion, low spirits, fatigue, weakness, palpitations, shortness of breath, excessive perspiration, night sweats, tender tongue with no coating and deficient and weak pulse.

EXCESS SYNDROME   This syndrome encompasses all diseases caused by an excess of pathogenic energy engaged in a violent struggle with body energy or an occurrence of energy congestion and blood coagulations due to an internal functional breakdown that may also lead to sputum and indigestion. The symptoms of the excess syndrome may include high fever, thirst, mental depression, delirium, abdominal fullness and pain that worsen with massage, constipation, short streams of reddish urine, "old" tongue with a yellowish, dry and rough coating and excess and forceful pulse, which are mostly seen in acute diseases.

## The Eight Grand Methods of Treatment

There are eight grand methods of treatment in Chinese medicine that have been established as the guiding principles in clinical practice. They are the methods of inducing perspiration, clearing heat, inducing bowel movements, striking a balance (or the harmonizing method), warming up coldness, tonification, eliminating and inducing vomiting.

### THE METHOD OF INDUCING PERSPIRATION

Inducing perspiration is also called initiating the superficial region in Chinese medicine. The objective of inducing perspiration is to induce the external pathogenic energies that have penetrated the human body to move outward by means of perspiration. In Chinese medicine, it is maintained that a pathogen will attack the human body from the outside and then it will penetrate into the

body, step by step. For this reason, when the pathogen is still residing in the superficial region (namely, the regions of the skin, hair and muscles), it is necessary to induce perspiration. This way, the pathogen will have a chance to get out of the body before it penetrates further into the body to cause a deep syndrome. The superficial syndrome, including such symptoms as dislike of cold, fever, headache, pain in the body and superficial pulse, should be treated by inducing perspiration. As each patient is different in terms of physical conditions and as each disease is also different, the superficial syndrome is further divided into the superficial cold syndrome and the superficial hot syndrome. However, the two syndromes are, in most cases, closely related to each other and, in clinical practice, they are usually treated together. Perspiration can be induced with pungent and warm herbs or with pungent and cold herbs.

In Chinese herbal therapy, herbs or foods with a pungent flavor and warm energy are used to treat a superficial cold syndrome, which displays the following symptoms: dislike of cold, fever, no perspiration, headache, nasal congestion, pain in the four limbs, thin and white coating of the tongue and superficial and tight pulse or superficial and relaxed pulse.

In Chinese herbal therapy, herbs or foods with a pungent flavor and cold energy are used to treat the superficial hot syndrome, which displays these symptoms: fever, headache, slight dislike of cold and wind, presence of perspiration, thirst, sore throat, red tongue with a thin, yellow and dry coating and superficial and rapid pulse.

### THE METHOD OF CLEARING HEAT

To clear heat means to clear and sedate the pathogenic heat for various kinds of deep and hot symptoms; clearing heat can also be used to treat deficiency heat or superficial heat. However, in clinical practice, a distinction must be made among the different types of heat, including energy heat, blood heat, yin heat, toxic heat, dampness-heat, heat in the internal organs, excess heat and deficiency heat. For instance, energy heat and excess heat should be treated by clearing heat and sedating fire at the same time, blood heat should be treated by clearing heat and cooling the blood at the same time, yin heat should be treated by clearing the heat and nourishing the yin at the same time, toxic heat in excess should be treated by clearing heat and counteracting toxic effects at the same time and heat in the internal organs should be treated by treating the organs involved.

TO CLEAR HEAT AND SEDATE FIRE   Basically, this means treating energy heat, which normally displays the following symptoms: high fever, thirst, dry tongue, yellowish and dry coating of the tongue and forceful and rapid pulse.

TO CLEAR HEAT AND COOL BLOOD   This involves treating blood heat, which normally displays the following symptoms: high fever, mental confusion, delirium, deep-red tongue and bleeding.

TO CLEAR HEAT AND COUNTERACT TOXIC EFFECTS
This involves treating various types of toxic heat, which usually displays the following symptoms: red swelling, fever, pain, pustulation and decomposition. Toxic heat includes the diseases caused by an attack of external energies, with such symptoms as sore throat, ulcers, vomiting of blood, nosebleed and delirium, all of which belong to the hot syndrome.

TO CLEAR HEAT IN THE INTERNAL ORGANS    This involves treating heat in the internal organs that display various symptoms. For instance, excess heat in the heart meridian will give rise to feeling depressed, thirst, ulcers in the mouth and on the tongue, short streams of reddish urine, difficulty in urination and pain on urination; excess fire in the liver meridian will give rise to pain in the upper abdomen, bitter taste in the mouth, pink eyes and pain in the eyes, wax in the ears, urinary straining, ulcers in the genitals and red swelling of the scrotum; heat in the lungs will give rise to cough and asthma; hot stomach or heat in the stomach will cause bad breath and swelling and bleeding of the gums, all of which may be treated by this method.

TO CLEAR HEAT AND TRANSFORM DAMPNESS    This involves treating dampness-heat, which generally displays the following symptoms: intermittent or prolonged fever, congested chest, abdominal swelling, sticky sensations in the mouth, nausea, poor appetite, reddish urine, watery stools and yellowish and greasy coating of the tongue. The same method can also be used to treat a syndrome called dampness-heat turning into fire, which generally gives rise to dysentery, jaundice, hot urinary straining, or discharge of yellowish fluids in skin diseases.

TO CLEAR HEAT AND LUBRICATE DRYNESS    This involves treating three syndromes:
1 the lungs-dryness syndrome, in which dryness impairs the lungs and the stomach, causing dry throat, thirst and dry cough with scant sputum;
2 the hot syndrome, particularly at its later stage when both energy and yin are impaired, causing such symptoms as dry mouth, mental depression, hiccups and poor appetite; and
3 the deficiency heat syndrome, which gives rise to such symptoms as hot sensations in the body as if they were coming from the bones, periodic fever, night sweats, or persistent low fever.

## THE METHOD OF INDUCING
## BOWEL MOVEMENTS

Inducing bowel movements relieves constipation and, for this reason, it can be used to treat a variety of syndromes as long as they involve constipation.

TO SEDATE EXCESS HEAT    This method involves treating the following three syndromes:
1 The stomach-heat syndrome, with such symptoms as periodic fever, delirium, abdominal fullness, abdominal pain worsening with massage, constipation, scorching and yellowish coating of the tongue with prickles or scorching, black, dry coating on a cleft tongue and slow and sliding pulse;
2 the toxic heat syndrome, with such symptoms as high fever, feeling depressed and hurried, mental confusion, twitching, dry mouth and throat, constipation, bleeding and skin eruptions; and
3 heat in the internal organs, which gives rise to sore and swollen throat, ulcers in the mouth and on the tongue, swollen gums, nosebleed, bad breath, constipation, hot sensations in the chest and diaphragm regions, headache, pink eyes, ringing in the ears, feeling hurried and jumpy and yellowish coating of the tongue.

TO ATTACK COLD ACCUMULATIONS    This method is used in treating the internal coldness syndrome. When a person consumes too much cold food with cold energy accumulating in the stomach and intestine, acute pain in the stomach and abdomen may occur that gets worse with massage. Or, when a person suffers from deficiency cold of the spleen and stomach, normal transformations and digestion are impaired, with the result that cold energy gets accumulated in the stomach and intestine, which may give rise to the following symptoms: abdominal pain that lessens with warmth, hardness felt with massage, thirst with craving for hot drink, constipation or difficult bowel movements, fear of the cold, cold limbs and white and sliding coating of the tongue.

TO LUBRICATE THE INTESTINE TO INDUCE BOWEL MOVEMENTS    This is used in treating the intestine-dryness syndrome for relief of constipation in older or weak patients or in pregnant women due to blood deficiency and shortage of fluids.

## THE METHOD OF STRIKING
## A BALANCE, OR HARMONIZING

This method of treatment can also be called "negotiating a settlement," because it is aimed at regulating and adjusting the relationships among the internal organs, meridians, energy and blood, for the purpose of removing external pathogenic energies to restore the normal functions of the body. This principle of treatment can be used in three different ways.

TO HARMONIZE THE SUPERFICIAL AND DEEP REGIONS
This involves treating the syndrome in between the superficial and deep, which normally displays the following symptoms: alternating cold and fever due to external causes, congested chest and discomfort in the upper-abdomen region, being

quiet with no appetite, feeling depressed, nausea, bitter taste in the mouth, dry throat, dizziness and wiry and rapid pulse.

### TO REGULATE AND HARMONIZE THE STOMACH AND THE INTESTINE
This involves treating the cold and deficient large-intestine syndrome. When external pathogenic energies reside in the stomach and intestine, one may display such symptoms as combination of chills and fever, dull sensations at the pit of the stomach, nausea, abdominal pain, watery stools or diarrhea and intestinal rumbling, which can be treated by this method.

### TO REGULATE AND HARMONIZE THE LIVER AND SPLEEN OR STOMACH
This is used in treating two syndromes: the liver-spleen disharmony syndrome and the liver-stomach disharmony syndrome. The liver-spleen disharmony syndrome involves two distinct syndromes: the liver energy congestion syndrome and the spleen deficiency syndrome. The two syndromes are very similar and may include the following symptoms: feeling depressed, abdominal swelling and pain, discomfort in the chest, intestinal rumbling and diarrhea or tension causing abdominal pain and diarrhea. The liver-stomach disharmony syndrome also involves two distinct syndromes: the liver energy congestion syndrome and the stomach energy upsurging syndrome. Likewise, both are very similar and may include such symptoms as congested chest, poor appetite, vomiting, belching, acid regurgitation and pain at the pit of the stomach.

## THE METHOD OF WARMING UP COLDNESS

Warming up coldness is also called expelling coldness and it is designed to tone up yang energy in order to expel the cold pathogen from the body. This method is used to treat the internal coldness syndrome, which is also called the deep coldness syndrome, as opposed to the superficial coldness syndrome. In Chinese herbal therapy, herbs to be used for warming up coldness are either warm or hot. The internal coldness syndrome is mostly due to a yang deficiency that has existed in one's physical conditions and generated coldness within the body or due to an attack of an external cold pathogen, resulting in a cold stroke, involving internal organs, that gives rise to a yang deficiency of the organs affected. Meridian coldness is mostly due to an accumulation of cold energy in the meridians causing a blockage of energy and blood within the meridians. There are a number of different methods of warming up coldness.

### TO WARM THE MIDDLE REGION AND DISPERSE COLDNESS
This involves treating the spleen-stomach yang deficiency syndrome, with such symptoms as cold pain at the pit of the stomach and in the intestine, vomiting, diarrhea, fat tongue with a white and sliding coating and deep and slow pulse or deep and tight pulse; the spleen yang deficiency syndrome, with abdominal pain, love of warmth, abdominal swelling, watery stools and cold limbs; and the cold stomach syndrome, with pain at the pit of the stomach that drags on and lessens with warmth or heat, vomiting of clear water and more. In clinical practice, the spleen-stomach yang deficiency syndrome is encountered most frequently, as the spleen and the stomach form a yin-yang relationship with each other, so their symptoms will also affect each other.

### TO RESTORE YANG AND RESCUE UPSURGING
This is used to treat yang prolapse syndrome, with the following symptoms: dislike of cold, lying down with body curled up, extremely cold limbs, vomiting and diarrhea, body temperature decreasing, pale complexion and fine and disappearing pulse or hollow and rapid pulse.

### TO WARM UP MERIDIANS AND DISPERSE COLDNESS
This is designed to treat the meridian coldness syndrome, with the following symptoms: cold pain in the four limbs, poor blood circulation, blue tips of the four limbs, rheumatism with coldness, cold pain in the muscles and difficulty in flexing and extending the joints.

## THE METHOD OF TONIFICATION

This treatment principle is an important one in Chinese medicine, as it can be applied to deal with inherent deficiency and acquired deficiency alike, so long as there are signs of yin or yang deficiency, energy deficiency, blood deficiency, shortage of semen, or shortage of fluids and so on. There are four methods of tonification: to tone up energy deficiency, blood deficiency, yin deficiency and yang deficiency.

### TO TONE UP ENERGY DEFICIENCY
This involves treating the energy deficiency syndrome, the lungs energy deficiency syndrome and the spleen energy deficiency syndrome. These syndromes may give rise to the following symptoms: fatigue, weakness, shortness of breath, too tired to talk, feeble and low voice, asthma triggered by labor or movements, whitish complexion, poor appetite, watery stools, excessive perspiration, edema, weak pulse, prolapse of the anus and prolapse of the uterus.

### TO TONE UP BLOOD DEFICIENCY
This is used to treat the blood deficiency syndrome, with the following symptoms: pale or withering and yellowish complexion, pale lips and nails, dizziness and spots in front of the eyes, palpitations, insomnia, irregular menstrual periods, scant menstrual flow in light color, numbness of hands and feet, pale tongue and fine pulse.

### TO TONE UP YIN DEFICIENCY
This is used to treat the yin deficiency syndrome, with the following symptoms: loss of weight, dry mouth and throat,

dizziness, ringing in the ears, sore loins and weak legs, red tongue with scant coating and fine pulse. The same treatment principle is also effective for the deficiency fire syndrome, with the following symptoms: red lips, reddish appearance in the zygoma, feeling depressed, insomnia, hot sensations in the middle of the palms and the soles of the feet, periodic fever, night sweats, seminal emission and discharge of blood from the mouth.

TO TONE UP YANG DEFICIENCY  This is used to treat the yang deficiency syndrome, with the following symptoms: fear of cold, cold limbs, sore loins, weak legs, cold pain across the loins or in the legs, impotence, sliding ejaculation, a long stream of plentiful clear urine, pale tongue and deep, fine and weak pulse. All of these symptoms are mostly seen in the *kidneys* yang deficiency syndrome. The heart yang deficiency syndrome and the *spleen* yang deficiency syndrome should be treated by the principle of warming up.

## THE METHOD OF ELIMINATING

This method of treatment is for such disorders as indigestion, swelling, accumulation, stones, ulcers and parasites. It can be broadly divided into two categories: to eliminate hardness and to eliminate coagulations.

TO ELIMINATE INDIGESTION  This treatment principle is designed to cope with symptoms arising from indigestion as follows: fullness of stomach, abdominal swelling, acid swallowing and belching of bad breath, nausea, vomiting, poor appetite, abdominal pain, constipation, diarrhea and thick and greasy coating of the tongue.

TO ELIMINATE SWOLLEN LUMPS AND EXPEL STONES
This principle can be applied in treating swollen lumps, such as of the liver and the spleen and hard symptoms and tumors as well as liver stone, gallstone, urinary stone and so on.

TO ELIMINATE CARBUNCLES AND DRAIN OFF PUS
This principle is designed for such external infections as carbuncles, abscesses, boils and furuncles. In clinical application, a further distinction between the yang syndrome and the yin syndrome is made. The yang syndrome includes the following symptoms: acute onset, redness, swelling, heat, pain and sticky fluids in cases of ulcers. The yin syndrome includes slow onset, white and spreading swelling, hardness with aching pain and clear and thin fluids in cases of ulcers.

TO ELIMINATE SPUTUM AND SOFTEN UP HARDNESS
This principle can be applied to deal with hard sputum in the meridians, with the following manifestations: lipoma, fibroma, tuberculosis lymph node, goiter, nodular goiter, carcinoma of the thyroid, simple goiter and so on.

## THE METHOD OF INDUCING VOMITING

Of the eight grand methods of treatment, inducing vomiting is the last. It is used to prevent poisoning and suffocation, consumption of toxic foods, presence of indigestible substances in the stomach, apoplexy and epilepsy.

# Herbology

In Chinese medicine, diseases are often treated with herbs. Applications of Chinese herbs in clinical practice are based upon the nature and capabilities of herbs and they in turn are based upon the energies, flavors, movements and meridian routes of herbs.

## THE FOUR ENERGIES

The four energies of herbs are cold, hot, warm and cool. These classifications are derived from the effects of herbs as originally observed from actual applications by the ancient Chinese. When an herb has proven effective in the treatment of a hot syndrome, that herb is considered to have a cold energy; when an herb has proven effective in the treatment of a cold syndrome, it is considered to have a hot energy. The four energies of herbs can be broadly divided into yin and yang, with cold and cool energies belonging to yin and hot and warm energies belonging to yang. Since the difference between cold and cool and between hot and warm is only a matter of degree, Chinese physicians are in the habit of using such expressions as "extremely warm" or "slightly warm" and "extremely cold" or "slightly cold."

## THE FIVE FLAVORS

The five flavors refer to pungent (or acrid), sweet, sour, bitter and salty, which are distinguished from each other by the sense of taste. The ancient Chinese distinguished various actions of herbs through a very long process of clinical experience and they came to the conclusion that pungent herbs can disperse, sour herbs can constrict, sweet herbs can slow down, bitter herbs can harden and salty herbs can soften up. This was clearly recorded in *The Yellow Emperor's Classics of Internal Medicine*. Subsequently, Chinese physicians have further discovered that pungent herbs can disperse and promote the flow of energy, sour herbs can constrict and obstruct, sweet herbs can tone up and harmonize, bitter herbs can dry up and cause diarrhea and salty herbs can soften up and promote downward movements. In addition, there is another classification called tasteless flavor, which can help dampness seep and promote urination. But, as tasteless flavor is similar to sweet flavor, the two are generally classified under the same flavor, which is why a celebrated Chinese herbalist has said, "Tasteless flavor is associated with sweet flavor."

*A formula may have, say, four common actions:
to clear the lungs, transform sputum, cool the blood
and counteract toxic effects.*

## THE FOUR MOVEMENTS

The four movements of herbs are to push upward, to push downward, to float and to sink. To push upward means that a given herb is capable of elevating falling symptoms, as with the prolapse of the anus and uterus or the internal organs. To push downward means the herb is capable of suppressing upsurging symptoms, as with hiccups and cough. To float means that the herb is capable of dispersing outward, as with inducing perspiration. And to sink means that the herb is capable of promoting diarrhea and directing energy downward. The herbs that can push upward and those that can float have the common functions of moving upward and outward, with such actions as inducing perspiration and vomiting as well as elevating yang energy. On the other hand, the herbs that can push downward and those that can sink have the common functions of moving downward and inward, with such actions as relieving vomiting, checking perspiration and inducing diarrhea.

## MERIDIAN ROUTES

The meridian routes refer to the meridians a given herb is capable of entering and travelling through, which accounts for two herbs with identical energy and flavor still displaying two different actions. In clinical application, herbs are selected that travel through the meridians in the diseased regions. For instance, a hot herb is used to treat a cold disease and a cold herb is used to treat a hot disease, which are standard procedures in Chinese herbal therapy. But two hot herbs may have different actions, with one herb being good for the cold *lungs* syndrome while the other being good for the cold *liver* syndrome. By the same token, one cold herb may be good for the hot *spleen* syndrome whereas another cold herb may be good for the hot lungs syndrome.

## ACTIONS

All important Chinese herbs or herbal formulas have a number of common actions, which is why they are considered important. In Western medicine, an antihistamine is used to counteract the effect of histamine, which is the action of an antihistamine. Similarly, Chinese herbs or herbal formulas have various actions, but they are expressed in different terminologies, such as to clear heat, sedate fire, or stop wind. The terminologies used for treatment principles and actions are identical. Thus, when a given formula can clear heat, its action is to clear heat, which may be used to treat the hot syndrome.

A formula may have, say, four common actions: to clear the lungs, transform sputum, cool the blood and counteract toxic effects. A doctor of Chinese medicine knows how to use this formula simply by identifying its common actions. Since this formula can cool the blood, we can use it to arrest bleeding, as in the case of

nosebleed; since it can clear the lungs, we can use it to suppress cough associated with the lungs; since it can transform sputum, we can use it to reduce mucous discharge in cough and asthma; and since it can counteract toxic effects, we can use it to heal swelling and boils in the skin.

Thus, the common actions of Chinese formulas are very important in clinical applications, but it takes quite a while for a person to fully understand the meaning of the common actions of formulas and learn how to apply them in the treatment of diseases. The basic reason is that in order to make use of common actions of formulas, one needs to know how to make diagnosis of a disease, which is not a very easy task. Even if we know, for example, that this particular formula can cool the blood, we still have a long way to go before we are able to apply it to arrest bleeding. There are many possible syndromes that account for bleeding, including the wind-cold syndrome, the spleen unable to govern the blood syndrome, external injuries, the large-intestine excess syndrome and the hot blood syndrome. If a formula can cool the blood, it can only be applied to treat nosebleed that falls within the scope of the hot blood syndrome in order to be effective. A doctor of Chinese medicine must make a diagnosis to determine if this particular case of nosebleed, for example, falls within the scope of the hot blood syndrome, before he or she can apply it to treat nosebleed. In addition, in order to determine the right syndrome of a nosebleed, the doctor needs to follow the standard procedures of Chinese diagnosis, which involve the theory of yin and yang as well as the Chinese organ theory.

## HERBAL FORMULAS

In most cases, a syndrome has more than one symptom that cannot be treated by one single herb. Thus, in Chinese herbal therapy, several herbs are used together in a formula in order to cope with the conditions of a disease. This is called compound therapy in Chinese medicine. Over the course of history, the Chinese have established more than 20,000 formulas, of which about 2,000 are currently in use. Although a physician of herbal therapy can use his or her own formulas to treat patients, established formulas have been proven effective in the past and, for this reason, they should be used for clinical applications whenever possible.

A standard herbal formula consists of a king herb, subject herb, assistant herb and servant herb. According to *The Yellow Emperor's Classics of Internal Medicine*, "The primary herb in a formula is called the king herb, the herb included in the formula to assist the king herb is called the subject herb in that formula and the herb included in the formula to be responsible to the subject herb is called the servant herb."

Every formula must have at least a king herb, but not every formula needs a subject herb, an assistant herb, or a servant herb. Sometimes a formula may have a king herb that also plays the role of a subject herb, just like a prime minister may also act as the finance minister in a cabinet. As a general rule, the king herb in a formula has the largest dose, followed by the subject herb, the assistant herb and the servant herb.

THE KING HERB   In a formula, the king herb is the herb that is primarily responsible for dealing with the syndrome under treatment. For instance, if the patient has been diagnosed as suffering from the cold syndrome, the king herb must be capable of warming up the body; if the patient has been diagnosed as suffering from the kidneys yang deficiency syndrome, the king herb must be capable of toning up the kidneys yang. Many formulas have more than one king herb, because a syndrome often contains two basic conditions that need to be treated simultaneously with two different herbs. Take the gallbladder dampness-heat syndrome for example. This syndrome contains two basic conditions, namely, gallbladder-dampness and gallbladder-heat, so the formula selected to treat this syndrome may contain one herb to remove gallbladder-dampness and a second herb to clear gallbladder-heat.

THE SUBJECT HERB   An herb in this category assists the king herb in two different ways: it reinforces the action of the king herb from a different angle and it treats the concurrent syndrome. For example, when the king herb in a formula is used to induce perspiration, a subject herb can be selected to produce body fluids to reinforce the function of the king herb in inducing perspiration. Sufficient body fluids will make perspiration easier, which means that the subject herb is helping the king herb achieve its objective indirectly. Another example is that when a person is suffering from two syndromes simultaneously, with one syndrome as the main one and the other syndrome as the concurrent one, the king herb will deal with the main syndrome while the subject herb will deal with the concurrent syndrome. As with king herbs, a formula can contain more than one subject herb.

THE ASSISTANT HERB   In a formula, the assistant herb can play one of the following three roles: it can assist the king herb or the subject herb in dealing with a relatively minor symptom, it can control the undesirable drastic actions of the king herb and the subject herb or reduce their toxic effects and it can play the role of an opposition to supplement the action of the king herb.

THE SERVANT HERB   In a formula, the servant herb plays two basic roles: it can direct the formula to the affected region and it can harmonize the herbs in the formula.

## HOW TO TAKE HERBS

After herbs are put together in a formula, they must be prepared for consumption. There are three common ways of taking a formula: decoction, powder and tablets.

DECOCTION   As many Chinese formulas have been made into tablets and many are also available in powder form, it has become less important for people to know how to decoct formulas. Nevertheless, the vast majority of Chinese formulas are still not available in either tablets or powder, which means that they need to be decocted. Moreover, herbal formulas that have been decocted are readily absorbed and take effect more quickly, which is beneficial for acute disorders. In order to produce the best therapeutic effects, formulas should be decocted according to established methods.

The pot used for decoction should be made of something other than iron or bronze in order to prevent chemical changes; usually, an earthenware pot is used instead. Place the herbs in the pot, add cold water just enough to cover all the herbs and then add one more cup, so that the water will be about half an inch higher than the herbs. Stir a little bit and let the herbs soak in the water for about 20 minutes. Then bring the water to boil; as soon as the water begins to boil, reduce the heat to low, both to keep the water from overflowing and to prevent its premature exhaustion. During the course of decoction, the pot should be covered and not opened too frequently in order to retain the volatile constituents of some herbs. The quantity of the water used varies with the herbs and the heat, because some herbs absorb more water than others and thus need more water for decoction and high heat consumes more water than low heat.

Before decoction, herbs should be soaked in water for about 20 minutes to make them soft and moist. The same water should be used for decoction to prevent any loss of the herbs' potency. The total decoction time depends upon the herbs being decocted. For instance, herbs for inducing perspiration can be decocted over high heat for less than 10 minutes after the water starts boiling and herbs for strengthening the body, traditionally called tonics, can be decocted for as long as an hour over low heat. After decoction, the herbs are strained.

When a Chinese patient gets a prescription from a doctor, he or she usually brings it to an herb shop for filling. The clerk at the herb shop will wrap up the herbs in small paper bags and give instructions for each bag to be decocted two to three times for oral administration. Normally, each decoction is to be taken all at once as one dosage, usually in one or two cups and two dosages are taken a day. The same bag of herbs can be decocted in the morning and then again in the late afternoon.

Sometimes it may be necessary to decoct the heavy or hard herbs, like wood or roots, over low heat for 10 to 20 minutes first, so that their constituents will become fully soluble in boiling water. Clinical experiences have shown that such heavy herbs can be decocted repeatedly to produce good results. After heavy and hard herbs have been boiled for 10 to 20 minutes, add the aromatic herbs and then the very light herbs, such as leaves and flowers, which should be decocted for only about five minutes or so in order to prevent evaporation of some constituents like essential oils.

POWDER   When herbs in a formula are ground into powder, they are easy to carry, take and preserve. Powder is also more economical than by decoction, because generally one bag of herbs supplying one day's consumption by decoction will supply four days of consumption in powder with the same effects. After the herbs have been ground into powder, filter the powder to make sure that it is fine enough for consumption. Here is how to take a formula in powder:

- The first thing you should do is mix up the powder thoroughly either in a jar or a bag to make sure that the powder is properly mixed, because herbal formulas contain different herbs which should be mixed up evenly.
- Put the powder in a cup and pour boiling water into the cup; then stir and drink it warm. If any residue remains at the bottom, repeat the same process and drink it again, so that you don't waste any powder.
- The quantity of powder you should take depends on how much you weigh, because the heavier you are, the more you should take. Assuming that you weigh 140 pounds, you should be taking 6 grams of powder (roughly one-third of the formula weight) each time (increase or decrease 1 gram for each 15 pounds of body weight). Therefore, if you weigh 155 pounds you should take 7 grams each time; if you weigh only 110 pounds, you should take only 4 grams each time, twice daily.
- The process of drinking Chinese herbal powder is similar to drinking instant coffee, except the powder may not dissolve in boiling water as quickly and easily as instant coffee and the powder may not taste as good as coffee. If you don't like the taste of it, you can also put it in empty capsules, which are available in health food stores. Alternatively, you can place the powder on your tongue, hold your breath and wash it down with a cup of warm water. Wash any residue down with another cup of water. This should be done twice daily.

TABLETS   Herbal powder can be made into tablets, which is normally done by manufacturers. Tablets have a number of advantages: they are easiest to take and carry; they are slow in absorption and therefore good for chronic and deficient diseases- and, since some formulas are very drastic in action, when they are taken as tablets, such drastic action can be slowed down. Follow the manufacturer's instructions on the quantity of tablets to take each time.

## THE THREE RULES FOR TAKING A FORMULA

There are three types of rule regarding taking an herbal formula, those specifying when the formula should be taken, whether it should be taken warm or cold and that it should be taken without tea.

WHEN TO TAKE A FORMULA   A formula can be taken before or after meals, depending on the formula and its effects. As a general rule, formulas that can disturb the digestive system and formulas for eye diseases should be taken after meals; formulas for malaria should be taken two hours prior to onset; formulas to induce sleep, as in insomnia, should be taken before bedtime; formulas for acute symptoms can be taken any time; formulas for chronic diseases should be taken according to a fixed schedule on a regular basis; and formulas taken as tonics to strengthen the body should be taken before meals. In addition, some formulas can be drunk like tea many times during the day without any fixed schedule.

The Chinese have this saying: "Withered plants will blossom and migratory birds return every year on schedule." When this principle is applied to taking formulas, it means that formulas should be taken regularly according to a fixed schedule or every day at the same time.

When formulas are used to treat disorders in the chest or above the chest, they should be taken after meals; when they are used to treat disorders below the heart, they should be taken before meals; when they are used to treat disorders of the four limbs and the blood vessels, they should be taken on an empty stomach; and when they are used to treat disorders of bones and marrow, they should be taken at night and after meals.

WHETHER THE FORMULA SHOULD BE TAKEN WARM OR COLD   Some formulas should be taken very warm, but others taken cold, depending on the disorder under treatment. Formulas taken to induce perspiration, as for the common cold, should be taken very warm or relatively hot. The patient should keep warm right after taking the formulas in order to induce light perspiration and, after taking such formulas, it is also wise to drink a little hot soup to reinforce the effects of the formulas.

When formulas are taken to treat a hot disease, they should be taken cold; when formulas are taken to treat a cold disease, they should be taken hot. However, certain formulas can cause vomiting when taken hot, in which case they should be taken cold.

TAKING THE FORMULA WITHOUT TEA   The third rule regarding taking formulas is to refrain from taking them with tea. Some people have a habit of taking formulas with tea for the sake of convenience, but this is definitely not advisable; warm water should be drunk instead. For one thing, tea is obstructive and it can obstruct the movements of herbs, reducing their effects. In the second place, tea has a cold energy, which can interfere with the warm energy of certain herbs. And thirdly, tea contains caffeine and theophylline, which can excite the central nervous system; so, when formulas used to treat insomnia, for example, are taken with tea, their effects will be cancelled out.

## Traditional Food Remedies

Is there such a thing as longevity food that we can eat in abundant quantities in order to live a long life? Many people, particularly those in the West, are in the habit of jumping from one magic solution to another, but unfortunately, no such foods exist. The basic reason for this is that people have differing physical constitutions and require different foods in order to stay in good health or to be immune from disease. However, in selecting foods in your quest for longevity, there is one fundamental concept that is helpful to keep in mind: Whether or not a given food contributes to longevity basically depends on whether your body needs it.

In 1747, for example, on board the *Salisbury*, a naval surgeon by the name of James Lind selected a few patients with scurvy and gave them lemons and oranges. These patients recovered in six days and the others who didn't consume any lemons and oranges made no progress. The seamen were in need of vitamin C, which proved beneficial to them. But it does not necessarily mean that consumption of vitamin C in great quantities is beneficial to all of us; on the contrary, it could be harmful to many of us, since we are not seamen and we eat lemons and oranges very frequently, if not every day.

If you are susceptible to, say, hypertension, you should try to eat those foods that can either prevent it or lower blood pressure. Likewise, if you are susceptible to hepatitis (inflammation of the liver), you should try to eat those foods that can prevent hepatitis. Many foods are good for people who are susceptible to hypertension—such as celery, peanuts, garlic, jellyfish and seaweed. Similarly, many foods are good for people susceptible to hepatitis—such as malt, pork gall bladder, tea and common button mushrooms.

The foods presented in this book are good for longevity, not because they will make you live a long life if you simply consume them in huge quantities, but because they are particularly conducive to longevity for a specific reason. In the

*"Withered plants will blossom and migratory birds return every year on schedule." When this principle is applied to taking formulas, it means that formulas should be taken regularly according to a fixed schedule or every day at the same time.*

discussion that follows, a number of important foods are singled out; many of them will be discussed in greater detail later in this book.

## SOYBEANS FOR MORE THAN QUALITY PROTEIN

Protein is an important source of heat and energy for the body and animal proteins are better than plant proteins in quality. But animal proteins have many other substances considered harmful to health, such as fat and cholesterol, particularly when they are consumed in large quantities. Thus, we are faced with a dilemma: We want proteins of high quality, but we do not want the undesirable substances found in meats.

Soybeans can resolve this dilemma. Soybeans have been grown in China for more than 3,000 years and they were first exported to Europe in the eighteenth century.

In 1960, when China was experiencing a severe economic recession with a critical food shortage, an increasing number of Chinese people were suffering from edema (a condition in which the body tissues retain an excessive amount of fluids). The Chinese government began to supply the people with soybeans in great quantities, which rapidly brought this widespread disease under control. How did the Chinese know about using soybeans to relieve edema? The medicinal uses of soybeans in China date all the way back to the third century B.C. when the first Chinese book of medicinal herbs, entitled *Agriculture Minister's Collection of Medicinal Herbs*, was published. This classic lists 365 medicinal herbs including soybean, clearly demonstrating the Chinese belief that soybeans are very important to health, whether used as a food or an herb.

In a subsequent book of medicinal herbs, entitled *Records of Celebrated Physicians*, published towards the end of the Han Dynasty (206 B.C.-A.D. 220), it says: "Soybeans can dispel retention of excessive tissue fluids." This statement by a professional herbalist marked the beginning of soybeans as a remedy for edema. Then later when the greatest herbalist in Chinese history named Shi-Chen Li (1518-1593) published his celebrated work in 1578, entitled *An Outline of Materia Medica*, he recommended soybeans as an effective remedy for "kidney diseases, water retention and poisoning."

As we have seen, the Chinese not only regard soybeans as food but also as an herb capable of healing many diseases. In addition to curing edema, they found soybeans to be helpful in treating the common cold, skin diseases, beriberi, diarrhea, toxemia of pregnancy (various symp-

*The foods presented in this book are good for longevity, not because they will make you live a long life if you simply consume them in huge quantities, but because they are particularly conducive to longevity for a specific reason.*

toms during pregnancy, such as vomiting, acute yellow atrophy of the liver and renal failure), habitual constipation, iron-deficiency anemia and leg ulcers. Small wonder that there is such a wide range of soybean products—from bean curd (or tofu) and soybean sprouts to flour, dried bean curd and bean drink—all of which are considered very beneficial to health.

Another important use of soybeans is to promote lactation. Chinese farmers know how to increase cow's milk secretion by feeding them soybean milk. And in old China, when life was very difficult, a nursing mother knew how to fry soybeans until they were aromatic and then steam them along with turnips and fresh ginger to eat at meals for promoting milk secretion. In the twentieth century, we know that during the period of lactation, the mother needs additional calcium to offset her loss of milk. But we must remember that the use of soybeans in a diet to increase milk secretion in nursing mothers dates back to over 1,000 years ago when no scientist in the West knew about calcium or any other nutrients. Soybeans are indeed a calcium-rich food as the Chinese have discovered in modern times and this shows that the ancient Chinese practice is consistent with that principle of modern nutrition but at least 10 centuries ahead of it.

In Japan, Dr. Y. Toyora has pointed out that most of the Japanese athletes who have won gold medals at Olympic Games have taken soybean proteins as their main source of heat and energy. He also noted that Chinese workers have demonstrated higher levels of energy and endurance than others, which may be attributed to their regular consumption of soybeans and soybean products. But is there any indication that soybeans directly contribute to longevity? Japanese researchers conducted an experiment in which animal proteins were used to feed one group of lab animals while plant proteins were used to feed another group. The results of the experiment show that the first group grew faster but with a shorter life and the second group grew more slowly but lived longer. And in his book, *Longevity and Eating Habits*, Professor Kondo Shoji of Tohoku University in Japan has pointed out that according to his research, the geographical regions in which soybeans are produced seem to have a higher percentage of longevous people.

At present, the majority of Chinese people living in big cities—particularly those with hypertension, arteriosclerosis, coronary heart disease and diabetes—are fully aware of the advantages of soybeans over meats and soybeans have become one of the essential foods in their diets.

The following is the food value of 100 grams of soybeans: protein, 36.3g; fat, 18.4g; carbohydrates, 25.3g; calories, 412; fiber, 5.0g; calcium, 564mg; phosphorus, 571mg; iron, 11mg; carotin, 0.40mg; vitamin B1, 0.79mg; vitamin B2, 0.25 mg; nicotinic acid, 2.5mg; and water, 10.2g.

No vitamin C is found in soybeans, but 100 grams of soybean sprouts contain 5 milligrams of vitamin C and soybean oil contains vitamin E. The food value of soybeans is comparable to that of meats, which is why the Chinese call soybeans "plant meats." According to one Chinese researcher, one pound of soybeans contains as much protein as 2 pounds of lean meat, 3 pounds of eggs, or 12 pounds of cow's milk. In addition, an average male requires a daily supply of 12 milligrams of iron, which can be supplied by 100 grams of soybeans. Some soybeans reportedly contain as much as 50 milligrams of iron, which is why soybeans have been used to treat iron-deficiency anemia.

There is no doubt that the greatest nutritional value of soybeans as judged from the standpoint of Western nutrition has to do with both the quantity and quality of the protein they contain. I have mentioned that soybeans contain more protein than lean meat or cow's milk, but how about its quality? First of all, the biological value (the proportion of nitrogen retained by the body) of soybean protein is very close to that of meat protein and the soybean amino acids are also very much like those of animal protein. The quality of soybean protein will equal that of eggs or cow's milk when a small quantity of eggs and meat is added to soybeans for consumption at meals.

In terms of fat, soybeans have a plentiful amount of unsaturated fatty acids, which are very easily digested and absorbed. Besides, soybeans also contain an essential fatty acid, called linolenic acid, which cannot be synthesized in the body and must be supplied by foods. For these reasons, the fats in soybeans are considered quality fats.

Were it not for the many harmful effects of animal foods, soybeans wouldn't have become such an important food in modern society. People in the developed nations have consumed animal foods in great amounts with the result that the so-called "civilized diseases"—including obesity, hypertension, arteriosclerosis (hardening of blood vessels) and coronary heart disease—have increased dramatically. These diseases have been found to be particularly related to the consumption of meat, eggs and milk—the primary foods consumed in the developed nations. The harmful effects of animal foods are generally attributed to the high cholesterol levels contained in them. Soybeans, on the other hand, have no cholesterol and the fats contained in them are unsaturated fats with essential fatty acids, which can lower the level of cholesterol in the blood and thereby minimize your chances of developing the diseases commonly attributed to eating animal foods. A few decades ago, the Chinese used to recommend regular consumption of soybeans primarily because they cost much less than animal foods although they have very high-quality proteins and fats, but now they have begun to see the many distinct advantages of eating soybeans beyond purely economic reasons.

TOFU    Besides soybeans, there are a few soybean products that are even more useful for regular consumption and for promoting good health; such products include bean curd (tofu), bean drink and soybean oil. Tofu has been a very popular food among the Chinese people from time immemorial. It is believed that the manufacturing of tofu in China dates back to over 2,000 years ago. The Chinese take great pride in this and regard it as a great invention in Chinese history. Tofu, which is now a staple of the modern health-food store, was not available in North America two decades ago.

To make tofu from soybeans, the first step is to soak the soybeans for about one day (but less time in the summer) and then grind them into a powder. Next, you add water to the powder and bring it to a boil and it will become bean drink. Add some coagulants to separate the beans from the water and this will give you tofu flowers. When the tofu flowers are squeezed and shaped, they become tofu. Tofu can be processed to become a variety of soybean products—such as dried, sliced and noodle tofu. The coagulant used in manufacturing tofu is mostly gypsum, which is a very common mineral containing hydrated calcium sulfate and that is what makes tofu a calcium-rich food.

From the point of view of Chinese medicine, tofu has three basic functions: First, it can increase body energy to make the body stronger; second, it can produce fluids and lubricate the system; and third, it can cool down the body, which is beneficial to many types of skin diseases. In addition, tofu may be boiled with vinegar to be eaten as soup for relief of periodic diarrhea. Tofu is also good for many "hot diseases," including fever, the common cold, inflammations and urination difficulties.

BEAN DRINK    Bean drink is another important soybean product that is very popular in China, as popular as milk is in the West. Often referred to as soybean milk, bean drink is widely used by Chinese people at breakfast, the same way many Western people drink milk every morning. One important advantage of bean drink over milk is that it can be consumed by everyone—adults and children, healthy people and patients—whereas many people have an intolerance to milk.

The quantity of protein in bean drink is about the same as that in milk, but the quality of the protein is slightly lower. Bean drink contains less fat than milk but more unsaturated fatty acids. Moreover, 250 grams of milk contain 33 milligrams of cholesterol, but bean drink has none. Milk has more vitamins than bean drink and in terms of minerals, milk contains more calcium, but bean drink contains more iron. Normally, a health-conscious Chinese family will mix bean drink

with eggs or milk to supplement missing nutrients. However, bean drink is very cool and sliding, which is why it's not recommended for those with gastroduodenal ulcers, chronic enteritis (inflammation of the intestines) and chronic diarrhea.

SOYBEAN SPROUTS    If you immerse soybeans in water and maintain an adequate temperature, the soybeans will absorb the water and gradually germinate; then within four to five days, they will become soybean sprouts that are ready to eat as a vegetable. Soybean sprouts retain all the nutrients of soybeans, only to a lesser degree, but every 100 grams of soybean sprouts contains 5 milligrams of vitamin C, which is not present in soybeans and soybean sprouts are also rich in fiber. Therefore, the Chinese make it a point to consume soybean sprouts in winter as their source of vitamin C when most other vegetables are not available. Moreover, soybean sprouts can be produced indoors, making them useful to seamen and to those living in cold climates since it may be difficult for them to grow other vegetables as a source of vitamin C.

Traditionally, soybean sprouts are used to cleanse toxins in the lungs and to suppress the production of sputum in the body. When patients cough with plenty of mucous discharge that appears yellowish and sticky, a Chinese physician will advise them to boil 4 or 5 pounds of soybean sprouts in abundant water over high heat for 4 to 5 hours and then to eat the soup and sprouts, which should relieve the symptoms quickly and effectively. In fact, soybean sprouts are considered good for any symptoms classified as "hot and dry," such as dry lips, cracked mouth, cankers, sore throat, pain in the chest and ribs and urination difficulties. Soybean sprouts are an excellent diuretic and can be used to correct various urination disorders, such as pain or burning sensations during urination and difficulty in passing urine.

## CHINESE YAMS, SWEET POTATOES AND UNPOLISHED GRAINS FOR YIN FLUIDS TO PROTECT THE BODY

Yin and yang are the two complementary principles of Chinese philosophy. Yin is negative, dark and feminine; yang is positive, bright and masculine. The interaction of these principles is thought to maintain the harmony of the universe. The theory of yin and yang is also fundamental to traditional Chinese medicine.

Chinese yams and sweet potatoes are the primary sources of sticky fluids for the body and such sticky fluids are the most precious yin energy in the body, according to traditional Chinese medicine. When the body lacks yin energy, it is called yin deficiency, which can cause a wide range of symptoms and diseases. Yin deficiency has been known to particularly cause consumptive diseases, like tuberculosis, but it also causes other disorders, such as hyperthyroidism, insomnia, fatigue, excessive perspiration, night sweat and constipation. In short, diseases characterized by weight loss and loss of strength are most likely due to yin deficiency, so patients with such diseases should consume more foods that can increase yin energy in the body.

Take hyperthyroidism, as an example. It is a condition due to excessive secretion of the thyroid gland. Patients with hyperthyroidism may increase their consumption of foods but still keep losing energy and weight. How do we account for this phenomenon? Normally, when people eat more food, they put on weight and increase their energy proportionally, but what happens to patients with hyperthyroidism seems to run counter to this general rule. The fundamental reason is that there's a shortage of yin energy in their body that creates an imbalance between their yin and yang energies. Yin energy nourishes the body to save its energy, whereas yang energy uses the body and spends its energy. Therefore, when yin energy is in short supply, yang energy will be in excess, causing these patients to keep losing energy and body weight while consuming nutritious foods in great amounts.

Some doctors tend to treat hyperthyroidism with large dosages of iodine; but, according to the Shanghai College of Chinese Medicine, large dosages of iodine will not do the job because iodine can merely inhibit the release of thyroxine (a principal thyroid hormone) but not inhibit its synthesis. A time-honored Chinese herbal formula that has proven very effective in the treatment of hyperthyroidism contains two categories of ingredients: iodine-rich foods, such as kelp and seaweed and foods and herbs rich in yin fluids.

Unlike water that flows quickly, yin energy consists of glutinous and sticky fluids that circulate throughout the body very slowly to perform a number of important functions. Many parts of the body are covered with mucous membranes full of glutinous fluids—from the mouth to the esophagus, stomach, small intestine, large intestine, rectum and anus, which is the digestive tract—and from the nose to the throat, trachea and bronchi, which belong to the respiratory system. Such glutinous fluids serve to protect different parts of the body from infections by lubricating them constantly the way oil lubricates an automobile engine. If we compare the human body to an automobile, then yang energy can be compared to gas, which runs out quickly and yin energy to oil, which lubricates different parts of the automobile slowly. Just as gas is consumed quickly in an automobile, so is yang energy in the body—and just as oil is consumed slowly, so is yin energy in the body. When the glutinous fluids are in short supply, the parts of the body affected will become more susceptible to infection, inflammation and cancer. No other foods seem to be able to supply the body with glutinous fluids as effectively as Chinese yams, sweet potatoes and unpolished grains.

Glutinous fluids also serve to retain the elasticity of the walls of blood vessels, lubricate the joints and cavities, prevent the atrophic degeneration of the connective tissues in the liver and kidneys and resist the attack of diseases related to a shortage of glutinous fluids. When an automobile runs out of oil, its engine will heat up and this is precisely what happens in the body. When people keep drinking water and still feel thirsty, as many diabetics do, it is because the yin energy in their lungs is inadequate. Consumption of water in great quantities will not help, however, because the water will be consumed by the excessive heat in their lungs. Likewise, when people keep eating and still feel hungry, as many diabetics do, it is because of a lack of yin energy in their stomach. And consuming food in large quantities will not help, because the food will be digested by the excessive heat in their stomach. What is needed is glutinous fluids to be supplied by appropriate foods, such as Chinese yams, sweet potatoes and unpolished grains.

Dr. T. Kawabara of Tokyo University of Dentistry has pointed out that from an anatomical point of view, glutinous fluids are an important ingredient in the functions of the pleural and articular cavities, the tendon sheath, the ligaments, the bones and the spinal disks. The body will break down as soon as glutinous fluids run out in those regions. Just imagine the parts of an automobile that will be affected if it runs out of oil. However, keep in mind that glutinous fluids do not refer to fats in the body. Although fats form an integral part of the cell membrane, they do not circulate to lubricate various parts of the body as glutinous fluids do.

A Japanese weight-lifting champion at the Olympic Games was said to consume 500 grams of salad and great amounts of soybeans and Chinese yams and sweet potatoes, on a daily basis. Small wonder that he became a champion, even though he was only 155 centimetres (5 feet) in height and 60 kilograms (132 pounds) in weight. A Japanese researcher on longevity lamented, "Since the Japanese people have changed their traditional eating habits rapidly in favor of Western life-styles and since the Japanese children have rushed to gobble up milk, cheese, meats and eggs, instead of eating traditional Japanese foods, many longevity villages in the past have gradually turned into villages of short-lived people."

CHINESE YAM   The Chinese yam is traditionally used both as an herb and a food and mainly serves to increase yin energy in the body. Four internal organs can benefit most from the Chinese yam: the lungs, spleen, pancreas and kidneys. That is why the Chinese yam is very frequently used to treat pulmonary tuberculosis, fatigue and diseases associated with the spleen and pancreas and the kidneys.

A number of disorders—including diarrhea, premature ejaculation and diabetes—are normally treated by the Chinese yam, with good results. Why are yams capable of stopping diarrhea? The reason is that yin energy moves slowly and diarrhea means quick bowel movements that should be slowed down—and yams, which are full of yin energy, can best do the job of slowing down bowel movements. The same reasoning holds true for premature ejaculation, which means quick movements of the seminal fluids from the male urethra and yams can slow them down due to their yin nature.

There are different ways of cooking the Chinese yam. For chronic diarrhea, take 60 grams of yams and grind them into a fine powder, add one glass of glutinous rice powder and mix thoroughly. Add 4 teaspoons of white sugar to the powder, form into balls and boil in water until they become very sticky. Eat at breakfast regularly. To heal chronic cough and asthma, particularly with mucous discharge, crush 100 grams of fresh yam and mix with a glass of sugarcane juice. Warm it up over a low heat and drink in two dosages in one day.

Perhaps the most important function of the yam in traditional Chinese medicine is to treat diabetes by boiling 120 grams of yam in water for daily consumption. Or, alternatively, yams can also be mixed with other foods to make a dish, or other herbs to make an herbal formula.

A Chinese chemist named Wu Yun-Chu, who started the monosodium glutamate manufacturing plant in Shanghai, was said to have suffered for many years from diabetes mellitus (a disorder of carbohydrate metabolism due to a shortage of insulin, according to Western medicine, but due to yin deficiency of the kidneys, according to Chinese medicine) and to have been treated by insulin injections without success. Subsequently, a doctor of traditional Chinese medicine gave him an herbal formula that contained two herbal ingredients, one of which was the Chinese yam. Being a chemist, Wu Yun-Chu took the two ingredients separately without mixing them. The first ingredient did not produce any change in his urine after one week of consumption. He then moved on to the second ingredient, which was the Chinese yam. After taking it for a while, he tested his urine and found that the sugar in it had been reduced considerably. He subsequently found that he had completely recovered from diabetes simply by taking the Chinese yam.

The following is the food value of 100 grams of the Chinese yam: protein, 1.9g; fat, 0.1g; carbohydrates, 19.9g; calories, 88, fiber, 0.4g; calcium, 44mg; phosphorus, 50mg; and iron, 1.1mg.

SWEET POTATOES   According to a Chinese book, "Seamen often enjoyed longevity, because they eat no other grains except sweet potatoes." Sweet potatoes are particularly good for the spleen, pancreas and kidneys and they are often used to treat chronic constipation, jaundice and diarrhea with blood in the stools. It may seem strange that

the same food can be used to treat both constipation and diarrhea, which are two opposing symptoms. However, sweet potatoes can treat constipation because they are full of yin energy, which can lubricate the intestine—and when the intestine is lubricated, bowel movements will occur. Sweet potatoes are particularly good for constipation due to the dryness of the large intestine. Sweet potatoes and the Chinese yam are effective for diarrhea for the same reason.

*People in the developed nations have consumed animal foods in great amounts with the result that the so-called "civilized diseases"—including obesity, hypertension, arteriosclerosis (hardening of blood vessels) and coronary heart disease—have increased dramatically.*

In traditional Chinese medicine, many herbs are equally good for two seemingly opposing symptoms. For example, one herb may be good for hypertension and hypotension at the same time. This is because herbs are used to regulate the conditions of the body and to regulate means to raise something that is too low and to lower something that is too high.

Sweet potatoes contain plenty of carotene, which is the precursor of vitamin A. Carotene is stored in the liver, where it is converted to vitamin A. That is why sweet potatoes are good for night blindness, which can also be treated by tender sweet potato leaves. You boil 60 to 90 grams of the leaves in water with 120 grams of sheep liver to be consumed for 2 to 3 days in a row as a course of treatment. Sweet potato leaves are said to contain an ingredient resembling insulin and when this ingredient is injected, it is twice as effective as an oral administration. As a remedy to get rid of blood in the stools, sweet potato leaves can be boiled in water, strained and then mixed with honey. As a remedy for diabetes and jaundice, boil some dried sweet potato leaves in water and then add seasoning. And for relieving constipation, fry 250 grams of sweet potato leaves with oil and salt and consume one dosage each day.

The following is the food value of 100 grams of sweet potatoes: protein, 0.9g; fat, 0.2 g; carbohydrates, 24g; calories 101; fiber, 0.5g; calcium, 77mg; carotene, 0.04mg; vitamin B2, 0.04mg; and nicotinic acid, 0.5mg.

UNPOLISHED GRAINS   There is a Chinese story about a little girl who was sold to another family to become the future wife of one of the sons, which was a common practice in China before the eighteenth century. Unfortunately, as it turned out, none of the family members liked her; so, at mealtimes, they all ate refined grains except this little girl who was only allowed to eat unpolished grains. Not long afterwards, all the members of the family had suffered vitamin-B deficiency diseases — such as diarrhea, stomatitis and indigestion — except this little girl. This is a simple story that illustrates how unpolished grains are more nutritious than refined ones.

In 1886, a Dutch physiologist named Christian Eijkman (1858-1930) had observed many prisoners in Indonesian jails developing beriberi (a disease characterized by pain and swelling of the limbs) due to a regular and high intake of refined rice. Subsequently, he discovered that beriberi and multiple neuritis are caused by a deficiency of vitamin B1 and was awarded a Nobel prize for the discovery. From that time on, nutritionists have attached great importance to eating unpolished grains as an important source of vitamin B.

*Unlike water that flows quickly, yin energy consists of glutinous and sticky fluids that circulate throughout the body very slowly to perform a number of important functions.*

Traditionally, the Chinese eat unpolished grains as yin tonics to treat yin deficiency in the body. Yin tonics are effective for the treatment of such symptoms as excessive perspiration, night sweats, diarrhea, diabetes and other disorders due to yin deficiency.

According to a story that has circulated widely among the Chinese, during the Second World War, the Chinese communist soldiers demonstrated great strength when they were waging guerrilla warfare against the Japanese; but after they had marched to the big cities to celebrate their victory over the Japanese, they began to weaken considerably. This was subsequently attributed to the fact that when the soldiers were hiding in the mountains to fight against the Japanese, they had virtually nothing else to eat except unpolished grains; but as soon as they came down to the big cities from the mountains, they began to enjoy the luxury of refined grains and consequently lost much of their strength.

However, the food value of unpolished grains is now regarded as beyond that of vitamin B because of the recent discovery that many other disorders can be treated by the consumption of unpolished grains. For example, unpolished grains are fiber-rich foods, which are found to reduce the risk of cancer of the colon. Many scientists have found that those who do not consume fiber-rich foods are many times more susceptible to cancer of the colon than those who regularly consume them. The scientists reason that a deficiency of fiber will slow down the passage of foods in the intestines and cause chronic constipation, which in turn will produce a toxin that can cause colon cancer. Therefore, a regular consumption of unpolished grains will improve elimination and reduce the chances of developing colon cancer.

Unpolished grains are also good for diabetes and high blood pressure, according to modern research. For example, in a study conducted in China between 1961 and 1962, it was found that among 13 diabetics treated with wheat bran, their blood sugar was significantly reduced in all cases and any symptoms of neuritis associated with diabetes were gone. In an experiment reported in a Chinese medical journal in 1974, lab animals were given wheat bran and other unpolished grains to make certain that their diet contained sufficient fiber; it was found that the cholesterol level in these animals was lowered considerably, in spite of the fact that they were also on a fat-rich diet during the experiment.

There is now general agreement among Chinese scientists that a high intake of unpolished grains will not only improve elimination, which is important in the prevention of colon cancer, but can also reduce the cholesterol level, which is important in preventing heart disease. A Chinese researcher has listed a number of "fiber-deficiency diseases" to run parallel with so-called "vitamin-deficiency diseases." Besides chronic constipation and heart disease, fiber-deficiency diseases include diabetes, varicose veins, hemorrhoids, colon cancer and intestinal oversensitivity syndrome.

## FOODS TO GENERATE YANG ENERGY IN THE BODY

Yin and yang are two opposing and yet mutually complementary energies in the body that interact to maintain a balance that is very fundamental to good health. At times, the body needs to be active — and at others, it needs to be inactive. Yang energy is responsible for being active, while yin energy is responsible for being inactive. I recall a taxi driver complaining that he found himself falling asleep while driving his cab, which is very dangerous indeed. When people feel sleepy too frequently, it is because they have accumulated excessive amounts of yin energy and it is necessary for them to introduce more yang foods in their diet to counteract the strength of their yin energy. An intake of yin foods can make you inactive; an intake of yang foods can make you active.

In addition, when one consumes yin foods, they have a tendency to stay in the body to serve as yin fluids; whereas when one consumes yang foods, the foods have a tendency to leave the body. For example, when you eat sweet potatoes, their fiber and residue will be excreted from the body, but the yin fluids that they generate will stay in the body to lubricate the joints and the cavities; on the other hand, when you eat ginger, which is a yang food, not only are fiber and residue excreted from the body, but ginger will cause perspiration and its energy will be eliminated along with it.

Therefore, yin foods increase input of energy while yang foods increase output of energy and both are necessary in the process of metabolism.

Metabolism involves two fundamental processes: an input process to assimilate and build up energy, which called "anabolism," and an output process to promote excretion of energy, which is called "catabolism." Thus, it is inaccurate to say unequivocally that the more you eat, the more you will gain weight, because putting on weight also depends to a large extent on whether you eat yin or yang foods.

Nowadays we often hear that in order to stay slim, we need more exercise. There is a great deal of truth to this statement because exercise is active, which is yang. This means that exercise will shift your body towards the yang side, which is another way of saying that exercise increases yang energy in the body to speed up the output process of metabolism. In Western medicine, there is something called "basal metabolism," which refers to energy expenditure when the body is at complete rest. An intake of yang foods will increase the basal metabolic rate even more effectively than exercise, because you are getting rid of that extra energy while you are at rest. This is why some people eat a lot but still remain slim or even underweight — that is, if they are not suffering from diabetes or hyperthyroidism and the like.

A retired man was complaining about his inability to calm down; he couldn't rest during the day, nor could he sleep at night. But worst of all, he couldn't even sit down for very long and had to keep moving around or even jogging, which was a serious problem. This man had become much too active as a result of accumulating great amounts of yang energy. Thus, it was necessary for him to reduce his intake of yang foods and increase his intake of yin foods to reverse the overactive tendency of his body.

Any foods that can increase the active state of the body are yang foods. Many of the foods we eat every day are yang foods, such as black and white pepper, chives, ginger, garlic, chili pepper and soybean oil; even tobacco and alcohol are considered yang foods. Consumption of alcohol often contributes to gaining weight, which may be attributed to the fact that alcohol increases a person's appetite so that more foods are consumed, whether yin or yang. Many smokers gain considerable weight very quickly after they quit smoking, which is another indication that yang foods can increase energy output in the metabolic process. Since tobacco and alcohol have many other harmful effects, they are not recommended for consumption even though there may be a deficiency of yang energy in the body.

FRESH GINGER    Fresh ginger is a typical yang food because it can stimulate many activities in the body. For example, it can speed blood circulation and secretion of stomach fluids, stimulate the intestinal tract and promote digestion. It can also increase blood pressure. It is reported that by chewing one gram of fresh ginger without swallowing it, systolic blood pressure rises as much as 11.2 millimetres of mercury and diastolic blood pressure as much as 14 millimetres of

mercury, with no apparent change in pulse rate. Fresh ginger extract has been found to stimulate the vasomotor and respiratory centers and the heart in laboratory cats. In fact, one type of hypertension is attributed to an excessive amount of yang energy in the liver and should be treated by an intake of yin energy to strike a balance. This, however, does not mean that all types of hypertension should be treated by yin foods, because hypertension has many different causes.

Here are a couple of fresh ginger recipes that may be helpful to use. The recipe that follows is a remedy to induce perspiration, which is good for both the common cold and its prevention, particularly when fever and chills are present. You grate 30 grams of fresh ginger, boil it in water, add one teaspoon of brown sugar and drink. The next recipe is for suppressing coughing due to the common cold. Grate 50 grams of fresh ginger and mix with 2 teaspoons of maltose, boil in 3 cups of water until the water is reduced to a half cup and then sip slowly.

Fresh ginger is a very popular condiment in China and is mostly used to improve the flavor and remove the bad odors of meats and fish. For example, in cooking vegetables, you can add a few small slices of fresh ginger to make a more delicious dish, in cooking fish, you can add a few slices of fresh ginger not only to improve the flavor but also to eliminate the fishy smell. From the standpoint of Chinese medicine, the most important use of fresh ginger in cooking is to increase the yang energy of foods. In other words, by adding slices of fresh ginger in cooking, yin foods will become less yin and more yang, while yang foods will increase in yang energy.

The following is the food value of 100 grams of fresh ginger: water, 87g; protein, 1.4g; fat, 0.7g; carbohydrates, 8.5g; calories, 46; crude fiber, 1g; ash, 1.4g; protein, 0.18mg; vitamin B1, 0.01mg; vitamin B2, 0.04mg; nicotinic acid, 0.4mg, vitamin C, 4mg; calcium, 20mg; phosphorus, 45mg; iron, 7mg; potassium, 387mg; and 0.25 to 3 percent of volatile oil.

GARLIC    Traditionally, garlic as a yang food has been used to promote energy circulation, warm the stomach and remove any accumulated toxic substances. This is consistent with the modern discovery of garlic being capable of killing germs, promoting digestion and improving appetite. But garlic has been found to have many more important therapeutic functions in recent years, such as being used as a remedy for hypertension, hepatitis and cancer. Garlic has been in popular use in Japan for a long time and a recent Japanese study has revealed that garlic contains a mineral called Ge that is reportedly capable of preventing stomach cancer. A team of doctors at the Hunan Medical College in China who call themselves the Research Group of Garlic as Anticancerous Agent have used a patented medicine made of garlic to treat 21 cases of nasopharyngeal carcinoma (cancer of the nose and throat) with significant results in most cases. In addition, the same group of physicians has also found garlic to be effective for pulmonary tuberculosis, whooping cough, bacillary and amebic dysentery, enteritis (inflammation of the intestine), oxyuriasis (pinworms), ancylostomiasis (hookworm disease), prevention of flu and epidemic encephalitis (inflammation of the brain) and external application for the treatment of trichomonas vaginitis.

There are a number of garlic recipes that may prove helpful. To treat bacillary dysentery and enteritis, boil two garlic cloves in water and consume as one dosage before meals three times daily for 2 to 3 days. To treat the early stages of the common cold, take 50 grams each of garlic, the white heads of green onion and fresh ginger and boil in water; then drink hot and cover yourself with a blanket so that you perspire. To treat whooping cough, immerse 60 grams of garlic in cold water for 5 to 6 hours, remove them from the water, add some white sugar to the water and drink one tablespoonful three times daily for a few days.

To treat trichomonas vaginitis, immerse a gauze in garlic juice until thoroughly wet and then squeeze the gauze inside the vagina. Change this gauze one to two times daily and use this course of treatment for 3 to 5 days. It is reportedly effective in over 95 percent of trichomonas cases. To treat oxyuriasis, crush 9 to 15 grams of garlic cloves and mix with petroleum jelly for external application to the anus and surrounding region. To get rid of germs in the mouth and to prevent the common cold and infections of the mouth and intestines, eat a few garlic cloves every day.

There are side effects of garlic, however and for that reason, it should be used with care. Garlic can make red blood cells become dark brown by contact and can also dissolve red blood cells when applied in high concentration. In addition, the volatile oil contained in garlic can inhibit the secretion of gastric juices and can also cause anemia. It is well known that garlic can cause bad breath, which can be reduced or eliminated by gargling with strong tea, eating some red dates, or drinking a few cups of tea.

The following is the food value of 100 grams of garlic: water, 69.8g; protein, 4.4g; fat, 0.2g; carbohydrates, 23.6g; calories, 113; crude fiber, 0.7g; ash, 1.3g; vitamin B1, 0.24mg; vitamin B2, 0.03mg; nicotinic acid, 0.9mg; vitamin C, 3mg; calcium, 5mg; phosphorus, 44mg; iron, 0.4mg; potassium, 130mg; sodium, 8.7mg; magnesium, 8.3mg; and chlorine, 35mg. In addition, every 100 grams of garlic leaves contain 77mg of vitamin C, which is over 20 times as much as in garlic.

WALNUTS   As a yang food, walnuts are traditionally used to boost sexual capacity in men, because when their sexual organs have insufficient yang energy, they will cool down and erection becomes difficult to achieve. For the purpose of improving sexual capacity in men, take 60 grams of crushed walnuts as a one-day dosage for one to two months.

Or, as an alternate treatment, fry a walnut with 6 grams of chive seeds and then boil the two ingredients in water; eat the walnut and chive seeds and drink the soup, once daily for 3 days.

Unlike fresh ginger and garlic, both of which are purely yang foods, walnuts are basically a yang food but also have a yin nature as well. Because of their yin nature, they can lubricate the intestine and that is why walnuts are traditionally used to treat constipation. As a food remedy to induce bowel movements, crush 60 grams of walnuts and 30 grams of sesame seeds into a powder and take one teaspoonful of this powder with warm water once a day, the first thing in the morning. Another method of treating chronic constipation, particularly in older or weaker people, is to chew 10 to 30 grams of walnuts slowly like chewing gum, twice a day, in the morning and the evening.

The food value of walnuts is as follows: fat, 40 to 50 percent; protein, 15.4 percent; carbohydrates, 10 percent; calcium, 0.119 percent; phosphorus, 0.369 percent; iron, 0.035 percent; carotene, 0.17 percent; and vitamin B2, 0.11 percent.

## VEGETABLES AND FRUITS FOR VITAMINS, MINERALS AND FIBER

Grains, meats and fish supply the body with carbohydrates, fats and proteins, but vegetables are the primary source of vitamins, minerals and fiber. There are many diseases associated with vitamin deficiencies and vegetables can help us avoid these diseases.

In recent years, it has been discovered that certain vitamins are anticancerous agents. One of them is vitamin C, which can be found in chili pepper, Chinese cabbage, kale, kohlrabi and parsley. One hundred grams of fresh chili pepper reportedly contain as much as 105 milligrams of vitamin C. Carotene and vitamin A have also been found to be anticancerous agents and they may be found in many vegetables, such as carrots, parsley, pumpkins, spinach and squash.

Vegetables and fruit are also primary sources of fiber, which has been found to be essential in promoting intestinal peristalsis, in aiding digestion, in inducing regular bowel movements and in reducing the quantities of coproporphyrin (a porphyrin present in feces with quantities altered in different diseases), as well as useful in preventing cancer of the colon.

In his article, "Research on Longevity," published in Japan in 1977, Dr. H. Y. Tora pointed out that as the Japanese economy continues to make headway, the Japanese people have had an excessive intake of animal foods at the expense of grains and vegetables. This has resulted in increased acidity and decreased alkalinity of the blood, leading to blood acidification, which accounts for the increased incidence of obesity, cancer, arteriosclerosis, heart disease, diabetes, hypertension, cerebral hemorrhage, coronary disease, arthritis and gout. In general, animal foods, fish and eggs are acidic foods (foods that produce acid after they have been digested), whereas fruits and vegetables are alkaline foods. Most fruits and vegetable can neutralize the effect of an excessive intake of acidic foods.

# Longevity and Conventional Chinese Wisdom

## SCIENCE VS. COMMON EXPERIENCE

Western nutrition as a science can be traced back to the father of chemistry, Antoine-Laurent Lavoisier (1743-1794), a French chemist who maintained that life is basically a chemical process. In point of fact, it is more accurate to say that life is an experience that may be enhanced through an understanding of the chemical processes involved. Throughout history, some people have managed to stay in good health and lived a long life whereas others have suffered poor health and lived a short life; through an understanding of life's chemical processes, it is possible to both promote and extend good health.

For example, by 1870, about one third of the children in London and Manchester were suffering from rickets. Subsequently, scientists discovered that the disease was caused by vitamin-D deficiency, so that people began to consume vitamin D to cure rickets. But science was only confirming what many people had discovered through common experience — that certain foods (containing what is now called vitamin D) cured rickets. While science was not developed until a few centuries ago, common knowledge has continued to expand and outstrip science in many areas. But much of this valid common experience in human health is often dismissed or ignored by modern scientists. Since scientists know so little about common nutritional lore and are inclined to dismiss what they do not understand, they are not the best guides in the search for foods that extend longevity.

Modern medical scientists have a universally skeptical attitude towards common experience, their thinking being that nothing is true until proven scientifically. A typical scientist will tell you, for example, that 100 grams of raw celery contain 17 calories, 0.9g of protein, 3.9g of carbohydrates, 39mg of calcium and 9mg of ascorbic acid. But he will shrug off the suggestion that celery can lower blood pressure, because he hasn't seen any research to that effect. In fact, celery has been proven effective for reducing blood pressure among the Chinese for many centuries and it has become the conventional Chinese wisdom.

Again, a typical scientist will tell you that 100 grams of dried fig contain 274 calories, 4.3g of protein, 1.3g of fat, 69g of carbohydrates, 126mg of calcium, 640mg of potassium and 80 I.U. of vitamin A, but he will shrug off the suggestion that figs can cure dysentery and hemorrhoids. In fact, the effects of fig have been verified in the common experiences of the Chinese for centuries and have become part of the conventional Chinese wisdom. Each culture has accumulated its own conventional wisdom, sometimes despite scientific denials.

Scientists, of course, do make new discoveries based on the common experience of people; but, unfortunately, sometimes they lag behind in the current understanding of human health. As long as people live, they struggle to find new ways of combating diseases and improving health. In the third century, the Chinese people were eating liver (which contains vitamin A, as we know it today) to cure night blindness. But scientists did not discover vitamin A until the early twentieth century. If those suffering with night blindness in the third century had chosen to wait for scientists to discover a cure, they would have been doomed to night blindness throughout their lives.

In the third century, the Chinese people were eating seaweed (which contains plenty of iodine) to cure simple goiter, but scientists did not discover iodine as a cure for goiter until the late eighteenth century. If those people with goiter in the third century had waited for scientists to invent a remedy, they would have suffered needlessly.

It may be possible for scientists to discover, sooner or later, a cure for every single disease and to eventually discover all the nutrients that will enable us to live forever, but it could take a very long time. There are three stages of truths regarding health, as well as in other fields of knowledge, which should be fully understood and distinguished from one another: first, something is true but nobody knows about it yet; second, something is true and some people know about it through experience; and third, something is true that has been verified by scientists.

That tea prevents scurvy is true today as it was true from time immemorial, even though nobody knew about it; this is truth at the first stage. When the truths have been discovered in human experience, they are truths at the second stage. In the middle of the eighteenth century, many seamen on board Western ships had become critically ill or even died from a disease now known as scurvy, but the same ordeal was a rare phenomenon among Chinese seamen, because they were drinking tea. That tea was beneficial to the health of seamen was discovered by the Chinese people through their common experience, which represents the truth at the second stage. When vitamin C was successfully isolated by Dr. Albert Szent-Gyorgyi in 1937 as a prevention of scurvy, it became truth at the third stage. There can be no doubt that there are far more truths at the first stage than at the second stage and there are equally far more truths at the second stage than at the third stage.

## CONVENTIONAL WISDOM OF CHINESE PHYSICIANS AS A GUIDE TO LONGEVITY

A physician of traditional Chinese medicine lives in the world of experience, in the truest sense of the word, to engage in the art of healing. To be sure, there's a great deal of abstract knowledge that a physician of traditional Chinese medicine must learn. There are also established clinical procedures he must become acquainted with, but once learned, he must strike out on his own in his clinical practice, not unlike a captain steering a vessel in a seaway. He knows that his abstract knowledge and standard procedures are useful to him only to the extent that they enable him to treat his patients successfully. His theoretical knowledge has to be tested in real life.

Unlike a physician of Western medicine who routinely applies the laboratory findings in his clinical practice as if laboratory animals and his patients were identical to one another, a physician of traditional Chinese medicine will try hard to establish his own experience of clinical practice. All good physicians of traditional Chinese medicine in the past have accumulated at least a few hundred successful clinical cases in their lifetime and towards the end of their careers, some of them wrote a few medical classics of their own to report on their successful experience in clinical practice. Undoubtedly, such physicians have something to offer us in the selection of foods for longevity, if for no other reason than that many of them had achieved unparalleled longevity themselves.

In the nineteenth century, a Chinese physician named Ding-Pu Lu observed, "Most outstanding Chinese physicians in the past have enjoyed longevity." This observation is supported by historical facts, because many outstanding physicians in Chinese history had indeed managed to live a longer life than the average Chinese person.

An outstanding Chinese physician named Meng Shen (621-713) had lived 92 years and was remembered in particular by the Chinese people for his remark, "A person who really knows how to nourish the body should always keep good foods and herbs handy." Another notable physician named Sun Shu Mao (581-682) had lived 101 years and once said, "Anyone over 40 years old should try to avoid laxatives, which will weaken his body and begin to take tonics. Anyone over 50 years old should take tonics all year round; such are the secrets of nourishing life to enjoy longevity." A Chinese physician at the Jin-Zhu Chinese Medical College by the name of Luo Ming Shan (1869-1982) had lived 113 years.

In a book entitled, *Outstanding Chinese Physicians in the Past and Their Medical Theories*, written by the staff of the Peking College of Chinese Medicine, published in 1964, a total of 37 of the most outstanding Chinese physicians in history (dating back as far as A.D. 581) are listed with their medical theories. Most of them had lived a much longer life than the average Chinese person. The average life span of these physicians was 80.56 years.

According to a survey conducted by the United Nations in 1977, the average life span of people in the world was 59 years, with people in industrialized nations averaging 70 years and in developing nations, 40 years. This means that the life span of outstanding Chinese physicians in the past was at least 36.53 percent longer than the average life span of people in 1977, 15 percent longer than the people in industrialized nations and 101 percent longer than the people in developing nations.

Do Western physicians live longer than the people in their own society? If so, how much longer? The data about the life span of Western physicians prior to the nineteenth century would be useful for comparison, but unfortunately, not many are available. However, from a list of outstanding Western physicians in the nineteenth century, we see that their average life span was 70.93 years.

The 10-year difference is even more significant when we take into consideration that many of the Chinese physicians listed lived before the eighteenth century, whereas virtually all the Western physicians lived after the eighteenth century. It is worth remembering that the life span of people has gradually increased over time. Thus, the Chinese physicians lived 21 years longer than the people in the world, on the average 10 years longer than those in industrialized nations and 40 years longer than the people in developing nations. Since China is a developing nation, it means that Chinese physicians live twice as long as people in their society. A similar conclusion cannot be drawn from the list of Western physicians.

When doctors are sick themselves, or when they wish to live a long life, they will usually follow prescriptions or a course of treatment based on their own medical knowledge. The fact that Chinese physicians of traditional medicine have managed to live a longer life than their Western counterparts demonstrates to what extent their medical knowledge is a reliable guide to longevity.

## Acupuncture

Although acupuncture and herbology are two different branches of Chinese medicine, with the former treating diseases by external methods and the latter by internal administration of herbs, they are frequently used simultaneously in clinical practice. Both are also based upon the theories of yin and yang, the five elements, the internal organs and the meridians. In addition, both are guided by the four methods of diagnosis and the eight classifications of disease.

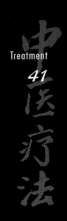

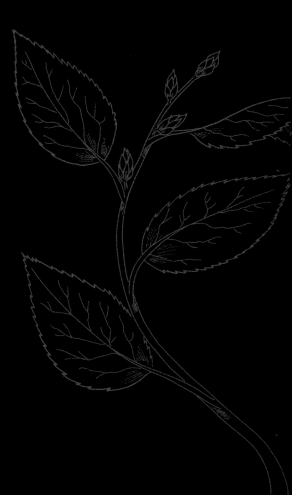

Treatment

# Clinical Diagnosis

What follow are a few clinical cases presented for making a diagnosis to illustrate how you can use this book for self-healing purposes. In each case, key symptoms are in boldface to indicate that they should be checked against the symptoms listed under the headings of Headache (pages 44-46) or Hyperthyroidism (pages 99-100), depending on the chief complaint. All the syndromes under the headings are taken into account and the ones with the highest score are used for diagnosis.

| *Clinical Case* | *No. 1* | *No. 2* |
|---|---|---|
| NAME OF PATIENT | Chen | Zhou |
| SEX | male | female |
| AGE | 29 | 36 |
| CHIEF COMPLAINT | headache | headache |
| HISTORY AND SYMPTOMS | The patient was **hit by a falling object** from the second floor while at work. He fainted on the spot and was sent to the hospital for treatment. On examination, he was found to have suffered skin injuries on the head and was experiencing sensations of aching pain. He was treated accordingly. Two weeks later, **prickling pain** occurred on the right side of the head that came in three or four attacks a day, worsening at night. | The patient has suffered **migraine headaches** since she was six years old and for more than 30 years. The **headache worsens with labor, fatigue, or use of the brain (thinking)**. The pain also gets worse each month during her menstrual period, which often occurs in a heavy flow, with **dizziness**, forcing her to lie down in bed for two or three days. Other symptoms include whirling sensations in the eyes, **palpitations**, poor memory, **withered complexion**, pale appearance of lips and nails, **fatigue** and dislike of talking. |
| DIAGNOSIS | To make a diagnosis of headache as the chief complaint, a total of nine syndromes should be taken into account, as can be seen on pages 44-46.<br><br>The symptoms in boldface are to be checked against those listed under each of the nine syndromes. The symptoms in boldface are found under "9. Blood coagulations syndrome." So, the diagnosis can be presented as follows:<br>1. Wind-cold syndrome (0) None<br>2. Wind-heat syndrome (0) None<br>3. Wind-dampness syndrome (0) None<br>4. Liver yang upsurging syndrome (0) None<br>5. Dampness-sputum syndrome (0) None<br>6. Energy deficiency syndrome (0) None<br>7. Blood deficiency syndrome (0) None<br>8. Kidneys energy deficiency syndrome (0) None<br>9. Blood coagulations syndrome (5)<br>    Headache caused by external injuries (4)<br>    Prickling pain in the head (1) | To make a diagnosis of headache as the chief complaint, a total of nine syndromes should be taken into account, as can be seen on pages 44-46.<br><br>The symptoms in boldface are to be checked against the symptoms listed under each of the nine syndromes.<br>1. Wind-cold syndrome (2)<br>    Dizziness (1)<br>    Headache with dizziness (1)<br>2. Wind-heat syndrome (2)<br>    Dizziness (1)<br>    Headache with dizziness (1)<br>3. Wind-dampness syndrome (0) — None<br>4. Liver yang upsurging syndrome (8)<br>    Dizziness (1)<br>    Headache (1)<br>    Headache in women (1)<br>    Headache on the side of head (migraine headache) (5)<br>5. Dampness-sputum syndrome (5)<br>    Dizziness (1)<br>    Headache with dizziness (3)<br>    Prolonged dizziness (1)<br>6. Energy deficiency syndrome (6)<br>    Dizziness (1)<br>    Fatigued eyes and spirits (fatigue) (1)<br>    Headache that occurs on fatigue after labor (2)<br>    Prolonged headache (2)<br>7. Blood deficiency syndrome (5)<br>    Dizziness (1)<br>    Fatigue (1)<br>    Headache with dizziness (3)<br>8. Kidneys energy deficiency syndrome (3)<br>    Dizziness (1)<br>    Fatigue (1)<br>    Prolonged dizziness (1)<br>9. Blood coagulations syndrome (0) None |
| CONCLUSIONS | Thus, the diagnosis is 9. blood coagulations syndrome, which has the highest score of 5. | Thus, the diagnosis is 4. Liver yang upsurging syndrome, which has the highest score of 8. |

| *Clinical Case* | *No. 3* | *No. 4* |
|---|---|---|
| NAME OF PATIENT | Jia | Li |
| SEX | female | female |
| AGE | 26 | 38 |
| CHIEF COMPLAINT | hyperthyroidism | hyperthyroidism |
| HISTORY AND SYMPTOMS | The patient was diagnosed with hyperthyroidism at a hospital of Western medicine. She came to the clinic later with **palpitations, excessive perspiration, jumpiness, fear of heat, hot sensations in hands and feet, increased appetite, fatigue, low fever, dry mouth, poor sleep** and **feeling as if some objects were in her throat**. | The patient came to the clinic with hyperthyroidism as diagnosed at a hospital of Western medicine. She displayed the following symptoms: **palpitations, excessive perspiration, misty vision, jumpiness, shaking of hands, good appetite with frequent hunger, weight loss, diarrhea** and **fatigue**. |
| DIAGNOSIS | To make a diagnosis of hyperthyroidism as the chief complaint, a total of six syndromes should be taken into account, as can be seen on pages 99-100.<br><br>The symptoms in boldface are the symptoms to be checked against those listed under the six syndromes.<br>1. Hot stomach syndrome (2)<br>    Getting hungry easily (1)<br>    Thirst (1)<br>2. Liver energy congestion syndrome (5)<br>    Insomnia (1)<br>    Psychological tension (jumpiness) (2)<br>    Subjective sensations of objects in the throat (2)<br>3. Sputum-fire syndrome (14)<br>    Dislike of heat (3)<br>    Eat a lot (2)<br>    Emotionally disturbed easily (3)<br>    Excessive perspiration (2)<br>    Palpitations (3)<br>    Sleeplessness (1)<br>4. Liver-kidneys yin deficiency syndrome (5)<br>    Fatigue (3)<br>    Palms of hands and soles of feet are both hot (1)<br>    Sleeplessness with forgetfulness (1)<br>5. Deficiency fire syndrome (9)<br>    Becoming angry easily (2)<br>    Excessive perspiration (2)<br>    Dry sensations in the mouth (1)<br>    Hot sensations in hands and feet (2)<br>    Low fever (1)<br>    Sleeplessness (1)<br>6. Simultaneous deficiency of yin and energy syndrome (8)<br>    Excessive perspiration (1)<br>    Fatigue (3)<br>    Hot sensations in hands and feet (1)<br>    Palpitations (2)<br>    "Tidal" fever in the afternoon (1) | To make a diagnosis of hyperthyroidism as the chief complaint, a total of six syndromes should be taken into account, as can be seen on pages 99-100.<br><br>The symptoms in boldface are the symptoms to be checked against those listed under the six syndromes.<br>1. Hot stomach syndrome (1)<br>    Getting hungry easily (1)<br>2. Liver energy congestion syndrome (0) None<br>3. Sputum-fire syndrome (7)<br>    Eat a lot (2)<br>    Excessive perspiration (2)<br>    Palpitations (3)<br>4. Liver-kidneys yin deficiency syndrome (3)<br>    Fatigue (3)<br>5. Deficiency fire syndrome (4)<br>    Becoming angry easily (2)<br>    Excessive perspiration (2)<br>6. Simultaneous deficiency of yin and yang syndrome (6)<br>    Excessive perspiration (1)<br>    Fatigue (3)<br>    Palpitations (2) |
| CONCLUSIONS | Thus, the diagnosis is 3. Sputum-fire syndrome, with the highest score of 14. | Thus, the diagnosis is 3. Sputum-fire syndrome, with the highest score of 7. |

Treatment of Complaints

## HEADACHE

| | *Wind-cold* | *Wind-heat* | *Wind-dampness* |
|---|---|---|---|
| SYMPTOMS | 1  Absence of perspiration<br>1  Breathing through the nose<br>1  Clear discharge from nose<br>1  Cough<br>1  Cough with heavy, unclear sounds and clear sputum<br>1  Diarrhea<br>1  Dislike of cold<br>1  Dizziness<br>1  Facial paralysis<br>1  Fever<br>2  Headache with stiff neck*<br>1  Headache with dizziness<br>1  Hoarseness at the beginning of illness<br>1  Loss of voice<br>1  Nosebleed<br>1  Pain in the body shifting around with no fixed region<br>1  Pain in the joints<br>1  Stuffed nose<br>1  Vomiting | 1  Asthma<br>1  Cough<br>1  Coughing out blood<br>1  Dizziness<br>3  Headache with swelling of the head*<br>1  Headache with dizziness<br>1  Intolerance of light in eyes with swelling and dislike of wind<br>1  Muddy discharge from nose<br>1  Nosebleed<br>1  Pain in the eyes<br>1  Pain in the throat<br>1  Red eyes<br>1  Ringing in ears and deafness<br>1  Tenesmus<br>1  Thirst<br>1  Toothache<br>1  Yellow urine<br>1  Yellowish discharge from the nose | 1  Chronic backache<br>1  Diarrhea<br>1  Eczema<br>1  Edema<br>1  Fever that becomes more severe in the afternoon<br>1  German measles<br>3  Headache with heavy or tight sensations in the head*<br>6  Heavy sensations in the body*<br>1  Itchy sores<br>1  Light swelling<br>1  Pain in all the joints<br>1  Pain shifting around with no fixed region<br>1  Scant urine |
| TREATMENT PRINCIPLE | to disperse wind and cold and stop headache | to disperse wind and heat and stop pain | to drive out wind, overcome dampness and relieve pain |
| TREATMENT FORMULA | *Chuan-Xiong-Cha-Tiao-San* | Sang-Ju-Yin | Qiang-Huo-Sheng-Shi-Tang |
| FOOD CURES | peppermint (including oil), spearmint, sweet basil, cayenne pepper, fennel, fresh ginger, mustard seed, star anise, prickly ash leaf, fresh ginger, green onion, chicken egg and red-beet sugar | banana, bitter endive, black fungus, salt, spinach, strawberry, bamboo shoot, cucumber, Job's-tears, liver, leaf beet, mung bean, peppermint, purslane, lily flower, salt and cattail | Job's-tears, orange peel, peppermint, spearmint, sweet basil, celery, coconut meat, green onion, jellyfish skin, prickly ash, rice, adzuki bean, rosin and tangerine |

| Liver Yang upsurging | Dampness-sputum | Energy deficiency | Blood deficiency |
|---|---|---|---|
| 1 Bitter taste in the mouth | 1 Cough | 1 Discharge of sticky, muddy stools or diarrhea | 1 Constipation |
| 1 Dizziness | 1 Discharge of sputum that can be coughed out easily | 1 Dizziness | 1 Dizziness |
| 1 Feeling insecure while asleep | 1 Discharge of white, watery sputum | 1 Edema in socket of eyeball | 1 Dry and cracked lips and mouth |
| 1 Headache | 1 Dizziness | 1 Fatigued eyes and spirits | 1 Dry sensations in the mouth |
| 1 Headache in women | 1 Excessive whitish vaginal discharge | 1 Feeble breath with a short and feeble voice | 1 Fatigue |
| 5 Headache on the side of the head* | 1 Frequent coughs during pregnancy that are prolonged and cause motion of fetus | 2 Headache (severe) that occurs with fatigue after labor* | 1 Fever |
| 1 Headache with dizziness | 3 Headache with dizzines* | 2 Headache at intervals* | 3 Headache as if being pulled by a string* |
| 1 Headache with severe pain and swelling | 1 Hiccups | 2 Headache in the morning* | 3 Headache in the afternoon* |
| 1 Heavy sensations in head and light sensations in feet | 1 Pain in the chest | 1 Lack of appetite | 3 Headache with dizziness* |
| 1 Misty vision | 1 Panting | 3 Pain may be relieved by massage* | 1 Lying down with an inability to sit up, which will cause dizziness |
| 1 Numbness | 1 Prolonged dizziness | 1 Perspiration on hands and feet | 1 Night sweats |
| 1 Numbness of fingers | 1 Sleep a lot | 2 Prolonged headache* | 1 Sleeplessness |
| 1 Pain and swelling in the ribs | 1 Sleeplessness | 1 Swallowing difficulty | 1 Underweight with dry skin |
| 1 Pain in the ribs | 1 Suppression of menses | 1 Tips of four limbs slightly cold | 1 White complexion |
| 1 Red complexion | 1 Vomiting | 1 Underweight with dry skin | |
| 1 Ringing in ears and deafness | 1 White, sliding sputum that can be cleared from throat easily | | |
| | 1 Whitish vaginal discharge | | |
| | 1 Women susceptible to morning sickness during pregnancy | | |
| to calm the liver and oppress the yang and to stop the wind and relieve pain | to transform sputum and mobilize the spleen and to relieve pain | to tone energy and elevate the yang and to nourish body energy | to nourish the blood, soften up the liver and stop the pain |
| Zhen-Gan-Xi-Feng-Tang | Ban-Xia-Xie-Xin-Tang | Bu-Zhong-Yi-Qi-Tang | Si-Wu-Tang |
| chicken egg yolk, cheese, kidney bean, abalone, cuttlefish, duck, duck egg, white fungus, oyster, pork, royal jelly and celery | peppermint, spearmint, sweet basil, celery, coconut meat, green onion, asparagus, bamboo shoot, date, leaf or brown mustard, mustard seed, black and white pepper, fresh ginger and crown daisy | grape, longan nuts, maltose, mandarin fish, Irish potato, sweet rice, apple cucumber, bog bean, gold carp, carrot, chestnut, ham, horse bean, hyacinth bean, Job's-tears, royal jelly, string bean, whitefish, yam, red and black date, mutton, squash and rock sugar | abalone, asparagus, cuttlefish, chicken egg, duck egg, white fungus, beef liver, grape, mandarin fish, oyster, milk, beef, cherry, blood clam and longan nuts |

| | HEADACHE (CONTINUED) | | DIZZINESS |
|---|---|---|---|
| | *Kidneys energy deficiency* | *Blood coagulations* | *Liver-fire upsurging* |
| SYMPTOMS | 1 Anuria (complete suppression of urination)<br>1 Asthma<br>1 Deafness<br>1 Dizziness<br>1 Fatigue<br>5 Headache as if a ball were inside the head*<br>5 Headache with ringing inside the head*<br>1 Impotence<br>1 Lumbago<br>1 Prolonged dizziness<br>1 Ringing in ears<br>1 Seminal emission | 2 Abdominal pain<br>2 Chest pain<br>1 Coughing out blood<br>4 Headache caused by external injuries*<br>3 Headache with fixed pain*<br>2 Lumbago<br>2 Pain in the upper abdomen or the ribs<br>1 Prickling pain in the head<br>2 Stomachache<br>1 Vomiting of blood | 2 Acute dizziness*<br>1 Bleeding from stomach<br>1 Congested chest<br>1 Deafness<br>1 Depressed and hot<br>1 Dim eyes<br>1 Dry sensations in the mouth<br>1 Getting angry easily<br>1 Headache on both sides of the head and in the corners of the eyes<br>3 Headache that is severe*<br>1 Hiccups<br>1 Nosebleed<br>1 Red eyes<br>1 Ringing in ears<br>1 Sleeplessness or sleep a lot<br>1 Vomiting of blood<br>1 Yellowish-red urine |
| TREATMENT PRINCIPLE | to improve the essence of the kidneys and stop pain | to activate the blood and remove coagulations | to clear the heat in the liver and nourish the yin |
| TREATMENT FORMULA | Shen-Qi-Wan | Tao-Hong-Si-Wu-Tang | Long-Dan-Xie-Gan-Tang |
| FOOD CURES | milk, millet, stamens, sword bean, wheat, black sesame seed, beef kidney, chestnut, chicken liver, lobster, perch, pork kidney, raspberry, sea cucumber, string bean and walnut | ambergris, brown sugar, chestnut, eggplant, peach, black soybean, sturgeon, sweet basil, crab, distillers' grains, papaya and saffron | spinach, chestnut, shepherd's purse, rye, black fungus, vinegar, abalone, asparagus, chicken egg, white fungus, pork and royal jelly |

| Yin deficiency with yang excess | Simultaneous deficiency of yin and yang | Spleen-sputum | Simultaneous deficiency of energy and blood |
|---|---|---|---|
| 1 Coughing out blood<br>5 Dizziness with ringing in the ears*<br>5 Dizziness that drags on (chronic dizziness)*<br>1 Excessive sex drive<br>1 Hot sensations in the body<br>1 Insomnia<br>1 Jumpiness<br>1 Night sweats<br>1 Red appearance in the zygomatic region<br>1 Seminal emission<br>1 "Tidal" fever<br>1 Underweight | 1 Cold limbs and cold sensations in the body<br>6 Dizziness with ringing in the ears*<br>5 Dizziness that worsens with fatigue*<br>1 Fatigue<br>1 Low energy<br>1 Palpitations<br>1 Perspiration with hot sensations in the body easily triggered by physical activities<br>1 Poor spirits<br>1 Ringing in ears<br>1 Too tired to talk<br>1 Underweight | 1 Abundant saliva<br>6 Dizziness with heavy sensations in the head*<br>6 Dizziness that causes inability to move*<br>1 Overweight, but eat only a small amount of food<br>1 Poor appetite<br>1 Slight fullness of the stomach<br>1 Suppression of menses in women<br>1 Weakened limbs | 1 Bleeding of various kinds with blood in light color, often seen in consumptive diseases<br>7 Dizziness that worsens with movement*<br>2 Fatigue<br>1 Flying objects seen in front of the eyes<br>2 Insomnia<br>1 Low energy<br>1 Low voice<br>1 Numbness of limbs<br>1 Pale complexion and lips<br>1 Pale nails<br>2 Palpitations |
| to tone the liver and kidneys and to oppress the liver yang | to tone the liver and kidneys and to warm and assist the original energy of the body | to dry up dampness, transform sputum and strengthen the spleen | to strengthen the spleen and nourish the heart and to tone up both the energy and the blood |
| Zhen-Gan-Xi-Feng-Tang | Shen-Qi-Wan | Ban-Xia-Bai-Zhu-Tian-Ma-Tang | Gui-Pi-Tang |
| peppermint, green onion, banana, bamboo shoot, bitter endive, celery, bird's nest, cheese, kidney bean, abalone, asparagus, chicken egg, cuttlefish, duck, duck egg, white fungus, oyster, pork and royal jelly | beef, cherry, bird's nest, butterfish, chicken, coconut meat, date, tofu, mustard seed, sweet rice, goose meat, mutton, jackfruit, squash, sweet potato, red and black date, rice, rock sugar, caraway seed, spearmint, common button mushroom, oregano, red bean, ambergris, dill seed, garlic, sweet basil, saffron, abalone, asparagus, cuttlefish, chicken egg, duck egg, white fungus, beef liver, grape, mandarin fish, oyster, milk, blood clam and longan nut | bamboo shoot, crown daisy, date, fresh ginger, leaf or brown mustard, black and white pepper, white or yellow mustard seed, asparagus and pear | abalone, asparagus, cuttlefish, chicken egg, duck egg, white fungus, beef liver, grape, mandarin fish, oyster, milk, beef, cherry, blood clam, longan nuts, maltose, Irish potato, sweet rice, apple cucumber, bog bean, gold carp, carrot, chestnut, ham, horse bean, hyacinth bean, Job's-tears, royal jelly, string bean, whitefish, yam, red and black date, mutton, squash and rock sugar |

## RINGING IN THE EARS AND DEAFNESS

| | *Wind-heat* | *Hot liver* | *Dampness-sputum* |
|---|---|---|---|
| SYMPTOMS | 1 Cough<br>1 Coughing out blood<br>1 Dizziness<br>1 Headache<br>1 Headache with dizziness<br>1 Intolerance of light in eyes with swelling and dislike of wind<br>1 Muddy discharge from nose<br>2 Nasal congestion*<br>1 Nosebleed<br>1 Pain in the eyes<br>1 Pain in the throat<br>1 Red eyes<br>3 Ringing in ears and deafness all of a sudden*<br>1 Thirst<br>1 Toothache<br>1 Yellow urine<br>1 Yellowish discharge from the nose | 1 Bitter taste in the mouth<br>1 Deafness<br>1 Dry throat<br>1 Head swelling<br>1 Haematuria (discharge of urine containing blood)<br>6 Loud ringing in ears*<br>1 Morning sickness<br>1 Pain in the ribs<br>1 Partial suppression of lochia<br>1 Pink eyes with swelling<br>1 Psychological depression<br>1 Sour taste in the mouth<br>1 Spasms<br>1 Twitching<br>1 Vaginal discharge with fishy and foul odors | 2 Cough<br>1 Discharge of sputum that can be coughed out easily<br>1 Discharge of white, watery sputum<br>1 Dizziness<br>1 Excessive whitish vaginal discharge<br>1 Frequent coughs during pregnancy that are prolonged and cause motion of fetus<br>1 Headache<br>1 Hiccups<br>1 Pain in the chest<br>2 Panting<br>1 Prolonged dizziness<br>2 Ringing in ears with dizziness*<br>2 Ringing in ears that comes and goes with varying degrees of volume*<br>1 Sleep a lot<br>1 Sleeplessness<br>1 Vomiting<br>1 White, sliding sputum that can be cleared from throat easily |
| TREATMENT PRINCIPLE | to clear heat and disperse wind and to expand the lungs | to clear heat and sedate fire | to transform sputum and clear fire and to harmonize the stomach |
| TREATMENT FORMULA | Yin-Qiao-San or Cang-Er-Zi-San | Long-Dan-Xie-Gan-Tang | Wen-Dan-Tang or Ban-Xia-Bai-Zhu-Tian-Ma-Tang |
| FOOD CURES | banana, bitter endive, black fungus, salt, spinach, strawberry, bamboo shoot, cucumber, Job's-tears, laver, leaf beet, mung bean, peppermint, purslane, spearmint, sweet basil, celery, coconut meat and green onion | cow's gallbladder, banana, bitter endive, black fungus, salt, spinach, strawberry, bamboo shoot, cucumber, Job's tears, leaf beet, mung bean, peppermint and purslane | peppermint, spearmint, sweet basil, celery, coconut meat, green onion, asparagus, bamboo shoot, date, leaf or brown mustard, mustard seed, black and white pepper, fresh ginger and crown daisy |

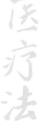

## LOSS OF VOICE

| *Kidneys deficiency* | *Wind-cold* | *Hot liver* | *Hot sputum* |
|---|---|---|---|
| 1  Chronic backache | 1  Absence of perspiration in hot weather | 1  Bitter taste in the mouth | 1  Asthma |
| 2  Deafness | 1  Asthma | 1  Deafness | 1  Coma |
| 2  Diarrhea | 1  Breathing through the nose | 1  Dry throat | 1  Cough |
| 1  Frequent miscarriage | 1  Clear discharge from nose | 1  Head swelling | 1  Discharge of hard, yellow sputum in lumps |
| 2  Hair falling out easily | 1  Cough | 1  Haematuria (discharge of urine containing blood) | 2  Discharge of sticky, turbid and thin stools |
| 1  Large quantities of urine with no thirst or drink | 1  Cough with heavy, unclear sounds and clear sputum | 6  Loud ringing in ears* | 2  Discharge of yellow, sticky sputum in lumps |
| 2  Love of lying down with desire to sleep | 1  Diarrhea | 1  Morning sickness | 1  Insanity |
| 1  Pain (falling) in the lower abdomen with desire for massage | 1  Dislike of cold | 1  Pain in the ribs | 1  Insomnia |
| 2  Ringing in ears and deafness | 1  Dizziness | 1  Partial suppression of lochia | 7  Loss of voice with heavy, unclear voice* |
| 2  Ringing in ears like the sound of a cicada that goes on and on | 1  Headache | 1  Pink eyes with swelling | 1  Stools with extremely bad smell |
| 2  Toothache | 1  Headache with dizziness | 1  Psychological depression | 1  Vomiting |
| 2  Urinary disorders | 1  Hoarseness at the beginning of illness | 1  Sour taste in the mouth | 3  Wheezing |
|  | 3  Loss of voice that occurs all of a sudden* | 1  Spasms |  |
|  | 1  Nosebleed | 1  Twitching |  |
|  | 1  Pain in the body shifting around with no fixed region | 1  Vaginal discharge with fishy and foul odors |  |
|  | 1  Stuffed nose |  |  |
|  | 1  Vomiting |  |  |
| to water yin and suppress yang and to tone the kidneys | to disperse wind and cold and to expand the lungs | .to clear heat and sedate fire | to clear heat in the lungs and transform sputum |
| Er-Long-Zuo-Ci-Wan or Da-Bu-Yin-Wan | Xing-Su-San | Long-Dan-Xie-Gan-Tang | Er-Mu-San or Sang-Ju-Yin |
| abalone, asparagus, chicken egg, white fungus, black sesame seed, beef kidney, chestnut, chicken liver, lobster, pork kidney, raspberry, scallop, sea cucumber, shrimp, string bean and walnut | peppermint (including oil), spearmint, sweet basil, cayenne pepper, fennel, fresh ginger, mustard seed, star anise and prickly ash leaf | cow's gallbladder, banana, bitter endive, black fungus, salt, spinach, strawberry, bamboo shoot, cucumber, Job's tears, leaf beet, mung bean, peppermint and purslane | banana, bitter endive, black fungus, salt, spinach, strawberry, bamboo shoot, cucumber, Job's-tears, laver, leaf beet, mung bean, peppermint, purslane, salt, cattail, agar, radish, bamboo shoot, crown daisy, date, fresh ginger, leaf or brown mustard, black and white pepper, white or yellow mustard seed, asparagus and pear |

LOSS OF VOICE (CONTINUED)                                     COUGH

| | *Lungs-dryness* | *Insufficient kidneys yin* | *Wind-cold* |
|---|---|---|---|
| **SYMPTOMS** | 2 Coughing out blood<br>2 Dry cough<br>1 Dry cough without sputum or coughing out slightly sticky fluids<br>1 Dry nose<br>1 Dry throat<br>1 Dryness in mouth and nose<br>2 Flaccidity syndrome<br>4 Loss of voice with hoarseness at the beginning, gradually becoming a complete loss of voice that drags on and on*<br>2 Morbid hunger<br>1 Thirst<br>2 Nosebleed<br>1 Pain in the throat<br>1 Presence of sputum that can't be<br>1 coughed out easily<br>1 Tickle in the throat | 2 Dizziness<br>2 Forgetfulness<br>2 Insomnia<br>4 Loss of voice with hoarseness at the beginning, gradually becoming a complete loss of voice that drags on and on*<br>2 Physical weakness<br>2 Ringing in ears<br>2 Seminal emission<br>2 Sore loins<br>2 Teeth as dry as withered bones | 1 Breathing through the nose<br>1 Clear discharge from nose<br>1 Cough<br>3 Cough with heavy, unclear sounds and clear sputum*<br>1 Diarrhea<br>1 Dislike of cold<br>1 Dizziness<br>1 Facial paralysis<br>1 Headache<br>1 Headache with dizziness<br>1 Hoarseness at the beginning of illness<br>1 Loss of voice<br>1 Nosebleed<br>3 Pain in the body shifting around with no fixed region*<br>1 Stuffed nose<br>1 Vomiting |
| **TREATMENT PRINCIPLE** | to clear heat and moisten dryness of the lungs | to water the yin, bring down fire and strengthen the lungs | to disperse wind and cold and to expand the lungs and stop cough |
| **TREATMENT FORMULA** | Yang-Yin-Qing-Fei-Yin | Mai-Wei-Di-Huang-Wan | Xing-Su-San |
| **FOOD CURES** | almond, apple, apricot, asparagus, white fungus, licorice, loquat, peanut, pear peel, rock sugar and tangerine | abalone, asparagus, chicken egg, cuttlefish, duck, duck egg, white fungus, oyster, pork, royal jelly, chestnut, chicken liver and pork kidneys | peppermint (including oil), spearmint, sweet basil, cayenne pepper, fennel, fresh ginger, mustard seed, star anise and prickly ash leaf |

| Wind-heat | Dryness-heat | Dampness-sputum | Liver-fire upsurging |
|---|---|---|---|
| 3 Coughing out sticky sputum* | 3 Constipation | 4 Cough that stops after sputum is cleared* | 1 Acute dizziness |
| 1 Coughing out blood | 4 Cough with no sputum* | 3 Discharge of abundant sputum that can be coughed out easily* | 2 Bleeding from stomach |
| 1 Dizziness | 4 Cough with a little sputum that is difficult to cough out* | 1 Discharge of white, watery sputum | 3 Cough with a sensation of some thing moving upward to the throat* |
| 1 Fever in children | 3 Diabetes mellitus | 1 Dizziness | 1 Depressed and hot |
| 1 German measles | 3 Dry nose or dry throat | 1 Frequent coughs during pregnancy that are prolonged and cause motion of fetus | 1 Dizziness |
| 1 Headache | 3 Thirst | 1 Headache | 1 Getting angry easily |
| 1 Headache with dizziness | | 1 Hiccups | 1 Headache on both sides of the head and in the corners of the eyes |
| 1 Intolerance of light in eyes with swelling and dislike of wind | | 1 Pain in the chest | 2 Headache that is severe |
| 1 Muddy discharge from nose | | 2 Panting | 2 Insanity |
| 1 Nosebleed | | 1 Prolonged dizziness | 1 Nosebleed |
| 1 Pain in the eyes | | 1 Sleep a lot | 1 Red eyes |
| 1 Pain in the throat | | 1 Sleeplessness | 1 Reddish-yellow urine |
| 1 Red eyes | | 2 Vomiting | 2 Ringing in ears |
| 1 Ringing in ears and deafness | | 1 White, sliding sputum that can be cleared from throat easily | 1 Sleeplessness or sleep a lot |
| 1 Tenesmus | | | |
| 1 Thirst | | | |
| 1 Toothache | | | |
| 1 Yellow urine | | | |
| 1 Yellowish discharge from the nose | | | |
| to disperse wind and heat and to expand the lungs and stop cough | to clear heat, moisten dryness, produce fluids and regulate the lungs | to strengthen the spleen and dry up dampness and to transform sputum and regulate the lungs | to calm the liver and sedate fire and to clear the lungs and stop cough |
| Sang-Ju-Yin | Sang-Xing-Tang or Qing-Zao-Jiu-Fei-Tang | Er-Chen-Tang | Ke-Xue-Fang |
| banana, bitter endive, black fungus, salt, spinach, strawberry, bamboo shoot, cucumber, Job's-tears, laver, leaf beet, mung bean, peppermint, purslane, spearmint, sweet basil, celery, coconut meat and green onion | asparagus, soya milk, bird's nest, cattail, chicken egg, honey, maltose, milk, pear, sesame oil, yellow soybean, banana, bitter endive, black fungus, salt, spinach, strawberry, bamboo shoot, cucumber, Job's-tears, laver, leaf beet, mung bean, peppermint and purslane | adzuki bean, ambergris, barley, common carp, cucumber, mung bean, seaweed, shepherd's purse, star fruit, bamboo shoot, crown daisy, date, fresh ginger, leaf or brown mustard, black and white pepper, white or yellow mustard seed, asparagus and pear | spinach, chestnut, shepherd's purse, rye, black fungus, vinegar, abalone, asparagus, chicken egg, white fungus, pork and royal jelly |

COUGH (CONTINUED)

# PALPITATIONS

| | *Yin deficiency* | *Simultaneous deficiency of energy and blood* | *Deficiency fire* |
|---|---|---|---|
| SYMPTOMS | 1 Bleeding from gums<br>1 Constipation<br>2 Dizziness<br>1 Dry and scant stools<br>3 Dry cough or dry throat with little sputum*<br>1 Dry sensations in the mouth<br>2 Fatigue<br>1 Headache in the afternoon<br>1 Light "tidal" fever that attacks in the afternoon<br>1 Night sweats<br>1 Nosebleed<br>1 Palms of hands and soles of feet are both hot<br>1 Sleeplessness<br>1 Swallowing difficulty<br>1 Toothache<br>1 Underweight | 1 Bleeding of various kinds with blood in light color, often seen in consumptive diseases<br>3 Dizziness<br>3 Fatigue<br>1 Flying objects seen in front of the eyes<br>3 Insomnia<br>1 Low energy<br>1 Low voice<br>1 Numbness of limbs<br>1 Pale complexion and lips<br>1 Pale nails<br>4 Palpitations with insecure feeling* | 1 Coughing out blood<br>1 Dry cough without sputum or coughing out slightly sticky fluids<br>1 Dry sensations in the mouth<br>1 Dry throat<br>4 Feeling miserable with palpitations*<br>1 Forgetfulness<br>1 Hot sensations in body<br>1 Illness attacks slowly but with a longer duration (chronic illness)<br>2 Night sweats<br>1 Pain in the throat<br>1 Ringing in ears<br>1 Seminal emission with dreams<br>1 Sleeplessness<br>1 Sore loins<br>1 Sputum with blood<br>1 Toothache |
| TREATMENT PRINCIPLE | to water the yin and clear fire and to moisten the lungs | to tone the blood and strengthen energy and to nourish the heart and secure the spirits | to water the yin and bring down the fire and to strengthen the kidneys and secure the heart |
| TREATMENT FORMULA | Bai-He-Gu-Jin-Tang | Gui-Pi-Tang | Bu-Xin-Dan |
| FOOD CURES | bird's nest, cheese, kidney bean, abalone, asparagus, chicken egg, cuttlefish, duck, duck egg, white fungus, oyster, pork and royal jelly | abalone, asparagus, cuttlefish, chicken egg, duck egg, white fungus, beef liver, grape, mandarin fish, oyster, milk, beef, cherry, blood clam, longan nuts, maltose, Irish potato, sweet rice, apple cucumber, bog bean, gold carp, carrot, chestnut, ham, horse bean, hyacinth bean, Job's-tears, royal jelly, string bean, whitefish, yam, red and black date, mutton, squash and rock sugar | banana, bitter endive, black fungus, salt, spinach, strawberry, bamboo shoot, cucumber, Job's-tears, liver, leaf beet, mung bean, peppermint, purslane, lily flower, salt, cattail, chicken egg, duck egg, asparagus, royal jelly, pork and oyster |

INSOMNIA

| Kidneys-water attacking the heart | Kidneys-water attacking the heart | Heart-spleen deficiency | Heart-kidneys unable to communicate with each other |
|---|---|---|---|
| 1 Congested chest with abdominal swelling<br>1 Cough<br>3 Dizziness*<br>3 Edema<br>1 Fingers and lips in blue-purple color<br>1 Inability to lie on back<br>1 Nervousness<br>5 Palpitations with a sensation of fullness below the heart*<br>3 Shortness of breath | 1 Congested chest with abdominal swelling<br>1 Cough<br>5 Dizziness*<br>3 Edema<br>1 Fingers and lips in blue-purple color<br>1 Inability to lie on back<br>1 Nervousness<br>5 Palpitations with a sensation of fullness below the heart*<br>3 Shortness of breath | 1 Abdominal swelling<br>1 Discharge of watery, thin stools<br>1 Eating very little<br>2 Fatigue<br>2 Forgetfulness<br>1 Impotence<br>1 Many dreams<br>1 Nervous spirits<br>2 Nervousness<br>1 Night sweats<br>2 Palpitations<br>3 Poor appetite*<br>1 Shortness of breath<br>1 Sleeplessness and wake up easily<br>1 Withering and yellowish complexion | 1 Deafness<br>1 Dizziness<br>1 Face becomes red when fatigued or working hard<br>1 Feeling miserable<br>2 Forgetfulness<br>1 Light but periodic fever not unlike the tide<br>2 Nervousness<br>1 Night sweats<br>2 Palpitations<br>1 Ringing in ears<br>2 Seminal emission<br>3 Sleeplessness due to stress or depression*<br>1 Sleeplessness with forgetfulness |
| to warm the heart and tone the energy and to promote water flow | to warm the heart and tone the energy and to promote water flow | to tone the heart and the spleen and to secure the heart and calm the spirits | to water yin and clear fire and to promote communication between the heart and the kidneys |
| Ling-Gui-Zhu-Gan-Tang | Ling-Gui-Zhu-Gan-Tang | Gui-Pi-Tang or Yang-Xin-Tang | Huang-Lian-E-Jiao-Tang |
| dried ginger, water spinach, cinnamon, longan nut, wheat, kidney, lobster, sardine, shrimp, sparrow, clove, dill seed, fennel, pistachio nut, sparrow egg, crab apple, raspberry and walnut | dried ginger, water spinach, cinnamon, longan nut, wheat, kidney, lobster, sardine, shrimp, sparrow, clove, dill seed, fennel, pistachio nut, sparrow egg, crab apple, raspberry and walnut | beef liver, chicken egg, cuttlefish, oyster, pork liver, sea cucumber, water spinach, longan nut, mandarin fish, apple cucumber, chestnut, horse bean, Job's-tears, Irish potato, rice, royal jelly and yam | asparagus, abalone, chicken egg, white fungus, bog bean, wheat, banana, bamboo shoot, bitter endive, oyster, royal jelly and pork |

INSOMNIA (CONTINUED)

| | *Heart-gallbladder deficiency* | *Sputum-fire* | *Indigestion* |
|---|---|---|---|
| **SYMPTOMS** | 3 Bitter taste in the mouth<br>3 Depressed with a desire to vomit<br>2 Feeling miserable with love of darkness and dislike of light<br>5 Insomnia due to nervousness*<br>2 Scared by events easily<br>5 Wake up at night easily due to shock* | 2 Difficult defecation or urination<br>2 Hungry with no appetite<br>3 Insanity<br>3 Ringing in ears and deafness<br>10 Sleeplessness due to congested chest* | 1 Abdominal pain<br>1 Abdominal pain with a desire for massage<br>1 Abdominal pain with an aversion to massage<br>5 Abdominal distension*<br>1 Belching of bad breath after meals<br>1 Chest and diaphragm congestion and discomfort<br>1 Diarrhea and constipation<br>1 Hot sensations in the middle of palms<br>1 Indigestion<br>1 Lack of appetite<br>1 Love of hot drink, but drink very little<br>1 Nausea<br>1 Pain in inner part of stomach with swelling and feeling of fullness<br>1 Stomachache<br>1 Stools with an extremely bad smell<br>1 Vomiting of clear water |
| **TREATMENT PRINCIPLE** | to strengthen energy, overcome nervousness and secure the spirits | to transform sputum and harmonize the middle region | to promote digestion and harmonize the middle region |
| **TREATMENT FORMULA** | An-Shen-Ding-Zhi-Wan | Wen-Dan-Tang | Bao-He-Wan |
| **FOOD CURES** | corn silk, cow's gallbladder, air bladder of shark, water spinach, abalone, asparagus, dried ginger and cinnamon | salt, cattail, agar, radish, bamboo shoot, crown daisy, date, fresh ginger, leaf or brown mustard, black and white pepper, white or yellow mustard seed, asparagus and pear | asafoetida, buckwheat, castor bean, jellyfish, peach, radish, water chestnut, cardamon seed, cayenne pepper, coriander, grapefruit, jackfruit, malt, sweet basil, tea and tomato |

# TICS

| Wind | Extreme heat generating wind | Blood deficiency generating wind | Simultaneous deficiency of energy and blood |
|---|---|---|---|
| 1 Diarrhea containing undigested food | 2 Convulsions | 2 Dizziness | 1 Bleeding of various kinds with blood in light color, often seen in consumptive diseases |
| 1 Discharge of watery, thin stools | 2 Fainting | 2 Fainting | 3 Dizziness |
| 1 Dislike of wind | 2 Feeling troubled, quick-tempered and insecure | 2 Muscular (spasmodic) contractions | 2 Fatigue |
| 1 Excessive perspiration | 6 High fever | 2 Muscular tightening | 1 Flying objects seen in front of the eyes |
| 1 Headache accompanied by fear of wind | 2 Muscular tightening | 2 Numbness of hands and feet | 2 Insomnia |
| 1 Headache with heavy sensations in the head | 2 Neck stiffness | 2 Pain in the upper abdomen | 1 Low energy |
| 1 Illness (acute) attacking all of a sudden | 2 Twitching or spasms of four limbs | ? Ringing in ears | 1 Low voice |
| 1 Itch | 2 Dry and shivering tongue | 2 Shaking of hands and feet | 5 Numbness of limbs* |
| 1 Itchy skin that becomes almost intolerable | | 2 Spots in front of the eyes | 1 Pale complexion and lips |
| 1 Light cough | | 2 Twitching | 1 Pale nails |
| 1 Nasal discharge | | | 2 Palpitations |
| 1 Numbness in the skin of the face | | | |
| 1 Pain in all the joints that attacks suddenly | | | |
| 1 Pain in the joints that shifts from one joint to another | | | |
| 1 Shaking of four limbs and body | | | |
| 1 Sneezing | | | |
| 1 Stiffness of muscles | | | |
| 1 Stuffed nose with heavy voice | | | |
| 1 Tickle in the throat | | | |
| 1 Dry mouth | | | |
| to expel wind and transform sputum and to relieve spasms and overcome convulsions | to clear heat and stop convulsions | to strengthen the liver and the kidneys and to stop convulsions | to tone energy in order to produce the blood and to nourish the blood in order to nourish the tendons |
| Wu-Hu-Zhui-Feng-San | An-Gong-Niu-Huang-Wan | Da-Ding-Feng-Zhu | Ba-Zhen-Tang |
| peppermint, spearmint, sweet basil, celery, coconut meat and green onion | peppermint, spearmint, sweet basil, celery, coconut meat, green onion, chicken egg, bitter endive, camellia, cattail, black fungus, salt, spinach, strawberry, banana, bamboo shoot, crab and water clam | egg, mulberry, abalone, liver, cuttlefish, grape, milk and brown sugar | abalone, asparagus, cuttlefish, chicken egg, duck egg, white fungus, beef liver, grape, mandarin fish, oyster, milk, beef, cherry, blood clam, longan nuts, maltose, Irish potato, sweet rice, apple cucumber, bog bean, gold carp, carrot, chestnut, ham, hors bean, hyacinth bean, Job's-tears, royal jelly, string bean, whitefish, yam, red and black date, mutton, squash and rock sugar |

## COUGHING OUT BLOOD

| | Heart-gallbladder deficiency | Wind-dryness | Liver-fire upsurging |
|---|---|---|---|
| **SYMPTOMS** | 4 Bitter taste in the mouth<br>2 Depressed with a desire to vomit<br>2 Feeling miserable with love of darkness and dislike of light<br>2 Insomnia<br>2 Scared by events easily<br>2 Sleeplessness<br>6 Trembling that is often triggered by nervousness* | 5 Blood in sputum*<br>1 Chest pain<br>1 Coughing with scant sputum<br>1 Dry nose<br>1 Dry skin with wrinkles<br>1 Dry throat<br>1 Dry, withered fingernails<br>1 Fever<br>1 Headache<br>4 Itch in the throat*<br>1 No perspiration<br>1 Pain in the upper abdomen<br>1 Symptoms attack or worsen in autumn or in a dry climate<br>1 Thirst | 1 Acute dizziness<br>1 Bleeding from stomach<br>3 Coughing out sputum with blood in it or coughing out fresh blood*<br>1 Deafness<br>1 Dim vision<br>1 Dizziness<br>1 Dry sensations in the mouth<br>1 Getting angry easily<br>1 Headache on both sides of the head and in the corners of the eyes<br>2 Headache that is severe<br>1 Nosebleed<br>1 Pain (falling) in the lower abdomen with desire for massage<br>1 Pain in the upper abdomen<br>1 Pink eyes with swelling<br>1 Reddish-yellow urine<br>1 Red eyes<br>1 Ringing in ears<br>1 Sleeplessness or sleep a lot |
| **TREATMENT PRINCIPLE** | to tone the energy of the heart and to overcome nervousness and secure the spirits | to disperse wind and heat and to lubricate the lungs | to sedate the liver, lubricate the lungs and stop bleeding |
| **TREATMENT FORMULA** | Gan-Mai-Da-Zao-Tang | Sang-Xing-Tang or Si-Sheng-Wan | Ke-Xue-Fang |
| **FOOD CURES** | corn silk, cow's gallbladder, air bladder of shark, water spinach, abalone, asparagus, dried ginger and cinnamon | peppermint, spearmint, sweet basil, celery, coconut meat, green onion, asparagus, egg, honey, pear, sesame oil, yellow soybean, spinach and tofu | spinach, chestnut, shepherd's purse, rye, black fungus, vinegar, abalone, asparagus, chicken egg, white fungus, pork and royal jelly |

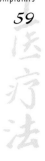

## VOMITING OF BLOOD

| *Yin deficiency* | *Hot stomach* | *Stomach-fire* | *Spleen unable to govern the blood* |
|---|---|---|---|
| 1 Bleeding from gums | 1 Bad breath | 1 Bitter taste in the mouth | 2 Blood in urine |
| 1 Constipation | 1 Bleeding from gums | 1 Bleeding from gums | 2 Discharge of blood from anus |
| 3 Coughing out abundant blood in light color* | 1 Foul breath from the mouth | 1 Constipation | 1 Discharge of sticky, muddy stools or diarrhea |
| 2 Dizziness | 1 Getting hungry easily | 1 Depressed, quick-tempered and insecure | 1 Dizziness |
| 1 Dry and scant stools | 1 Gums swelling | 1 Dry sensations in the mouth | 1 Mentally fatigued |
| 1 Dry sensations in the mouth or the throat | 1 Hiccups | 1 Eating a lot and still feeling hungry | 2 Nosebleed |
| 2 Fatigue | 1 Morning sickness | 1 Fever | 1 Palpitations |
| 1 Headache in the afternoon | 1 Nosebleed | 1 Headache | 2 Poor appetite |
| 1 Night sweats | 2 Pain in the gums with swelling | 1 Hiccups | 2 Pure-white complexion |
| 1 Pain in the throat, also red and swollen | 1 Pain in the throat | 1 Hungry with good appetite and eat lot but still under-weight | 1 Shortness of breath |
| 1 Palms of hands and soles of feet are both hot | 1 Perspiring on the head | 1 Nosebleed | 1 Stomach and abdomen swelling and fullness |
| 1 Short and reddish streams of urine | 2 Stomachache | 1 Pain in the gums with swelling | 3 Vomiting of dark- and light-colored blood that recurs frequently* |
| 1 Sleeplessness | 1 Thirst and craving for cold | 1 Pain in the throat, also red and swollen | 1 Withering and yellowish complexion |
| 1 Swallowing difficulty | 3 Vomiting of fresh blood or blood mixed with foods* | 1 Screaming during sleep in children | |
| 1 Toothache | 1 Vomiting right after eating | 1 Toothache | |
| 1 Underweight | 1 Vomiting with stomach discomfort as if hungry, empty, or hot | 2 Vomiting of blood that occurs all of a sudden and in hug amounts* | |
| | | 2 Vomiting of red or dark blood* | |
| | | 1 Vomiting right after eating | |
| to water the yin, clear heat, lubricate dryness and stop bleeding | to clear the heat in the stomach, sedate fire, cool the blood and stop bleeding | to clear the heat in the liver, cool the blood and stop bleeding | to tone the energy and the blood and to constrict the blood and stop bleeding |
| Bai-He-Gu-Jin-Tang | Xie-Xin-Tang | Yu-Nü-Jian | Huang-Tu-Tang |
| bird's nest, cheese, kidney bean, abalone, asparagus, chicken egg, cuttlefish, duck, duck egg, white fungus, oyster, pork and royal jelly | salt, lily flower, bitter endive, camellia, cattail, black fungus, spinach, strawberry, banana, cucumber and licorice | areca nuts, buckwheat, common carp, banana, bitter endive, black fungus, salt, spinach, strawberry, bamboo shoot, cucumber, Job's-tears, liver, leaf beet, mung bean, peppermint, purslane, lily flower, salt and cattail | chicken, grape, longan nuts, maltose, mandarin fish, Irish potato, sweet rice, apple cucumber, bog bean, gold carp, carrot, chestnut, ham, horse bean, hyacinth bean, Job's-tears, royal jelly, string bean, whitefish, yam, red and black date, mutton, squash, rock sugar and chicken egg yolk |

## NOSEBLEED

| | Hot lungs | Hot stomach | Hot liver |
|---|---|---|---|
| SYMPTOMS | 1 Acute panting in high-pitched sound with rapid expiration<br>1 Bitter taste in the mouth<br>1 Cough with subdued and oppressed sounds<br>1 Coughing out and vomiting of pus and blood with a fishy smell<br>1 Coughing out yellow and sticky sputum<br>1 Discharge of dry stools<br>3 Dry nose*<br>1 Dry sensations in the mouth<br>1 Flickering of nostrils<br>1 Hot sensations in the body<br>1 Light but periodic fever not unlike the tide<br>3 Nosebleed with fresh blood*<br>1 Pain in the chest or in the throat<br>1 Presence of sputum that can't be coughed out easily<br>1 Psychological depression<br>1 Urgent panting | 3 Bad breath*<br>1 Bleeding from gums<br>2 Dry nose*<br>2 Nosebleed with blood in fresh red color*<br>2 Pain in the gums with swelling<br>1 Pain in the throat<br>1 Perspiring on the head<br>2 Stomachache<br>1 Thirst and craving for cold<br>2 Vomiting<br>2 Vomiting of blood<br>1 Vomiting right after eating | 1 Bitter taste in the mouth<br>1 Blood in urine<br>1 Deafness<br>1 Dry throat<br>3 Head swelling or headache*<br>4 Nosebleed with abundant blood in fresh red color*<br>3 Pain in the upper abdomen*<br>1 Partial suppression of lochia<br>1 Pink eyes with swelling<br>1 Psychological depression<br>1 Sour taste in the mouth<br>1 Spasms<br>1 Twitching<br>1 Vaginal discharge with fishy and foul odors |
| TREATMENT PRINCIPLE | to sedate the lungs and clear the heat in the lungs and to cool the blood and stop bleeding | to clear the heat in the stomach, nourish the yin and cool the blood and stop bleeding | to calm the liver and clear the heat in the liver and to cool the blood and stop bleeding |
| TREATMENT FORMULA | Sang-Xing-Tang or He-Ye-Wan | Yu-Nü-Jian | Long-Dan-Xie-Gan-Tang |
| FOOD CURES | apple, apple cucumber, apricot, white fungus, ham, jackfruit, lemon, maltose, mandarin orange, mulberry, olive, peach, pear, sweet potato, red and black date, tomato, white sugar, mung bean and eggplant | salt, lily flower, bitter endive, camellia, cattail, black fungus, spinach, strawberry, banana, cucumber and licorice | cow's gallbladder, banana, bitter endive, black fungus, salt, spinach, strawberry, bamboo shoot, cucumber, Job's tears, leaf beet, mung bean, peppermint and purslane |

# BLOOD IN URINE

| Heart-fire | Dampness-heat flowing downward | Simultaneous deficiency of energy and blood | Kidneys deficiency |
|---|---|---|---|
| 1 Bleeding from gums<br>3 Burning sensations on urination*<br>1 Cold hands and feet<br>1 Discharge of blood from the mouth<br>1 Dribbling after urination<br>1 Feeling miserable<br>1 Hot sensations in the middle of palms<br>1 Morning sickness<br>1 Mouth canker<br>1 Not alert<br>1 Pain on urination<br>1 Palpitations<br>1 Pulpy and decayed tongue and mouth<br>1 Reddish-yellow urine<br>1 Seminal emission<br>1 Short streams of urine<br>1 Sleeplessness<br>1 Urine blood in fresh red color | 1 Abdominal pain<br>4 Burning sensations and itch in the genitals*<br>1 Congested chest<br>1 Diarrhea<br>1 Fever that doesn't appear high<br>1 Jaundice<br>3 Urine blood in fresh red color*<br>1 Perspiration on hands and feet<br>1 Reddish and scant urine<br>1 Retention of urine<br>1 Short and reddish streams of urine<br>1 Swollen body of the tongue<br>1 Thirst | 1 Bleeding of various kinds with blood in light color, often seen in consumptive diseases<br>3 Dizziness<br>3 Fatigue<br>1 Flying objects seen in front of the eyes<br>3 Insomnia<br>1 Low energy<br>1 Low voice<br>1 No burning sensation on urination<br>1 Numbness of limbs<br>1 Pale complexion and lips<br>1 Pale nails<br>3 Palpitations | 1 Asthma<br>2 Chronic backache<br>1 Clear, watery and whitish vaginal discharge<br>2 Deafness<br>2 Diarrhea<br>2 Hair falling out easily<br>1 Large quantities of urine with no thirst or drink<br>1 Love of lying down with desire to sleep<br>2 No burning sensation on urination<br>1 Pain (falling) in the lower abdomen with desire for massage<br>1 Ringing in ears<br>2 Ringing in ears and deafness<br>1 Seminal emission<br>1 Toothache |
| to clear the heat in the heart and to cool the blood and stop bleeding | to clear the heat in the bladder and promote urination and to cool the blood and stop bleeding | to tone the energy and the blood and to constrict the blood and stop bleeding | to water the yin and strengthen the kidneys and to constrict the blood and stop bleeding |
| Xiao-Ji-Yin-Zi | Ba-Zheng-San | Gui-Pi-Tang or Huang-Tu-Tang | Liu-Wei-Di-Huang-Wan or Da-Bu-Yin-Wan |
| asparagus, pear peel, banana, bitter endive, black fungus, salt, spinach, strawberry, bamboo shoot, cucumber, Job's tears, liver, leaf beet, mung bean, peppermint, purslane, lily flower, salt and cattail | carp, celery, horse bean, jellyfish skin, Job's-tears, prickly ash, hyacinth bean, oregano, sweet basil, adzuki bean, bamboo shoot, soybean sprouts, rosin, banana, bitter endive, black fungus, salt, spinach, strawberry, cucumber, leaf beet, mung bean, peppermint and purslane | abalone, asparagus, cuttlefish, chicken egg, duck egg, white fungus, beef liver, grape, mandarin fish, oyster, milk, beef, cherry, blood clam, longan nuts, maltose, Irish potato, sweet rice, apple cucumber, bog bean, gold carp, carrot, chestnut, ham, horse bean, hyacinth bean, Job's-tears, royal jelly, string bean, whitefish, yam, red and black date, mutton, squash and rock sugar | abalone, asparagus, chicken egg, white fungus, black sesame seed, beef kidney, chestnut, chicken liver, lobster, pork kidney, raspberry, scallop, sea cucumber, shrimp, string bean and walnut |

| | BLOOD IN STOOL | | VOMITING |
| --- | --- | --- | --- |
| | *Spleen unable to govern the blood* | *Large-intestine dampness-heat* | *Cold-dampness* |
| **SYMPTOMS** | 1 Blood in urine<br>4 Bowel movements, followed by bleeding*<br>4 Discharge of blood from anus with blood in dark color*<br>1 Discharge of sticky, muddy stools or diarrhea<br>1 Dizziness<br>1 Mentally fatigued<br>2 Nosebleed<br>1 Palpitations<br>1 Poor appetite<br>1 Pure-white complexion<br>1 Shortness of breath<br>1 Stomach and abdomen swelling and fullness<br>68 Withering and yellowish complexion | 2 Abdominal Pain<br>3 Bleeding, following by bowel movement*<br>4 Blood in fresh-red color*<br>1 Damp, glossy and reddened anus in children<br>2 Diarrhea with stools containing pus and blood<br>1 Discharge of blood from anus<br>2 Dysentery<br>3 Hemorrhoids<br>2 Pain in anus with swelling and burning sensations<br>1 Short and reddish streams of urine | 1 Absence of perspiration in hot weather<br>1 Cold sensations in lower abdomen-genitals region<br>1 Cough<br>1 Coughing out sputum with a low sound<br>2 Diarrhea<br>1 Discharge of sputum that can be coughed out easily<br>2 Dysentery<br>1 Edema in the four limbs<br>1 Headache<br>1 Movement difficulty<br>4 Nausea*<br>1 Pain in the body<br>1 Pain in the joints<br>1 Scant and clear urine<br>1 Stomachache |
| **TREATMENT PRINCIPLE** | to strengthen the spleen and warm the middle region and to constrict the blood and stop bleeding | to clear the dampness-heat in the large intestine and to cool the blood and stop bleeding | to disperse cold, dry up dampness, harmonize the stomach and stop vomiting |
| **TREATMENT FORMULA** | Gui-Pi-Tang or Huang-Tu-Tang | Chi-Xiao-Dou-Dang-Gui-San, Huai-Hua-San | Huo-Xiang-Zheng-Qi-San |
| **FOOD CURES** | chicken, grape, longan nuts, maltose, mandarin fish, Irish potato, sweet rice, apple cucumber, bog bean, gold carp, carrot, chestnut, ham, horse bean, hyacinth bean, Job's-tears, royal jelly, string bean, whitefish, yam, red and black date, mutton, squash, rock sugar and chicken egg yolk | hyacinth bean, mackerel, sweet basil, day lily, abalone, adzuki bean, celery, chicken egg white, mung bean, Job's-tears, jellyfish and eggplant | cayenne pepper, dill seed, fennel, fresh ginger, mustard seed, prickly ash, star anise, white or yellow mustard, wine, carp, celery, horse bean, jellyfish skin, Job's-tears, hyacinth bean, oregano, sweet basil, adzuki bean, bamboo shoot, soybean sprouts and rosin |

| Indigestion | Dampness-sputum | Stomach energy upsurging | Yang deficiency |
|---|---|---|---|
| 1 Abdominal pain | 1 Cough | 2 Dysphagia | 1 Clear and long streams of urine |
| 1 Abdominal pain with a desire for massage | 1 Discharge of sputum that can be coughed out easily | 2 Dry vomiting | 1 Cold hands and feet |
| 1 Abdominal pain with an aversion to massage | 1 Discharge of white-watery sputum | 2 Eating in the evening and vomiting in the morning | 1 Constipation |
| 3 Belching of bad breath after meals* | 1 Dizziness | 2 Eating in the morning and vomiting in the evening | 1 Diarrhea |
| 1 Chest and diaphragm congestion and discomfort | 1 Headache | 2 Hiccups in short sounds | 1 Diminished urination |
| 1 Diarrhea and constipation | 1 Hiccups | 2 Nausea | 1 Discharge of watery, thin stools |
| 1 Diarrhea in children | 1 Pain in the chest | 3 Upset stomach | 1 Edema |
| 1 Hot sensations in the middle of palms | 3 Panting | 3 Vomiting of foods, watery sputum, or acidic and bitter water* | 1 Fatigue with lack of power |
| 1 Indigestion | 2 Prolonged dizziness | 2 Vomiting right after eating | 1 Fear of cold |
| 1 Lack of appetite | 2 Sleep a lot | | 1 Fingertips often cold |
| 1 Love of hot drink, but drink only a little | 2 Sleeplessness | | 1 Frequent fear of cold both in hands and feet |
| 1 Malaria | 3 Vomiting of watery sputum | | 1 Frequent illness and love of sleep |
| 1 Nausea | 2 White, sliding sputum that can be cleared from throat easily | | 1 Head and body curled up while lying down |
| 1 Pain in inner part of stomach with swelling and feeling of fullness | | | 1 Headache in the morning |
| 1 Stomachache | | | 1 Palpitations |
| 1 Stools with an extremely bad smell | | | 1 Perspiration like cold water |
| 2 Vomiting of clear water or rotten acid* | | | 1 Scant energy and too tired to talk |
| | | | 1 Sleep a lot |
| | | | 1 Vomiting of clear water* |
| | | | 1 Vomiting right after a full meal* |
| to promote digestion, harmonize the stomach and stop vomiting | to warm and transform sputum and to harmonize the stomach and stop vomiting | to harmonize the stomach, regulate stomach energy and stop vomiting | to warm the middle region and strengthen the spleen and to strengthen the stomach and stop vomiting |
| Bao-He-Wan | Xiao-Ban-Xia-Tang | Xuan-Fu-Dai-Zhe-Tang | Li-Zhong-Tang or Wu-Zhu-Yu-Tang |
| asafoetida, buckwheat, castor bean, jellyfish, peach, radish, water chestnut, cardamon seed, cayenne pepper, coriander, grapefruit, jackfruit, malt, sweet basil, tea and tomato | adzuki bean, ambergris, barley, common carp, cucumber, mung bean, seaweed, shepherd's purse, star fruit, bamboo shoot, crown daisy, date, fresh ginger, leaf or brown mustard, black and white pepper, white or yellow mustard seed, asparagus and pear | almond, areca nut, sugar beet, brake, buckwheat, common carp, cashew nut, coriander, loquat, malt, pea, black and white pepper, radish, rice bran and sword bean | kidneys, lobster, sardine, shrimp, star anise and red and black date |

| | VOMITING (CONTINUED) | HICCUPS | |
|---|---|---|---|
| | *Yin deficiency* | *Cold* | *Hot* |
| **SYMPTOMS** | 1 Bleeding from gums<br>1 Constipation<br>2 Dizziness<br>1 Dry sensations in the mouth<br>1 Dry throat<br>3 Dry vomiting*<br>1 Fatigue<br>1 Headache in the afternoon<br>1 Light fever in the afternoon<br>1 Night sweats<br>1 Nosebleed<br>1 Pain in the throat<br>1 Short and reddish streams of urine<br>1 Sleeplessness<br>1 Swallowing difficulty<br>1 Toothache<br>1 Underweight | 1 Constipation<br>1 Coughing out and vomiting bubbles of saliva<br>1 Dislike of cold or dislike of talking<br>1 Dizziness with objects appearing in front of eyes<br>1 Dry throat<br>1 Hands and feet extremely cold<br>1 Heavy and unclear voice with high-pitched and rough tone<br>2 Hiccups with loud and forceful sounds*<br>2 Hiccups with cold hands and feet and easily started by cold air*<br>1 Love of hot drink<br>1 Pain in inner part of stomach, getting better after meals<br>1 Pain shifting around with no fixed region<br>1 Pale complexion<br>1 Plenty of saliva<br>1 Severe pain in the joints<br>1 Sore loins and weak legs<br>1 Thinking about water but with no desire to drink it<br>1 Whitish urine | 1 Constipation or diarrhea<br>1 Depressed, quick-tempered and insecure<br>1 Diminished urination<br>1 Discharge of copious, yellow, sticky sputum<br>1 Dry lips or dry teeth<br>1 Escape of gas from the anus with noise<br>2 Hiccups that make loud and short sound, with dryness and thirst*<br>2 Hiccups that make quick sound and occur quite frequently*<br>1 Light fever<br>1 Light sensations in the body that can turn easily<br>1 Limbs are warm<br>1 Little saliva<br>1 Love of cold or cold drink<br>1 Stools with an extremely bad smell<br>1 Thirst with an incessant desire to drink<br>1 Throat swelling and red, producing rotten liquid<br>1 Urine with an extremely bad smell<br>1 Vomiting of sour, bad-smelling foods, with a love of cold drink |
| **TREATMENT PRINCIPLE** | to water the yin and nourish the stomach and to lubricate dryness and stop vomiting | to warm the middle region and disperse cold and to harmonize the stomach and stop hiccups | to clear the heat and sedate the fire and to harmonize the stomach and stop hiccups |
| **TREATMENT FORMULA** | Sha-Shen-Mai-Dong-Tang | Ding-Xiang-Shi-Di-Tang | Zhu-Ye-Shi-Gao-Tang |
| **FOOD CURES** | bird's nest, cheese, kidney bean, abalone, asparagus, chicken egg, cuttlefish, duck, duck egg, white fungus, oyster, pork and royal jelly | cayenne pepper, dill seed, fennel, fresh ginger, mustard seed, prickly ash, star anise, white or yellow mustard and wine | banana, bitter endive, black fungus, salt, spinach, strawberry, bamboo shoot, cucumber, Job's-tears, laver, leaf beet, mung bean, peppermint and purslane |

| Indigestion | Yin deficiency | Yang deficiency | Large-intestine heat |
|---|---|---|---|
| 1  Abdominal pain | 1  Bleeding from gums | 1  Clear and long streams of urine | 2  Abdominal pain |
| 1  Abdominal pain with a desire for massage | 1  Constipation | 1  Cold hands and feet | 5  Constipation with bad breath* |
| 1  Abdominal pain with an aversion to massage | 1  Dizziness | 1  Constipation or diarrhea | 1  Discharge of blood from anus |
| 2  Bad taste in the mouth* | 1  Dry and scant stools | 1  Diminished urination | 5  Discharge of solid, dry and hard stools* |
| 2  Belching of bad breath after meals* | 1  Dry sensations in the mouth | 1  Discharge of watery, thin stools | 1  Discharge of sticky, muddy stools with a rotten and bad smell |
| 1  Chest and diaphragm congestion and discomfort | 1  Dry throat | 1  Fatigue | 1  Dry sensations in the mouth |
| 1  Diarrhea and constipation | 1  Fatigue | 1  Fear of cold | 1  Gums swelling |
| 2  Hiccups with loud and forceful sound* | 1  Headache in the afternoon | 1  Fingertips often cold | 1  Lips are scorched |
| 1  Hot sensations in the middle of palms | 2  Hiccups that occur more readily on an empty stomach* | 1  Frequent fear of cold both in hands and feet | 1  Pain in anus with swelling and burning sensations |
| 1  Indigestion | 2  Hiccups with weak and low sound* | 1  Headache in the morning | 1  Short and reddish streams of urine |
| 1  Lack of appetite | 1  Light fever in the afternoon | 2  Hiccups that occur more readily on an empty stomach* | 1  Yellow stools like rice pulp with bad smell |
| 1  Love of hot drink, but drink only a little | 1  Night sweats | 3  Hiccups with weak and low sound* | |
| 1  Nausea | 1  Nosebleed | 1  Palpitations | |
| 1  Pain in inner part of stomach with swelling and feeling of fullness | 1  Short and reddish streams of urine | 1  Perspiration due to hot weather or putting on warm clothes | |
| 1  Stomachache | 1  Sleeplessness | 1  Perspiration like cold water | |
| 1  Stool with an extremely bad smell | 1  Swallowing difficulty | 1  Scant energy and too tired to talk | |
| 1  Vomiting | 1  Toothache | 1  Sleep a lot | |
| | 1  Underweight | | |

| | | | |
|---|---|---|---|
| to promote digestion, regulate the stomach and stop hiccups | to produce fluids and strengthen the stomach and to lubricate dryness and stop hiccups | to tone the spleen and the kidneys and to harmonize the stomach and stop hiccups | to clear heat and lubricate the large intestine |
| Bao-He-Wan | Yi-Wei-Tang | Li-Zhong-Tang | Ma-Zi-Ren-Wan or Zeng-Yi-Cheng-Qi-Tang |
| asafoetida, buckwheat, castor bean, jellyfish, peach, radish, water chestnut, cardamon seed, cayenne pepper, coriander, grapefruit, jackfruit, malt, sweet basil, tea and tomato | bird's nest, cheese, kidney bean, abalone, asparagus, chicken egg, cuttlefish, duck, duck egg, white fungus, oyster, pork and royal jelly | kidneys, lobster, sardine, shrimp, star anise and red and black date | preserved duck egg, flour, banana, bitter endive, black fungus, salt, spinach, strawberry, bamboo shoot, cucumber, Job's-tears, laver, leaf beet, mung bean, peppermint, purslane, sesame oil and apple |

CONSTIPATION (CONTINUED)

| | Energy congestion | Cold large-intestine | Energy deficiency |
|---|---|---|---|
| SYMPTOMS | 2 Abdominal pain<br>1 Chest and ribs discomfort<br>2 Chest pain<br>5 Constipation with a desire to empty the bowel*<br>1 Pain in inner part of stomach with prickling sensation and swelling<br>2 Pain in the upper abdomen<br>1 Retention of urine<br>1 Ringing in ears and deafness<br>2 Stomachache<br>1 Subjective sensation of lump in the throat<br>1 Swallowing difficulty<br>1 Swelling and congestion after eating | 4 Abdominal pain*<br>2 Abdominal pain with abdominal rumbling<br>2 Abdominal rumbling<br>2 Clear and long streams of urine<br>2 Cold hands and feet<br>5 Difficult bowel movements*<br>3 Discharge of sticky, muddy stools not unlike dung of a goose | 1 Abdominal pain<br>1 Constipation with discharge of soft stools*<br>1 Discharge of sticky, turbid stools or diarrhea*<br>1 Dizziness<br>1 Fatigued following bowel movment*<br>1 Headache (severe) that occurs with fatigue after labor<br>1 Headache at intervals, headache in the morning, or prolonged headache<br>1 Lying down with an inability to sit up, which will cause dizziness<br>1 Misty vision<br>1 Numbness<br>1 Palpitations with insecure feeling<br>1 Perspiration on hands and feet<br>1 Prolonged headache<br>1 Ringing in ears that causes deafness<br>1 Shaking of hands<br>1 Shortness of breath<br>1 Swallowing difficulty<br>1 Talking in weak voice<br>1 Tips of four limbs slightly cold<br>1 Underweight with dry skin |
| TREATMENT PRINCIPLE | to promote energy flow | to warm the large intestine and promote bowel movements | to strengthen the energy and promote bowel movement |
| TREATMENT FORMULA | Liu-Mo-Yin | Ji-Chuan-Jian | Bu-Zhong-Yi-Qi-Tang |
| FOOD CURES | beef, cherry, bird's nest, butterfish, chicken, coconut meat, date, tofu, mustard seed, sweet rice, goose meat, mutton, jackfruit, squash, sweet potato, red and black date, rice, rock sugar, caraway seed, spearmint, common button mushroom, oregano, red bean, ambergris, dill seed, garlic, sweet basil and saffron | capers, cayenne pepper, fresh ginger, prickly ash, star anise, white or yellow mustard seed, white or yellow mustard, wine, chicken, clove, herring, nutmeg and black and white pepper | grape, longan nuts, maltose, mandarin fish, Irish potato, sweet rice, apple cucumber, bog bean, gold carp, carrot, chestnut, ham, horse bean, hyacinth bean, Job's-tears, royal jelly, string bean, whitefish, yam, red and black date, mutton, squash and rock sugar |

## DIARRHEA

| Blood deficiency | Cold-dampness | Superficial dampness-heat | Indigestion |
|---|---|---|---|
| 1 Abdominal pain | 1 Absence of perspiration in hot weather | 1 Burning sensation and itch in the genitals or burning sensation in the anus | 3 Abdominal pain that lessens following bowel movement* |
| 1 Constipation with discharge of hard stool* | 1 Cold sensations in lower abdomen-genitals region | 5 Diarrhea with forceful discharge of stools* | 1 Belching of bad breath after meals |
| 1 Difficult bowel movement* | 1 Cough | 1 Discharge of yellowish-red, turbid stools with bad smell | 1 Chest and diaphragm congestion and discomfort |
| 1 Dizziness | 1 Coughing out sputum with a low sound | 1 Excessive perspiration | 1 Diarrhea and constipation |
| 1 Dry and cracked lips and mouth | 6 Diarrhea with discharge of soft stools with an offensive smell* | 1 Feeling miserable | 3 Diarrhea with an unusually offensive smell* |
| 1 Fatigue | 1 Discharge of sputum that can be coughed out easily | 1 Itch and pain in the vulva frequently | 1 Hot sensations in the middle of palms |
| 1 Fever | 2 Dysentery | 1 Low fever | 1 Indigestion |
| 1 Feeling miserable | 1 Edema in the four limbs | 1 Pain in the joints of four limbs, with swelling and heaviness | 1 Lack of appetite |
| 1 Headache in the afternoon or with dizziness | 1 Headache | 1 Paralysis | 1 Love of hot drink, but drink only a little |
| 1 Lips lightly colored | 1 Movement difficulty | 1 Perspiration on hands and feet or the head | 1 Malaria |
| 1 Lying down with an inability to sit up, which will cause dizziness | 1 Pain in the body | 1 Reddish and scant streams of urine | 1 Nausea |
| 1 Misty vision | 1 Pain in the joints | 1 Retention of urine | 1 Pain in inner part of stomach with swelling and feeling of fullness |
| 1 Muscles jumping that cannot be controlled | 1 Scant and clear urine | 1 Short and reddish streams of urine | 1 Stomachache |
| 1 Night sweats | 1 Stomachache | 1 Swollen body of the tongue | 1 Stools with an extremely bad smell |
| 1 Palpitations with insecure feeling | | 1 Thirst | 1 Vomiting |
| 1 Sleeplessness | | 1 Yellowish color of body | 1 Vomiting of clear water |
| 1 Spasms | | | |
| 1 Tics of four limbs | | | |
| 1 Underweight with dry skin | | | |
| 1 White complexion | | | |
| to nourish the blood and lubricate the large intestine | to remove dampness with aromatic herbs and to disperse cold and dry dampness | to clear heat and remove dampness and to regulate the stomach and the intestine | to promote digestion and regulate the stomach and intestine |
| Run-Chang-Wan | Huo-Xiang-Zheng-Qi-San | Ge-Gen-Qin-Lian-Tang | Mu-Xiang-Bing-Lang-Wan |
| abalone, asparagus, cuttlefish, chicken egg, duck egg, white fungus, beef liver, grape, mandarin fish, oyster, milk, beef, cherry, blood clam and longan nuts | cayenne pepper, dill seed, fennel, fresh ginger, mustard seed, prickly ash, star anise, white or yellow mustard, wine, carp, celery, horse bean, jellyfish skin, Job's-tears, hyacinth bean, oregano, sweet basil, adzuki bean, bamboo shoot, soybean sprouts and rosin | carp, celery, horse bean, jellyfish skin, Job's-tears, prickly ash, hyacinth bean, oregano, sweet basil, adzuki bean, bamboo shoot, soybean sprouts, rosin, banana, bitter endive, black fungus, salt, spinach, strawberry, cucumber, leaf beet, mung bean, peppermint and purslane | asafoetida, buckwheat, castor bean, jellyfish, peach, radish, water chestnut, cardamon seed, cayenne pepper, coriander, grapefruit, jackfruit, malt, sweet basil, tea and tomato |

DIARRHEA (CONTINUED)

| | Liver offending the spleen | Spleen-dampness | Spleen-kidneys yang deficiency |
|---|---|---|---|
| SYMPTOMS | 3 Abdominal enlargement<br>3 Abdominal pain<br>1 Abdominal rumbling<br>1 Chronic diarrhea<br>8 Diarrhea occurs right after abdominal pain starts*<br>1 Fatigued spirits<br>2 Hungry with no appetite<br>1 Thirst with no desire for drink | 1 Chest discomfort without appetite<br>5 Diarrhea that comes and goes*<br>5 Diarrhea with discharge of watery stools*<br>1 Edema<br>1 Heavy sensations in head as if the head were covered with something<br>1 Heavy sensations in the body with discomfort<br>1 Jaundice<br>1 Love of hot drink<br>1 Nausea and vomiting<br>1 Stomach fullness and discomfort<br>1 Sweet, sticky taste in mouth<br>1 Too tired to talk or move | 1 Ascites<br>1 Being physically weak and too tired to talk<br>1 Cold hands and feet<br>1 Cold loins<br>2 Diarrhea before dawn*<br>2 Diarrhea right after pain occurs*<br>1 Diarrhea with sticky and muddy stools<br>1 Dysentery<br>1 Eating only a little<br>1 Edema<br>1 Edema that occurs all over the body<br>1 Fatigue<br>1 Fear of cold<br>1 Feeling comfortable after bowel movement<br>1 Four limbs weakness<br>1 Frequent urination with clear or white urine<br>1 Mentally fatigued<br>1 Sputum rumbling with panting |
| TREATMENT PRINCIPLE | to regulate energy and oppress the liver and to harmonize the stomach and support the spleen | to tone the energy and strengthen the spleen and to help dampness seep and stop diarrhea | to warm the spleen and the kidneys and to solidify the intestine and stop diarrhea |
| TREATMENT FORMULA | Tong-Xie-Yao-Fang | Shen-Ling-Bai-Zhu-San or Bu-Zhong-Yi-Qi-Tang | Si-Shen-Wan |
| FOOD CURES | brown sugar, kumquat, mandarin orange, apple cucumber, bog bean, gold carp, carrot, chestnut, corncob, horse bean, hyacinth bean, Job's-tears, Irish potato, royal jelly, string bean, whitefish and yam | gold carp, corncob, horse bean, Job's-tears, prickly ash, adzuki bean and bamboo shoot | air bladder of shark, chicken, cayenne pepper, fennel, nutmeg, black and white pepper, prickly ash, mutton, sword bean, white or yellow mustard, kidney, lobster, sardine, shrimp, sparrow, clove, dill seed, fennel, pistachio nut, sparrow egg, crab apple, raspberry and walnut |

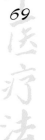

## CHEST PAIN

| *Cold* | *Dampness-sputum* | *Blood coagulations* | ## PAIN IN THE UPPER ABDOMEN<br>*Wind-cold* |
|---|---|---|---|

| | | | |
|---|---|---|---|
| 1 Abdominal pain | 3 Chest pain that affects the back of shoulders* | 1 Abdominal pain | 1 Absence of perspiration in hot weather |
| 1 Absence of perspiration in hot weather | 2 Chest pain that is dull and mild* | 2 Chest pain in a fixed region without shifting around* | 1 Clear discharge from nose |
| 1 Absence of thirst in mouth | 2 Cough | 2 Chest pain that is caused by injuries* | 1 Cough |
| 1 Abundant watering of eyes | 1 Discharge of sputum that can be coughed out easily | 2 Chest pain that worsens on pressure* | 1 Diarrhea |
| 1 Chest pain that affects the back of shoulders | 1 Discharge of white, watery sputum | 1 Coughing up blood | 1 Dislike of cold |
| 2 Chest pain often triggered or intensified by cold* | 1 Dizziness | 1 Pain in the upper abdomen | 1 Dizziness |
| 1 Clear and long streams of urine in large amounts | 1 Headache | 2 Palpitations with insecure feeling* | 1 Facial paralysis |
| 1 Cold chest, cold hands and feet, or cold bodily sensations | 1 Hiccups | 1 Partial suppression of lochia | 1 Fever or hot and cold sensations that come and go |
| 1 Constipation | 2 Panting | 2 Spasm* | 1 Headache |
| 1 Contraction of tendons and muscles | 1 Prolonged dizziness | 2 Stomachache* | 1 Headache with dizziness |
| 1 Diarrhea with watery stools containing undigested food or with sticky and muddy stool | 1 Sleep a lot | 2 Stroke* | 1 Hoarseness at the beginning of illness |
| | 1 Sleeplessness | 1 Swelling and congestion after eating | 1 Loss of voice |
| 1 Dizziness with objects appearing in front of eyes | 2 Vomiting | 1 Vomiting of blood | 1 Nausea |
| 1 Dry throat | 1 White, sliding sputum that can be cleared from throat easly | | 1 Nosebleed |
| 1 Hands and feet extremely cold | | | 1 Pain in the body shifting around with no fixed region |
| 1 Heavy and unclear voice in high pitched and rough tone | | | 2 Pain in the upper abdomen with chest congestion* |
| 1 Hiccups with cold hands and feet and mild taste in mouth, triggered by cold air | | | 1 Pain in the joints |
| 1 Love of hot drink | | | 1 Stuffed nose |
| 1 Pain in the throat | | | 1 Vomiting |
| 1 Pain shifting around with no fixed region | | | |
| 1 Pale complexion | | | |
| 1 Perspire heavily | | | |

| | | | |
|---|---|---|---|
| to warm the internal region and disperse cold | to transform sputum and remove dampness | to remove blood coagulations and promote blood circulation | to reduce the heat in the gallbladder |
| Zhi-Gan-Cao-Tang or Gua-Lou-Xic-Bai-Bai-Jiu-Tang | Gua-Lou-Xie-Bai-Ban-Xia-Tang | Shen-Tong-Zhu-Yu-Tang | Xiao-Chai-Hu-Tang |
| cayenne pepper, dill seed, fennel, fresh ginger, mustard seed, prickly ash, star anise, white or yellow mustard and wine | adzuki bean, ambergris, barley, common carp, cucumber, mung bean, seaweed, shepherd's purse, star fruit, bamboo shoot, crown daisy, date, fresh ginger, leaf or brown mustard, black and white pepper, white or yellow mustard seed, asparagus and pear | ambergris, brown sugar, chestnut, eggplant, peach, black soybean, sturgeon, sweet basil, crab, distillers' grains, papaya and saffron | peppermint (including oil), spearmint, sweet basil, cayenne pepper, fennel, fresh ginger, mustard seed, star anise and prickly ash leaf |

PAIN IN THE UPPER ABDOMEN (CONTINUED)

| | Superficial dampness-heat | Liver-fire upsurging | Energy congestion |
|---|---|---|---|
| **SYMPTOMS** | 1 Abdominal pain<br>1 Burning sensation and itch in the genitals or burning sensation in the anus<br>1 Congested chest<br>1 Diarrhea with forceful discharge of stools<br>1 Discharge of yellowish-red, turbid stools with bad smell<br>1 Edema<br>1 Excessive perspiration<br>1 Itch and pain in the vulva frequently<br>1 Jaundice<br>1 Low fever<br>2 Pain in the upper abdomen that worsens with massage*<br>1 Pain in the joints of the four limbs, with swelling and heaviness<br>1 Perspiration on hands and feet or the head<br>1 Reddish and scant urine<br>1 Retention of urine<br>2 Severe pain in the upper abdomen*<br>1 Short streams of reddish urine<br>1 Swollen body of the tongue<br>1 Thirst | 1 Acute dizziness<br>1 Bleeding from stomach<br>1 Deafness<br>1 Dim vision<br>1 Dizziness<br>1 Dry sensations in the mouth<br>1 Getting angry easily<br>1 Headache on both sides of the head and in the corners of the eyes<br>1 Headache that is severe<br>1 Hiccups<br>1 Nosebleed<br>1 Pain (falling) in the lower abdomen with desire for massage<br>1 Pain in the chest and the ribs<br>1 Pain in the upper abdomen triggered by anger or emotional upset*<br>1 Pink eyes with swelling<br>1 Red eyes<br>1 Ringing in ears<br>1 Severe pain in the upper abdomen*<br>1 Sleeplessness or sleep a lot<br>Vomiting of blood | 2 Abdominal pain<br>1 Chest and ribs discomfort<br>2 Chest pain<br>3 Constipation with a desire to empty the bowel*<br>1 Pain in inner part of stomach with pricking sensations and swelling<br>3 Pain in the upper abdomen that moves around*<br>1 Poor appetite<br>1 Retention of urine<br>1 Ringing in ears and deafness<br>2 Stomachache<br>1 Subjective sensation of lump in the throat<br>1 Swallowing difficulty<br>1 Swelling and congestion after eating |
| **TREATMENT PRINCIPLE** | to clear dampness-heat in the liver and the gallbladder | to calm the liver and sedate fire in the liver | to relax the liver and regulate the energy of the liver and to strengthen the spleen and nourish the blood |
| **TREATMENT FORMULA** | Yin-Chen-Hao-Tang or Long-Dan-Xie-Gan-Tang | Qing-Gan-Tang | Xiao-Yao-San or Chai-Hu-Shu-Gan-San |
| **FOOD CURES** | carp, celery, horse bean, jellyfish skin, Job's-tears, prickly ash, hyacinth bean, oregano, sweet basil, adzuki bean, bamboo shoot, soybean sprouts, rosin, banana, bitter endive, black fungus, salt, spinach, strawberry, cucumber, leaf beet, mung bean, peppermint and purslane | spinach, chestnut, shepherd's purse, rye, black fungus, vinegar, abalone, asparagus, chicken egg, white fungus, pork and royal jelly | beef, cherry, bird's nest, butterfish, chicken, coconut meat, date, tofu, mustard seed, sweet rice, goose meat, mutton, jackfruit, squash, sweet potato, red and black date, rice, rock sugar, caraway seed, spearmint, common button mushroom, oregano, red bean, ambergris, dill seed, garlic, sweet basil, saffron, sweet potato, red and black date, Chinese chive, brown sugar, mandarin orange and garlic |

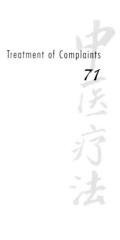

| *Blood coagulations* | *Dampness* | *Yin deficiency* | *Liver energy congestion* |
|---|---|---|---|
| 1 Abdominal pain | 1 Abdominal pain with abdominal rumbling | 1 Bleeding from gums | 2 Abdominal obstruction |
| 1 Bleeding from gums | 1 Diarrhea | 1 Constipation | 2 Abdominal pain |
| 1 Chest pain | 1 Diminished urination | 1 Dizziness | 1 Belching |
| 1 Coughing out blood | 1 Discharge of hard stool followed by sticky, turbid stool | 1 Dry and scant stool | 1 Convulsions |
| 1 Headache | 1 Dry sensations in the mouth | 1 Nausea |
| 1 Jaundice | 1 Dizziness | 1 Dry throat | 1 Numbness |
| 1 Lumbago | 1 Headache as if the head were being wrapped up | 2 Fatigue | 5 Stomachache that affects the upper abdomen and gets slightly better with massage* |
| 2 Pain in the upper abdomen as if being pricked by a sharp needle* | 1 Headache in the afternoon |
| 1 Heavy sensation in body with intestinal rumbling and watery stools | 1 Jaundice | 6 Stomachache that worsens with anger * |
| 2 Pain in the upper abdomen in a fixed region without moving around* | 1 Light fever in the afternoon |
| 1 Heavy sensations and stagnation of lower limbs | 1 Night sweats | 3 Subjective sensations of objects in the throat |
| 1 Pain in the loins as if being pierced with an awl | 1 Nosebleed | 1 Vomiting of blood |
| 1 Heavy sensations in head as if head were wrapped up | 1 Pain in the throat, also red and swollen |
| 1 Pain in the ribs | 1 Heavy sensations in the body | 1 Palms of hands and soles of feet are both hot |
| 1 Palpitations with insecure feeling | 1 Illness starts mostly from lower regions of the body |
| 1 Partial suppression of lochia | 1 Palpitations with insecure feeling |
| 1 Spasm | 1 Itch | 1 Severe pain in the body that attacks all of a sudden |
| 1 Stomachache | 1 Love of hot drink |
| 1 Stroke | 1 Love of sleep and heavy sensations in the body | 1 Short streams of reddish urine |
| 1 Swelling and congestion after eating | 1 Sleeplessness |
| 1 Pain always in same joints with heavy sensations in the body | 1 Swallowing difficulty |
| 1 Vomiting of blood | 1 Toothache |
| 1 Pain in the loins as if sitting in water with heaviness in body | 1 Underweight |
| 1 Quick bowel movements |
| 1 Stomach and abdomen swollen and full |
| 1 Toes extremely itchy |
| 1 White, small granular pimples in the skin |
| to transform blood coagulations and regulate energy | to strengthen the spleen, dry dampness and regulate the liver | to water the yin and nourish the blood and to soften up the liver | to disperse energy congestion, regulate energy conditions and harmonize the stomach and relieve pain |
| Ge-Xia-Zhu-Yu-Tang | Bu-Huan-Jin-Zheng-Qi-San or Shen-Ling-Bai-Zhu-San | Yi-Guan-Jian or Liu-Wei-Di-Huang-Wan | Si-Ni-San |
| ambergris, brown sugar, chestnut, eggplant, peach, black soybean, sturgeon, sweet basil, crab, distillers' grains, papaya and saffron | carp, celery, horse bean, jellyfish skin, Job's-tears, prickly ash, hyacinth bean, oregano, sweet basil, adzuki bean, bamboo shoot, soybean sprouts and rosin | bird's nest, cheese, kidney bean, abalone, asparagus, chicken egg, cuttlefish, duck, duck egg, white fungus, oyster, pork and royal jelly | brown sugar, garlic, turmeric, kumquat, beef, cherry, bird's nest, butterfish, chicken, coconut meat, date, tofu, mustard seed, sweet rice, goose meat, mutton, jackfruit, squash, sweet potato, red and black date, rice, rock sugar, caraway seed, spearmint, common button mushroom, oregano, red bean, ambergris, dill seed, garlic, sweet basil and saffron |

STOMACHACHE (CONTINUED)

| | Blood coagulations | Indigestion | Deficiency and cold |
|---|---|---|---|
| **SYMPTOMS** | 1 Abdominal pain | 1 Abdominal pain | 2 Abdominal pain on the right and left sides of navel (umbilicus) |
| | 1 Bleeding from gums | 1 Belching of bad breath after meals | 2 Cold hands and feet |
| | 1 Chest pain | 1 Chest and diaphragm congestion and discomfort | 1 Cold sensations in lower abdomen-genitals region |
| | 1 Coughing out blood | 1 Diarrhea and constipation | 2 Diarrhea containing undigested food |
| | 1 Headache | 1 Diarrhea in children | 1 Fatigue |
| | 1 Jaundice | 1 Hot sensations in the middle of palms | 2 Fear of cold |
| | 1 Lumbago | 1 Indigestion | 1 Fingerprint appears light red |
| | 1 Pain (acute) around umbilicus resisting massage and hard spots felt by hands | 1 Lack of appetite | 3 Love of hot drink* |
| | 1 Pain in region between navel and pubic hair with feeling of hardness | 1 Love of hot drink, but drink only a little | 1 Love of sighing |
| | 1 Pain in the upper abdomen as if being pricked by a needle | 1 Malaria | 1 Night sweats |
| | 2 Pain in the upper abdomen that worsens after eating* | 1 Nausea | 1 Palpitations |
| | 1 Pain in the loins as if being pierced with an awl | 1 Pain in inner part of stomach with swelling and feeling of fullness | 1 Run-down feeling |
| | 1 Pain in the ribs | 2 Stomachache that worsens with massage* | 1 Shortness of breath |
| | 1 Palpitations with insecure feeling | 3 Stomachache that occurs all of a sudden with dislike of foods* | 1 Vomiting slowly with a feeble sound |
| | 1 Spasm | 1 Stools with an extremely bad smell | 1 White complexion |
| | 1 Stomachache | 1 Vomiting | |
| | 1 Stroke | 1 Vomiting of clear water | |
| | 1 Swelling and congestion after eating | | |
| | 1 Vomiting of blood | | |
| **TREATMENT PRINCIPLE** | to activate the blood and transform coagulations and to harmonize the stomach and relieve pain | to promote digestion and harmonize the stomach | to strengthen the spleen and the stomach and to warm the internal region and disperse cold |
| **TREATMENT FORMULA** | Shi-Xiao-San | Bao-He-Wan | Li-Zhong-Tang or Xiang-Sha-Liu-Jun-Zi-Tang |
| **FOOD CURES** | ambergris, brown sugar, chestnut, eggplant, peach, black soybean, sturgeon, sweet basil, crab, distillers' grains, papaya and saffron | asafoetida, buckwheat, castor bean, jellyfish, peach, radish, water chestnut, cardamon seed, cayenne pepper, coriander, grapefruit, jackfruit, malt, sweet basil, tea and tomato | cayenne pepper, dill seed, fennel, fresh ginger, mustard seed, prickly ash, star anise, white or yellow mustard, wine, grape, longan nuts, maltose, mandarin fish, Irish potato, sweet rice, apple cucumber, bog bean, gold carp, carrot, chestnut, ham, horse bean, hyacinth bean, Job's-tears, royal jelly, string bean, whitefish, yam, red and black date, mutton, squash and rock sugar |

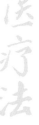

## ABDOMINAL PAIN

| *Yin deficiency* | *Cold spleen* | *Deficiency and cold* | *Excess and hot* |
|---|---|---|---|
| 1 Bleeding from gums | 3 Abdominal pain that attacks all of a sudden* | 2 Abdominal pain that drags on and on* | 6 Abdominal pain that gets worse when hot and better when cold* |
| 1 Burning pain in the stomach | 1 Abdominal pain that drags on and on | 2 Abdominal pain that gets worse when cold and better when warm* | 5 Abdominal pain that gets worse with massage* |
| 1 Constipation | 4 Abdominal pain that gets worse when cold and better when warm* | 3 Abdominal pain that gets worse when hungry* | 5 Abdominal pain with burning sensations* |
| 1 Dry and scant stools | 1 Cold hands and feet | 1 Cold hands and feet | 1 Constant desire for drink, but drink only a little |
| 1 Dry sensations in the mouth | 1 Dark-yellow ski | 1 Cold sensations in lower abdomen-genitals region | 1 Hiccups that make loud and forceful sound |
| 1 Dry throat | 1 Diarrhea with a feeling of coolness | 1 Diarrhea containing undigested food | 1 Pain in the throat, also red and swollen |
| 1 Fatigue | 1 Discharge of watery, thin stools | 1 Fatigue | 1 Vomiting that comes on rather forcefully, with a strong sound |
| 1 Headache in the afternoon | 1 Edema | 1 Fear of cold | |
| 1 Light fever in the afternoon | 1 Indigestion | 1 Love of hot drink | |
| 1 Night sweats | 1 Lips lightly colored | 1 Love of sighing | |
| 1 Nosebleed | 1 Pleasant taste in the mouth | 1 Night sweats | |
| 1 Pain in the throat | 1 Poor appetite | 1 Palpitations | |
| 1 Pain in the throat, also red and swollen | 1 Prolonged diarrhea | 1 Run-down feeling | |
| 1 Palms of hands and soles of feet are both hot | 1 Runny, thin saliva | 1 Shortness of breath | |
| 1 Short streams of reddish urine | 1 Vomiting | 1 Vomiting slowly with a feeble sound | |
| 1 Sleeplessness | | 1 White complexion | |
| 2 Stomachache that worsens when the stomach is empty* | | | |
| 1 Toothache | | | |
| 1 Underweight | | | |
| to tone the yin and strengthen the stomach and to clear the heat in the stomach | to disperse cold and warm the spleen | to strengthen energy and warm the internal region | to sedate heat and regulate energy |
| Mai-Men-Dong-Tang | Wen-Pi-Tang | Li-Zhong-Tang | Hou-Pu-San-Wu-Tang |
| bird's nest, cheese, kidney bean, abalone, asparagus, chicken egg, cuttlefish, duck, duck egg, white fungus, oyster, pork and royal jelly | cinnamon, clove oil, dill seed, garlic, pistachio nut, cayenne pepper, fennel, fresh ginger, mustard seed, prickly ash, star anise, white or yellow mustard and wine | cayenne pepper, dill seed, fennel, fresh ginger, mustard seed, prickly ash, star anise, white or yellow mustard, wine, grape, longan nuts, maltose, mandarin fish, Irish potato, sweet rice, apple cucumber, bog bean, gold carp, carrot, chestnut, ham, horse bean, hyacinth bean, Job's-tears, royal jelly, string bean, whitefish, yam, red and black date, mutton, squash and rock sugar | banana, bitter endive, black fungus, salt, spinach, strawberry, bamboo shoot, cucumber, Job's-tears, laver, leaf beet, mung bean, peppermint and purslane |

ABDOMINAL PAIN (CONTINUED)

| | Indigestion | Energy congestion | Blood coagulations |
|---|---|---|---|
| SYMPTOMS | 4 Abdominal pain that gets worse with massage and better after bowel movement*<br>1 Belching of bad breath after meals<br>1 Diarrhea and constipation<br>1 Dislike of foods<br>1 Hot sensations in the middle of palms<br>1 Indigestion<br>1 Lack of appetite<br>1 Love of hot drink, but drink only a little<br>1 Nausea<br>1 Pain in inner part of stomach with swelling and feeling of fullness<br>4 Stomachache*<br>1 Stools with an extremely bad smell<br>1 Vomiting<br>1 Vomiting of clear water | 2 Abdominal pain that reduces after flatulence*<br>2 Belching or hiccups*<br>1 Chest and ribs discomfort<br>1 Chest pain<br>2 Constipation with a desire to empty the bowel*<br>1 Pain in inner part of stomach with prickling sensation and swelling<br>2 Pain in the upper abdomen*<br>1 Retention of urine<br>1 Ringing in ears and deafness<br>2 Stomachache*<br>1 Subjective sensation of lump in the throat<br>1 Swallowing difficulty<br>1 Swelling and congestion after eating | 2 Abdominal pain as if being pricked by a needle*<br>1 Abdominal pain in a fixed region without moving around<br>1 Bleeding from gums<br>1 Chest pain<br>1 Coughing out blood<br>1 Headache<br>1 Jaundice<br>1 Lumbago<br>1 Pain (acute) around umbilicus resisting massage & hard spots felt by hands<br>1 Pain in region between navel & pubic hair with feeling of hardness<br>1 Pain in the upper abdomen<br>1 Pain in the loins as if being pierced with an awl<br>1 Pain in the ribs<br>1 Palpitations with insecure feeling<br>1 Spasm<br>1 Stomachache<br>1 Stroke<br>1 Swelling and congestion after eating<br>1 Vomiting of blood |
| TREATMENT PRINCIPLE | to promote digestion and harmonize the stomach | to regulate energy and promote energy circulation | to activate the blood and transform coagulations and to promote energy circulation and relieve pain |
| TREATMENT FORMULA | Bao-He-Wan or Zhi-Shi-Dao-Zhi-Wan | Mu-Xiang-Shun-Qi-San | Shao-Fu-Zhu-Yu-Tang |
| FOOD CURES | asafoetida, buckwheat, castor bean, jellyfish, peach, radish, water chestnut, cardamon seed, cayenne pepper, coriander, grapefruit, jackfruit, malt, sweet basil, tea and tomato | beef, cherry, bird's nest, butterfish, chicken, coconut meat, date, tofu, mustard seed, sweet rice, goose meat, mutton, jackfruit, squash, sweet potato, red and black date, rice, rock sugar, caraway seed, spearmint, common button mushroom, oregano, red bean, ambergris, dill seed, garlic, sweet basil and saffron | ambergris, brown sugar, chestnut, eggplant, peach, black soybean, sturgeon, sweet basil, crab, distillers' grains, papaya and saffron |

# LUMBAGO

| Wind-dampness | Cold-dampness | Superficial dampness-heat | Blood coagulations |
|---|---|---|---|
| 1  Chronic backache<br>1  Diarrhea<br>1  Eczema<br>1  Edema<br>1  Fever that becomes more severe in the afternoon<br>1  German measles<br>1  Headache with heavy sensations in the head<br>1  Itchy sores<br>1  Light swelling<br>4  Lower-back pain affecting the lower limbs*<br>4  Lower-back pain that gets worse on rainy days*<br>1  Pain in all the joints<br>1  Pain shifting around with no fixed region<br>1  Scant urine | 1  Absence of perspiration in hot weather<br>5  Cold lower-back pain*<br>1  Cold sensations in lower abdomen-genitals region<br>1  Cough<br>1  Coughing out sputum with a low sound<br>2  Diarrhea<br>1  Discharge of sputum that can be coughed out easily<br>2  Dysentery<br>1  Edema in the four limbs<br>1  Headache<br>1  Movement difficulty particularly in turning around<br>1  Pain in the body or in the joints<br>1  Scant and clear urine<br>1  Stomachache | 1  Abdominal pain<br>1  Burning sensation & itch in the genitals or burning sensation in the anus<br>1  Congested chest<br>1  Diarrhea with forceful discharge of stools*<br>1  Discharge of yellowish-red, turbid stools with bad smell<br>1  Edema<br>1  Excessive perspiration<br>1  Feeling miserable<br>1  Jaundice<br>1  Low fever<br>1  Lower-back pain with a weak back or burning sensations*<br>1  Pain in the joints of four limbs, with swelling and heaviness<br>1  Paralysis<br>1  Perspiration on hands and feet or the head<br>1  Reddish and scant urine<br>1  Retention of urine<br>1  Short streams of reddish urine<br>1  Swollen body of the tongue<br>1  Thirst<br>1  Yellowish color of body | 1  Abdominal pain<br>1  Bleeding from gums<br>1  Chest pain<br>1  Coughing out blood<br>1  Headache<br>1  Jaundice<br>1  Lower-back pain as sharp as being cut by a knife*<br>1  Lower-back pain that worsens with massage*<br>1  Lower-back pain that occurs in a fixed region without moving around*<br>1  Pain (acute) around umbilicus resisting massage and hard spots felt by hands<br>1  Pain in region between navel & pubic hair with feeling of hardness<br>1  Pain in the upper abdomen<br>1  Pain in the loins as if being pierced with an awl<br>1  Pain in the ribs<br>1  Palpitations with insecure feeling<br>1  Partial suppression of lochia<br>1  Spasm<br>1  Stomachache<br>1  Stroke<br>1  Swelling & congestion after eating<br>1  Vomiting of blood |
| to expel wind and disperse cold and to remove dampness and relieve pain | to expel cold and remove dampness and to warm the internal region | to clear heat and remove dampness and to promote energy circulation | to activate the blood and transform coagulations and to regulate energy and relieve pain |
| Du-Huo-Ji-Sheng-Tang | Shen-Zhuo-Tang | San-Miao-Wan | Shen-Tong-Zhu-Yu-Tang |
| peppermint, spearmint, sweet basil, celery, coconut meat, green onion, jellyfish skin, prickly ash, rice, adzuki bean, rosin and tangerine | cayenne pepper, dill seed, fennel, fresh ginger, mustard seed, prickly ash, star anise, white or yellow mustard, wine, carp, celery, horse bean, jellyfish skin, Job's-tears, hyacinth bean, oregano, sweet basil, adzuki bean, bamboo shoot, soybean sprouts and rosin | carp, celery, horse bean, jellyfish skin, Job's-tears, prickly ash, hyacinth bean, oregano, sweet basil, adzuki bean, bamboo shoot, soybean sprouts, rosin, banana, bitter endive, black fungus, salt, spinach, strawberry, cucumber, leaf beet, mung bean, peppermint and purslane | ambergris, brown sugar, chestnut, eggplant, peach, black soybean, sturgeon, sweet basil, crab, distillers' grains, papaya and saffron |

| | LUMBAGO (CONTINUED) | | JAUNDICE |
|---|---|---|---|
| | *Kidneys yin deficiency* | *Kidneys yang deficiency* | *Superficial damp-ness-heat with more heat than dampness* |
| SYMPTOMS | 1 Cold hands and feet<br>1 Cough with sputum containing blood or coughing out fresh blood<br>1 Dizziness<br>1 Dry sensations in the mouth<br>1 Dry throat<br>1 Fatigue<br>1 Feeling miserable and hurried, with fever<br>1 Hot sensations in body<br>1 Hot sensations in the middle of palms or soles of feet<br>1 Lower-back pain that drags on and on*<br>1 Lower-back pain that worsens with fatigue*<br>1 Lower-back pain with weakness of the back*<br>1 Night sweats<br>1 Pain in the heels<br>1 Retention of urine<br>1 Ringing in ears<br>1 Seminal emission with dreams<br>1 Sleeplessness<br>1 Spots in front of the eyes<br>1 Thirst | 1 Cold feet, cold loins & legs, cold sensations in the genitals, or cold sensations in the muscles<br>1 Cough and panting<br>1 Diarrhea before dawn<br>1 Diarrhea with sticky, muddy stools<br>1 Discharge of watery, thin stools<br>1 Dizziness<br>1 Edema<br>1 Fatigue<br>1 Frequent urination at night<br>1 Impotence<br>1 Infertility<br>1 Lack of appetite<br>1 Panting<br>1 Perspiration on the forehead<br>1 Retention of urine<br>1 Ringing in ears<br>1 Seminal emission<br>1 Shaky teeth<br>1 Shortness of breath<br>1 Swelling of body<br>1 Wheezing | 1 Abdominal pain<br>1 Burning sensation and itch in the genitals or burning sensation in the anus<br>1 Congested chest<br>1 Diarrhea with forceful discharge of stools<br>2 Discharge of dry stools*<br>1 Edema<br>1 Excessive perspiration<br>1 Feeling miserable<br>2 Hot sensations in the body*<br>1 Low fever<br>1 Pain in the joints of four limbs, with swelling and heaviness<br>1 Perspiration on hands and feet or the head<br>2 Reddish and scant urine*<br>1 Retention of urine<br>1 Short streams of reddish urine<br>2 Thirst * |
| TREATMENT PRINCIPLE | to tone the yin and clear fire and to nourish the blood | to warm the kidney yang | to clear heat, sedate fire, remove dampness and relax the liver |
| TREATMENT FORMULA | Zuo-Gui-Yin | You-Gui-Yin | Yin-Chen-Hao-Tang |
| FOOD CURES | abalone, asparagus, chicken egg, cuttlefish, duck, duck egg, white fungus, oyster, pork, royal jelly, chestnut, chicken liver and pork kidneys | kidney, lobster, sardine, shrimp, sparrow, clove, dill seed, fennel, pistachio nut, sparrow egg, crab apple, raspberry and walnut | carp, celery, horse bean, jellyfish skin, Job's-tears, prickly ash, hyacinth bean, oregano, sweet basil, adzuki bean, bamboo shoot, soybean sprouts, rosin, banana, bitter endive, black fungus, salt, spinach, strawberry, cucumber, leaf beet, mung bean, peppermint and purslane |

EDEMA

| Superficial damp-ness-heat with more dampness than heat | Hot | Cold-dampness | Wind-water syndrome |
|---|---|---|---|
| 1 Abdominal pain | 2 Acute jaundice* | 1 Absence of perspiration in hot weather | 3 Cold or hot symptoms |
| 2 Burning sensation and itch in the genitals or burning sensation in the anus* | 2 Both the body and eyes are fresh yellowish color* | 5 Body and eyes in dark-yellowish color* | 3 Cough |
| 2 Diarrhea with forceful discharge of stools* | 1 Burning sensation and itch in the genitals | 1 Clear urine | 4 Discharge of scant urine* |
| 2 Discharge of watery stools* | 1 Constipation | 1 Cough | 6 Puffiness of eyelids or face, gradually extending towards the four limbs and the whole body at relatively high rate* |
| 1 Edema | 2 Discharge of blood from the anus* | 1 Coughing out sputum with a low sound | 4 Soreness in the joints with heavy sensations* |
| 1 Excessive perspiration | 1 Dry lips or dry teeth | 2 Diarrhea | |
| 2 Heavy sensations in the body* | 2 High fever* | 1 Discharge of sputum that can be coughed out easily | |
| 1 Itch and pain in the vulva frequently | 1 Limbs are warm | 1 Dysentery | |
| 1 Low fever | 1 Love of cold drink | 1 Edema in the four limbs | |
| 2 No thirst* | 2 Nosebleed* | 1 Headache | |
| 1 Pain in the joints of the four limbs, with swelling and heaviness | 1 Pain in inner part of stomach becoming acute after meals and fond of cold | 1 Movement difficulty | |
| 1 Perspiration on hands and feet or the head | 1 Psychological depression | 1 Pain in the body | |
| 2 Poor appetite* | 1 Reddish complexion, eyes, or urine | 1 Pain in the joints | |
| 1 Retention of urine | 1 Stools with an extremely bad smell | 1 Soft stools | |
| | 1 Thirst with an incessant desire to drink | 1 Stomachache | |
| | 1 Urine with an extremely bad smell | | |
| to remove dampness and clear heat | to clear toxic heat, cool the blood and rescue the yin | to warm the yang and expel dampness and to relax the liver and transform blood coagulations | to expel wind and promote water flow |
| Yin-Chen-Wu-Ling-San | Qian-Jin-Xi-Jiao-San or Ju-Fang-Zhi-Bao-Dan | Yin-Chen-Zhu-Fu-Tang | Yue-Bi-Jia-Zhu-Tang |
| carp, celery, horse bean, jellyfish skin, Job's-tears, prickly ash, hyacinth bean, oregano, sweet basil, adzuki bean, bamboo shoot, soybean sprouts, rosin, banana, bitter endive, black fungus, salt, spinach, strawberry, cucumber, leaf beet, mung bean, peppermint and purslane | banana, bitter endive, black fungus, salt, spinach, strawberry, bamboo shoot, cucumber, Job's-tears, laver, leaf beet, mung bean, peppermint and purslane | cayenne pepper, dill seed, fennel, fresh ginger, mustard seed, prickly ash, star anise, white or yellow mustard, wine, carp, celery, horse bean, jellyfish skin, Job's-tears, hyacinth bean, oregano, sweet basil, adzuki bean, bamboo shoot, soybean sprouts and rosin | carp, celery, horse bean, jellyfish skin, Job's-tears, prickly ash, hyacinth bean, oregano, sweet basil, bamboo shoot, soybean sprouts, rosin, adzuki bean, ambergris, barley, common carp, cucumber, mung bean, seaweed, shepherd's purse, star fruit, peppermint, spearmint, coconut meat and green onion |

| | Stoppage of internal water | Flooding of water-dampness | Spleen yang deficiency |
|---|---|---|---|
| SYMPTOMS | 1 Chest congestion<br>1 Cold sensations in the back<br>1 Deep and wiry pulse<br>1 Dizziness<br>1 Edema in the face<br>5 Edema that fails to recover after being depressed by finger pressure*<br>1 Intestinal rumbling<br>1 Pain in the upper abdomen<br>1 Pain induced by cough or spitting<br>6 Severe edema in the limbs*<br>1 Vomiting of bubbles<br>1 Water noise in the stomach<br>1 White and greasy coating on tongue<br>1 Wiry pulse | 1 Ascites<br>2 Diminished urination<br>1 Chest congestion<br>2 Difficult bowel movements<br>2 Heavy sensations in the body<br>9 Edema all over the body*<br>1 Light edema in the eye socket as if just getting up from bed<br>2 Thirst | 2 Abdominal pain<br>1 Cold in the forehead that does not warm up<br>2 Diarrhea<br>2 Dysentery<br>5 Edema that appears most severe in the lower half of the body*<br>5 Edema that fails to return after being depressed by finger pressure*<br>2 Stomachache |
| TREATMENT PRINCIPLE | to increase energy and promote water flow | to remove water drastically | to warm and mobilize the spleen yang and to transform dampness and promote water flow |
| TREATMENT FORMULA | Wu-Ling-San or Wu-Pi-Yin | Shu-Zao-Yin-Zi | Shi-Pi-Yin |
| FOOD CURES | adzuki bean, ambergris, barley, bamboo shoot, common carp, cucumber, mung bean, seaweed, shepherd's purse and star fruit | carp, celery, horse bean, jellyfish skin, Job's-tears, prickly ash, hyacinth bean, oregano, sweet basil, bamboo shoot, soybean sprouts, rosin, adzuki bean, ambergris, barley, common carp, cucumber, mung bean, seaweed, shepherd's purse and star fruit | air bladder of shark, chicken, cayenne pepper, fennel, nutmeg, black and white pepper, prickly ash, mutton, sword bean and white or yellow mustard |

## DIMINISHED URINATION

| Kidneys yang deficiency | Hot lungs | Heart-fire | Superficial dampness-heat |
|---|---|---|---|
| 1 Cold feet, cold loins and legs, cold sensations in the genitals, or cold sensations in the muscles | 1 Acute panting in high-pitched sound with rapid expiration | 1 Bleeding from gums | 1 Burning sensation & itch in the genitals or burning sensation in the anus |
| 1 Cough and panting | 1 Bitter taste in the mouth | 1 Cold hands and feet | 2 Burning sensation on urination* |
| 1 Diarrhea before dawn | 1 Coughing out and vomiting of pus and blood with a fishy smell | 3 Difficult urination with reddish or very yellowish urine* | 1 Diarrhea with forceful discharge of stools |
| 1 Diarrhea with sticky, muddy stools | 1 Coughing out yellow, sticky sputum | 2 Discharge of blood from the mouth | 1 Discharge of yellowish-red, turbid stools with bad smell |
| 1 Discharge of watery, thin stools | 1 Discharge of dry stools | 1 Dribbling after urination | 1 Edema |
| 1 Dizziness | 1 Discharge of yellow, sticky sputum in lumps | 1 Feeling miserable | 1 Excessive perspiration |
| 3 Edema that appears most severe in the lower half of the body* | 2 Dripping of urine with difficult urination* | 1 Hot sensations in the middle of palms | 1 Feeling miserable |
| 2 Edema that fails to return after being depressed by finger pressure* | 1 Dry sensations in the mouth | 2 Mouth canker | 1 Frequent itch and pain in the vulva |
| 1 Fatigue | 1 Flickering of nostrils | 1 Not alert | 1 Jaundice |
| 1 Frequent urination at night | 1 Hot sensations in the body | 1 Pain on urination | 1 Low fever |
| 1 Lack of appetite | 1 Light but periodic fever not unlike the tide | 2 Palpitations | 1 Pain in the joints of the four limbs, with swelling & heaviness |
| 1 Pain in the loins (lumbago) | 1 Nosebleed | 1 Pulpy and decayed tongue and mouth | 1 Paralysis |
| 1 Palpitations | 1 Pain in the chest | 1 Seminal emission | 1 Perspiration on hands and feet or the head |
| 1 Panting | 1 Pain in the throat | 2 Sleeplessness | 1 Reddish and scant urine |
| 1 Perspiration on the forehead | 1 Pain in throat with dry sensations & exhaling hot air from nose | 1 Thirst | 1 Retention of urine |
| 1 Ringing in ears | 1 Paralysis | | 1 Scant, turbid urine |
| 1 Wheezing | 1 Presence of sputum that can't be coughed out easily | | 1 Short streams of reddish urine |
| | 1 Psychological depression | | 1 Swollen body of the tongue |
| | 1 Throat swelling and red | | 1 Thirst |
| | 1 Urgent panting | | |
| to warm the kidneys yang and promote water flow | to clear the heat in the lungs | to clear the heat in the heart and sedate the fire | to clear the heat and remove the dampness and to promote urination |
| Shen-Qi-Wan or Zhen-Wu-Tang | Huang-Qin-Qing-Fei-Yin | Dao-Chi-San | Jia-Wei-Si-Ling-San |
| kidney, lobster, sardine, shrimp, sparrow, clove, dill seed, fennel, pistachio nut, sparrow egg, crab apple, raspberry and walnut | apple, apple cucumber, apricot, white fungus, ham, jackfruit, lemon, maltose, mandarin orange, mulberry, olive, peach, pear, sweet potato, red and black date, tomato, white sugar, mung bean and eggplant | asparagus, pear peel, banana, bitter endive, black fungus, salt, spinach, strawberry, bamboo shoot, cucumber, Job's-tears, liver, leaf beet, mung bean, peppermint, purslane, lily flower, salt and cattail | carp, celery, horse bean, jellyfish skin, Job's-tears, prickly ash, hyacinth bean, oregano, sweet basil, adzuki bean, bamboo shoot, soybean sprouts, rosin, banana, bitter endive, black fungus, salt, spinach, strawberry, cucumber, leaf beet, mung bean, peppermint and purslane |

DIMINISHED URINATION (CONTINUED)

| | Energy deficiency | Excessive heat in the bladder | Blood coagulations |
|---|---|---|---|
| SYMPTOMS | 1 Abdominal pain<br>1 Constipation with discharge of soft stools<br>1 Discharge of sticky, turbid stools or diarrhea<br>1 Dizziness<br>1 Fatigued following bowel movement<br>1 Headache (severe) that occurs with fatigue after labor<br>1 Headache at intervals, headache in the morning, or prolonged headache<br>1 Lying down with an inability to sit up, which will cause dizziness<br>1 Misty vision<br>1 Numbness<br>1 Palpitations with insecure feeling<br>1 Perspiration on hands and feet<br>1 Prolonged headache<br>1 Ringing in ears that causes deafness<br>1 Shaking of hands<br>1 Shortness of breath<br>1 Swallowing difficulty<br>1 Talking in weak voice<br>1 Tips of four limbs slightly cold<br>1 Under-weight with dry skin | 3 Discharge of urine containing pus and blood<br>3 Hot pain inside the genitals on passing urine<br>2 Muddy, unclear urine<br>3 Obstructed and diminished urination in short streams<br>3 Pain in lower abdomen with swollen feeling that is hard and full<br>3 Urinary gravel<br>3 Yellowish-red urine | 1 Abdominal pain<br>1 Bleeding from gums<br>1 Chest pain<br>1 Coughing out blood<br>1 Headache<br>1 Jaundice<br>1 Lumbago<br>1 Pain (acute) around umbilicus resiting massage & hard spots felt by hands<br>1 Pain in region between navel & pubic hair with feeling of hardness<br>1 Pain in the upper abdomen<br>2 Pain in the loins as if being pierced with an awl<br>1 Pain in the ribs<br>1 Palpitations with insecure feeling<br>1 Partial suppression of lochia<br>1 Spasm<br>1 Stomachache<br>1 Stroke<br>1 Swelling & congestion after eating<br>1 Vomiting of blood |
| TREATMENT PRINCIPLE | to strengthen energy and elevate the yang | to remove the heat from the bladder and promote urination | to break up the blood and remove coagulations |
| TREATMENT FORMULA | Bu-Zhong-Yi-Qi-Tang | Tong-Guan-Wan | Dai-Di-Dang-Wan |
| FOOD CURES | grape, longan nuts, maltose, mandarin fish, Irish potato, sweet rice, apple cucumber, bog bean, gold carp, carrot, chestnut, ham, horse bean, hyacinth bean, Job's-tears, royal jelly, string bean, whitefish, yam, red and black date, mutton, squash and rock sugar | flour, duck, kelp, water spinach, banana, bitter endive, black fungus, salt, spinach, strawberry, bamboo shoot, cucumber, Job's-tears, leaf beet, mung bean, peppermint and purslane | ambergris, brown sugar, chestnut, eggplant, peach, black soybean, sturgeon, sweet basil, crab, distillers' grains, papaya and saffron |

## INCONTINENCE OF URINATION

| *Kidneys yang deficiency* | *Spleen-lungs energy deficiency* | *Kidneys energy deficiency* | *Looseness of kidneys energy* |
|---|---|---|---|
| 1 Chronic diarrhea | 1 Abdominal swelling | 2 Deafness | 5 Bed-wetting* |
| 1 Cold feet, cold loins and legs, cold sensations in the genitals, or cold sensations in the muscles | 1 Coughing out and spitting of sputum and saliva | 1 Dizziness | 1 Clear and long streams of urine |
| 1 Cough and panting | 1 Decreased appetite | 4 Dribbling after urination* | 1 Dizziness |
| 1 Diarrhea before dawn | 1 Diarrhea with sticky, muddy stools | 1 Fatigue | 1 Dribbling of urine |
| 1 Diarrhea with sticky, muddy stools | 1 Discharge of copious, clear, watery sputum | 4 Frequent urination with scant streams* | 1 Fatigue |
| 1 Discharge of water, thin stools | 1 Eating only a little with indigestion | 1 Headache | 1 Frequent urination particularly at night |
| 1 Dizziness | 1 Fatigue of the four limbs | 2 Impotence | 1 Incontinence of urination |
| 1 Edema | 1 Fatigue with lack of power | 2 Lumbago | 1 Pain and softness in the loins and the knees |
| 1 Fatigue | 4 Frequent desire to pass urine* | 1 Prolonged dizziness | 1 Premature ejaculation |
| 1 Frequent urination at night | 1 Prolonged cough | 1 Ringing in ears | 1 Ringing in ears |
| 1 Hands and feet not warm | 1 Rapid panting | 1 Seminal emission | 2 Seminal emission |
| 1 Impotence | 1 Shortness of breath | | 2 Seminal emission without erotic dreams |
| 1 Infertility | 1 Underweight | | 2 Vaginal discharge or bleeding |
| 1 Lack of appetite | 4 Urine dribbling* | | |
| 1 Pain in the loins (lumbago) | | | |
| 1 Palpitations | | | |
| 1 Panting) | | | |
| 1 Perspiration on the forehead | | | |
| 1 Ringing in ears | | | |
| 1 Scant urine | | | |
| to warm and tone the kidneys yang | to strengthen energy and elevate the yang | to warm and strengthen the kidneys and control urination | to strengthen energy and reinforce the kidneys |
| Shen-Qi-Wan | Bu-Zhong-Yi-Qi-Tang | Suo-Niao-Wan or Shen-Qi-Wan | Sang-Piao-Xiao-San |
| kidney, lobster, sardine, shrimp, sparrow, clone, dill seed, fennel, pistachio nut, sparrow egg, crab apple, raspberry and walnut | grape, longan nuts, maltose, mandarin fish, Irish potato, sweet rice, apple cucumber, bog bean, gold carp, carrot, chestnut, ham, horse bean, hyacinth bean, Job's-tears, royal jelly, string bean, whitefish, yam, red and black date, mutton, squash, rock sugar, chicken egg yolk and cheese | milk, millet, stamens, sword bean, wheat, black sesame seed, beef kidney, chestnut, chicken liver, lobster, perch, pork kidney, raspberry, sea cucumber, string bean and walnut | longan fruit, chicken, walnuts, stamens, crab apple, yam, raspberry and strawberry |

## SEMINAL EMISSION AND PREMATURE EJACULATION IN MEN

| | Deficiency fire | Superficial dampness-heat | Kidneys yin deficiency |
|---|---|---|---|
| **SYMPTOMS** | 2 Coughing out blood<br>1 Dry cough without sputum or coughing out slightly sticky fluids<br>1 Dry sensations in the mouth<br>1 Dry throat<br>1 Feeling miserable<br>1 Forgetfulness<br>1 Hot sensations in body<br>1 Illness attacks slowly but with a longer duration (chronic illness)<br>1 Light but periodic fever not unlike the tide<br>1 Night sweats<br>1 Pain in the throat<br>1 Ringing in ears<br>2 Seminal emission with erotic dream*<br>1 Sleeplessness<br>1 Sore loins<br>1 Sputum with blood<br>2 Toothache | 1 Abdominal pain<br>1 Burning sensation & itch in the genitals or burning sensation in the anus<br>1 Congested chest<br>1 Diarrhea with forceful discharge of stool<br>1 Discharge of yellowish-red, turbid stools with bad smell<br>1 Edema<br>2 Ejaculates running out along with urine*<br>1 Excessive perspiration<br>1 Jaundice<br>1 Low fever<br>1 Pain in the joints of the four limbs, with swelling & heaviness<br>2 Pain inside the penis*<br>1 Perspiration on hands & feet or the head<br>1 Reddish and scant urine<br>1 Retention of urine<br>2 Seminal emission that occurs very frequently*<br>1 Thirst | 1 Cold hands and feet<br>1 Cough with sputum containing blood or coughing out fresh blood<br>1 Deafness<br>1 Dizziness<br>1 Dry sensations in the mouth or dry throat<br>1 Fatigue<br>1 Feeling miserable and hurried, with fever<br>1 Fever at night with burning sensations in internal organs<br>1 Hot sensations in any part of the body<br>1 Night sweats<br>1 Pain in the heels<br>1 Pain in the loins (lumbago)<br>1 Pain in the tibia<br>1 Ringing in ears<br>1 Seminal emission mostly without dreams*<br>1 Sleeplessness<br>1 Sore loins and weak legs<br>1 Spots in front of the eyes<br>1 Thirst<br>1 Toothache or loose teeth |
| **TREATMENT PRINCIPLE** | to water the yin and sedate fire and to secure the heart and control emission | to clear dampness-heat and reinforce the kidneys energy to control semen | to strengthen the kidneys yin to control ejaculation |
| **TREATMENT FORMULA** | Feng-Sui-Dan or Zhi-Bai-Di-Huang-Wan | Bei-Xie-Fen-Qing-Yin | Liu-Wei-Di-Huang-Wan or Zuo-Gui-Wan |
| **FOOD CURES** | banana, bitter endive, black fungus, salt, spinach, strawberry, bamboo shoot, cucumber, Job's-tears, liver, leaf beet, mung bean, peppermint, purslane, lily flower, salt, cattail, chicken egg, duck egg, asparagus, royal jelly, pork and oyster | carp, celery, horse bean, jellyfish skin, Job's-tears, prickly ash, hyacinth bean, oregano, sweet basil, adzuki bean, bamboo shoot, soybean sprouts, rosin, banana, bitter endive, black fungus, salt, spinach, strawberry, cucumber, leaf beet, mung bean, peppermint and purslane | abalone, asparagus, chicken egg, cuttlefish, duck, duck egg, white fungus, oyster, pork, royal jelly, chestnut, chicken liver and pork kidneys |

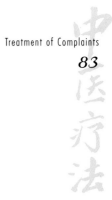

## IMPOTENCE IN MEN

| *Kidneys energy deficiency* | *Deficiency fire* | *Spleen deficiency* | *Kidneys yang deficiency* |
|---|---|---|---|
| 3 Cold sensations in the genitals* <br> 2 Deafness <br> 2 Dizziness <br> 2 Fatigue <br> 2 Headache <br> 2 Impotence <br> 2 Lumbago <br> 1 Prolonged dizziness <br> 2 Ringing in ears <br> 2 Seminal emission that occurs spontaneously as if semen were just sliding out* | 1 Coughing out blood <br> 1 Dry cough without sputum or coughing out slightly sticky fluids <br> 1 Dry sensations in the mouth or dry throat <br> 1 Feeling miserable <br> 1 Forgetfulness <br> 1 Hot sensations in body <br> 1 Illness attacks slowly but with a longer duration (chronic illness) <br> 1 Light but periodic fever not unlike the tide <br> 1 Night sweats <br> 1 Pain in the throat <br> 1 Ringing in ears <br> 1 Seminal emission with dreams <br> 1 Sleeplessness <br> 1 Sore loins <br> 1 Sputum with blood <br> 5 Strong sexual desire with very quick ejaculation* <br> 1 Toothache | 2 Chronic diarrhea <br> 2 Chronic dysentery <br> 6 Lack of firm erection* <br> 1 Poor appetite <br> 6 Prolapse of any internal organ* <br> 2 Prolapse of anus <br> 1 Shortness of breath | 1 Cold feet, cold loins and legs, or cold sensations in the genitals <br> 2 Diarrhea before dawn <br> 1 Diarrhea with sticky, muddy stools <br> 1 Dizziness <br> 2 Edema <br> 1 Excessive perspiration <br> 2 Fatigue <br> 1 Frequent urination at night <br> 2 Panting <br> 1 Perspiration on the forehead <br> 1 Retention of urine <br> 1 Ringing in ears <br> 1 Scant urine <br> 2 Seminal emission <br> 1 Shortness of breath |
| to tone the kidneys energy and control the semen gate | to sedate fire and tone the kidneys yin | to tone energy and strengthen the spleen | to warm the kidneys and reinforce kidneys yang energy |
| You-Gui-Wan or Jin-Suo-Gu-Jing-Wan | Zhi-Bai-Di-Huang Wan | Bu-Zhong-Yi-Qi-Tang | You-Gui-Wan |
| milk, millet, stamens, sword bean, wheat, black sesame seed, beef kidney, chestnut, chicken liver, lobster, perch, pork kidney, raspberry, sea cucumber, string bean and walnut | banana, bitter endive, black fungus, salt, spinach, strawberry, bamboo shoot, cucumber, Job's-tears, liver, leaf beet, mung bean, peppermint, purslane, lily flower, salt, cattail, chicken egg, duck egg, asparagus, royal jelly, pork and oyster | longan nuts, mandarin fish, apple cucumber, gold carp, carrot, chestnut, corncob, Job's-tears, Irish potato, rice, royal jelly, string bean, yam, beef and red and black date | kidney, lobster, sardine, shrimp, sparrow, clove, dill seed, fennel, pistachio nut, sparrow egg, crab apple, raspberry and walnuts |

# INFERTILITY IN WOMEN

| | Simultaneous deficiency of energy and blood | Yin deficiency | Cold and deficient womb |
|---|---|---|---|
| **SYMPTOMS** | 1 Bleeding of various kinds with blood in tight color, often seen in consumptive diseases<br>1 Dizziness<br>1 Fatigue<br>1 Flying objects seen in front of 1 the eyes<br>1 Insomnia<br>1 Irregular menstruation<br>1 Low energy<br>1 Low voice<br>4 Menstrual flow in light-red color*<br>1 Mentally depressed<br>3 Regular menstruation, but with very scant flow, lasting for one or two days only*<br>1 Numbness of limb<br>1 Pale complexion and lips<br>1 Pale nails<br>1 Palpitations | 1 Bleeding from gums<br>1 Constipation<br>1 Dizziness<br>1 Dry & scant stools, dry sensations in the mouth, or dry throat<br>1 Fatigue<br>1 Headache in the afternoon<br>1 Low fever in the afternoon<br>1 Menstrual flow in dark color*<br>1 Night sweats<br>1 Nosebleed<br>1 Pain in the throat, also red and swollen<br>1 Palms of hands and soles of feet are both hot<br>1 Palpitations with insecure feeling<br>1 Regular menstruation with scant flow, lasting for half day or one day*<br>1 Short & reddish streams of urine<br>1 Sleeplessness<br>1 Swallowing difficulty<br>1 Toothache<br>1 Underweight<br>1 Vomiting of blood or nosebleed during menstrual periods | 10 Cold pain or cold sensations in the lower abdomen or cold sensations in the genitals*<br>1 Dark, blackish menstrual flow<br>1 Failure of the fetus to grow<br>1 Fetus motion<br>1 Frequent miscarriage<br>1 Functional disturbances of the ovary<br>1 Habitual miscarriage<br>1 Pale complexion<br>1 Poor appetite<br>1 Thin and watery menstrual flow in light color<br>1 Underdevelopment of the womb |
| **TREATMENT PRINCIPLE** | to tone the energy and the blood simultaneously and to tone the kidneys | to water the yin and clear the heat and to nourish the blood and regulate menstruation | to warm the womb |
| **TREATMENT FORMULA** | Ba-Zhen-Yi-Mu-Wan | Yang-Jing-Zhong-Yu-Tang, Qing-Gu-Zi-Shen-Tang, or Qing-Xue-Yang-Yin-Tang | Ai-Fu-Nuan-Gong-Wan |
| **FOOD CURES** | abalone, asparagus, cuttlefish, chicken egg, duck egg, white fungus, beef liver, grape, mandarin fish, oyster, milk, beef, cherry, blood clam, longan nuts, maltose, Irish potato, sweet rice, apple cucumber, bog bean, gold carp, carrot, chestnut, ham, horse bean, hyacinth bean, Job's-tears, royal jelly, string bean, whitefish, yam, red and black date, mutton, squash and rock sugar | bird's nest, cheese, kidney bean, abalone, asparagus, chicken egg, cuttlefish, duck, duck egg, white fungus, oyster, pork and royal jelly | cinnamon, kidneys, lobster, sheep's milk, sardine, shrimp, star anise, red and black date and sword bean |

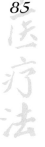

| Hot blood | Liver energy congestion | Dampness-sputum | Spleen-dampness |
|---|---|---|---|
| 1 Abdominal pain that occurs at onset of menstrual periods<br>1 Deep-red or violet menstrual flow<br>1 Discharge of blood from anus before periods<br>1 Fever after childbirth<br>1 Irregularity of menstrual periods<br>1 Menstrual flow somewhat heavy<br>1 Menstrual flow with a bad smell<br>1 Nosebleed<br>1 Plentiful menstrual flow<br>7 Premature menstrual periods, which may be more than 10 days early or two periods within one month*<br>1 Red and plentiful menstrual flow<br>1 Skin ulcers<br>1 Vaginal bleeding<br>1 Vomiting of blood or nosebleed during menstrual periods | 1 Abdominal pain<br>1 Convulsions<br>1 Irregularity of menstrual periods<br>5 Menstrual pain*<br>1 Morning sickness<br>1 Numbness<br>2 Pain in the upper abdomen<br>1 Premature periods or overdue period<br>1 Shortage of milk secretion after childbirth<br>2 Stomachache<br>2 Subjective sensations of objects in the throat<br>1 Vomiting of blood<br>1 Whitish vaginal discharge | 1 Discharge of sputum that can be coughed out easily or discharge of white, watery sputum<br>1 Dizziness<br>1 Excessive whitish vaginal discharge<br>1 Frequent coughs during pregnancy that are prolonged and cause motion of fetus<br>1 Headache<br>1 Hiccups<br>1 Light-red menstrual flow<br>1 Menstrual periods overdue frequently<br>1 Morning sickness<br>1 Turbid and sticky menstrual flow<br>1 Pain in the chest<br>1 Panting<br>1 Plentiful menstrual flow<br>1 Prolonged dizziness<br>1 Sleep a lot or sleeplessness<br>1 Susceptible to morning sickness during pregnancy<br>1 Suppression of menses<br>1 Vomiting<br>1 White, sliding sputum that can be cleared from throat easily<br>1 Whitish vaginal discharge | 1 Chest discomfort without appetite<br>1 Diarrhea<br>1 Edema<br>4 Feeling sleepy all day long*<br>1 Heavy sensations in head as if the head were covered with something<br>5 Heavy sensations in the body with a desire to lie down*<br>1 Jaundice<br>1 Love of hot drink<br>1 Nausea and vomiting<br>1 Plentiful vaginal discharge<br>1 Stomach fullness and discomfort<br>1 Sweet, sticky taste in mouth<br>1 Too tired to talk or move |
| to clear the heat in the blood | to relax the liver and disperse energy congestion | to strengthen the spleen and dry up dampness | to dry up dampness, strengthen the spleen and wake up the spirits |
| Qing-Jing-Tang | Xiao-Yao-San or De-Sheng-Dan | Qi-Gong-Wan | Tai-Wu-Shen-Zhu-San, Hou-Pu-Xia-Ling-Tang, Wei-Ling-Tang, or San-Ren-Tang |
| bitter endive, camellia, cattail, black fungus, salt, spinach, strawberry, banana, cucumber and licorice | brown sugar, garlic, turmeric, kumquat, beef, cherry, bird's nest, butterfish, chicken, coconut meat, date, tofu, mustard seed, sweet rice, goose meat, mutton, jackfruit, squash, sweet potato, red and black date, rice, rock sugar, caraway seed, spearmint, common button mushroom, oregano, red bean, ambergris, dill seed, garlic, sweet basil and saffron | adzuki bean, ambergris, barley, common carp, cucumber, mung bean, seaweed, shepherd's purse, star fruit, bamboo shoot, crown daisy, date, fresh ginger, leaf or brown mustard, black and white pepper, white or yellow mustard seed, asparagus and pear | gold carp, corncob, horse bean, Job's-tears, prickly ash, adzuki bean and bamboo shoot |

SLEEPINESS (CONTINUED)

| | Dampness-sputum | Spleen energy deficiency | Yang deficiency |
|---|---|---|---|
| **SYMPTOMS** | 1 Cough<br>1 Discharge of sputum that can be coughed out easily<br>1 Discharge of white, watery sputum<br>1 Dizziness<br>1 Excessive whitish vaginal discharge<br>1 Frequent coughs during pregnancy that are prolonged and cause motion of fetus<br>1 Headache<br>1 Hiccups<br>1 Pain in the chest<br>2 Panting<br>1 Prolonged dizziness<br>3 Sleep a lot*<br>1 Sleeplessness<br>1 Suppression of menses<br>2 Vomiting<br>1 White, sliding sputum that can be cleared from throat easily | 2 Abdominal Pain<br>2 Diarrhea<br>1 Edema<br>3 Fatigue*<br>4 Feeling sleepy particularly after meals*<br>1 Lips rolled up<br>3 Loud snoring during sleep*<br>1 Stiff tongue<br>2 Stomachache<br>1 Vomiting of blood | 1 Clear and long streams of urine<br>1 Cold hands and feet<br>1 Constipation<br>1 Diarrhea<br>1 Diminished urination<br>1 Discharge of watery, thin stools<br>1 Edema<br>1 Fatigue<br>1 Fear of cold<br>1 Fingertips often cold<br>1 Forgetfulness<br>1 Frequent fear of cold in hands and feet<br>1 Headache in the morning<br>2 Older patients*<br>1 Palpitations<br>1 Perspiration due to hot weather or putting on warm clothes<br>1 Perspiration like cold water<br>1 Scant energy and too tired to talk<br>1 Sleep a lot |
| **TREATMENT PRINCIPLE** | to transform sputum and wake up the spirits | to strengthen the spleen and energy | to strengthen energy and warm the yang |
| **TREATMENT FORMULA** | Wen-Dan-Tang | Xiang-Sha-Liu-Jun-Zi-Tang or Cang-Er-Zi-San with Er-Chen-Tang | Fu-Zi-Li-Zhong-Wan with Shen-Qi-Wan |
| **FOOD CURES** | adzuki bean, ambergris, barley, common carp, cucumber, mung bean, seaweed, shepherd's purse, star fruit, bamboo shoot, crown daisy, date, fresh ginger, leaf or brown mustard, black and white pepper, white or yellow mustard seed, asparagus and pear | grape, longan nuts, maltose, mandarin fish, Irish potato, sweet rice, apple cucumber, bog bean, gold carp, carrot, chestnut, ham, horse bean, hyacinth bean, Job's-tears, royal jelly, string bean, whitefish, yam, red and black date, mutton, squash, rock sugar and chicken egg yolk | kidneys, lobster, sardine, shrimp, star anise and red and black date |

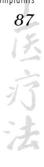

OBESITY

| Blood coagulations | Liver energy congestion | Heart energy deficiency | Spleen-dampness |
|---|---|---|---|
| 1 Abdominal pain | 2 Abdominal obstruction | 2 Chest pain | 1 Chest discomfort without appetite |
| 1 Chest pain | 2 Abdominal pain | 2 Epilepsy | 1 Diarrhea |
| 1 Coughing out blood | 3 Bitter taste in the mouth* | 2 Fatigue | 3 Edema* |
| 1 Headache | 1 Convulsions | 2 Forgetfulness | 1 Heavy sensations in head as if the head were covered with something |
| 2 History of past injuries* | 1 Dizziness | 2 Insomnia | |
| 1 Jaundice | 1 Numbness | 2 Nervousness | |
| 1 Lumbago | 2 Pain in the upper abdomen | 2 Pain in the heart | 1 Heavy sensations in the body with discomfort |
| 1 Pain in the upper abdomen | 3 Sleep a lot normally* | 2 Palpitations | 1 Jaundice |
| 1 Pain in the loins as if being pierced with an awl | 2 Stomachache | 3 Spells of sleep mostly* | 1 Love of hot drink |
| 1 Palpitations with insecure feeling | 2 Subjective sensations of objects in the throat | 1 White complexion | 1 Nausea and vomiting |
| 2 Sleep for about 10 minutes each time* | 1 Vomiting of blood | | 4 Poor appetite* |
| 1 Spasm | | | 3 Scant urine* |
| 2 Stomachache | | | 1 Stomach fullness and discomfort |
| 2 Symptoms worsening in the afternoon and at night* | | | 1 Sweet, sticky taste in mouth |
| 1 Vomiting of blood | | | 1 Too tired to talk or move |

| | | | |
|---|---|---|---|
| to activate the blood and remove blood coagulations | to disperse liver energy congestion | to strengthen heart energy and secure the spirits | to strengthen the spleen and remove dampness |
| Tong-Qiao-Huo-Xue-Tang or Fu-Yuan-Huo-Xue-Tang | Dan-Zhi-Xiao-Yao-San | Yang-Xin-Tang | Fang-Ji-Huang-Qi-Tang with Ling-Gui-Zhu-Gan-Tang |
| ambergris, brown sugar, chestnut, eggplant, peach, black soybean, sturgeon, sweet basil, crab, distillers' grains, papaya and saffron | brown sugar, garlic, turmeric, kumquat, beef, cherry, bird's nest, butterfish, chicken, coconut meat, date, tofu, mustard seed, sweet rice, goose meat, mutton, jackfruit, squash, sweet potato, red and black date, rice, rock sugar, caraway seed, spearmint, common button mushroom, oregano, red bean, ambergris, dill seed, sweet basil and saffron | air bladder of shark, water spinach, abalone, asparagus, dried ginger and cinnamon | gold carp, corncob, horse bean, Job's-tears, prickly ash, adzuki bean and bamboo shoot |

OBESITY (CONTINUED)

|  | Spleen and stomach heat and dampness | Liver energy congestion | Simultaneous energy congestion and blood coagulations |
|---|---|---|---|
| SYMPTOMS | 1 Abdominal swelling*<br>1 Bad breath<br>1 Bleeding from gums<br>1 Dizziness*<br>1 Constipation*<br>1 Foul breath from the mouth<br>1 Getting hungry easily<br>1 Gums swelling<br>1 Hiccups<br>1 Light taste in the mouth<br>1 Nosebleed<br>1 Pain in the gums with swelling<br>1 Pain in the throat<br>1 Perspiring on the head<br>1 Stomachache<br>1 Thirst and craving for cold<br>1 Vomiting<br>1 Vomiting of blood<br>1 Vomiting right after eating<br>1 Vomiting with stomach discomfort as if hungry, empty, or hot | 2 Abdominal obstruction<br>2 Abdominal pain<br>3 Bitter taste in the mouth*<br>1 Convulsions<br>1 Dry tongue<br>3 Getting angry easily*<br>1 Numbness<br>2 Pain in the upper abdomen<br>2 Poor appetite*<br>2 Stomachache<br>2 Subjective sensations of objects in the throat<br>1 Vomiting of blood | 2 Abdominal swelling<br>1 Chronic hepatitis<br>1 Cirrhosis<br>1 Congested chest<br>1 Irregular menstruation with blood clots in women<br>1 Love of sighing<br>1 Lump in the abdomen that stays in the same region<br>4 Pain in the upper abdomen*<br>4 Palpitations*<br>4 Shortness of breath* |
| TREATMENT PRINCIPLE | to clear the heat in the stomach and remove dampness from the stomach | to disperse liver energy congestion | to regulate energy and remove blood coagulations |
| TREATMENT FORMULA | Fang-Feng-Tong-Sheng-San | Da-Chai-Hu-Tang | Tao-Hong-Si-Wu-Tang |
| FOOD CURES | carp, celery, horse bean, jellyfish skin, Job's-tears, prickly ash, hyacinth bean, oregano, sweet basil, adzuki bean, bamboo shoot, soybean sprouts, rosin, banana, bitter endive, black fungus, salt, spinach, strawberry, cucumber, leaf beet, mung bean, peppermint and purslane | brown sugar, garlic, turmeric, kumquat, beef, cherry, bird's nest, butterfish, chicken, coconut meat, date, tofu, mustard seed, sweet rice, goose meat, mutton, jackfruit, squash, sweet potato, red and black date, rice, rock sugar, caraway seed, spearmint, common button mushroom, oregano, red bean, ambergris, dill seed, sweet basil and saffron | beef, cherry, bird's nest, butterfish, chicken, coconut meat, date, tofu, mustard seed, sweet rice, goose meat, mutton, jackfruit, squash, sweet potato, red and black date, rice, rock sugar, caraway seed, spearmint, common button mushroom, oregano, red bean, ambergris, dill seed, garlic, sweet basil, saffron, ambergris, brown sugar, chestnut, eggplant, peach, black soybean, sturgeon, crab, distillers' grains, papaya and saffron |

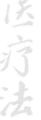

| *Internal sputum* | *Spleen-kidneys yang deficiency* |
|---|---|
| 1 Abdominal swelling or rumbling | 1 Abdominal swelling |
| 1 Congested chest | 1 Cold hands and feet or cold loins |
| 3 Dizziness* | 1 Diarrhea before dawn |
| 1 Headache | 1 Diarrhea with sticky, muddy stools |
| 3 Heaviness in the body* | 1 Dysentery |
| 1 Love of hot drink | 1 Eating very little |
| 2 Love of sweet or greasy foods* | 1 Edema |
| 2 Numbness* | 1 Edema that occurs all over the body |
| 1 Pain in the chest or upper abdomen | 1 Fatigue |
| 1 Palpitations | 1 Fear of cold |
| 1 Stomachache | 1 Four limbs weakness |
| 1 Swollen body of the tongue | 1 Frequent urination with clear or white urine |
| 2 Vomiting or coughing out watery sputum in large amounts* | 1 Mentally fatigued |
| | 2 Poor appetite* |
| | 2 Scant urine* |
| | 1 Sputum rumbling with panting |
| | 2 Watery stools* |

to strengthen the spleen and transform sputum

to warm the kidneys and strengthen the spleen

Wen-Dan-Tang

Zhen-Wu-Tang with Huang-Ji-Huang-Qi-Tang

bamboo shoot, crown daisy, date, fresh ginger, leaf or brown mustard, mustard seed, black and white pepper, white or yellow mustard seed, asparagus and pear

air bladder of shark, chicken, cayenne pepper, fennel, nutmeg, black and white pepper, prickly ash, mutton, sword bean, white or yellow mustard, kidney, lobster, sardine, shrimp, sparrow, clove, dill seed, fennel, pistachio nut, sparrow egg, crab apple, raspberry and walnut

# Treatment of Diagnosed Disorders

Hypertension

Hypotension

High Cholesterol

Diabetes Mellitus

Coronary Heart Disease

Urinary Stones

Anemia

Epilepsy

Hyperthyroidism

Hypothyroidism

Arthritis and rheumatoid arthritis

Common Cold and Flu

Bacillary Dysentery:

Bronchitis

Bronchial asthma

Pneumonia

Acute Gastroenteritis

Chronic gastritis and peptic ulcers

Nephritis

Cerebrovascular Accident

Neurosis

Dementia, including Alzheimer's Disease

Allergies

The normal blood pressure is the systolic pressure between 90 and 140mm of mercury and the diastolic pressure between 60 and 90mm of mercury. Hypertension means that the systolic pressure is over 140 and the diastolic pressure is over 90mm of mercury. Hypotension means that the systolic pressure is lower than 90 and the diastolic pressure is lower than 60mm of mercury.

## HYPERTENSION

| | *Liver-fire* | *Liver & kidneys yin deficiency with liver yang upsurging* | *Both yin & yang are deficient with deficient yang moving upward* |
|---|---|---|---|
| **SYMPTOMS** | 2 Bitter taste in the mouth<br>4 Blood pressure rises readily with anger or stress*<br>2 Discharge of yellowish and scant urine<br>2 Dry mouth<br>2 Hot temper<br>2 Red eyes<br>2 Red face<br>2 Severe headache<br>2 Vertigo | 4 Blood pressure rises readily with fatigue and stress<br>2 Discharge of reddish and scant urine<br>1 Hot temper<br>2 Insomnia<br>2 Lumbago<br>2 Many dreams<br>2 Numbness of the four limbs<br>2 Pain in the legs<br>2 Ringing in the ears<br>2 Seminal emission in men<br>2 Vertigo | 1 Blurred vision<br>2 Cold limbs<br>1 Dry mouth<br>2 Frequent urination at night<br>2 Heavy breathing on walking<br>1 Insomnia<br>1 Light headache<br>1 Lumbago<br>1 Many dreams<br>1 Perspiration<br>2 Ringing in the ears<br>1 Slightly red face<br>2 Twitching of muscles<br>1 Vertigo<br>1 Weak legs |
| **TREATMENT PRINCIPLE** | to reduce liver-fire and nourish the yin | to nourish liver yin and kidney yin and to suppress liver yang | to tone both the yin and the yang |
| **TREATMENT FORMULA** | Long-Dan-Xie-Gan-Tang | Zhen-Gan-Xi-Feng-Tang | Shen-Qi-Wan |
| **FOOD CURES** | 1. Boil 100g seaweed to eat every day;<br>2. wash and cut up 60g celery to boil with 60g rice for one-day consumption and continue for 10 days<br>3. boil 30g fresh water chestnut with 30g jellyfish skin (with salt washed off) in water for consumption two times daily;<br>4. boil kelp and mung bean, 60g each, until both are extremely soft and then season with brown sugar to drink once daily for one week.<br>spinach, chestnut, shepherd's purse, rye, black fungus, vinegar, abalone, asparagus, chicken egg, white fungus, pork and royal jelly. | 1. Prepare a pork gallbladder, squeeze as many black soybeans as possible into the gallbladder, steam it until cooked and dry it under the sun; eat 20 to 30 black soybeans each time, twice daily, for one week.<br>2. Wash and soak 250g fresh celery in hot water for 20 minutes, cut up the celery to squeeze juice, season with white sugar to drink like tea, once daily for a few days.<br>bird's nest, cheese, chicken egg, kidney bean, brown sugar, mussel, abalone, asparagus, chicken egg, cuttlefish, duck, duck egg, white fungus, oyster, pork, royal jelly, chestnut, chicken liver and pork kidneys. | Boil 300g fresh celery with five red dates until cooked; drink the soup and eat celery and dates once daily for one week.<br>chicken egg yolk, cheese, kidney bean, abalone, cuttlefish, duck, duck egg, white fungus, oyster, pork, royal jelly and celery. |

## HYPOTENSION

| | Spleen-kidneys deficiency | Simultaneous deficiency of yin and energy | Heart-kidneys yang deficiency |
|---|---|---|---|
| **SYMPTOMS** | 1 Deafness<br>1 Diarrhea<br>1 Difficult urination<br>9 Dizziness*<br>1 Fatigue of the four limbs<br>1 Forgetfulness<br>1 Insomnia<br>1 Misty vision<br>1 Palpitations<br>1 Ringing in the ears<br>1 Shortness of breath<br>1 Yellowish complexion | 1 Constipation<br>1 Dizziness<br>1 Dry cough with scant sputum<br>1 Dry mouth<br>1 Discharge of dry stools<br>2 Excessive perspiration<br>1 Fatigue<br>1 Fever<br>1 Frequent vomiting<br>1 Hot sensations in the palms of hands and soles of feet<br>2 Light stomachache with swelling<br>2 Palpitations<br>1 Poor appetite<br>1 Scant urine<br>1 Sore throat<br>1 Thirst<br>1 Too tired to talk | 1 Cold limbs<br>1 Cold sweats<br>1 Discharge of watery, thin stools<br>2 Edema<br>1 Frequent urination particularly at night<br>4 Heavy head with light feet sensations*<br>3 Orthostatic hypotension (hypotension occurring when a person assumes an erect position)*<br>2 Pain in the chest<br>2 Palpitations<br>2 Nervousness<br>1 Shock |
| **TREATMENT PRINCIPLE** | to tone the spleen and the kidneys | to tone the energy and the yin simultaneously | to tone the heart yang and the kidney yang |
| **TREATMENT FORMULA** | Shen-Huang-Gan-Qi-Tang | Sheng-Mai-San | Shen-Fu-Tang |
| **FOOD CURES** | chicken egg yolk, common button mushroom, wheat bran, rice, beef, cherry, bird's nest, coconut meat, date, tofu, mustard seed, sweet potato, red and black date, rock sugar, apple cucumber, carrot, chestnut, Irish potato, abalone, asparagus, chicken egg, white fungus, black sesame seed, beef kidney, chicken liver, lobster, pork kidney, raspberry, scallop, sea cucumber, shrimp, string bean and walnut | bird's nest, cheese, kidney bean, abalone, asparagus, chicken egg, cuttlefish, duck, duck egg, white fungus, oyster, pork, royal jelly, grape, longan nuts, maltose, mandarin fish, Irish potato, sweet rice, apple cucumber, bog bean, gold carp, carrot, chestnut, ham, horse bean, hyacinth bean, Job's-tears, royal jelly, string bean, whitefish, yam, red and black date, mutton, squash and rock sugar | dried ginger, cinnamon, wheat, water spinach, kidneys, star anise, red and black date, lobster, sardine, shrimp, sparrow, clove, dill seed, fennel, pistachio nut, sparrow egg, crab apple, raspberry and walnut |

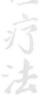

## HIGH CHOLESTEROL

| *Superficial dampness-heat* | *Spleen-sputum* | *Hot stomach* | *Liver-fire upsurging* |
|---|---|---|---|
| | | | |
| 2 Abdominal swelling or pain* | 1 Abdominal swelling | 1 Bad breath | 1 Acute dizziness |
| 1 Burning sensation & itch in the geni-tals or burning sensation in the anus | 3 Abundant saliva | 1 Bleeding from gums | 1 Bleeding from stomach |
| 1 Congested chest | 6 Coughing out watery sputum* | 1 Foul breath from the mouth | 1 Congested chest |
| 1 Diarrhea with forceful discharge of stools | 4 Fatigue* | 1 Getting hungry easily | 1 Deafness |
| 1 Discharge of yellowish-red, turbid stools with bad smell | 1 Overweight, but eat only a small amount of food | 1 Gums swelling | 1 Dim eyes |
| 2 Edema* | 1 Poor appetite | 1 Hiccups | 1 Dizziness |
| 1 Excessive perspiration | 2 Slight fullness of the stomach | 1 Morning sickness | 1 Dry sensations in the mouth |
| 1 Feeling miserable | 1 Suppression of menses | 1 Nosebleed | 1 Feeling hurried and quick tempered or feeling insecure about sleep |
| 1 Itch and pain in the vulva frequently | 1 Weakened limbs | 2 Pain in the gums with swelling | 1 Getting angry easily |
| 1 Jaundice | | 1 Pain in the throat | 1 Headache on both sides of the head and in the corners of the eyes |
| 1 Pain in the joints of the four limbs, with swelling and heaviness | | 1 Perspiring on the head | 1 Headache that is severe |
| 1 Perspiration on hands and feet or the head | | 2 Stomachache | 1 Hiccups |
| 1 Reddish and scant urine, reten-tion of urine, or short streams of reddish urine | | 1 Thirst and craving for cold | 1 Insanity |
| 1 Swollen body of the tongue | | 1 Vomiting | 1 Nosebleed |
| 1 Thirst | | 2 Vomiting of blood | 1 Pain in the chest and the upper abdomen |
| 1 Yellowish body color | | 1 Vomiting right after eating | 1 Red eyes |
| | | 1 Vomiting with stomach discom-fort as if hungry, empty, or hot | 1 Ringing in ears |
| | | | 1 Sleeplessness or sleep a lot |
| | | | 1 Vomiting of blood |
| | | | 1 Yellowish-red urine |
| | | | |
| to clear heat and remove dampness | to strengthen the spleen, harmonize the stomach, remove sputum and transform dampness | to clear the internal heat and promote bowel movements | to clear the heat and sedate the fire in the liver |
| | | | |
| Xiao-Zhi-Tang | Jia-Wei-Er-Chen-Tang | Da-Cheng-Qi-Tang | Long-Dan-Xie-Gan-Tang |
| | | | |
| carp, celery, horse bean, jellyfish skin, Job's-tears, prickly ash, hyacinth bean, oregano, sweet basil, adzuki bean, bamboo shoot, soybean sprouts, rosin, banana, bitter endive, black fungus, salt, spinach, strawberry, cucumber, leaf beet, mung bean, peppermint and purslane | bamboo shoot, crown daisy, date, fresh ginger, leaf or brown mustard, black and white pepper, white or yellow mustard seed, asparagus and pear | salt, lily flower, bitter endive, camellia, cattail, black fungus, spinach, strawberry, banana, cucumber and licorice | spinach, chestnut, shepherd's purse, rye, black fungus, vinegar, abalone, asparagus, chicken egg, white fungus, pork and royal jelly |

| | Spleen-kidneys yang deficiency | Simultaneous deficiency of energy and blood | Lungs-fire |
|---|---|---|---|
| HIGH CHOLESTEROL (CONTINUED) | | | DIABETES MELLITUS |
| SYMPTOMS | 1 Abdominal swelling<br>1 Cold hands and feet or cold loins<br>1 Diarrhea before dawn<br>1 Diarrhea with sticky, muddy stools<br>1 Eating only a little<br>1 Edema<br>1 Edema that occurs all over the body<br>1 Fatigue<br>1 Fear of cold<br>3 Flying objects seen in front of the eyes*<br>1 Four limbs weakness<br>1 Frequent urination with clear or white urine<br>1 Lumbago<br>1 Mentally fatigued<br>3 Over 65 years old*<br>1 Sputum rumbling with panting | 2 Arteriosclerosis patient*<br>1 Bleeding of various kinds with blood in light color, often seen in consumptive diseases<br>2 Chest pain or congestion*<br>2 Dizziness<br>2 Fatigue<br>1 Flying objects seen in front of the eyes<br>2 Insomnia<br>1 Low energy<br>1 Low voice<br>1 Numbness of limbs<br>1 Pale complexion and lips<br>1 Pale nails<br>2 Palpitations<br>1 Ringing in the ears | 4 Dry nose and mouth<br>3 Frequent urination<br>3 Normal bowel movements<br>4 Pain in the throat, also red and swollen<br>3 Very thirsty and drink a lot<br>3 Vomiting of blood |
| TREATMENT PRINCIPLE | to tone the kidneys and the spleen yang | to regulate energy and activate the blood | To produce fluids and clear heat |
| TREATMENT FORMULA | Qing-Zhi-Tang | Guan-Xin-Er-Hao-Fang | Xiao-Ke-Fang and Jiang-Tang-Yi-Hao-Fang |
| FOOD CURES | air bladder of shark, chicken, cayenne pepper, fennel, nutmeg, black and white pepper, prickly ash, mutton, sword bean, white or yellow mustard, kidney, lobster, sardine, shrimp, sparrow, clove, dill seed, fennel, pistachio nut, sparrow egg, crab apple, raspberry and walnuts | abalone, asparagus, cuttlefish, chicken egg, duck egg, white fungus, beef liver, grape, mandarin fish, oyster, milk, beef, cherry, blood clam, longan nuts, maltose, Irish potato, sweet rice, apple cucumber, bog bean, gold carp, carrot, chestnut, ham, horse bean, hyacinth bean, Job's-tears, royal jelly, string bean, whitefish, yam, red and black date, mutton, squash and rock sugar<br><br>Another formula called Dan-Tian-Jiang-Zhi-Wan has been found to lower cholesterol. According to a relatively recent research project involving 251 subjects with high cholesterol, after treatment with this formula 33 percent showed significant improvement. Take 4g of this herbal powder each day in two doses (one in the morning and one in the afternoon) for three months for best results.**<br><br>**  *Journal of Traditional Chinese Medicine*, 1986:39. | lily flower, salt, cattail, asparagus, soya milk, duck egg and olive |

## CORONARY HEART DISEASE

| Stomach-fire | Kidneys yin deficiency | Heart-blood coagulations | Simultaneous energy congestion & blood coagulations |
|---|---|---|---|
| 1 Bitter taste in the mouth<br>1 Bleeding from gums<br>1 Bleeding from space between teeth with pain<br>1 Constipation with dry stools<br>1 Dry sensations in the mouth<br>1 Eating a lot and still feeling hungry<br>1 Fever<br>1 Headache<br>1 Hiccups<br>1 Hungry with good appetite and eat a lot, but still underweight<br>1 Incapable of sound sleep in children<br>1 Morning sickness<br>1 Nosebleed<br>1 Pain in the gums with swelling<br>1 Pain in the throat, also red and swollen<br>1 Toothache<br>2 Underweight*<br>1 Vomiting of blood<br>1 Vomiting right after eating | 1 Cough with sputum containing blood or coughing out fresh blood<br>1 Dry sensations in the mouth particularly at night<br>1 Dry throat<br>1 Fatigue<br>2 Frequent urination*<br>1 Hot sensations in any part of the body<br>1 Night sweats<br>1 Pain in the heels<br>2 Pain in the loins (lumbago)*<br>1 Retention of urine<br>1 Ringing in ears<br>1 Seminal emission with dreams<br>1 Sleeplessness<br>1 Spots in front of the eyes<br>1 Thirst<br>1 Toothache or shaky teeth<br>2 Urine as thick as fat* | 5 Chest congestion*<br>1 Chronic backache<br>1 Cold hands and feet<br>1 Excessive perspiration<br>1 Pain in the chest<br>6 Pain in the heart and chest as if being pricked with a needle*<br>1 Pale complexion<br>1 Palpitations<br>1 Perspire a lot<br>1 Poor appetite<br>1 Shortness of breath | 1 Abdominal swelling<br>5 Chest pain affecting the back*<br>7 Chest pain that comes and goes as if being pricked by a needle*<br>2 Congested chest<br>1 Liver disease<br>1 Love of sighing<br>1 Lump in the abdomen that stays in the same region<br>1 Shortness of breath<br>1 Ulcers |
| to sedate fire and nourish the yin and to lubricate dryness | to strengthen the semen and the kidney yin | to warm the heart yang and promote blood circulation | to activate the blood and promote energy circulation |
| Shi-Gao-Zhi-Mu-Jia-Ren-Shen-Tang and Jiang-Tang-Er-Hao-Fang | Liu-Wei-Di-Huang-Wan, Wu-Wei-Di-Huang-Wan, or Jiang-Tang-San-Hao-Fang | Gua-Lou-Xie-Bai-Gui-Zhi-Tang | Xue-Fu-Zhu-Yu-Tang |
| areca nuts, buckwheat, common carp, banana, bitter endive, black fungus, salt, spinach, strawberry, bamboo shoot, cucumber, Job's-tears, liver, leaf beet, mung bean, peppermint, purslane, lily flower, salt and cattail | abalone, asparagus, chicken egg, cuttlefish, duck, duck egg, white fungus, oyster, pork, royal jelly, chestnut, chicken liver and pork kidneys | ambergris, brown sugar, chestnut, eggplant, peach, black soybean, sturgeon, sweet basil, crab, distillers' grains, papaya and saffron | beef, cherry, bird's nest, butterfish, chicken, coconut meat, date, tofu, mustard seed, sweet rice, goose meat, mutton, jackfruit, squash, sweet potato, red and black date, rice, rock sugar, caraway seed, spearmint, common button mushroom, oregano, red bean, ambergris, dill seed, garlic, sweet basil, saffron, brown sugar, chestnut, eggplant, peach, black soybean, sturgeon, sweet basil, crab, distillers' grains, papaya and saffron |

Urinary stones usually display pain across the loins, abdominal pain, prickling pain on urination and blood in urine

CORONARY HEART DISEASE (CONTINUED)

## URINARY STONES

| | *Liver-kidneys yin deficiency* | *Simultaneous deficiency of yin and yang* | *Lower burning space dampness-heat* |
|---|---|---|---|
| **SYMPTOMS** | 3 Chest pain particularly at night*<br>1 Difficulty with both defecation and urination<br>1 Dizziness<br>3 Dry eyes, throat, or mouth*<br>1 Fatigue<br>1 Headache with pain in the brow<br>1 Lumbago<br>1 Menstrual pain<br>1 Night blindness<br>1 Night sweats<br>1 Pain in the upper abdomen<br>1 Palms of hands and soles of feet are both hot<br>1 Paralysis<br>1 Sleeplessness with forgetfulness<br>1 Weak loins and tibia<br>1 Withering complexion | 1 Cold limbs and cold sensations in the body<br>1 Fatigue<br>4 Frequent urination at night*<br>1 Low energy<br>3 Pain in the heart*<br>1 Palpitations<br>1 Perspiration with hot sensations in the body easily triggered by physical activities<br>1 Poor appetite<br>1 Poor spirits<br>1 Ringing in ears<br>1 Too tired to talk<br>1 Underweight<br>3 Wake up at night due to pain* | 3 Pain affecting the lower abdomen or shooting pain towards the genitals*<br>3 Colic pain in the abdomen and across the loins*<br>3 Dribbling after urination*<br>2 Frequent desire to pass urine*<br>1 Frequent urination in short reddish streams<br>1 Low fever in the afternoon<br>1 Nausea or vomiting<br>2 Pain on urination*<br>1 Poor appetite<br>1 Seminal emission<br>1 Thirst with no desire for drink<br>2 Yellowish and turbid urine* |
| **TREATMENT PRINCIPLE** | to strengthen the kidneys and liver yin and to activate the blood and transform blood coagulations | to regulate and strengthen both the yin and yang and to strengthen the energy and the blood simultaneously | to clear the heat and remove dampness and to expel stones |
| **TREATMENT FORMULA** | Yang-Yiri-Tong-Bi-Tang | Zhi-Gan-Cao-Tang | Dao-Chi-San |
| **FOOD CURES** | bird's nest, cheese, chicken egg, kidney bean, brown sugar, mussel, abalone, asparagus, chicken egg, cuttlefish, duck, duck egg, white fungus, oyster, pork, royal jelly, chestnut, chicken liver and pork kidneys | beef, cherry, bird's nest, butterfish, chicken, coconut meat, date, tofu, mustard seed, sweet rice, goose meat, mutton, jackfruit, squash, sweet potato, red and black date, rice, rock sugar, caraway seed, spearmint, common button mushroom, oregano, red bean, ambergris, dill seed, garlic, sweet basil, saffron, abalone, asparagus, cuttlefish, chicken egg, duck egg, white fungus, beef liver, grape, mandarin fish, oyster, milk, beef, blood clam and longan nuts | mung bean sprouts, ambergris, kiwi fruits, sturgeon, adzuki bean, Chinese cabbage, mango, pea and watermelon |

ANEMIA

| Simultaneous energy congestion & blood coagulations | Spleen-kidneys yang deficiency | Heart-spleen deficiency | Liver-kidneys yin deficiency |
|---|---|---|---|
| 1 Abdominal swelling | 6 Chronic stone* | 1 Abdominal swelling | 1 Difficulty in both defecation and urination |
| 2 Aching pain in the lower abdomen* | 1 Cold hands and feet | 2 Bleeding symptoms* | 2 Dizziness |
| 3 Chronic stones* | 1 Cold loins | 1 Discharge of watery, thin stools | 1 Dry eyes or throat |
| 2 Colic pain on urination* | 2 Diarrhea before dawn | 1 Dizziness | 2 Fatigue |
| 1 Congested chest | 1 Diarrhea with sticky, muddy stools | 1 Eating very little | 1 Headache with pain in the brow |
| 3 Dribbling after urination* | 1 Eating very little | 1 Fatigue | 2 Lumbago |
| 1 Love of sighing | 1 Edema that occurs all over the body | 1 Fatigue with a lack of power | 1 Night blindness |
| 1 Lump in the abdomen that stays in the same region | 2 Fatigue | 1 Forgetfulness | 1 Night sweats |
| 3 Pain across the loins* | 1 Fear of cold | 1 Impotence | 2 Pain in the upper abdomen |
| 3 Pain on urination* | 1 Four limbs weakness | 1 Low voice | 1 Palms of hands and soles of feet are both hot |
| | 1 Frequent urination with clear or white urine | 2 Nervousness | 1 Red eyes |
| | 1 Mentally fatigued | 1 Night sweats | 1 Ringing in the ears |
| | 1 Sputum rumbling with panting | 2 Palpitations | 1 Sleeplessness with forgetfulness |
| | | 1 Poor appetite | 1 Weak loins and tibia |
| | | 1 Shortness of breath | 1 Withering complexion |
| | | 2 Sleeplessness | 1 Zygomatic regions on both sides appear tender and red |
| | | 1 Withering and yellowish complexion | |
| to regulate energy and remove blood coagulations | to strengthen the spleen and the kidneys and to promote urination and expel stones | to strengthen the spleen & the heart and to tone the blood and the energy | to water the liver yin and the kidney yin and to nourish the blood and strengthen the essence of the kidneys |
| Tao-Hong-Si-Wu-Tang | Shen-Ling-Bai-Zhu-San | Gui-Pi-Tang | Gui-Shao-Di-Huang-Tang |
| beef, cherry, bird's nest, butterfish, chicken, coconut meat, date, tofu, mustard seed, sweet rice, goose meat, mutton, jackfruit, squash, sweet potato, red and black date, rice, rock sugar, caraway seed, spearmint, common button mushroom, oregano, red bean, ambergris, dill seed, garlic, sweet basil, saffron, brown sugar, chestnut, eggplant, peach, black soybean, sturgeon, crab, distillers' grains, papaya & saffron | air bladder of shark, chicken, cayenne pepper, fennel, nutmeg, black and white pepper, prickly ash, mutton, sword bean, white or yellow mustard, kidney, lobster, sardine, shrimp, sparrow, clove, dill seed, fennel, pistachio nut, sparrow egg, crab apple, raspberry and walnut | beef liver, chicken egg, cuttlefish, oyster, pork liver, sea cucumber, water spinach, longan nut, mandarin fish, apple cucumber, chestnut, horse bean, Job's-tears, Irish potato, rice, royal jelly and yam | bird's nest, cheese, chicken egg, kidney bean, brown sugar, mussel, abalone, asparagus, chicken egg, cuttlefish, duck, duck egg, white fungus, Oyster, pork, royal jelly, chestnut, chicken liver and pork kidneys |

## EPILEPSY

| | *Spleen-kidneys yang deficiency* | *Wind-sputum* | *Sputum-fire* |
|---|---|---|---|
| **SYMPTOMS** | 2 Cold hands and feet<br>2 Cold loins<br>2 Diarrhea before dawn<br>1 Diarrhea with sticky and muddy stools<br>1 Eating very little<br>2 Edema<br>1 Edema that occurs all over the body<br>2 Fatigue<br>1 Fear of cold<br>1 Four limbs weakness<br>1 Frequent urination with clear or white urine<br>1 Mentally fatigued<br>1 Pale complexion<br>1 Palpitations<br>1 Poor appetite<br>1 Puffy face<br>1 Sputum rumbling with panting | 1 Convulsions<br>1 Discharge of clear sputum with lots of bubbles<br>1 Dizziness<br>1 Numbness of the four limbs<br>2 Seizures that occur very frequently*<br>2 Seizures with a shrill cry*<br>2 Seizures with incontinence of both urination and bowel movements*<br>2 Seizures with lockjaw or both eyes looking straight up*<br>2 Seizures preceded by headache, dizziness and congested chest*<br>1 Sputum noise in the throat<br>1 Stiffness of the tongue and unable to talk<br>1 Sudden fainting<br>1 Tics<br>1 Vomiting of clear or white, watery sputum<br>1 Dry mouth and eyes | 2 Bitter taste in the mouth<br>2 Constipation<br>1 Hungry with no appetite<br>1 Insanity<br>2 Insomnia<br>2 Jumpiness<br>4 Presence of sputum difficult to spit out*<br>1 Ringing in cars and deafness<br>2 Seizures with a shrill cry<br>3 Seizures with fainting, convulsions and vomiting of sputum* |
| **TREATMENT PRINCIPLE** | to strengthen the spleen and the kidneys and to tone the energy and the blood | to expel sputum and relieve seizures | to clear the heat in the liver and sedate fire and to transform sputum and open the cavities |
| **TREATMENT FORMULA** | Ren-Shen-Yang-Ying-Tang | Ding-Xian-Wan or Xie-Gan-An-Shen-Wan | Long-Dan-Xie-Gan-Tang with Tiao-Tan-Tang |
| **FOOD CURES** | air bladder of shark, chicken, cayenne pepper, fennel, nutmeg, black and white pepper, prickly ash, mutton, sword bean, white or yellow mustard, kidney, lobster, sardine, shrimp, sparrow, clove, dill seed, fennel, pistachio nut, sparrow egg, crab apple, raspberry and walnut | peppermint, spearmint, sweet basil, celery, coconut meat, green onion, asparagus, bamboo shoot, date, leaf or brown mustard, mustard seed, black and white pepper, fresh ginger and crown daisy | salt, cattail, agar, radish, bamboo shoot, crown daisy, date, fresh ginger, leaf or brown mustard, black and white pepper, white or yellow mustard seed, asparagus and pear |

## HYPERTHYROIDISM

| Heart-kidneys yang deficiency | Hot stomach | Liver energy congestion | Sputum-fire |
|---|---|---|---|
| 1 Discharge of watery, thin stools<br>1 Edema<br>4 Epilepsy with a long history*<br>3 Forgetfulness*<br>1 Frequent urination<br>2 Pain in the chest<br>2 Palpitations<br>1 Poor appetite<br>2 Nervousness<br>1 Shock<br>1 Speech not clear<br>1 Sputum | 2 Bad breath<br>1 Bleeding from gums<br>1 Foul breath from the mouth<br>1 Getting hungry easily<br>1 Gums swelling<br>1 Hiccups<br>1 Nosebleed<br>2 Pain in the gums with swelling<br>1 Pain in the throat<br>1 Perspiring on the head<br>2 Stomachache<br>1 Thirst and craving for cold drink<br>1 Underweight<br>2 Vomiting<br>2 Vomiting of blood<br>1 Vomiting right after eating | 2 Abdominal obstruction<br>2 Abdominal pain<br>1 Convulsions<br>2 Insomnia*<br>1 Numbness<br>2 Pain in the upper abdomen<br>2 Psychological tension*<br>2 Stomachache<br>2 Subjective sensations of objects in the throat*<br>2 Swollen tonsils*<br>1 Vomiting of blood<br>1 Worry a lot | 3 Dislike of heat*<br>2 Eat a lot*<br>3 Emotionally disturbed easily*<br>2 Excessive perspiration*<br>1 Hungry with no appetite<br>1 Insanity<br>3 Palpitations*<br>1 Ringing in ears and deafness<br>1 Sleeplessness<br>3 Swollen tonsils* |
| to tone the heart and the kidneys and to strengthen the spleen and transform sputum | to clear the heat in the stomach and disperse the energy in the liver | to regulate the energy of the liver and to remove sputum and relieve congestion | to sedate sputum-fire and to nourish the heart and secure the spirits |
| He-Che-Wan or Da-Bu-Yuan-Jian with Liu-Jun-Zi-Tang | Dao-Chi-Cheng-Qi-Tang | Si-Hai-Shu-Yu-Wan | Er-Yin-Jian with Ding-Zhi-Wan |
| dried ginger, cinnamon, wheat, water spinach, kidneys, star anise, red and black date, lobster, sardine, shrimp, sparrow, clove, dill seed, fennel, pistachio nut, sparrow egg, crab apple, raspberry and walnut | salt, lily flower, bitter endive, camellia, cattail, black fungus, spinach, strawberry, banana, cucumber and licorice | brown sugar, garlic, turmeric, kumquat, beef, cherry, bird's nest, butterfish, chicken, coconut meat, date, tofu, mustard seed, sweet rice, goose meat, mutton, jackfruit, squash, sweet potato, red and black date, rice, rock sugar, caraway seed, spearmint, common button mushroom, oregano, red bean, ambergris, dill seed, sweet basil and saffron | salt, cattail, agar, radish, bamboo shoot, crown daisy, date, fresh ginger, leaf or brown mustard, black and white pepper, white or yellow mustard seed, asparagus and pear |

| | *Liver-kidneys yin deficiency* | *Deficiency fire* | *Simultaneous deficiency of yin and energy* |
|---|---|---|---|
| SYMPTOMS | 1 Difficulty in both defecation and urination<br>3 Dizziness<br>1 Dry eyes or dry throat<br>3 Fatigue<br>1 Headache with pain in brow<br>3 Lumbago<br>1 Night blindness<br>1 Night sweats<br>3 Pain in the upper abdomen<br>1 Palms of hands and soles of feet are both hot<br>1 Sleeplessness with forgetfulness<br>1 Withering complexion | 2 Becoming angry easily*<br>1 Coughing out blood<br>1 Dry cough without sputum or coughing out slightly sticky fluids<br>1 Dry sensations in the mouth<br>1 Dry or sore throat<br>2 Excessive perspiration*<br>1 Feeling miserable<br>1 Forgetfulness<br>2 Hot sensations in body, including hands and feet*<br>1 Light but periodic fever not unlike the tide<br>1 Night sweats<br>2 Red complexion*<br>1 Ringing in ears<br>1 Seminal emission with dreams<br>1 Sleeplessness<br>1 Sputum with blood | 1 Constipation<br>1 Dry cough with scant sputum or dry mouth<br>1 Discharge of dry stools<br>1 Excessive perspiration<br>3 Fatigue*<br>1 Hot sensations in the palms of hand and soles of feet<br>2 Light stomachache with swelling<br>2 Palpitations<br>1 Poor appetite<br>1 Ringing in ears<br>1 Scant urine<br>1 Sore throat<br>3 Thirst*<br>1 "Tidal" fever in the afternoon |
| TREATMENT PRINCIPLE | to tone the energy & the yin and to water the kidneys & nourish the liver | to water the yin, increase body fluids and clear the stomach and nourish the lung | to strengthen the energy and nourish the yin and to tone the lungs and water the kidneys |
| TREATMENT FORMULA | Sheng-Mai-San with Yi-Guan-Jian | Yu-Nü-Jian with Zeng-Yi-Tang | Di-Huang-Yin-Zi |
| FOOD CURES | bird's nest, cheese, chicken egg, kidney bean, brown sugar, mussel, abalone, asparagus, chicken egg, cuttlefish, duck, duck egg, white fungus, oyster, pork, royal jelly, chestnut, chicken liver & pork kidneys | banana, bitter endive, black fungus, salt, spinach, strawberry, bamboo shoot, cucumber, Job's-tears, liver, leaf beet, mung bean, peppermint, purslane, lily flower, salt, cattail, chicken egg, duck egg, asparagus, royal jelly, pork and oyster | bird's nest, cheese, kidney bean, abalone, asparagus, chicken egg, cuttlefish, duck, duck egg, white fungus, oyster, pork, royal jelly, grape, longan nuts, maltose, mandarin fish, Irish potato, sweet rice, apple cucumber, bog bean, gold carp, carrot, chestnut, ham, horse bean, hyacinth bean, Job's-tears, royal jelly, string bean, whitefish, yam, red and black date, mutton, squash and rock sugar |

## HYPOTHYROIDISM

| *Spleen-kidneys yang deficiency* | *Heart-kidneys yang deficiency* | *Spleen-kidneys yang deficiency* | *Simultaneous deficiency of kidneys yin & kidneys yang* |
|---|---|---|---|
| 1 Being physically weak and too tired to talk<br>1 Cold hands and feet<br>1 Cold loins<br>2 Diarrhea before dawn<br>1 Diarrhea with sticky and muddy stools<br>2 Dysentery<br>1 Eating very little<br>2 Edema<br>1 Edema that occurs all over the body<br>2 Fatigue<br>1 Fear of cold<br>1 Four limbs weakness<br>1 Frequent urination with clear or white urine<br>4 Impotence in men and irregular menstruation in women*<br>1 Mentally fatigued<br>1 Sputum rumbling with panting | 2 Chest pain*<br>2 Cold limbs*<br>1 Discharge of watery, thin stools<br>2 Edema<br>1 Frequent urination<br>2 History of hydropericardium and cardiac insufficiency*<br>2 Love of lying down*<br>2 Pain in the chest<br>2 Palpitations<br>2 Nervousness<br>1 Shock<br>1 Sputum | 1 Being physically weak and too tired to talk<br>1 Cold hands and feet<br>1 Cold loins<br>2 Diarrhea before dawn<br>1 Diarrhea with sticky and muddy stools<br>1 Dysentery<br>1 Eating very little<br>1 Edema that occurs all over the body<br>1 Fatigue<br>1 Fear of cold<br>2 Feeble breath*<br>1 Frequent urination with clear or white urine<br>2 History of myxedema*<br>2 Low body temperature*<br>1 Mentally fatigued<br>1 Sputum rumbling with panting | 1 Cough<br>1 Decreased sexual desire in men<br>2 Dry mouth*<br>1 Edema<br>2 Fatigue<br>1 Grey hair and falling out of hair<br>1 Impotence in men<br>1 Infertility in women<br>1 Lumbago<br>1 Mental fatigue<br>2 Panting<br>2 Thirst<br>1 Weakened legs<br>3 Yellowish urine* |
| to warm the kidneys and strengthen the spleen | to warm the heart yang and strengthen the kidneys energy | to strengthen the yang energy and to warm th kidneys and the spleen | to tone both the yin and the yang |
| You-Gui-Wan | Ling-Gui-Zhu-Gan-Tang with Shen-Qi-Wan | Si-Ni-Jia-Ren-Shen-Tang | Zuo-Gui-Wan |
| air bladder of shark, chicken, cayenne pepper, fennel, nutmeg, black and white pepper, prickly ash, mutton, sword bean, white or yellow mustard, kidneys, lobster, sardine, shrimp, sparrow, clove, dill seed, pistachio nut, sparrow egg, crab apple, raspberry and walnut | dried ginger, cinnamon, wheat, water spinach, kidneys, star anise, red and black date, lobster, sardine, shrimp, sparrow, clove, dill seed, fennel, pistachio nut, sparrow egg, crab apple, raspberry and walnut | air bladder of shark, chicken, cayenne pepper, fennel, nutmeg, black and white pepper, prickly ash, mutton, sword bean, white or yellow mustard, kidneys lobster, sardine, shrimp, sparrow love, dill seed, pistachio nut, sparrow egg, crab apple, raspberry and walnuts | abalone, asparagus, chicken egg, cuttlefish, duck, duck egg, white fungus, oyster, pork, royal jelly, chestnut, chicken liver, pork kidneys, lobster, sardine, shrimp, sparrow, clove, dill seed, fennel, pistachio nut, sparrow egg, crab apple, raspberry and walnut |

ARTHRITIS AND RHEUMATOID ARTHRITIS

| | *Wind-predominating type* | *Cold-predominating type* | *Dampness-predominating type* |
|---|---|---|---|
| SYMPTOMS | 1 Diarrhea containing undigested food<br>1 Discharge of watery, thin stools<br>1 Dislike of wind<br>1 Headache accompanied by fear of wind<br>1 Headache with heavy sensations in the head<br>1 Itchy skin that becomes almost intolerable<br>1 Light cough<br>1 Nasal discharge<br>1 Numbness in the skin of the face<br>3 Pain in all the joints that attacks suddenly*<br>3 Pain in the joints that shifts from one joint to another*<br>1 Shaking of four limbs and body<br>1 Sneezing<br>1 Stiffness of muscles<br>1 Stuffed nose with heavy voice<br>1 Tickle in the throat | 1 Abdominal pain<br>1 Absence of perspiration in hot weather<br>1 Absence of thirst in mouth<br>1 Abundant watering of eyes<br>1 Clear and long streams of urine in large amounts<br>1 Cold chest or cold hands and feet<br>1 Cold sensations in the body<br>1 Contraction of tendons and mucles<br>1 Coughing out and vomiting bubbles of wate<br>1 Diarrhea with sticky and muddy stools<br>1 Dislike of cold<br>1 Hands and feet extremely cold<br>1 Headache with pain in back of neck<br>1 Love of hot drink<br>1 Pale complexion<br>5 Severe pain in the joints* | 1 Abdominal pain with abdominal rumbling<br>1 Diarrhea<br>1 Diminished urination<br>1 Discharge of hard stool followed by sticky, turbid stool<br>1 Discharge of watery pus through openings of carbuncles<br>1 Discharge of yellow, sticky fluids from blisters that break open<br>1 Dizziness<br>1 Eczema<br>1 Edema on the dorsum of foot<br>1 Four limbs weakness<br>1 Headache as if the head were being wrapped up<br>1 Heavy sensation in body or in any part of the body<br>1 Love of hot drink<br>1 Love of sleep and heavy sensations in the body<br>2 Pain always in same joints with heavy sensations of the body*<br>2 Pain in the loins as if sitting in water with heaviness in body*<br>2 Pain starts mostly from lower regions of the body* |
| TREATMENT PRINCIPLE | to expel the wind, disperse cold and remove dampness | to warm the body and disperse cold and to remove wind and dampness | to strengthen the spleen and remove dampness and to expel wind and disperse cold |
| TREATMENT FORMULA | Fang-Feng-Tang | Wu-Tou-Tang | Yi-Yi-Ren-Tang |
| FOOD CURES | peppermint, spearmint, sweet basil, celery, coconut meat and green onion | cayenne pepper, dill seed, fennel, fresh ginger, mustard seed, prickly ash, star anise, white or yellow mustard and wine | carp, celery, horse bean, jellyfish skin, Job's-tears, prickly ash, hyacinth bean, oregano, sweet basil, adzuki bean, bamboo shoot, soybean sprouts and rosin |

## RHEUMATOID ARTHRITIS

| *Heat-predominating type* | *Wind-cold-dampness type* | *Heat-excess yin-deficiency type* | *Deficiency type* |
|---|---|---|---|
| 1 Acute onset of pain in the joints | 5 Joints neither red nor burning* | 3 Bitter taste in the mouth | 1 Breathing with a low sound and feeble breath |
| 1 Constipation | 5 Pain affected by change in weather* | 3 Dry mouth | 2 Chronic pain in the joints over a long duration* |
| 1 Diminished urination | 2 Pain gets worse when cold and better when warm | 3 Joints swollen and painful with burning sensations | 1 Eating very little |
| 1 Discharge of copious, yellow, sticky sputum | 5 Pain involving one or two joints only* | 5 Arthritis with a longer history* | 1 Feeble voice with intermittent speech |
| 1 Dry lips or teeth | 2 Arthritis with a shorter history | 3 Pain gets better with coolness at the beginning, then gradually gets better with warmth | 1 Hiccups that are slow and occur infrequently |
| 1 Escape of gas from the anus with noise | 1 Stiffness of joints more severe in the morning | 3 Stiffness of joints | 1 Hoarseness |
| 1 Light fever | | | 1 Light and clear voice with low and feeble tone |
| 1 Love of cold drink | | | 1 Little power |
| 2 Pain in the joints that shifts around* | | | 1 Pain in inner part of stomach that lessens after meals and desire for massage |
| 2 Pain in the joints with burning sensations* | | | 3 Pain in the joints that is more severe at night* |
| 2 Pain very severe with inability to extend or flex the joints* | | | 1 Prolonged dizziness |
| 1 Red complexion, red eyes, or red urine | | | 1 Retention of urine |
| 1 Short streams of scant urine | | | 1 Scant and handicapped breathing |
| 1 Stools with an extremely bad smell | | | 1 Scant breathing that becomes intermittent when talking too much |
| 1 Thirst with an incessant desire to drink | | | 1 Small breaths |
| 1 Throat swollen & red, producing rotten liquid | | | 1 Talking in weak voice |
| 1 Urine with an extremely bad smell | | | 1 Underweight |
| to clear heat and to expel wind and remove dampness | to warm the body & disperse cold & to expel dampness & disperse wind | to disperse cold and remove dampness and to transform sputum and activate the blood | to strengthen the kidneys and the body energy and to promote energy and blood circulation to relieve pain |
| Bai-Hu-Jia-Gui-Zhi-Tang | Juan-Bi-Tang | Gui-Zhi-Shao-Yao-Zhi-Mu-Tang | Juan-Bi-Tang |
| banana, bitter endive, black fungus, salt, spinach, strawberry, bamboo shoot, cucumber, Job's-tears, laver, leaf beet, mung bean, peppermint and purslane | peppermint, (including oil), spearmint, sweet basil, cayenne pepper, fennel, fresh ginger, mustard seed, star anise and prickly ash leaf | banana, bitter endive, black fungus, salt, spinach, strawberry, bamboo shoot, cucumber, Job's-tears, laver, leaf beet, mung bean, peppermint and purslane | soya milk, goose meat, milk, royal jelly, grape, longan nuts, mandarin fish, milk, maltose and Irish potato |

## COMMON COLD AND FLU

| | Wind-cold | Wind-heat | Summer heat |
|---|---|---|---|
| SYMPTOMS | 1 Absence of perspiration in hot weather<br>1 Breathing through the nose<br>1 Clear discharge from nose<br>1 Cough with heavy, unclear sounds and clear sputum<br>1 Diarrhea<br>3 Dislike of cold*<br>1 Dizziness<br>1 Headache with dizziness<br>1 Hoarseness at the beginning of illness<br>1 Itch in the throat<br>2 Light fever*<br>1 Loss of voice<br>1 Nosebleed<br>1 Pain in the body shifting around with no fixed region<br>1 Pain in the joints<br>1 Stuffed nose<br>1 Vomiting | 2 Coughing out yellowish sputum<br>2 Fever appears more severe than chills*<br>1 Headache with dizziness<br>1 Intolerance of light in eyes with swelling and dislike of wind<br>1 Muddy discharge from nose<br>1 Nosebleed<br>1 Pain in the eyes<br>2 Pain in the throat*<br>4 Perspiration*<br>1 Red eyes<br>1 Thirst<br>1 Toothache<br>1 Yellow urine<br>1 Yellowish discharge from the nose | 1 Chest discomfort<br>1 Constipation<br>1 Cough<br>2 Dizziness*<br>1 Dry lips or dry sensations in the mouth<br>1 Fatigue<br>1 Feeling miserable and thirsty<br>1 Heavy sensations in the head<br>2 High fever*<br>1 Nausea and vomiting<br>2 No perspiration*<br>1 Obstructed urination with red urine<br>1 Oppressed and rapid breath<br>1 Perspiration due to hot weather or putting on warm clothes<br>1 Perspire a lot<br>1 Scant and reddish urine<br>1 Thirst |
| TREATMENT PRINCIPLE | to induce perspiration and expand the lungs and to disperse cold | to induce perspiration and clear heat | to clear summer heat and transform dampness with aromatic herbs |
| TREATMENT FORMULA | Jing-Fang-Bai-Du-San | Yin-Qiao-San | Xin-Jia-Xiang-Ru-Yin |
| FOOD CURES | peppermint (including oil), spearmint, sweet basil, cayenne pepper, fennel, fresh ginger, mustard seed, star anise and prickly ash leaf | banana, bitter endive, black fungus, salt, spinach, strawberry, bamboo shoot, cucumber, Job's-tears, laver, leaf beet, mung bean, peppermint, purslane, spearmint, sweet basil, celery, coconut meat and green onion | apple, apple cucumber, cantaloupe, coconut liquid, hyacinth bean, lemon, watermelon, banana, bamboo shoot, bitter endive, bitter gourd, celery, chicken egg white, crab, mung bean, peppermint and purslane |

## BACILLARY DYSENTERY
Acute

Chronic

## BRONCHITIS
Acute

| Superficial dampness-heat | Heat poisoning penetrating into the deep regions | Spleen yang deficiency | Cold-wind restricting the lungs |
|---|---|---|---|

| | | | |
|---|---|---|---|
| 2 Abdominal pain* | 2 Acute abdominal pain* | 3 Abdominal pain* | 2 Common cold |
| 2 Congested chest* | 2 Acute onset of symptoms* | 3 Chronic bowel movement difficulty* | 3 Cough with heavy, unclear sounds and clear sputum* |
| 1 Diarrhea with forceful discharge of stools | 1 Breathing difficulty | 1 Cold in the forehead that does not warm up | 1 Dislike of cold |
| 1 Discharge of yellowish-red, turbid stools with bad smell | 1 Cold and hot sensations together | 3 Dysentery with discharge of pus and blood* | 3 Fever* |
| 1 Excessive perspiration | 2 Discharge of pus and blood from anus* | 2 Edema | 1 Headache |
| 2 Greasy taste in the mouth* | 1 Discharge of blood from the mouth | 3 Hot sensations with nausea* | 1 Itch in the throat |
| 2 Jaundice | 1 Headache that is severe | 3 Intermittent diarrhea* | 1 Lack of perspiration |
| 1 Low fever | 2 High fever* | 2 Stomachache | 3 Nasal congestion* |
| 1 Pain in the joints of the four limbs, with swelling & heaviness | 1 Misty vision | | 3 Nasal discharge* |
| 1 Perspiration on hands and feet or the head | 1 Nosebleed | | 2 Panting |
| 1 Reddish and scant urine | 1 Not alert | | |
| 1 Retention of urine | 1 Severe pain in whole body | | |
| 1 Swollen body of the tongue | 1 Twitching | | |
| 2 Thirst with no desire for drink* | 2 Very difficult bowel movements* | | |
| 1 Yellowish body | 1 Vomiting of blood | | |

| | | | |
|---|---|---|---|
| to clear heat and remove dampness and to regulate energy and harmonize the blood | to clear heat and remove dampness and to cool the blood and counteract poisoning | to warm the spleen yang and to clear heat and remove dampness | to disperse wind and cold and to expand the lungs and stop cough |

| | | | |
|---|---|---|---|
| Shao-Yao-Tang | Ge-Gan-Qin-Lian-Tang | Huang-Lian-Tang | Xing-Su-San |

| | | | |
|---|---|---|---|
| carp, celery, horse bean, jellyfish skin, Job's-tears, prickly ash, hyacinth bean, oregano, sweet basil, adzuki bean, bamboo shoot, soybean sprouts, rosin, banana, bitter endive, black fungus, salt, spinach, strawberry, cucumber, leaf beet, mung bean, peppermint and purslane | adzuki bean, banana, bitter endive, bitter gourd, chicken egg white, chicken gallbladder, cucumber, fig, mung bean, black and white pepper, peppermint, squash and strawberry | air bladder of shark, chicken, cayenne pepper, fennel, nutmeg, black and white pepper, prickly ash, mutton, sword bean and white or yellow mustard | almond, rock sugar, asparagus, peppermint (including oil), spearmint, sweet basil, cayenne pepper, fennel, fresh ginger, mustard seed, star anise, prickly ash leaf, leaf or brown mustard, walnut, common button mushroom and tangerine |

|  | *Wind-heat offending the lungs* | *Lungs-dryness* | *Spleen-dampness offending the lungs* |
|---|---|---|---|
| **SYMPTOMS** | 1 Common cold<br>2 Coughing out yellow and sticky sputum*<br>1 Dislike of wind<br>3 Fever*<br>1 Flickering nostrils<br>1 Headache<br>1 Pain in the chest<br>1 Pain in the throat<br>3 Perspiration*<br>3 Sore throat*<br>2 Sputum with blood<br>1 Thirst in the mouth with a desire for drink | 1 Coughing out blood<br>3 Dry cough*<br>3 Dry cough without sputum or coughing out slightly sticky fluid*<br>1 Dry nose<br>1 Dry throat<br>1 Dryness in mouth and nose<br>1 Loss of voice<br>2 Morbid hunger<br>2 Thirst<br>2 Nosebleed<br>1 Pain in the throat<br>1 Presence of sputum that can't be coughed out easily<br>1 Tickle in the throat | 3 Cough<br>1 Discharge of sputum that can be coughed out easily<br>2 Discharge of white, watery sputum<br>2 Fatigue of the four limbs<br>2 Heavy sensations in head as if head were wrapped up<br>2 Heavy sensations in the limbs and trunk<br>2 Inability to lie on back<br>2 Poor appetite<br>2 Short breath<br>1 Swelling of hands and feet<br>1 Vomiting |
| **TREATMENT PRINCIPLE** | to expel wind and clear heat and to expand the lungs and stop cough | to clear heat and produce fluids and to lubricate dryness-lungs and rescue the lungs | to strengthen the spleen, dry dampness, transform sputum and regulate the lungs |
| **TREATMENT FORMULA** | Sang-Ju-Yin (1) | Qing-Re-Jiu-Fei-Tang | Er-Chen-Tang |
| **FOOD CURES** | apple, apple cucumber, sweet rice, lemon, sweet potato, tofu, tomato, white sugar, coriander and parsley | almond, apple, apricot, asparagus, white fungus, licorice, loquat, peanut, pear peel, rock sugar and tangerine | gold carp, corncob, horse bean, Job's-tears, prickly ash, adzuki bean, bamboo shoot, cheese, ambergris, barley, common carp, cucumber, mung bean, seaweed, shepherd's purse and star fruit |

## BRONCHIAL ASTHMA

| Liver-fire attacking the lungs | Cold sputum obstructing the lungs | Sputum-heat accumulated in the lungs | Lungs-dampness |
|---|---|---|---|
| 5 Cough that causes pain in the upper abdomen* | 1 Cold limbs | 2 Acute respiration and gasping for air | 2 Congested chest |
| 1 Cough with sticky sputum | 1 Congested chest with a choking sensation | 7 Cough out yellowish or sticky sputum* | 4 Copious, sticky sputum* |
| 2 Coughing out blood | 5 Cough out thin and watery sputum* | 3 Panting | 2 Cough with gasping for air |
| 1 Dry throat | 1 Love of hot or warm drink | 3 Swelling of the lungs | 2 Insomnia |
| 1 Painful sensations running through chest and ribs | 1 No perspiration | 1 Thirst with craving for cold drink | 2 Nausea |
| 1 Rapid breath | 3 Pain in the chest | 4 Wheezing | 2 Palpitations |
| 2 Red face | 3 Panting | | 2 Poor appetite |
| 2 Sputum with blood | 1 Swelling of the lungs | | 2 Vomiting |
| 1 Thirst | 4 Wheezing* | | 2 Underweight |
| 4 Vomiting of blood | | | |
| to calm the liver, sedate fire and clear the heat in the lungs and stop cough | to warm the lungs and expel cold and to remove sputum | to expand the lungs, clear heat, transform sputum and push down the lungs energy | to push down lungs energy, transform sputum, promote energy circulation and stop panting and cough |
| Ke-Xue-Fang | She-Gan-Ma-Huang-Tang | Ma-Xing-Shi-Gan-Tang | San-Zi-Tang with Er-Chen-Tang |
| asparagus, soya milk, duck egg, olive, spinach, chestnut, shepherd's purse, rye, black fungus, vinegar, abalone, asparagus, chicken egg, white fungus, pork and royal jelly | fresh ginger, leaf or brown mustard, black and white pepper and white or yellow mustard seed | apple peel, common button mushroom, grapefruit peel, radish and pear | cheese, Job's-tears, adzuki bean, ambergris, barley, bamboo shoot, common carp, cucumber, mung bean, seaweed, shepherd's purse and star fruit |

| | *Lungs unable to push down energy* | *Lungs energy deficiency* | *Loss of the kidneys capacity for absorbing inspiration* |
|---|---|---|---|
| SYMPTOMS | 1 Cough<br>3 Discharge of copious, whitish and sticky sputum*<br>1 Dislike of cold<br>1 Dry throat but without thirst<br>1 Inability to lie on back<br>3 More exhaling than inhaling*<br>1 Pain in the throat<br>1 Palpitations<br>1 Short streams of reddish urine<br>1 Swelling of the lower abdomen<br>3 Wheezing that persists or occurs all of a sudden*<br>3 Wheezing triggered or intensified by moving around* | 1 Breathing difficulty<br>1 Cold limbs<br>2 Common cold<br>1 Copious, clear and watery sputum<br>2 Cough<br>1 Excessive perspiration<br>2 Fatigue<br>1 Fear of cold<br>1 Dislike of wind<br>2 Light wheezing<br>1 Low and weak voice<br>1 Shortness of breath<br>1 Smooth urination<br>2 Swelling of the lungs<br>1 Too tired to talk | 1 Breathing difficulty<br>1 Cold limbs<br>1 Fear of cold<br>1 Frequent fear of cold both in hands and feet<br>3 Frequent urination*<br>2 More inhaling than exhaling*<br>3 Panting that is triggered or intensified by moving around*<br>1 Perspiration due to hot weather or putting on warm clothes<br>1 Shortness of breath<br>2 Swelling of the lungs<br>2 Wheezing<br>2 Whitish sputum* |
| TREATMENT PRINCIPLE | to push down upsurging lungs energy, transform sputum and relieve panting | to strengthen lungs energy, solidify the superficial region and relieve panting and cough | to tone and warm the kidneys |
| TREATMENT FORMULA | Shen-Zhe-Zhen-Qi-Tang | Bu-Fei-Tang | Shen-Qi-Wan |
| FOOD CURES | adzuki bean, ambergris, barley, bamboo shoot, seaweed, black soybean, almond, areca nut, buckwheat, common carp, cashew nut, coriander, grapefruit peel, loquat, malt, nutmeg, pea, black and white pepper, radish, rice bran, sword bean and clove | cheese, Job's-tears, yam grape, longan nut, maltose, mandarin fish, Irish potato, sweet rice, apple cucumber, bog bean, gold carp, carrot, chestnut, ham, horse bean, hyacinth bean, royal jelly, string bean, whitefish, yam, red and black date, mutton, squash and rock sugar | abalone, asparagus, chicken egg, cuttlefish, duck, duck egg, white fungus, milk, lobster, oyster, pork, royal jelly, chestnut, chicken liver, pork kidneys, sardine, shrimp, sparrow, clove, dill seed, fennel, pistachio nut, sparrow egg, crab apple, raspberry and walnut |

中
医
疗
法

## PNEUMONIA

| Wind-warm-superficial | Sputum energy heat | Heat enters the pericardium | Extreme heat generating wind |
|---|---|---|---|
| 4 Acute onset of symptoms* <br> 2 Cough <br> 4 Dry mouth or thirst* <br> 1 Fear of cold <br> 4 High fever* <br> 1 Light thirst <br> 1 Nasal discharge <br> 1 Slight dislike of cold <br> 1 Stuffy nose <br> 1 Wheezing from the throat | 1 Cough and panting <br> 1 Coughing out sputum containing silky blood <br> 1 Discharge of copious, yellow and sticky sputum <br> 1 Dry mouth with desire to wash mouth, not to drink <br> 2 High fever that does not go down for a prolonged period of time* <br> 1 Light cough <br> 1 Oppressed and rapid breath <br> 1 Scanty urine <br> 3 Shivering* <br> 2 Sputum of a rusty color* <br> 2 Thirst* <br> 3 Wheezing with sputum noise* | 2 Being slow and dull in response <br> 3 Chest pain* <br> 1 Difficulty in speech <br> 3 High fever* <br> 1 Illusive hearing <br> 1 Illusive vision <br> 1 Incontinence of both bowel movements and urination <br> 1 Indifferent in expression <br> 1 Mental dizziness <br> 3 Slightly cold limbs* <br> 3 Sputum noise in the throat* <br> 1 Twitching | 3 Convulsions* <br> 1 Fainting <br> 1 Feeling troubled, quick-tempered and insecure <br> 3 High feve* <br> 1 Muscular tightening <br> 1 Neck stiffness <br> 3 Red complexion* <br> 3 Stiff neck and limbs* <br> 3 Twitching or spasms of the four limbs* <br> 1 Dry and shivering tongue |
| to induce perspiration with pungent and cool herbs, to expand the lungs and transform sputum | to clear heat and expand the lungs and to transform sputum and push down the upsurging energy of the lungs | to expand the lungs & transform sputum & to clear the heat in the heart & promote blood circulation throughout the whole body | to nourish the yin and clear heat and to calm the liver and stop the internal wind |
| Yin-Qiao-San | Ma-Xing-Shi-Gan-Tang with Wei-Jing-Tang | Wei-Jing-Tang with Qing-Gong-Tang | Ling-Jiao-Gou-Teng-Tang with Qing-Ying-Tang |
| apple, apple cucumber, sweet rice, lemon, sweet potato, tofu, tomato, white sugar, coriander and parsley | banana, bitter endive, black fungus, salt, spinach, strawberry, bamboo shoot, cucumber, Job's-tears, laver, leaf beet, mung bean, peppermint, purslane, salt, cattail, agar, radish, crown daisy, date, fresh ginger, leaf or brown mustard, black and white pepper, white or yellow mustard seed, asparagus and pear | asparagus, pear peel, banana, bitter endive, black fungus, salt, spinach, strawberry, bamboo shoot, cucumber, Job's-tears, liver, leaf beet, mung bean, peppermint, purslane, lily flower, salt and cattail | peppermint, spearmint, sweet basil, celery, coconut meat, green onion, chicken egg, bitter endive, camellia, cattail, black fungus, salt, spinach, strawberry, banana, bamboo shoot, crab and water clam |

## ACUTE GASTROENTERITIS

| | Cold-dampness | Summer heat and dampness | Stomach indigestion |
|---|---|---|---|
| **SYMPTOMS** | 2 Abdominal pain with rumbling*<br>1 Absence of perspiration in hot weather<br>2 Acute attack of vomiting and diarrhea*<br>1 Clear and watery vaginal discharge with fishy smell<br>1 Cold sensations in lower abdomen-genitals region<br>1 Cough<br>1 Coughing out sputum with a low sound<br>3 Diarrhea with discharge of watery stool without offensive smell*<br>1 Discharge of sputum that can be coughed out easily<br>1 Edema in the four limbs<br>1 Headache<br>1 Movement difficulty<br>1 Pain in the body<br>1 Pain in the joints<br>1 Scant and clear urine<br>1 Stomachache | 1 Abdominal fullness<br>2 Burning sensation in the anus*<br>1 Chest discomfort<br>1 Diarrhea<br>2 Fever*<br>3 Forceful discharge of stools during defecation*<br>1 Lack of appetite<br>1 Perspiration due to hot weather or putting on warm clothes<br>1 Reddish urine<br>3 Sudden attack of vomiting and diarrhea*<br>1 Thirst<br>2 Vomiting of substances with acid*<br>1 Yellowish and watery stools | 3 Abdominal pain or swelling that lessens after bowel movement*<br>2 Acid swallowing and belching of bad breath<br>3 Belching with poor appetite*<br>1 Discharge of watery, thin stools<br>1 Insomnia<br>1 Sour and bad breath from mouth<br>2 Stomachache<br>3 Stools with an extremely bad smell*<br>3 Vomiting and diarrhea simultaneously*<br>1 Vomiting of sour and badsmelling foods, with a love of cold drink |
| **TREATMENT PRINCIPLE** | to transform dampness-sputum with aromatic herbs and to disperse cold and dry dampness | to clear heat and remove dampness and to regulate the stomach and intestines | to promote digestion and regulate the stomach and intestine |
| **TREATMENT FORMULA** | Huo-Xiang-Zheng-Qi-San | Ge-Gen-Qin-Lian-Tang | Bao-He-Wan |
| **FOOD CURES** | cayenne pepper, dill seed, fennel, fresh ginger, mustard seed, prickly ash, star anise, white or yellow mustard, wine, carp, celery, horse bean, jellyfish skin, Job's-tears, hyacinth bean, oregano, sweet basil, adzuki bean, bamboo shoot, soybean sprouts and rosin | banana, bamboo shoot, bitter endive, bitter gourd, celery, chicken egg white, crab, cucumber, mung bean, peppermint, purslane, carp, horse bean, jellyfish skin, Job's-tears, prickly ash, hyacinth bean, oregano, sweet basil, adzuki bean, soybean sprouts and rosin | asafoetida, buckwheat, castor bean, jellyfish, malt, peach, radish, water chestnut, cardamon seed, cayenne pepper, coriander, grapefruit, jackfruit, malt, sweet basil, tea and tomato |

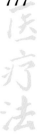

## CHRONIC GASTRITIS AND PEPTIC ULCERS

| *Spleen-stomach yang deficiency syndrome* | *Stomach indigestion* | *Liver energy offending the stomach* | *Stomach yin deficiency* |
|---|---|---|---|
| 2 Abdominal pain* | 3 Abdominal pain or swelling that lessens after bowel movement* | 1 Abdominal rumblin | 1 Burning pain in stomach |
| 2 Clear urine* | 1 Acid swallowing and belching of bad breath | 3 Belching | 1 Constipation |
| 1 Cold limbs | 2 Belching with poor appetite* | 1 Chest discomfort | 1 Dry cough |
| 2 Diarrhea and vomiting that occur frequently* | 1 Discharge of watery, thin stools | 3 Hiccups | 1 Dry lips |
| 1 Fatigue | 2 Dry stools* | 1 Irregular bowel movements | 2 Dry sensations in the mouth with craving for drink* |
| 1 Intermittent hiccups with low sound | 1 Hot sensations in the body | 2 Pain in inner part of stomach | 1 Dysphagia |
| 1 Love of warmth and massage | 1 Insomnia | 2 Painful sensations running through ribs on both sides | 1 Hiccups |
| 1 Pain gets worse with fatigue and hunger and better with rest and eating | 1 Red complexion | 6 Stomachache that worsens with emotional disturbances* | 1 Hot sensations in the limbs |
| 1 Pale complexion | 1 Sour and bad breath from mouth | 1 Vomiting of acid or blood | 1 Indigestion |
| 2 Perspiration with cold limbs* | 2 Stomachache that worsens on pressure of hand* | | 1 Insomnia |
| 1 Poor appetite | 2 Stools with an extremely bad smell* | | 1 Light but periodic fever not unlike the tide |
| 1 Shortness of breath | 2 Vomiting and diarrhea simultaneously* | | 1 Low fever |
| 1 Stomachache | 1 Vomiting of sour and bad-smelling foods, with a love of cold drink | | 1 No appetite |
| 1 Upset stomach | | | 1 Palpitations |
| 1 Vomiting of undigested foods | | | 2 Stomachache that worsens on an empty stomach* |
| 1 Water noise in the stomach | | | 2 Vomiting* |
| | | | 1 Vomiting of blood |
| to warm the middle region and disperse cold and to strengthen the spleen and the stomach | to promote digestion and harmonize the stomach | to disperse the liver energy and harmonize the stomach | to strengthen the stomach & tone the stomach yin energy & to clear the heat in the stomach & push down the upsurging energy of the stomach |
| Fu-Zi-Li-Zhong-Wan | Bao-He-Wan | Si-Ni-San | Mai-Men-Dong-Tang |
| air bladder of shark, chicken, cayenne pepper, fennel, nutmeg, black and white pepper, prickly ash, mutton, sword bean, white or yellow mustard, cardamon seed, carp, cinnamon, garlic and beef | asafoetida, buckwheat, castor bean, jellyfish, malt, peach, radish, water chestnut, cardamon seed, cayenne pepper, coriander, grapefruit, jackfruit, malt, sweet basil, tea and tomato | carp, celery, corn silk, brown sugar, sweet orange, kumquat, barley, peanut, red and black date, chestnut and white fungus | alfalfa, ginseng leaf, bird's nest, cheese, kidney bean, abalone, asparagus, chicken egg, cuttlefish, duck, duck egg, white fungus, oyster, pork, royal jelly |

CHRONIC GASTRITIS AND PEPTIC ULCERS (CONTINUED)

NEPHRITIS
Acute

| | Spleen-stomach yang deficiency | Stomach blood-coagulations | Cold-wind restricting the lungs |
|---|---|---|---|
| **SYMPTOMS** | 1 Abdominal pain<br>2 Cold limbs*<br>1 Diarrhea<br>1 Fatigue<br>1 Intermittent hiccups with low sound<br>2 Love of warmth and massage*<br>1 Pain worsens with fatigue and hunger<br>1 Pain improves with rest and eating<br>1 Poor appetite<br>1 Shortness of breath<br>2 Stomachache with dull pain*<br>1 Upset stomach<br>3 Vomiting of undigested foods, acid, or clear water*<br>1 Water noise in the stomach<br>1 Withered and yellowish complexion | 2 Feeling of emptiness and sickness in abdomen<br>2 Pain worsens with massage<br>5 Pain in inner part of stomach with prickling sensation and swelling*<br>2 Pain in inner part of stomach that is acute after meals, with aversion to massage<br>6 Pain in fixed region without shifting around*<br>3 Vomiting of blood | 2 Common cold<br>1 Cough with heavy, unclear sounds and clear sputum<br>3 Dislike of cold*<br>1 Dry stools<br>2 Edema in the head, face and four limbs*<br>2 Fever*<br>1 Headache<br>1 Itch in the throat<br>1 Lack of perspiration<br>1 Nasal congestion<br>1 Nasal discharge<br>2 Panting<br>1 Scant and yellowish urine<br>1 Thirst |
| **TREATMENT PRINCIPLE** | to strengthen the spleen and the stomach and to warm the middle region and expel cold | to activate the blood and transform blood coagulations and to harmonize the stomach and relieve pain | to expand the lungs, induce perspiration and promote energy circulation |
| **TREATMENT FORMULA** | Li-Zhong-Tang | Jia-Wei-Shi-Xiao-San | Yue-Bi-Tang |
| **FOOD CURES** | air bladder of shark, chicken, cayenne pepper, fennel, nutmeg, black and white pepper, prickly ash, mutton, sword bean, white or yellow mustard, cardamon seed, carp, cinnamon, garlic and beef | saffron, ambergris, brown sugar, chestnut, eggplant, peach, black soybean, sturgeon, sweet basil, crab, distillers' grains and papaya | almond, rock sugar, asparagus, peppermint (including oil), spearmint, sweet basil, cayenne pepper, fennel, fresh ginger, mustard seed, star anise, prickly ash leaf, leaf or brown mustard, walnut, common button mushroom and tangerine |

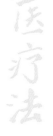

Chronic

| Wind-heat offending the lungs | Dampness heat | Spleen-dampness offending the lungs | Spleen-kidneys yang deficiency |
|---|---|---|---|
| 1 Common cold<br>1 Cough<br>1 Coughing out yellow and sticky sputum<br>1 Dry stools<br>2 Fever*<br>1 Flickering of nostrils<br>2 Headache*<br>2 Light edema in the four limbs, gradually becoming more severe*<br>1 Pain in the chest<br>1 Pain in the throat<br>2 Scant and reddish urine*<br>2 Sputum with blood<br>2 Sore throat*<br>1 Thirst in the mouth with a desire for drink | 2 Dry mouth<br>2 Frequent urination in short, red dish streams<br>5 Light edema*<br>5 Sore throat with pus in the back of the throat*<br>6 Swollen tonsils* | 1 Abdominal swelling with watery stools<br>1 Cough<br>1 Discharge of sputum that can be coughed out easily<br>1 Discharge of white, watery sputum<br>1 Fatigue of the four limbs<br>2 Fear of cold*<br>1 Heavy sensations in head as if head were wrapped up<br>1 Heavy sensations in the limbs and trunk<br>1 Inability to lie on back<br>2 Perspiration or light perspiration*<br>1 Poor appetite<br>3 Severe edema particularly in the head and face and the upper half of body*<br>1 Shortness of breath<br>1 Sore throat<br>1 Swelling of hands and feet<br>1 Vomiting | 2 Abdominal swelling like a drum*<br>1 Ascites<br>1 Being physically weak and too tired to talk<br>1 Cold hands and feet<br>1 Cold loins<br>2 Diarrhea before dawn<br>1 Diarrhea with sticky and muddy stools<br>2 Edema that occurs all over the body<br>2 Fatigue<br>1 Fear of cold<br>1 Four limbs weakness<br>1 Frequent urination in clear or white streams<br>1 Mentally fatigued<br>1 Poor appetite<br>1 Scant and clear urine<br>1 Sputum rumbling with panting |
| to expand the lungs and clear the heat in the lungs and to promote urination | to water and nourish the kidney yin and to clear heat and detoxicate | to expand the lungs, strengthen the spleen and reduce edema | to warm the spleen and kidneys yang and to promote energy circulation and urination |
| Yin-Qiao-San | Xiao-Ji-Yin-Zi | Yue-Bi-Jia-Zhu-Tang with Ma-Huang-Lian-Qiao-Chi-Xiao-Dou-Tang | Shi-Pi-Yin |
| apple, apple cucumber, sweet rice, lemon, sweet potato, tofu, tomato, white sugar, coriander and parsley | mung bean sprouts, ambergris, kiwi fruit, sturgeon, adzuki bean, Chinese cabbage, mango, pea and watermelon | gold carp, corncob, horse bean, Job's-tears, prickly ash, adzuki bean, bamboo shoot, cheese, ambergris, barley, common carp, cucumber, mung bean, seaweed, shepherd's purse and star fruit | air bladder of shark, chicken, cayenne pepper, fennel, nutmeg, black and white pepper, prickly ash, mutton, sword bean, white or yellow mustard, kidneys, lobster, sardine, shrimp, sparrow, clove, dill seed, pistachio nut, sparrow egg, crab apple, raspberry and walnut |

NEPHRITIS, CHRONIC (CONTINUED)

| | Simultaneous deficiency of energy and blood | Spleen-kidneys yang deficiency | Liver-kidneys yin deficiency |
|---|---|---|---|
| **SYMPTOMS** | 3 Abdominal swelling followed by severe edema*<br>1 Bleeding of various kinds with blood in light color, often seen in consumptive diseases<br>1 Dizziness<br>2 Edema that appears only slightly depressed on finger pressure*<br>2 Fatigue<br>1 Flying objects seen in front of the eyes<br>2 Insomnia<br>1 Low energy<br>1 Low voice<br>2 Numbness of limbs*<br>1 Pale complexion and lips<br>1 Pale nails<br>1 Palpitations<br>1 Scant urine | 1 Ascites<br>1 Being physically weak and too tired to talk<br>1 Cold hands and feet<br>1 Cold loins<br>1 Diarrhea before dawn<br>1 Diarrhea with sticky and muddy stools<br>2 Dysentery<br>1 Eating very little<br>1 Edema<br>1 Edema that occurs all over the body<br>1 Fatigue<br>1 Fear of cold<br>1 Four limbs weakness<br>1 Frequent urination in clear or white streams<br>1 Mentally fatigued<br>3 Proteins in the urine*<br>1 Sputum rumbling with panting | 2 Blurred vision*<br>1 Difficulty in both defecation and urination<br>1 Dizziness<br>1 Dry eyes<br>1 Dry throat<br>1 Fatigue<br>2 Headache with pain in the brow*<br>1 Lumbago<br>1 Night blindness<br>1 Night sweats<br>1 Pain in the upper abdomen<br>2 Palms of hands and soles of feet are both hot*<br>1 Paralysis<br>1 Ringing in the ears<br>1 Sleeplessness with forgetfulness<br>1 Weak loins and tibia<br>1 Withering complexion |
| **TREATMENT PRINCIPLE** | to tone energy & blood simultaneously | to strengthen the spleen and the kidneys yang | to water the liver and the kidneys yin |
| **TREATMENT FORMULA** | Shi-Quan-Da-Bu-Wan | Shen-Qi-Wan with Wu-Zi-Yan-Zong-Wan | Jian-Ling-Tang |
| **FOOD CURES** | abalone, asparagus, cuttlefish, chicken egg, duck egg, white fungus, beef liver, grape, mandarin fish, oyster, milk, beef, cherry, blood clam, longan nut, maltose, Irish potato, sweet rice, apple cucumber, bog bean, gold carp, carrot, chestnut, ham, horse bean, hyacinth bean, Job's-tears, royal jelly, string bean, whitefish, yam, red and black date, mutton, squash and rock sugar | air bladder of shark, chicken, cayenne pepper, fennel, nutmeg, black and white pepper, prickly ash, mutton, sword bean, white or yellow mustard, kidneys, lobster, sardine, shrimp, sparrow, clove, dill seed, pistachio nut, sparrow egg, crab apple, raspberry and walnuts | bird's nest, cheese, chicken egg, kidney bean, brown sugar, mussel, abalone, asparagus, chicken egg, cuttlefish, duck, duck egg, white fungus, oyster, pork, royal jelly, chestnut, chicken liver and pork kidneys. |

## UREMIA

## CEREBROVASCULAR ACCIDENT Cerebral Hemorrhage

| *Stomach energy upsurging* | *Kidneys yang deficiency* | *Spleen-kidneys deficiency* | *Yang closure type* |
|---|---|---|---|
| 3 Dysphagia<br>2 Dry vomiting<br>2 Eating in the evening and vomiting in the morning<br>2 Eating in the morning and vomiting in the evening<br>1 Fatigue<br>3 Hiccups in short sounds<br>1 Nausea<br>1 Sleepiness<br>3 Upset stomach<br>1 Vomiting of foods, watery sputum, or acidic and bitter water<br>1 Vomiting right after eating | 1 Cold feet or cold loins and legs<br>1 Cold sensations in the genitals or the muscles<br>1 Cough and panting<br>1 Diarrhea before dawn<br>1 Diarrhea with sticky and muddy stools<br>1 Edema<br>1 Fatigue<br>1 Frequent urination at night<br>1 Hair falling out easily<br>1 Impotence<br>1 Infertility<br>1 Lack of appetite<br>1 Pain in the loins (lumbago)<br>1 Palpitations<br>1 Panting<br>1 Perspiration on the forehead<br>1 Retention of urine<br>1 Ringing in cars<br>1 Shortness of breath<br>1 Wheezing | 3 Diarrhea<br>2 Difficult urination<br>2 Dizziness<br>3 Fatigue of the four limbs<br>2 Insomnia<br>2 Misty vision<br>2 Palpitations<br>2 Shortness of breath<br>2 Yellowish complexion | 2 Both fists closed tightly<br>4 Breathe heavily*<br>4 Loud sputum sound like the sound of sawing*<br>4 Neither urination nor bowel movement*<br>3 Red complexion*<br>2 Lockjaw<br>1 Sudden fainting with complete unconsciousness |
| to harmonize the stomach and push down the upsurging stomach energy | to warm the kidneys yang and strengthen the true yin of the kidneys | to strengthen the spleen and the kidneys simultaneously | to wake up the patient by acupuncture or other forms of first aid |
| Xiao-Ban-Xia-Jia-Fu-Ling-Tang | Di-Huang-Yin-Zi | Ren-Shen-Yang-Ying-Tang | |
| almond, areca nut, sugar beet, brake, buckwheat, common carp, cashew nut, coriander, loquat, malt, pea, black and white pepper, radish, rice bran and sword bean | kidneys, lobster, sardine shrimp, sparrow, clove, dill seed, fennel, pistachio nut, sparrow egg, crab apple, raspberry and walnut | chicken egg yolk, common button mushroom, wheat bran, rice, beef, cherry, bird's nest, coconut meat, date, tofu, mustard seed, sweet potato, red and black date, rock sugar, apple cucumber, carrot, chestnut, Irish potato, abalone, asparagus, chicken egg, white fungus, black sesame seed, beef kidneys, chicken liver, lobster, pork kidneys, raspberry, scallop, sea cucumber, shrimp, string bean and walnut | Use Kai-Guan-San to open the lockjaw first and then use 1 tablet of Zhi-Bao-Dan (crush into powder first) mixed with warm water and fresh ginger juice to administer to the patient through either the mouth or the nose; afterwards, use Zhen-Gan-Xi-Feng-Tang. |

|  | *Yin closure type* | *Prolapse type* | *Aftereffects* |
|---|---|---|---|
| SYMPTOMS | 3 Both fists closed tightly<br>4 Cold limbs*<br>3 Lockjaw<br>4 Low but heavy sputum sound*<br>2 Sudden fainting with complete unconsciousness<br>4 Whitish or pale complexion* | 3 Both eyes are closed<br>2 Cold limbs<br>3 Hands are stretched after fainting<br>3 Incontinence of urination<br>3 Mouth remains open<br>3 Perspiration<br>3 Snoring | 1 Hemiplegia |
| TREATMENT PRINCIPLE | to wake up the patient by acupuncture or other forms of first aid | to wake up the patient by acupuncture or other forms of first aid | to tone the blood and energy simultaneously and to remove blood coagulations |
| TREATMENT FORMULA |  |  | Bu-Yang-Huan-Wu-Tang |
| FOOD CURES | Use 1 tablet of Su-He-Xiang-Wan (crush into powder first) mixed with warm water and fresh ginger juice to administer to the patient through either the mouth or the nose; afterwards, use Dao-Tan-Tang. | Use the formula Shen-Fu-Tang (crush it into powder first) mixed with warm water and fresh ginger juice to administer to the patient through either the mouth or the nose; afterwards, use Di-Huang-Yin-Zi. |  |

| | | | |
|---|---|---|---|
| 1   Speechlessness | 1   Dry eyes and mouth | 1   Incontinence of urination | 1   Cerebral Thrombosis |
| to expel wind and remove sputum and to tone the yin and the yang | to expel wind and remove sputum and to promote energy circulation | to tone the middle region and strengthen energy and to strengthen the bladder and control urination | to expel wind and remove sputum and to activate the blood and promote blood circulation |
| Di-Huang-Yin-Zi for weaker patients and Tiao-Tan-Tang for stronger patients | Qian-Zheng-San | Bu-Zhong-Yi-Qi-Tang | Da-Qin-Jiao-Tan |

| | CEREBROVASCULAR ACCIDENT, CEREBRAL HEMORRHAGE (CONTINUED) | NEUROSIS Neurasthenia | |
|---|---|---|---|
| | | *Liver-fire upsurging* | *Heart-spleen deficiency* |
| **SYMPTOMS** | 1 Subarachnoid Hemorrhage | 1 Acute dizziness<br>1 Bleeding from stomach<br>1 Dim eyes<br>1 Dry sensations in the mouth<br>2 Feeling hurried and quick-tempered*<br>2 Getting angry easily*<br>1 Headache that is severe<br>1 Hiccups<br>2 Many dreams*<br>1 Nosebleed<br>1 Pain in the upper abdomen<br>1 Red eyes<br>1 Ringing in ears<br>2 Sleeplessness or sleep a lot*<br>1 Vomiting of blood<br>1 Yellowish-red urine | 1 Abdominal swelling<br>1 Discharge of watery, thin stools<br>1 Eating very little<br>1 Fatigue<br>1 Fatigue with lack of power<br>1 Forgetfulness<br>1 Impotence<br>1 Nervous spirits<br>1 Nervousness<br>1 Night sweats<br>1 Palpitations<br>1 Shortness of breath<br>3 Sleeplessness with many dreams*<br>1 Underweight<br>3 Wake up easily at night*<br>1 Withering and yellowish complexion |
| **TREATMENT PRINCIPLE** | to water the yin and cool the blood and to oppress the yang and stop the wind | to sedate the liver-fire and nourish the heart | to strengthen the spleen and energy and to tone the blood and nourish the heart |
| **TREATMENT FORMULA** | Ling-Jiao-Gou-Teng-Tang | Long-Dan-Xie-Gan-Tang | Gui-Pi-Tang |
| **FOOD CURES** | | spinach, chestnut, shepherd's purse, rye, black fungus, vinegar, abalone, asparagus, chicken egg, white fungus, pork and royal jelly | beef liver, chicken egg, cuttlefish, oyster, pork liver, sea cucumber, water spinach, longan nut, mandarin fish, apple cucumber, chestnut, horse bean, Job's-tears, Irish potato, rice, royal jelly and yam |

| | HYSTERIA | | DEMENTIA<br>Including Alzheimer's Disease |
|---|---|---|---|
| *Heart-kidneys unable to communicate with each other or heart-kidneys yin deficiecy* | *Heart-spleen deficiency* | *Liver energy congestion* | *Spleen-sputum* |
| 1 Deafness<br>1 Dizziness<br>1 Face becomes red when fatigued or working hard<br>1 Feeling miserable<br>1 Feeling miserable with love of darkness and dislike of light<br>4 Forgetfulness*<br>1 Light but periodic fever not unlike the tide<br>1 Nervousness<br>4 Night sweats*<br>2 Palpitations<br>1 Ringing in ears<br>1 Sleeplessness with forgetfulness<br>1 Sore loins and weak legs | 1 Abdominal swelling<br>1 Discharge of watery, thin stools<br>1 Eating very little<br>2 Fatigue<br>1 Fatigue without power<br>1 Forgetfulness<br>3 Frequent yawning*<br>1 Nervousness<br>1 Night sweats<br>1 Palpitations<br>3 Sadness with a desire to cry*<br>2 Shortness of breath<br>2 Sleeplessness<br>1 Withering and yellowish complexion | 1 Abdominal obstruction<br>1 Abdominal pain<br>1 Convulsions<br>3 Feeling very depressed*<br>3 Frequent sighing*<br>2 Pain in the upper abdomen<br>1 Premature menstrual periods<br>1 Shortage of milk secretion after childbirth<br>2 Stomachache<br>3 Subjective sensations of objects in the throat*<br>1 Vomiting of blood<br>1 Whitish vaginal discharge | 2 Abundant saliva<br>4 Being silent all day long*<br>1 Bronchiectasis<br>4 Loss of memory*<br>1 Overweight, but eat only a small amount of food<br>1 Poor appetite<br>1 Slight fullness of the stomach<br>4 Sudden crying and sudden laughing*<br>2 Weakened limbs |
| to nourish the yin and clear internal heat and to promote communication between the heart and the kidneys | to tone the energy and blood simultaneously and to lubricate dryness and slow down progression of symptoms | to relieve the liver energy congestion, transform sputum and push down the upsurging energy | to strengthen the spleen and remove sputum |
| Liu-Wei-Di-Huang-Wan with Huang-Lian-E-Jiao-Tang | Gan-Mai-Da-Zao-Tang | Ban-Xie-Hou-Pu-Tang | Liu-Jun-Zi-Tang or Xi-Xin-Tang |
| asparagus, abalone, chicken egg, white fungus, bog bean, wheat, banana, bamboo shoot, bitter endive, oyster, royal jelly and pork | beef liver, chicken egg, cuttlefish, oyster, pork liver, sea cucumber, water spinach, longan nut, mandarin fish, apple cucumber, chestnut, horse bean, Job's-tears, Irish potato, rice, royal jelly and yam | Brown sugar, garlic, turmeric, kumquat, beef, cherry, bird's nest, butterfish, chicken, coconut meat, date, tofu, mustard seed, sweet rice, goose meat, mutton, jackfruit, squash, sweet potato, red and black date, rice, rock sugar, caraway seed, spearmint, common button mushroom, oregano, red bean, ambergris, dill seed, sweet basil and saffron | bamboo shoot, crown daisy, date, fresh ginger, leaf or brown mustard, black and white pepper, white or yellow mustard seed, asparagus and pear |

DEMENTIA, INCLUDING ALZHEIMER'S (CONTINUED)

| | Simultaneous occurrence of sputum congestion and blood coagulations | Hot sputum | Spleen-kidneys yang deficiency |
|---|---|---|---|
| SYMPTOMS | 2 Alternating illogical talking and silence*<br>3 Alternating silence & jumpiness*<br>2 Chest pain<br>1 Heavy sensations<br>2 Insanity<br>2 Lumpy spots in the body that do not shift<br>2 Numbness<br>2 Prickling and chronic pain in a fixed region that does not shift<br>2 Symptoms get worse in cold weather and better in warm weather<br>2 Unclear consciousness | 1 Asthma history<br>4 Chronic dementia now getting worse*<br>1 Coma<br>1 Cough<br>1 Discharge of hard, yellow sputum in lumps<br>1 Discharge of sticky, turbid and thin stools<br>1 Discharge of yellow, sticky sputum in lumps<br>2 Insanity<br>3 Insomnia<br>1 Stools with an extremely bad smell<br>1 Vomiting<br>3 Wheezing | 2 Being silent all day or speechlessness*<br>2 Clear signs of aging*<br>1 Cold hands and feet or cold loins<br>1 Diarrhea before dawn<br>1 Diarrhea with sticky and muddy stools<br>1 Edema that occurs all over the body<br>1 Fatigue<br>1 Fear of cold<br>1 Frequent urination in clear or white streams<br>2 Incontinence of urination and bowel movement*<br>2 Loss of memory*<br>2 Paralysis of limbs*<br>2 Slow movement*<br>1 Sputum rumbling with panting |
| TREATMENT PRINCIPLE | to disperse the liver energy congestion and to transform blood coagulations and remove sputum | to clear hot sputum | to warm the kidneys and the spleen and to transform sputum and remove blood coagulations |
| TREATMENT FORMULA | Chen-Shi-Yi-Zhuan-Dai-Dan | Wen-Dan-Tang | Shen-Qi-Wan with Er-Chen-Tang |
| FOOD CURES | bamboo shoot, crown daisy, date, fresh ginger, leaf or brown mustard, black and white pepper, white or yellow mustard seed, asparagus and pear | banana, bitter endive, black fungus, salt, spinach, strawberry, bamboo shoot, cucumber, Job's-tears, laver, leaf beet, mung bean, peppermint, purslane, salt, cattail, agar, radish, crown daisy, date, fresh ginger, leaf or brown mustard, black and white pepper, white or yellow mustard seed, asparagus and pear | air bladder of shark, chicken, cayenne pepper, fennel, nutmeg, black and white pepper, prickly ash, mutton, sword bean, white or yellow mustard, kidneys, lobster, sardine, shrimp, sparrow, clove, dill seed, pistachio nut, sparrow egg, crab apple, raspberry and walnuts |

## ALLERGIES
Food

| Liver-kidneys yin deficiency | Simultaneous energy congestion and blood coagulations | Liver offending the spleen | Spleen-stomach deficiency |
|---|---|---|---|
| 1 Dizziness | 2 Abdominal swelling | 2 Abdominal enlargement | 1 Abdominal pain |
| 1 Dry eyes or throat | 3 Being indifferent or pathetic emotionally* | 2 Abdominal pain | 4 Allergic to cold foods and greasy foods in particular* |
| 2 Explosive laughter and crying* | 2 Congested chest | 1 Abdominal rumbling | 4 History of chronic enteritis, chronic gastritis, or chronic hepatitis* |
| 1 Fatigue | 2 Forgetfulness | 2 Chronic diarrhea | |
| 1 Headache with pain in the brow | 3 Hallucination* | 5 Diarrhea with watery stools often triggered by foods* | 1 Diarrhea |
| 2 Hemiplegia* | 1 Love of sighing | 5 Digestive breakdown often intensified by emotional upset* | 4 Dysentery alternating with very soft stools* |
| 2 Loss of speech* | 1 Lump in the abdomen that stays in the same region | 1 Fatigued spirits | 1 Edema |
| 1 Lumbago | 3 Slow response* | 1 Hungry with no appetite | 1 Falling of stomach (gastroptosis) |
| 1 Night blindness | 3 Sudden fear and nervousness* | 1 Thirst with no desire for drink | 1 Hiccups |
| 1 Night sweats | | | 1 Plenty of saliva |
| 1 Pain in the upper abdomen | | | 1 Rickets |
| 1 Palms of hands and soles of feet are both hot | | | 1 Stomachache |
| 1 Poor memory | | | |
| 2 Shaking of hands* | | | |
| 1 Sleeplessness with forgetfulness | | | |
| 1 Weak loins and tibia | | | |

| | | | |
|---|---|---|---|
| to water the yin and soften up the liver and to transform blood coagulations and stop the internal wind | to activate the blood and transform coagulations and to promote energy circulation | to inhibit the liver and support the spleen and to regulate energy and dry up dampness | to strengthen the spleen and the stomach |
| Liu-Wei-Di-Huang-Wan or Sang-Nu-San-Jia-Tang | Tao-Ren-Fu-Sang-Fang | Tong-Xie-Yao-Fang with Ping-Wei-San | Shen-Ling-Bai-Zhu-San |
| bird's nest, cheese, chicken egg, kidney bean, brown sugar, mussel, abalone, asparagus, chicken egg, cuttlefish, duck, duck egg, white fungus, oyster, pork, royal jelly, chestnut, chicken liver and pork kidneys | beef, cherry, bird's nest butterfish, chicken, coconut meat date, tofu, mustard seed, sweet rice, goose meat, mutton, jackfruit, squash, sweet potato, red and black date, rice, rock sugar, caraway seed, spearmint, common button mushroom, oregano, red bean, ambergris, dill seed, garlic, sweet basil, saffron, brown sugar chestnut, eggplant, peach, black soybean, sturgeon, crab, distillers' grains, papaya and saffron | brown sugar, kumquat, mandarin orange, apple cucumber, bog bean, gold carp, carrot, chestnut, corncob, horse bean, hyacinth bean, Job's-tears, Irish potato, royal jelly, string bean, whitefish and yam | star anise, cayenne pepper, fresh ginger, chicken, clove, black and white pepper, apple cucumber, chestnut, ham, horse bean, Irish potato, rice, royal jelly, beef, red and black date, garlic, pistachio nut, barley and rock sugar |

ALLERGIES, FOOD (CONTINUED)

Environmental Allergies, including allergies
Allergies of the Eyes, including spring
allergic reactions of the eyes

| | *Cold-dampness large-intestine* | *Energy congestion* | *Wind-heat* |
|---|---|---|---|
| **SYMPTOMS** | 2 Abdominal pain<br>2 Abdominal pain with abdominal rumbling<br>2 Abdominal rumbling<br>1 Clear and long streams of urine<br>1 Cold hands and feet<br>1 Congested chest<br>4 Discharge of pure-white substances*<br>1 Discharge of sticky, muddy stools not unlike goose dung<br>4 Heavy sensations in the body*<br>2 Poor appetite | 2 Abdominal pain<br>1 Belching<br>1 Chest and ribs discomfort<br>2 Chest pain<br>2 Constipation with a desire to empty the bowel*<br>2 Discharge of stools like sheep dung*<br>1 Pain in inner part of stomach with prickling sensation and swelling<br>2 Pain in the upper abdomen<br>1 Retention of urine<br>1 Ringing in ears and deafness<br>2 Stomachache<br>1 Subjective sensation of lump in the throat<br>1 Swallowing difficulty<br>1 Swelling and congestion after eating | 2 Burning sensation and uncomfortable dryness in the eyes*<br>1 Coughing out blood<br>1 Dizziness<br>1 Headache<br>1 Headache with dizziness<br>2 Intolerable itch in the eyes*<br>1 Intolerance of light in eyes with swelling and dislike of wind<br>1 Muddy discharge from nose<br>1 Nosebleed<br>2 Pain in the eyes*<br>2 Red eyes*<br>1 Ringing in ears and deafness<br>1 Tenesmus<br>1 Thirst<br>1 Toothache<br>1 Yellow urine<br>1 Yellowish discharge from the nose |
| **TREATMENT PRINCIPLE** | to warm and transform cold and dampness | to promote energy circulation and disperse energy congestion | to expel wind & activate the blood & to clear heat & nourish the blood |
| **TREATMENT FORMULA** | Wei-Ling-Tang | Liu-Mo-Yin or Wu-Mo-Yin-Zi | Xi-Gan-San |
| **FOOD CURES** | capers, cayenne pepper, fresh ginger, prickly ash, star anise, white or yellow mustard seed, white or yellow mustard, wine, chicken, clove, herring, nutmeg and black and white pepper | banana, bitter endive, black fungus, salt, spinach, strawberry, bamboo shoot, cucumber, Job's-tears, laver, leaf beet, mung bean, peppermint, purslane, salt, cattail, agar, radish, crown daisy, date, fresh ginger, leaf or brown mustard, black and white pepper, white or yellow mustard seed, asparagus and pear | banana, bitter endive, black fungus, salt, spinach, strawberry, bamboo shoot, cucumber, Job's-tears, laver, leaf beet, mung bean, peppermint, purslane, spearmint, sweet basil, celery, coconut meat and green onion |

caused by pollution, plants and animals catarrh, spring conjunctivitis and other

Allergies of the Nose, including hay fever, pollen rhinitis, allergic rhinitis and other allergic reactions of the nose

| *Wind-dampness-heat* | *Lungs energy deficiency and cold* | *Spleen-lungs energy deficiency* | *Kidneys yang deficiency* |
|---|---|---|---|
| 1 Chronic backache | 1 Breathing difficulty | 1 Abdominal swelling | 1 Allergies all year round* |
| 1 Diarrhea | 1 Common cold | 3 Clear and white nasal discharge* | 1 Cold feet or cold loins and legs |
| 1 Eczema | 1 Copious, clear and watery sputum | 1 Cough | 1 Cold sensations in the genitals or |
| 1 Edema | 1 Cough | 1 Coughing out and spitting of | the muscles |
| 3 Eyes in dark-red color* | 1 Excessive perspiration | sputum and saliva | 1 Diarrhea before dawn |
| 1 Fever that becomes more severe | 1 Fatigue | 1 Decreased appetite | 1 Diarrhea with sticky and |
| in the afternoon | 1 Fear of cold | 3 Decreased sense of smell* | muddy stools |
| 1 Headache with heavy sensations | 2 Frequent sneezing* | 1 Diarrhea with sticky and | 1 Discharge of watery, thin stools |
| in the head | 2 Impaired sense of smell* | muddy stools | 1 Edema |
| 3 Itch in the eyes not very severe* | 1 Light wheezing | 1 Discharge of copious, clear, | 1 Fatigue |
| 1 Itchy sores | 1 Low and weak voice | watery sputum | 1 Frequent urination at night* |
| 1 Light swelling | 2 Nasal congestion* | 1 Eating only a little and | 1 Frequent sneezing with clear |
| 2 Pain in all the joints | 2 Severe itch in the nose* | with indigestion | nasal discharge* |
| 1 Pain shifting around with no | 1 Shortness of breath | 1 Fatigue of the four limbs | 1 Impotence in men |
| fixed region | 1 Smooth urination | 1 Fatigue with lack of power | 1 Infertility in women |
| 1 Scant urine | 1 Too tired to talk | 1 Prolonged cough | 1 Lack of appetite |
| 2 Whites of the eyes not very | | 1 Rapid panting | 1 Palpitations |
| clear as if covered with a | | 1 Shortness of breath | 1 Panting |
| colloid substance* | | 2 Underweight and weak | 1 Perspiration on the forehead |
| | | | 1 Retention of urine |
| | | | 1 Ringing in ears |
| | | | 1 Shortness of breath |
| | | | 1 Wheezing |
| to expel wind and clear heat and to remove dampness and stop itch | to warm and strengthen the lungs and to expel cold and drive out wind | to strengthen the spleen and to tone up the energy and the lungs | to tone the lungs and warm the kidneys |
| Xiao-Feng-San | Wen-Fei-Zhi-Liu-Dan or Yu-Ping-Feng-San with Cang-Er-Zi-San | Si-Jun-Zi-Tang with Shen-Ling-Bai-Zhu-San | Shen-Qi-Wan or Wen-Fei-Zhi-Liu-Dan |
| peppermint, spearmint, sweet basil, celery, coconut meat, green onion, jellyfish skin, prickly ash, rice, adzuki bean, rosin and tangerine | cheese, Job's-tears, yam, grape, longan nuts, maltose, mandarin fish, Irish potato, sweet rice, apple cucumber, bog bean, gold carp, carrot, chestnut, ham, horse bean, hyacinth bean, royal jelly, string bean, whitefish, yam, red and black date, mutton, squash and rock sugar | grape, longan nuts, maltose, mandarin fish, Irish potato, sweet rice, apple cucumber, bog bean, gold carp, carrot, chestnut, ham, horse bean, hyacinth bean, Job's-tears, royal jelly, string bean, whitefish, yam, red and black date, mutton, squash, rock sugar, chicken egg yolk, cheese and bean | kidneys, lobster, sardine, shrimp, sparrow, clove, dill seed, fennel, pistachio nut, sparrow egg, crab apple, raspberry and walnut |

## Kidneys yin deficiency

**SYMPTOMS**

2 Allergies all year round*
1 Cold hands and feet
1 Cough with sputum containing blood or coughing out fresh blood
1 Deafness
1 Dizziness
1 Dry sensations in the mouth particularly at night
1 Dry throat
1 Fatigue
1 Feeling miserable and hurried, with fever
1 Fever at night with burning sensations in internal organs
1 Hot sensations in the middle of palms or soles of feet
1 Night sweats
1 Pain in the heels
1 Pain in the loins (lumbago)
1 Retention of urine
1 Ringing in ears
1 Sleeplessness
2 Spots in front of the eyes
2 Thirst

**TREATMENT PRINCIPLE**

to water the kidneys yin

**TREATMENT FORMULA**

Zuo-Gui-Wan

**FOOD CURES**

abalone, asparagus, chicken egg, cuttlefish, duck, duck egg, white fungus, oyster, pork, royal jelly, chestnut, chicken liver and pork kidneys

中医疗法

Herbology

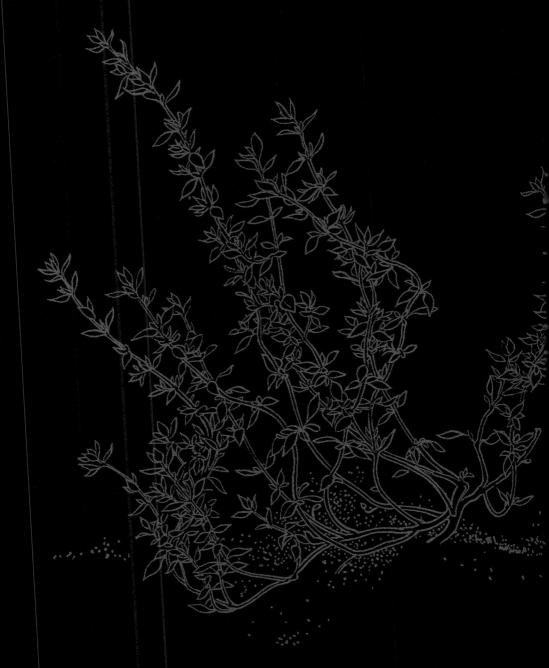

The classification of various items under study marked the beginning of science and has continued into modern times. In botany, for example, we classify plants into different families to further our understanding of them. Chinese herbs are as old as Chinese history and the ancient Chinese classified herbs according to their basic actions—in other words, what they could do to the human body. There are a total of 20 major classifications within Chinese herbalism today, each of which represents a number of important actions.

is not desirable for patients suffering from chronic diseases of the internal organs. Second, symptoms that have already dehydrated the body, such as vomiting, diarrhea and bleeding, should not be treated by this class of herbs. Third, after taking this class of herbs, it is desirable to stay calm and keep warm so that perspiration will occur to a suitable degree, being neither excessive nor insufficient. Fourth, when a rather weak patient such as an older person takes this class of herbs to heal an illness, it is wise for him or her to consume some herbs under the classification of herbs to treat deficiencies, namely, class 16.

# Classification of Chinese Herbs

## CLASS OF HERBS TO INDUCE PERSPIRATION

The herbs that fall under this classification have one thing in common, namely, that they can induce perspiration, which is their major action. For this reason, an illness that can be alleviated by perspiration can be treated with this class of herbs. Conversely, a patient with an illness that can be intensified by perspiration should avoid this class of herbs. If, for example, you catch a cold, herbs in this class would benefit you, because in order to overcome the common cold or the flu, it is necessary to induce perspiration. On the other hand, if you suffer from night sweats, excessive perspiration, or chronic diarrhea, which will have already drained off a great deal of water from your body, you should avoid herbs in this class as much as possible.

Herbs that induce perspiration are divided into two subclasses: herbs for symptoms characterized by cold sensations (namely, Chinese ephedra, lily-flowered magnolia and purple perilla) and herbs for symptoms characterized by fever (namely, hare's ear, kudzu vine and mulberry-leaved chrysanthemum). Thus, if you are suffering from the common cold with chills, the first subclass of herbs should be used; but once you display high fever, the second subclass is recommended.

All classes of herbs have specific uses and also entail a few measures of precaution. The major uses for the class of herbs that induce perspiration are the common cold and the flu as well as many related symptoms, such as headache, fever, pain in the body and a cough. In addition, this class of herbs is also frequently used to treat bronchitis, bronchial asthma, measles at an early stage, acute glomerulonephritis and acute rheumatic fever.

There are four measures of precaution in using this class of herbs. First, herbs in this class are not good for chronic symptoms involving the internal organs. This is partly because such symptoms cannot be treated simply by inducing perspiration and partly because a prolonged consumption of these herbs will weaken the body, which

From the point of view of modern medicine, the class of herbs to induce perspiration performs two basic functions. First, the herbs in this class can expand blood capillaries in the superficial region of the body and activate the secretion of the sweat gland in order to reduce fever, get rid of toxin, inhibit bacteria and strengthen the body's ability to ingest and destroy bacteria and defend itself against foreign invasion. Second, this class of herbs can increase glomerular filtration to remove excessive water in the body.

## CLASS OF HERBS TO REDUCE EXCESSIVE HEAT INSIDE THE BODY

Many diseases are due to the presence of excessive heat inside the body. This class of herbs is capable of reducing excessive heat inside the body and is used for those diseases that are mostly characterized by inflammation or infection. This class is divided into three subclasses: herbs to reduce the "heat of fire" (namely, carrizo, cork tree, goldthread, purslane, selfheal, skullcap and wind weed), herbs to reduce heat in the blood (namely, Chinese pulsatilla and white rose) and herbs to reduce heat and detoxicate at the same time (namely, Asian dandelion, chicken-bone grass, Chinese violet, Japanese honeysuckle and puff ball).

The concept of heat is a unique concept in Chinese medicine, as heat is believed to be the cause of many so-called hot symptoms. Herbs that can reduce "heat of fire" are used to treat acute inflammatory and infectious diseases, because acute diseases can be said to attack as fast as fire burning down a building. Such acute diseases include encephalitis, which is inflammation of the brain; pneumonia, which is inflammation of the lungs; and acute bronchitis, which is inflammation of the bronchial mucous membrane. Herbs that can reduce heat in the blood are used to arrest bleeding, such as with nosebleeds, discharge of blood from the mouth and vaginal bleeding. Herbs that can reduce heat and detoxicate simultaneously are normally used to treat inflammatory and infectious diseases that are suppurative, such as many skin diseases, mumps, lymphangitis, mastitis and appendicitis.

A few measures of precaution should be taken in using this class of herbs. First, symptoms related to the common cold or the flu and to fever or excessive heat in the body due to constipation should not be treated by this class of herbs. Second, herbs in this class tend to be bad for the stomach, because they are not easily digested; for this reason, they can be taken with the class of herbs for promoting digestion, if necessary (class 9). Third, this class of herbs can dehydrate the body and for this reason, they can be taken with yin tonics, which consist of herbs to treat yin deficiency (class 16).

From the viewpoint of modern medicine, this class of herbs can be used to heal inflammation, counteract bacteria, arrest bleeding, reduce body temperature, increase urination and activate the ureter, which explains why such herbs can treat urinary stones effectively.

## CLASS OF HERBS
## TO COUNTERACT RHEUMATISM

Most of the herbs in this class can be used to relieve pain and they are especially effective for the treatment of muscular pain and pain of arthritis and rheumatism. The herbs included under this classification are Chinese clematis, mistletoe and slender acanthopanax root bark.

Arthritis and rheumatism, at the beginning stage, should be treated by herbs in this class along with those in the class to induce perspiration (class 1). As these illnesses enter the intermediate stage, they should be treated by this class of herbs along with the class of herbs to promote blood circulation (class 12).

The Chinese believe that rheumatism is caused by three factors, or any combination of them. These three factors are wind, cold and dampness. When rheumatism is caused by wind, the pain travels around the entire body, which is why it is called wandering pain and is difficult for the patient to pinpoint. Chinese clematis and mistletoe are particularly good for arthritis and rheumatism caused by wind. When rheumatism is caused by dampness, the pain will stay in a fixed region, so that the patient can easily point to where the pain is occurring. Slender acanthopanax root bark is especially good for this type of rheumatism.

## CLASS OF HERBS TO REDUCE
## COLD SENSATIONS INSIDE THE BODY

This class of herbs is used to warm the body in the treatment of ailments associated with cold sensations inside the body, such as vomiting, diarrhea, cold abdominal pain, cold stomachache and poor appetite. Some people feel a need to vomit because of cold sensations in the stomach and others develop diarrhea due to cold sensa-tions in the bowel. One herb in this class is called evodia; it is a warm herb and is frequently used to stop vomiting and relieve cold pain.

If you have a cold symptom such as vomiting or diarrhea and you have also caught a cold and are not completely recovered, you can take this class of herbs along with the class of herbs to induce perspiration (class 1). As herbs that reduce cold sensations inside the body are warm and dry, they are not to be taken by people with a hot disease or by those whose water content in the body is in short supply.

From the standpoint of modern medicine, this class of herbs can improve the functions of the cardiovascular system, increase heart action, excite the vasomotor center and the sympathetic nervous system, elevate blood pressure and improve blood circulation. In addition, these herbs have been found to improve the hypothalamo-hypophysial function and the function of the endocrine glands, as well as elevate the effects of the neurohumoral regulation for better coordination among various vital internal organs that will in turn improve metabolism.

## CLASS OF HERBS TO REDUCE
## DAMPNESS IN THE BODY

When dampness accumulates in the body, it can cause many ailments, including abdominal swelling, swelling of the stomach, puffiness in the limbs, diarrhea, jaundice and a few skin diseases. This class is divided into two subclasses: herbs to transform or absorb dampness (namely, buyuryo, grey atractylodes and Korean mint) and herbs to promote urination (namely, Asiatic plantain, coin grass and evergreen artemisia).

To transform dampness means to stimulate the action of the spleen so that it can speed up the excretion of water from the body. The Chinese believe that one reason why dampness continues to accumulate in the body is that the spleen is not strong enough to make water flow. The herbs that can transform dampness are able to correct the conditions of the spleen. Another way of getting rid of dampness inside the body is through promoting urination. The herbs for promoting urination are often used to treat many urination disturbances and related symptoms, such as edema, stones in the urinary system and acute nephritis. In addition, many obese people have accumulated an excessive quantity of water in the body, which is why this class of herbs is often used for weight reduction.

Along with reducing dampness inside the body, this class of herbs, at the same time, can also reduce yin energy in the body. For this reason, people with dry conditions and thin and weak people should not use this class of herbs.

From the point of view of modern medicine, this class of herbs has been proven effective for cardiac-renal edema, nutritional edema, prostato-megaly urinary retention and other symptoms associated with gastroenteric disturbances, such as nausea, vomiting, poor appetite and diarrhea. These usages are attributed to the following three functions performed by this class of herbs: First, this class of herbs can enhance the functions of the heart, lungs and kidneys; second, it can regulate the functions of the stomach and the intestines to stop many digestive disturbances; and third, it can adjust the neurohumoral regulation, which contributes to excretion of excessive water in the body.

## CLASS OF HERBS FOR LUBRICATING DRY SYMPTOMS

A dry disease should be lubricated. Dry diseases can be either internal or external and this class of herbs is used for treating both categories. Internal dryness may give rise to dry skin, constipation, discharge of dry and solid stools, discharge of scanty urine, thirst, dry throat with cracked lips and sleeplessness; external dryness may give rise to absence of perspiration in hot weather, blood in sputum, dry cough, dry nose and dry skin.

This class of herbs is divided into three subclasses. The first subclass consists of herbs for lubricating the lungs. Herbs in this subclass are used to treat dryness of the lungs and yin deficiency of the lungs, which can manifest in the following ailments: loss of voice, coughing up blood, dry cough, atrophic rhinitis, the common cold, influenza, bronchitis, diabetes insipidus, throat pain, dry nose and throat and tickle in the throat. The second subclass consists of herbs for producing fluids and strengthening the stomach. These herbs are used to produce fluids in the stomach, mostly for the treatment of yin deficiency of the stomach, manifesting as diabetes mellitus, morbid hunger, dry lips, or stomachache. The third subclass consists of herbs for watering the yin (to increase yin energy in the body, as in watering a plant) and lubricating dryness of the intestines. These herbs are mostly used to treat yin exhaustion, dryness of the intestines and dry constipation.

Herbs in this class can slow down movements inside the body, including energy circulation, blood circulation and digestion. So, for this reason, those with poor energy circulation, poor blood circulation, or chronic indigestion, should avoid this class of herbs.

## CLASS OF HERBS TO INDUCE VOMITING

Most of the herbs in this class are very strong, which is why they can induce vomiting. Among them is the herb called black false hellebore, which is often used to induce vomiting of sputum and undigested foods, particularly in patients of epilepsy, apoplexy, thyroiditis and lymphadenitis, in order to remove substances that may block the throat and obstruct breathing. Normally herbs in this class are available in powdered form.

If a patient fails to vomit within 10 to 20 minutes, he or she should use a finger to penetrate the throat to induce vomiting. If a patient continues to vomit without stop, some ginger juice, cold rice soup, or cold water can be administered to stop the vomiting. After vomiting, the patient should have some soup or semiliquid food and avoid greasy food and other food difficult to digest.

This class of herbs should not be consumed by patients with swallowing difficulty, asthma, a cough, pulmonary tuberculosis, aneurysm, arteriosclerosis, hypertension, or heart disease. Young and old patients, pregnant women and weak patients should also avoid it.

## CLASS OF HERBS TO INDUCE BOWEL MOVEMENTS

Herbs in this class, such as rhubarb, are most commonly used to treat constipation. However, many other diseases can also by treated by it, according to two treatment principles in Chinese medicine.

One treatment principle states that symptoms that occur in the upper region of the body can be treated by inducing bowel movements. Thus, inflammation of the eyes, ears, nose, mouth and skin and facial acne can be treated by this class of herbs as long as constipation or poor bowel movements are also indicated. The other treatment principle states that when smooth bowel movements are obstructed, abdominal pain and swelling may occur. These symptoms can be treated by this class of herbs so long as constipation or poor bowel movements are also indicated.

It's important to note that inducing bowel movements is a temporary measure in the treatment of an acute condition.

## CLASS OF HERBS TO PROMOTE DIGESTION

This class of herbs is used to treat indigestion, swelling of the stomach, abdominal swelling, belching, nausea, vomiting, abdominal pain, diarrhea and poor appetite. As a general rule, the symptoms to be treated by this class of herbs must be due to indigestion. Chinese hawthorn is an herb in this class.

Sometimes it may be necessary to use this class of herbs along with the class of herbs to regulate energy (class 11), because indigestion and poor energy circulation are often associated with each other. When the herbs to promote digestion fail to work, it may be necessary to induce bowel movements as well, but both the herbs to promote digestion and the herbs to induce bowel movements (class 8) can only be used temporarily, as neither of them will contribute to the long-term health of the patient.

## CLASS OF HERBS TO SUPPRESS COUGH AND REDUCE SPUTUM

This class of herbs can perform two actions simultaneously, namely, suppress coughing and reduce sputum. However, it is also frequently used to treat asthma, tuberculosis of the lymph node, goiter, epilepsy and convulsions. This class of herbs is divided into three subclasses: First, herbs to reduce hot sputum (including antipyretic dichroa, snake gourd and tendril-leaved fritillary bulb); second, herbs to suppress coughing and relieve asthma (including momordica fruit, sweet apricot, zuccarini's buttercup and white cynanchum); and third, herbs to reduce cold sputum (such as jimson weed). Hot sputum appears yellowish whereas cold sputum appears white.

Herbs to reduce hot sputum are often used to treat tuberculosis of the lymph node and goiter; herbs to reduce cold sputum are often used to treat aching pain in the joints, as in arthritis; and herbs to suppress coughing and relieve asthma are often used to treat bronchitis, bronchial asthma, chronic cough, pulmonary tuberculosis and tracheitis.

Since there are many different causes of sputum, the precise cause should be determined in order to treat it effectively. A cough with discharge of blood should not be treated by large dosages of herbs in this class in order to avoid additional bleeding. A cough associated with the common cold should be treated by this class of herbs along with the class of herbs to induce perspiration (class 1).

## CLASS OF HERBS TO REGULATE ENERGY

Energy is a very fundamental concept in Chinese medicine, often compared with the blood. The energy in the body circulates the same way as blood circulates and as with blood, energy can circulate too slowly, too quickly, or irregularly. When energy keeps flowing upwards, it can cause hiccups and vomiting; when it keeps flowing downwards, it can cause prolapse of the anus, the uterus, or the stomach. When energy flows too slowly, it can cause chest pain and depression. The class of herbs to regulate energy is used to make energy circulate smoothly in the body and one such herb is yellow jasmine.

The ailments often treated by this class of herbs include chest pain, pain in the ribs, abdominal pain, vomiting, hiccups, prolapse of the anus, prolapse of the uterus, prolapse of the stomach, menstrual pain, enteritis and acute bronchitis.

However, herbs in this class travel very fast in the body, so they can use up a great deal of energy, not unlike a car that runs fast using up a great deal of gas and oil. For this reason, this class of herbs should not be used for a prolonged period of time.

The Chinese classify energy as yang and blood as yin. They are sister and brother, with energy as brother and blood as sister and they travel in the body hand in hand. In order to ensure that they travel together smoothly, the herbs to regulate energy and the herbs to regulate blood (class 12) are often used together.

## CLASS OF HERBS TO REGULATE BLOOD

This class of herbs can regulate the blood in two different ways, which is why it is divided into two subclasses: first, herbs to promote blood circulation (including Siberian motherwort and two-toothed amaranthus) and second, herbs to arrest bleeding (including agrimony and pseudo-ginseng).

When the blood fails to circulate smoothly, one major result can be blood coagulation, which is responsible for many ailments. For example, blood coagulation can cause the suppression of menstruation, menstrual pain, abdominal pain after childbirth and chest pain. External factors can also result in blood coagulation, such as injuries from an automobile accident, a fall from a high place, or lifting a heavy object in an improper manner. Some people experience pain in the chest, for example, long after an accident, which could be due to blood coagulation caused by the accident. Since blood coagulation occurs in many diseases, including thromboangiitis obliterans, coronary heart disease and erythema nodosum, herbs in this class can be effective in their treatment. Herbs to arrest bleeding are used to treat bleeding of various kinds, including vomiting of blood, nosebleeds, discharge of blood from the anus, blood in the urine, vaginal bleeding and bleeding from external causes.

## CLASS OF HERBS TO REGAIN CONSCIOUSNESS

Sudden fainting often occurs in patients of apoplexy or epilepsy and with those suffering from convulsions or high fever. In apoplexy, for example, in order to arouse a patient who has fainted, it may be necessary to administer the herb by hand, which is one reason why this class of herbs comes in tablets and powder.

There are two different ways of suffering from loss of consciousness; one is called the "closed type" and the other is called the "prolapse type," and each should be treated differently. When a patient faints with closed fists, a locked jaw, rough breathing and a strong pulse, it is a closed type and should be treated by herbs in this class, such as benzoin. But when a patient faints with open hands, a pale complexion and a weak pulse, it is a prolapse type, which should be treated by ginseng, an herb in class 16.

## CLASS OF HERBS TO REDUCE ANXIETY

This class of herbs is often used to treat insomnia, excessive dreaming, forgetfulness, palpitations, epilepsy, convulsions, dizziness, depression, night sweats, excessive perspiration and a congested chest. Oriental arborvitae seed belongs to this class of herbs. However, when these ailments are due to blood deficiency, they should be treated by this class of herbs along with the class of herbs to treat blood deficiency, also referred to as blood tonics (class 16).

## CLASS OF HERBS TO STOP INVOLUNTARY MOVEMENTS

Involuntary movements are often manifested as a shaking of the head or of the hands, or muscular twitching, as observed in apoplexy. Tuber of elevated gastrodia belongs to this class of herbs. Herbs in this class are often used along with herbs in other classes, because frequently patients with involuntary movement problems also display other symptoms as well. For example, when a patient also suffers from insomnia and palpitations, the class of herbs to reduce anxiety (class 14) should be used in combination.

## CLASS OF HERBS TO CORRECT DEFICIENCIES

This class of herbs plays a fundamental role in Chinese medicine and its major function is to make the body stronger. In the terminology of Western medicine, this class of herbs could be called the class of herbs to enhance the body's immune function, but there is a basic difference between the Chinese and the Western approaches in this connection. Western scientists believe that if something can enhance the body's immune function, it must be good for everybody, but it is maintained in Chinese medicine that the body can be strengthened only in accordance with the nature of its weaknesses. A person may be strong in certain respects and weak in others and it is essential to determine exactly what the weak aspects are of each individual before this class of herbs can be used effectively.

In Chinese medicine, when a person has a weakness, it is called a "deficiency." There are four types of deficiencies: energy deficiency, which means low energy; yang deficiency, which means weak kidneys in general and low sexual capacity in particular; blood deficiency, which means either shortage or poor quality of blood; and yin deficiency, which means shortage of body fluids.

This class of herbs is divided into four subclasses based on the four types of deficiency. The first subclass consists of herbs to treat energy deficiency and they are called energy tonics. Chinese ginseng, Chinese yam, licorice, membraneous milk vetch and red date, belong to this subclass. The second subclass consists of herbs to treat yang deficiency, which are called yang tonics and dodder, eucommia bark, longspur epimedium, morinda root, snake-bed seed, snow lotus and teasel belong to this subclass. The third subclass consists of herbs to treat blood deficiency, which are called blood tonics and danggui, glutinous rehmannia and tuber of multiflower knotweed belong to it. And the fourth subclass consists of herbs to treat yin deficiency, which are called yin tonics; lily, matrimony vine, sealwort, sesame, tremella, wax tree and white peony belong to it.

Herbs for treating energy deficiency are effective for shortness of breath, asthma, fatigue, low body weight, poor appetite, indigestion, diarrhea, abdominal swelling, puffiness, prolapse of the uterus and the anus and prolapse of the stomach. Herbs for treating yang deficiency are effective for lumbago, cold limbs, frequent urination, impotence, seminal emission, chronic diarrhea, abdominal pain, infertility and blurred vision. Herbs for treating blood deficiency are effective for palpitations, forgetfulness, insomnia, headaches, dizziness, ringing in the ears, irregular menstruation, muscular twitching, opisthotonos, night sweats and diabetes. Herbs for treating yin deficiency are effective for a chronic cough, night sweats, seminal emission, hoarseness, constant thirst, a chronic sore throat, a dry cough, excessive perspiration, lumbago, blurred vision, ringing in the ears and diabetes.

According to a report published in 1983 by the Chinese Academy of Medical Science, this class of herbs can be effectively used in the treatment of chronic tracheitis, atherosclerosis, coronary heart disease, glomerulonephritis, hyperthyroidism, chronic atrophic gastritis, hepatitis B, rheumatoid arthritis, lupus erythematosus, scleroderma, pulseless disease, Behcet's disease, tumors, organic transplantation and aging, as well as in the prevention of the common cold.

## CLASS OF HERBS TO CONSTRICT AND OBSTRUCT MOVEMENTS

To constrict means to tighten up, thus making movements more difficult and to obstruct means to slow down the movements by making the passage rougher. This class of herbs is divided into two subclasses. The first subclass consists of herbs that can constrict and obstruct the movement of semen in men and of urination (such as cherokee rose). The second subclass consists of herbs that can constrict and obstruct bowel movements (such as water lily). Herbs that can constrict and obstruct the movement of semen in men and of urination, are used to treat premature ejaculation during sexual intercourse, seminal emission, enuresis and frequent urination. Herbs that can constrict and obstruct bowel movements are mostly used to check diarrhea.

However, this class of herbs is only used to deal with these problems symptomatically, which means that it cannot be used as a fundamental cure. For instance, when diarrhea occurs, this class of herbs should be used only when the real cause of it cannot be identified; otherwise, the herbal treatment should be directed towards the cause. If the diarrhea is caused by indigestion, it should be treated by the class of herbs that promote digestion (class 9); if it is caused by cold sensations in the bowel, it should be treated by the class of herbs that warm the body, (class 4).

## CLASS OF HERBS TO EXPEL OR DESTROY PARASITES

Parasites can cause intermittent abdominal pain, vomiting of bubbles, grinding of teeth at night, poor appetite, morbid hunger, love of strange foods, itch in the anus or the ears or the nose, a withered and yellowish complexion and puffiness all over the body. Such problems should be treated by this class of herbs according to the types of parasites involved.

The herbs to expel or destroy parasites should be administered on an empty stomach, so that they will produce stronger effects on the parasites. The patient taking such herbs should rest well and avoid greasy foods and after the parasites have been expelled, should take some tonics (class 16) to facilitate early recovery.

This class of herbs should not be administered to pregnant women, young or weak patients and patients with high fever or acute abdominal pain.

## CLASS OF HERBS FOR ULCERS AND TUMORS

The Chinese have developed three basic strategies against ulcers and tumors. The first strategy is to boost the patient's immune system, particularly if the patient is weak or old, so that the body can fight off the disease. The second strategy is to attack the ulcers and tumors by clearing toxic heat in the body. And the third strategy is to make certain that blood and energy are circulating properly.

The herbs to boost the immune system are presented under class 16, the herbs to promote blood circulation are presented under class 11 and the herbs to promote energy circulation are presented under class 12. The herbs that attack ulcers and tumors by clearing toxic heat are in this class and are fairly strong herbs that should be used with great care.

This class of herbs is divided into six subclasses. The first subclass consists of herbs for reducing heat, counteracting toxic effects and healing swelling. The second subclass consists of herbs for reducing heat, benefitting water metabolism and removing dampness. The third consists of herbs for removing sputum and dispersing coagulations. The fourth consists of herbs for transforming sputum and softening up hardness. The fifth consists of herbs for opening up the passages of meridians and activating them. And the sixth consists of other miscellaneous herbs for ulcers and tumors.

## CLASS OF HERBS
## FOR EXTERNAL APPLICATIONS

Herbs in this class are used for boils, carbuncles, fractures and bleeding due to external injuries. Such herbs can counteract toxic effects, heal swelling, remove pus and relieve pain. Although some of these herbs can also be consumed internally, most of them are toxic and should be taken with caution.

This class of herbs is divided into six subclasses. The first subclass consists of herbs for destroying worms and counteracting toxic effects. The second consists of herbs for healing swelling, dispersing coagulations and softening up hardness. The third consists of herbs for expelling pus and transforming decay. The fourth consists of herbs for activating the blood and removing wind (for more about the ill effects of wind, turn to page 13). The fifth consists of herbs for the arrestment of bleeding through constrictive effects. And the sixth is made up of other miscel-laneous herbs for external application.

For each of the herbs discussed in this chapter, information in the following categories is included.

# Herbs and Their Legends

### Chinese

This is the Romanization of the name of the herb under discussion. Commonly called pinyin, it is also the Chinese pronunciation of the name of the herb.

### Re

This is the reference number of the herb, based upon An Encyclopedic Dictionary of Chinese Herbs, compiled by the Jiangsu College of Traditional Chinese Medicine and published in two volumes by the Shanghai Scientific Technology Press in 1977. This publication lists over 5,000 Chinese herbs, with their assigned reference numbers.

### Common name

A Chinese herb may have more than one common name. However, the common names listed in this book are the ones most frequently used. The common name of an herb should not be used for identification purposes.

### Family

In biology, this is used to refer to a major subdivision in the classification of plants and animals.

### Chinese name

Chinese is an ideogramic language, which means that Chinese words represent ideas or objects, rather than speech sounds, as in English. So, when Chinese words are used to name an herb, the words represent an idea or ideas; the Chinese name of an herb listed here is usually the English translation of those ideas.

### Scientific Name

This is the scientific or botanical name of the herb under discussion.

### Pharmaceutical Name

This is the pharmaceutical name of the herb. It normally consists of two or more words—with the first word representing the part of the plant being used as the herb and the remaining word or words denoting the overall plant. For example, "radix ginseng" means that the root of the plant is used as the herb, because "radix" means root; "ginseng" refers to the plant called Panax Ginseng C. A. Mey.

### Part used

Different parts of a plant can be used as herbs with different functions, such as leaves, roots, stems, fruit, or seeds.

### Dosage

The indicated dosages are for one-day consumption for an adult, when the herb is decocted and used as a single ingredient. Dosages should be reduced by half for children between 6 and 13 years old, by one third for children between 3 and 5 years old and by one quarter for children under 3 years old.

### Flavor

An herb may taste sweet, bitter, pungent, salty, sour, light, or constrictive.

### Energy

An herb may be cold, cool, warm, hot, or neutral in energy.

### Class

There is a total of 20 classes of herbs; a given herb can belong to one or more classes. (The classes are described in pages 126-131.)

### Meridians

There is a total of 12 meridians through which herbs may travel after they have been digested. When an herb travels through a meridian, it means the herb is acting on that meridian and related organ.

### Actions

The actions of herbs are important to remember, because they often give us evidence for their applications.

### Indications

These are the symptoms and diseases that are treated by a given herb. However, a disorder may be due to different causes, which means that it should be treated differently; for this reason, the actions of herbs should be taken into account before the herbs are used to treat the disorders in this category.

### Notes

This includes additional information about the herb in question, including modern experiments.

*Medicinal Cornel Fruit, Shanzhuyu (Sour Mountain Date) and Morinda Root, Bajitian (Never-Withering-and-Falling)*

# Eleven Longevity Herbs

Throughout Chinese history, most Chinese emperors lived a relatively short life, partly because of their involvements in hectic politics and partly because of their excessive indulgence in sex. Both took their toll, physically and emotionally, at least from the point of view of Chinese medicine. However, an emperor named Qian Long of the Manchu Dynasty (1644-1911) was recorded to have lived the longest life of all the Chinese emperors prior to his time, dying at the age of 89. Emperor Qian Long was said to have frequently boasted about the secret methods he used to achieve longevity and had called himself "the long-life emperor."

That Qian Long had managed to stay youthful and had lived a long life is a historical fact. The British ambassador to China at that time was said to have written something like this in his diary, "When I met Emperor Qian Long, he was already at the age of 83, but he looked as if he was only 60 years old. He was in perfect good health and surpassed young men in energy and spirits." Many Chinese physicians have attributed Qian Long's longevity to his regular consumption of many herbs, but most notably, medicinal cornel fruit and morinda root.

The fruit of medicinal cornel looks like a date, tastes sour and is found mostly in the mountains, which is why the Chinese call it "sour mountain date."

But what makes this sour mountain date capable of promoting longevity? The story behind this is that the flowers of this plant appear as early as May, but its fruit do not become ripe until November, which means that it takes a longer period of time than other plants to bear fruit. Moreover, in November when most other plants have died, the sour mountain date has not only survived, but its fruit are hanging from it elegantly. The fact that it takes a long time for the sour mountain date to bear fruit signifies that the fruit must have a certain element of long life in them and the fact that this plant can resist the assault of severe winter cold means that there must be a quality of toughness in it.

The fruit of medicinal cornel was used as the "king ingredient" in a celebrated Chinese herbal formula, called "the eight-flavoured tablets," during the third century A.D. This formula was used to treat many serious disorders, including diabetes, chronic nephritis and sexual weaknesses. A "king ingredient" means that the ingredient plays a very important role in the formula. A report prepared by the National Peking Research Institute indicates that the fruit of medicinal cornel can promote urination and lower blood pressure for many hours.

What follows are standard, modern descriptions of this herb.

# 山茱萸

| Chinese | Shanzhuyu (Sour Mountain Date) |
|---|---|
| RE | 0370 |
| COMMON NAME | medicinal cornel fruit |
| FAMILY | Cornaceae |
| CHINESE NAME | wild date (so named because of its shape like a date) |
| SCIENTIFIC NAME | Cornus officinalis Sieb et Zucc |
| PHARMACEUTICAL NAME | Fructus Corni |
| PART USED | fruit |
| DOSAGE | 5g |
| FLAVOR | sour |
| ENERGY | slightly warm |
| CLASS | 17, herbs to constrict and obstruct movements |
| MERIDIANS | liver and kidneys |
| ACTIONS | to tone up the liver and kidneys, constrict semen and check perspiration |
| INDICATIONS | seminal emission, excessive perspiration, lumbago, dizziness, ringing in ears and insomnia |
| NOTES | Experiments have shown shanzhuyu to be effective in inhibiting gastrointestinal peristalsis and in reducing blood sugar. Since this herb is obstructive, it is not recommended for those with constipation. |

Morinda root is called "never-withering-and-falling" in Chinese, because it is a creeping vine that hangs on persistently and "never withering and falling" means longevity in Chinese. The root of this plant, which is used for medicinal purposes, contains vitamin C and carbohydrates.

Shanzhuyu and jinyingzi, which will be discussed later, are both constrictive with the effects of tonification. So, they can be used to treat seminal emission, seminal sliding, enuresis, excessive urination, excessive menstrual flow and vaginal discharge due to kidney deficiency.

Shanzhuyu can be decocted with renshen (radix ginseng), which will be discussed later, to treat patients with extremely cold sensations after profuse perspiration.

To treat insomnia, fry 20g shanzhuyu quickly over low heat until it is dry, grind into powder to soak in 5 cups of wine and seal in bottle. Leave for one month, shaking the bottle once a day. Then strain it to drink the wine, twice a day, in the morning and in the evening. To treat other diseases, decoct 10g shanzhuyu in water for consumption in a standard manner (see Chapter 3).

*Glutinous Rehmannia,
Shengdi (New Place) and
Shudihuang (Old Place)*

# 巴戟天

| Chinese | Bajitian (Never-Withering-and-Falling) |
|---|---|
| RE | 1034 |
| COMMON NAME | morinda root |
| FAMILY | Rubiaceae |
| CHINESE NAME | morinda root |
| SCIENTIFIC NAME | Morinda officinalis How |
| PHARMACEUTICAL NAME | Radix Morindae Officinalis |
| PART USED | root |
| DOSAGE | 7 to 18g |
| FLAVOR | pungent and sweet |
| ENERGY | warm |
| CLASS | 16, herbs to correct deficiencies |
| MERIDIANS | kidneys |
| ACTIONS | to warm up the kidneys, strengthen yang and strengthen tendons and bones |
| INDICATIONS | kidney yang deficiency, impotence, lumbago, dizziness and ringing in ears |
| NOTES | Bajitian is effective for treating impotence, lumbago and cold-damp rheumatism due to kidney yang deficiency |

A Chinese government official in the Ming Dynasty (1368-1644), known as Mayor Lin, was said to have fathered a baby girl at the age of 104 and he was believed to be in the habit of taking glutinous rehmannia. The Chinese have a famous riddle: "I have visited a new place and returned to an old one simultaneously, what herb am I?" The answer is: "I am glutinous rehmannia." When glutinous rehmannia is used in raw form, it is called "new place," because the Chinese ideograms for raw glutinous rehmannia and "new place" are identical; but when rehmannia is processed by steaming and drying in the sun, it is called "old place," because the Chinese ideograms for processed glutinous rehmannia and "old place" are identical. The Chinese traditionally process raw glutinous rehmannia by steaming it 10 times and drying it in the sun nine times, in order to make it shiny and black as if it were painted with black ink. But why do the Chinese bother to go to such great lengths in processing it? There is a good reason underlying their efforts.

Raw glutinous rehmannia can reduce heat in the blood, whereas processed glutinous rehmannia can treat blood deficiency. Thus, in Chinese herbalism, the raw and the processed forms of glutinous rehmannia are regarded as two entirely different herbs. They belong to two different classes and there's a world of difference between them in terms of their clinical uses.

A report published in the *Chinese Medical Journal* indicates that raw glutinous rehmannia has been shown to be effective in the treatment of rheumatic and rheumatoid arthritis. Also, glutinous rehmannia and licorice have been shown to be a good combination. A report published in the *Medical Technology Reporter* indicates that in the treatment of bronchial asthma, injections of processed glutinous rehmannia and processed licorice have produced very positive results. Another report, published in the *New Pharmacological Journal*, indicates obvious improvements in cases of contagious hepatitis treated by injections of raw glutinous rehmannia and raw licorice.

# 生地　　熟地

| Chinese | Shengdi (New Place) | Shudihuang (Old Place) |
|---|---|---|
| RE | 5370 | 5517 |
| COMMON NAME | glutinous rehmannia (raw) | steamed glutinous rehmannia |
| FAMILY | Berberidaceae | Scrophulariaceae |
| CHINESE NAME | fresh earth's yellowness (literal translation) | cooked earth's yellowness (literal translation) |
| SCIENTIFIC NAME | Rehmannia glutinosa Libosch | Rehmannia glutinosa Libosch |
| PHARMACEUTICAL NAME | Radix Rehmanniae | Radix Rehmanniae praeparatae |
| PART USED | dried tuberous root | tuberous root |
| DOSAGE | 10 to 90g | 20g |
| FLAVOR | sweet and bitter | sweet |
| ENERGY | cold | slightly warm |
| CLASS | herbs to reduce excessive heat inside the body (class 2) and herbs for lubricating dry symptoms (class 6) | 16, herbs to correct deficiencies |
| MERIDIANS | heart, liver and kidneys | liver and kidneys |
| ACTIONS | to increase yin energy to a moderate degree, bring down fire, cool down the blood, lubricate the intestine and produce fluids | to tone up blood, water kidneys, nourish yin and make grey hair return to former color |
| INDICATIONS | sore throat, vomiting of blood, coughing up blood, nosebleed, discharge of urine containing blood and diabetes | blood deficiency, grey hair, ringing in ears, night sweats, vaginal bleeding, diabetes and seminal emission |
| NOTES | Experiments have shown shengdi to be an effective heart tonic and an effective coagulant | Experiments have shown that shudihuang can protect the liver and reduce blood sugar. |

Shengdi is sticky and contains moisture. So, when it is decocted with other herbs, it should be decocted first for 10 minutes before adding the other herbs.

Shudihuang is good for kidney yin deficiency with dizziness and vertigo. It is an effective blood tonic and is also effective for the arrestment of bleeding due to blood deficiency and can thus be used to treat such symptoms as palpitations, excessive menstrual flow and blood in urine.

## Matrimony Vine, Gouqizi (Thorny Stalk Seed)

There is a story about a Chinese traveller who, while passing through a village called Xihe, happened to witness a young lady beating an old man with grey hair all over his head. The young lady looked about 15 or 16 years old and the old man somewhere between 80 and 90. The traveller asked the young lady why she was beating the old man and she explained that she was his granddaughter and she was angry with him for failing to take his longevity herbs. That was why he looked so old, she said. The traveller asked her age and was told that she was 372 years old. Rather taken aback, he asked her how she had managed to live that long and she replied that she consumed matrimony vine all year around.

China's greatest herbalist, Shih-Chen Li, who wrote the celebrated *Outline of Materia Medica*, published in 1578, pointed out in this book that the people in the village of Nan-Qiu were in the habit of eating matrimony vine and that a very high percentage of them lived a long life. And a famous Chinese poet in the Tang Dynasty (618-907) by the name of Yu-Xi Liu wrote a poem in praise of the wonderful effects of matrimony vine, which said that even the water from a well near the plant can make people live a long life.

In fact, matrimony vine is not only good for longevity, but it is often associated with beauty as well. For instance, a Chinese writer reported that he knew a beautiful woman from a wealthy family who had always made it a point to drink matrimony vine tea and eat the seeds every day, which was why, he said, she looked 20 years younger than her age.

Matrimony vine is a trailing shrub with thorny stalks. Its seeds are the most valuable part for medicinal purposes, although the roots of this plant are beneficial as well.

Another story relates how a scholar spotted some beautiful flowers on the plant, so out of curiosity he began to dig out the roots. To his amazement, the roots were shaped like two dogs bound together. But he washed them anyway and boiled them in water. After having eaten the roots for a few days, the scholar all of a sudden felt very light in his body, as if he could fly away.

枸杞子

| Chinese | Gouqizi (Thorny Stalk Seed) |
|---|---|
| RE | 3163 |
| COMMON NAME | matrimony vine fruit |
| FAMILY | Solanaceae |
| CHINESE NAME | aspen-willow fruit (so named because this herb is as thorny as an aspen, its stems resemble those of a willow and its fruit is used) |
| SCIENTIFIC NAME | Lycium barbarum L. |
| PHARMACEUTICAL NAME | Fructus Lycii |
| PART USED | ripe fruit |
| DOSAGE | 6g |
| FLAVOR | sweet |
| ENERGY | neutral |
| CLASS | 16, herbs to correct deficiencies |
| MERIDIANS | liver, lungs and kidneys |
| ACTIONS | to tone up kidneys, nourish the liver, nourish blood and sharpen vision |
| INDICATIONS | blood deficiency with dizziness and blurred vision, lumbago, seminal emission and diabetes |
| NOTES | Experiments have shown that gouqizi can protect the liver and reduce blood sugar |

Gouqizi can tonify the kidneys. It is good for dizziness, vertigo and lumbago, due to kidney deficiency, as well as for dizziness and vertigo, due to liver deficiency. It is also good for nourishing the liver to sharpen vision.

Gouqizi can be decocted with juhua to nourish the liver and sharpen vision. This combination is considered very beneficial for people suffering from dizziness and blurred vision.

中医疗法

# Momordica Fruit, Luohanguo (Arhat Fruit)

羅漢果

**M**omordica fruit is one of the few fruits that cannot be eaten until it is dried by fire. For the last few centuries, this fruit has almost exclusively been a product of the province of Guangxi in southern China. The people of this region have called this fruit "longevity fruit" because they have believed that a prolonged consumption of it would make people live a long life. This fruit is said to resemble the stomach of a Buddha, which is why its official Chinese name is "arhat fruit," since "arhat" refers to a Buddhist who has attained Nirvana.

Momordica fruit has traditionally been used for a number of common ailments, such as cough with sputum, constipation, chronic laryngitis, hoarseness and chronic bronchitis. But it has also recently emerged as an important herb in the curing and prevention of cancer. According to a Japanese report, this fruit contains an unnamed substance that makes it taste 300 times sweeter than ordinary sugar. Although it tastes so sweet, the Chinese nevertheless believe that it is good for diabetes.

| *Chinese* | *Luohanguo (Arhat Fruit)* |
|---|---|
| RE | 2806 |
| COMMON NAME | fruit of Grosvenor Momordica |
| FAMILY | Cucurbitaceae |
| CHINESE NAME | big fellow's fruit |
| SCIENTIFIC NAME | Momordica grosvenori Swingle |
| PHARMACEUTICAL NAME | Fructus Momordicae |
| PART USED | fruit |
| DOSAGE | 10 to 16g |
| FLAVOR | sweet |
| ENERGY | cool |
| CLASS | herbs to suppress coughing and reduce sputum (class 10) and herbs to induce bowel movements (class 8) |
| MERIDIANS | lungs and spleen |
| ACTIONS | to clear lungs and lubricate intestines |
| INDICATIONS | whooping cough, cough with sputum fire and constipation due to dry blood. |

## Baiziren (Oriental Arborvitae Seed)

柏子仁

A notorious Chinese emperor in the Qin Dynasty (221-207 B.C.) called himself "the first emperor of China," meaning that, after his death, his son would be the second emperor and his grandson the third and on and on without interruption. Not only had the emperor built the Great Wall to head off possible foreign invasion from the North, but he had also kept over 3,000 concubines in his palace to satisfy his fantasies. But no sooner had the emperor died than his palace was burned down and the empire he had built came to a total collapse. All the concubines either escaped or were sent away from the palace by the new conqueror and one was later found in the woods.

After this concubine escaped from the palace, she hid in the woods, where there was little to eat. After a while, she met an old man, who advised her to eat Oriental arborvitae seeds. Since they were not pleasing to the taste, she hesitated at first, but finally came to realize that she had no choice. And so, she began to eat them, gradually becoming used to their taste. As it turned out, she developed great strength in resisting the severe winter cold as well as the extreme summer heat.

It wasn't until a century and a half later that a group of hunters found her in the woods; she was naked and had long black hair and was seen escaping as fast as a monkey. The hunters were very curious and ran after her in pursuit. Once they finally captured her, they questioned her and were shocked to find that the black-haired woman used to be a concubine of the first emperor of China and that she was now 200 years old.

From the point of view of modern medicine, Oriental arborvitae seed contains 14 percent fat, volatile oil and saponin. It can reduce cholesterol level and prevent cardiovascular diseases.

| Chinese | Baiziren (Oriental Arborvitae Seed) |
|---|---|
| RE | 3154 |
| COMMON NAME | Oriental arborvitae kernel |
| FAMILY | Cupressaceae |
| CHINESE NAME | lateral cypress kernel (so named because its leaves are flat and grow laterally) |
| SCIENTIFIC NAME | Biota orientalis (L.) Endl |
| PHARMACEUTICAL NAME | Semen Biotae |
| PART USED | ripe kernel |
| DOSAGE | 6g |
| FLAVOR | sweet |
| ENERGY | neutral |
| CLASS | 14, herbs to reduce anxiety |
| MERIDIANS | heart and spleen |
| ACTIONS | to secure the heart, check perspiration, lubricate dryness and induce bowel movements |
| INDICATIONS | insomnia, palpitations, constipation and night sweats |
| NOTES | Experiments have shown that baiziren can sedate and inhibit. |

# Sesame, Heizhima (Barbarian's Hemp)

A Chinese woman in ancient China was said to have consumed sesame for more than 80 years on end, which made her live to over 90 years of age and still look like a young lady. At 90, she could still walk 300 miles a day and run as fast as a deer.

A Chinese document relates that sesame can be boiled and made into tablets as big as bullets. By taking one tablet each day for one year, you will get a shiny complexion. By taking the same dosage for 2 years, the grey hair will go away; for 3 years, lost teeth will grow back; for 4 years, you will have complete freedom from disease; for 5 years, you will be able to run as fast as a horse; and for life, you will achieve longevity. From the point of view of modern medicine, sesame contributes to longevity primarily because it contains vitamin E.

Sesame can also increase the beauty of the skin and the Chinese often make use of a combination of sesame and rice powder as a beauty formula. First, fry sesame in an oil-free pan and, after a while, add a little water and mix thoroughly. Next, strain the sesame and add a little rice powder to the sesame fluid. Then bring the fluid to a boil over low heat. Remove from heat and add a little honey or sugar or other condiments to taste.

The Chinese believe that the skin can be made beautiful, not by vegetables or fruits alone, but also by an adequate amount of vegetable oils, particularly sesame. The combination of sesame and rice powder is also effective for treating constipation, which is a symptom that needs to be corrected if the skin is to become beautiful.

Sesame is called barbarian's hemp in Chinese, because it looks like hemp and it was originally imported from a foreign country on the western border of China by a Chinese general named Zhang Qian, when he was sent by the Chinese emperor to conquer that country in 119 B.C. It must be pointed out that the Chinese regarded all foreigners as barbarians during that period of Chinese history.

黑芝麻

| Chinese | Heizhima (Barbarian's Hemp) |
|---|---|
| RE | 4955 |
| COMMON NAME | sesame |
| FAMILY | Pedaliaceae |
| CHINESE NAME | wild sesame |
| SCIENTIFIC NAME | Sesamum indicum L. |
| PHARMACEUTICAL NAME | Semen Sesami |
| PART USED | seed |
| DOSAGE | 3 to 12g |
| FLAVOR | sweet |
| ENERGY | neutral |
| CLASS | herbs for lubricating dry symptoms (class 6) and herbs to correct deficiencies (class 16) |
| MERIDIANS | liver and kidneys |
| ACTIONS | to tone up the liver and kidneys and lubricate the five viscera |
| INDICATIONS | liver-kidney deficiency, headaches, dizziness, ringing in the ears, constipation and shortage of milk secretion in women |
| NOTES | Heizhima can tonify and nourish the liver and the kidneys. It is an effective herb for blurred vision and dizziness, ringing in the ears and numbness of the arms and legs. It is associated with yin deficiency of the liver and the kidneys. |

## Slender Acanthopanax Root Bark, Wujiapi (Thorny Ginseng)

五加皮

According to a story told by China's most celebrated herbalist, Shih-Chen Li, half a dozen Chinese politicians and scholars prior to his time had lived to be over 300 years old as a result of consuming slender acanthopanax root bark soaked in rice wine, traditionally known as "thorny ginseng wine." Legends of this sort are taken so seriously by some Chinese people that one famous poet declared that he would "rather have a taste of thorny ginseng wine than be in possession of a cartful of gold."

When I visited China in 1983, I bought a few bottles of liquid made from this plant and the label said, "good for neurasthenia, insomnia, many dreams, forgetfulness, dizziness, poor appetite, palpitation, coronary heart disease, angina pectoris and a prolonged consumption will cure leukopenia caused by physiotherapy and chemotherapy and will slow down aging."

A report prepared by the Seventh Shanghai Pharmaceutical Factory said that of the 43 cases of leukopenia treated with this herb, 70.4 percent showed effective results, with a rise in white blood cells to normal within an average of 2 weeks. Among the patients treated, 37 cases were caused by chemotherapy and radiation of tumors, three cases were caused by hypersplenism and three cases were due to other causes. The treatment involved an oral administration of 3.6g of this herb each day, for a period of 3 to 15 days. It was also indicated that the treatment showed better results in those cases caused by chemotherapy and among them, two cases underwent a marrow test, which showed signs of proliferation. And according to a statistical report compiled by 10 Chinese hospitals, of the 113 cases of tumor patients with leukopenia caused by chemotherapy and radiation treated by this herb, 13.7 percent showed obviously effective results with an overall effective rate of 74.5 percent. In another report, 100 cases of chronic tracheitis were treated with this herb. The results showed improvements in symptoms, in physical strength and in frequency of attack, with the effect of increasing the function of the adrenal cortex.

Slender acanthopanax root bark comes from a shrub with many fine thorns on small branches and belongs to the same family as Chinese ginseng, which is why the Chinese call it "thorny ginseng."

| Chinese | Wujiapi (Thorny Ginseng) |
|---|---|
| RE | 0767 |
| COMMON NAME | Acanthopanax root bark |
| FAMILY | Araliaceae |
| CHINESE NAME | five plus bark |
| SCIENTIFIC NAME | Acanthopanax gracilistylus W. W. Smith |
| PHARMACEUTICAL NAME | Cortex Acanthopanacis Radicis |
| PART USED | dry root bark |
| DOSAGE | 6 to 12g |
| FLAVOR | pungent |
| ENERGY | warm |
| CLASS | 3, herbs to counteract rheumatism |
| MERIDIANS | liver and kidneys |
| ACTIONS | to remove wind and dampness and strengthen bones and tendons. |
| INDICATIONS | rheumatism, beriberi and weak limbs |
| NOTES | Experiments have shown wujiapi to be an effective heart tonic, as it can produce adrenocortical hormones and also to be an effective herb for the relief of pain and rheumatism. |
| | Wujiapi is especially effective in treating rheumatism in the lower half of the body due to dampness. |

Tianxingren
(Sweet Apricot)
and Chicken Head
Kernel, Qianshi
(Water Lily)

甜杏仁

A 60-year-old woman in the Wen Feng Commune suffered from a severe illness and was very overweight. Seeing that nothing could help her, her family started preparing her funeral. Meanwhile, an old Chinese doctor of traditional Chinese medicine told her to grind 450 g of sweet apricot and 450 g of water lily into a fine powder and to take the powder regularly. No sooner had she finished all the powder, than the woman recovered from her illness; continuing to take this powder, she was free from illness thereafter. The water lily fruit looks like the head of a chicken, which is why the Chinese call it "chicken head kernel."

There are two kinds of apricot kernel: bitter apricot kernel, called kuxingren and sweet apricot kernel, called tianxingren. Tianxingren is larger than kuxingren. Kuxingren can expel sputum, suppress coughing and lubricate the intestines and is good for coughing and asthma and abundant sputum due to the common cold, as well as for constipation. Tianxingren can lubricate the lungs, suppress coughing and make the intestines smooth; it is better for a chronic cough or a dry cough without sputum due to yin deficiency of the lungs.

In his celebrated classic, entitled *One Thousand Ounces Gold Classic*, published in 682, Sun Shu Mao (581-682) presented a formula for longevity called "sweet apricot mixture." You fry 5kg of sweet apricot kernel quickly over low heat until dry, grind it into powder and immerse it in rice wine. Next, you strain it and mix the liquid with 2.5kg of honey to make a 7.5kg mixture, which you boil over low heat again, until it becomes as thick as jelly. Then you put it in a container and seal it tightly. Take 20 to 35g of this liquid per dosage to recover from an illness and achieve longevity.

| Chinese | Tianxingren (Sweet Apricot) |
|---|---|
| RE | 4495 |
| COMMON NAME | sweet apricot seed |
| FAMILY | Rosaceae |
| CHINESE NAME | sweet apricot seed (so named because it tastes sweet) |
| SCIENTIFIC NAME | Prunus armeniaca Linne |
| PHARMACEUTICAL NAME | Semen Armeniacae Dulcis |
| PART USED | ripe seed |
| DOSAGE | 10g |
| FLAVOR | sweet |
| ENERGY | neutral |
| CLASS | herbs for lubricating dry symptoms (class 6) and herbs to suppress cough and reduce sputum (class 10) |
| MERIDIANS | lungs and large intestine |
| ACTIONS | to lubricate lungs, expel sputum, suppress cough and relieve asthma |
| INDICATIONS | dry cough, asthma and constipation |

# 苦杏仁 芡實

| Chinese | Kuxingren (Bitter Apricot) | Qianshi (Water Lily) |
|---|---|---|
| RE | 2240 | 2183 |
| COMMON NAME | bitter apricot kernel | gorgon fruit |
| FAMILY | Rosaceae | Nymphaceae |
| CHINESE NAME | bitter apricot kernel | gorgon fruit |
| SCIENTIFIC NAME | Prunus armeniaca L. var. ansu Maxim, prunus sibirica L, Prunus mandshurica (Maxim) Koehne & Prunus armeniaca L. | Euryale ferox Salisb |
| PHARMACEUTICAL NAME | Semen Armeniacae Amarum | Semen Euryales |
| PART USED | ripe kernel | kernel |
| DOSAGE | 6g | 6 to 10g |
| FLAVOR | bitter | sweet |
| ENERGY | warm | neutral |
| CLASS | 10, herbs to suppress cough and reduce sputum | 17, herbs to constrict and obstruct movements |
| MERIDIANS | lungs and large intestine | spleen and kidneys |
| ACTIONS | to suppress cough, expel sputum, expand lungs and calm down asthma | to strengthen the spleen, benefit the kidneys, solidify semen and relieve diarrhea |
| INDICATIONS | cough in the common cold, asthma with copious sputum and constipation due to exhaustion of fluids | diarrhea due to spleen deficiency, seminal emission and vaginal discharge |
| NOTES | Bitter apricot is slightly toxic. It contains cyanic glycosides that can suppress cough. Experiments have shown it to be effective for suppression of cough and also for asthma. | Qianshi is obstructive and thus should be avoided by those with constipation. |

中医疗法

## Tuber of Multiflower Knotweed, Heshouwu (Mr. He's Black Hair)

何首烏

In 812, a 56-year-old man by the name of He was pruning his trees when two plants a few metres apart suddenly caught his attention. He thought it was very strange that the vines of these plants were crossing each other not unlike a man and a woman embracing each other in love. "There's got to be a good reason for these plants to be doing this kind of thing," he thought. He then dug out the roots of the plants and brought them home to cook and eat as food.

He had been so weak since childhood that he had never married. However, after consuming the roots for seven days, he began to have a desire for marriage. After consuming the roots for a few months, he began to feel much stronger; and after one year of consumption, his grey hair had all returned to black and he began to look like a young man. At that point, He got married and then fathered a baby boy. Both the father and the son lived to over 130 years of age. The Chinese have called tuber of multiflower knotweed "He's black hair" ever since.

From the point of view of modern medicine, the effects of tuber of multiflower knot-weed are similar to those of an adrenocortical hormone. In a medical experiment, two groups of animals were placed in a –5°C refrigerator for 17½ hours; before being placed in the refrigerator, one group was fed the herb for two weeks. The results showed that 32.3 percent of the animals in the group fed the herb died compared with the 67.7 percent death rate in the other group. In another experiment on the treatment of chronic tracheitis, one group of patients was treated by a standard herbal formula while another group was treated by the same herbal formula plus tuber of multiflower knotweed. The second group showed obviously better results, with both local symptoms and fear of wind and cold, cold sensations in the back and shortness of breath considerably improved.

| Chinese | Heshouwu (Mr. He's Black Hair) |
|---|---|
| RE | 2310 |
| COMMON NAME | multiflower knotweed tuber |
| FAMILY | Polygonaceae |
| CHINESE NAME | Mr. He's black hair |
| SCIENTIFIC NAME | Polygonum multiflorum Thunb |
| PHARMACEUTICAL NAME | Radix Polygoni Multiflori |
| PART USED | tuberous root |
| DOSAGE | 10 to 25g |
| FLAVOR | bitter and sweet |
| ENERGY | slightly warm |
| CLASS | 16, herbs to correct deficiencies |
| MERIDIANS | liver and kidneys |
| ACTIONS | to tone up the liver and kidneys and to benefit semen and blood |
| INDICATIONS | seminal emission, vaginal discharge, lumbago and premature grey hair |
| NOTES | According to experiments, heshouwu can treat fatty liver, increase red blood cells and reduce blood fat. |

# Agrimony

One summer two Chinese officials were making a long trip to Peking to take a national examination for promotion. Seeing that time was almost running out, they hastened their journey, only to find themselves in a desert without any village in sight. They were hungry and thirsty and physically exhausted, but they could find neither water to drink, food to eat, nor a place to rest. One of the officials suddenly developed a nosebleed and the bleeding wouldn't stop, so his fellow traveller ripped a sheet of paper from an old book and squeezed it into his friend's nose. But it was in vain, as the blood continued to flow from his nose.

The official with the nosebleed said, "I wish I had some water." "Where could I possibly get water for you?" responded his nervous friend. "We are on a wide desert now. We're in dire straits. I wish someone would help us."

At that moment, a bird few past them with a loud cry. The official with the nosebleed looked up and saw a red-crowned crane circling over his head. "Dear bird, I wish I could borrow your wings to fly out of this desert," shouted the official, with both arms outstretched and his mouth wide open. Shocked by the official's loud shouting, the red-crowned crane suddenly opened its beak and a blade of grass dropped from it to the ground. The official picked it up and murmured with a smile, "Even if I can't borrow your wings, I can still use this grass to moisten my mouth for some relief." And so, he put the grass in his mouth and started chewing it as if it were a piece of gum. Oddly enough, the nosebleed stopped after a short while and both officials started jumping with joy. "The bird gave us a magic grass," one of them said jokingly.

The two Chinese officials made it to the examination hall in the capital just in time for the examination and both of them passed and got promoted. When the two officials got together again some time later, they recalled the event on the desert and began to wonder about the grass that stopped the nosebleed. They started making inquiries about the name of the grass, but no herbalists knew anything about it. The two then drew pictures of the grass from their recollections and ordered their subordinates to search for it.

Finally, many years later, the grass was found growing along some hillsides. It was a perennial herb with long soft hairs over the entire plant. Discovering that the plant still had no name, the officials named it after the red-crowned crane.

中医疗法

# 仙鶴草

| Chinese | Xianhecao (Red-Crowned Crane's Herb) |
|---|---|
| RE | 1372 |
| COMMON NAME | agrimony |
| FAMILY | Rosaceae |
| CHINESE NAME | red-crowned crane plant (literal translation) |
| SCIENTIFIC NAME | Agrimonia pilosa Ledeb |
| PHARMACEUTICAL NAME | Herba Agrimoniae |
| PART USED | whole plant |
| DOSAGE | 30g |
| FLAVOR | bitter |
| ENERGY | neutral |
| CLASS | 12, herbs to regulate blood |
| MERIDIANS | lung, spleen, stomach & large intestine |
| ACTIONS | to constrict and arrest bleeding |
| INDICATIONS | vomiting of blood, coughing up blood, nosebleeds and vaginal bleeding |
| NOTES | Since xianhecao is obstructive, it should be avoided by those with constipation.<br><br>Experiments have shown that xianhecao can increase and protect blood platelets and that it is an effective coagulant and can arrest bleeding (as a hemostatic). |

Agrimony is an important Chinese herb used for the arrestment of bleeding and its effects have been proven by modern research. In one study, 20 cases of bleeding, including bleeding from external causes and bleeding caused by intracranial and thoracic and abdominal surgeries, were treated by the hemostatic powder made from this herb. The results of this study showed that the bleeding stopped within 1 to 2 minutes in all cases. Agrimony produced in the Soviet Union has been found to contain plenty of tannin and a small quantity of vitamin K-1, both of which are believed to be responsible for the hemostatic effects of the herb.

# Changshan (Mount Eternity)

# Antipyretic Dichroa

On a mountain in China called Mount Eternity, there was an old temple where a poor monk lived. This monk was so poor that he had to go all the way to a village to beg for food.

One day the monk was attacked by malaria and he experienced intermittent fever and chills nearly once every day thereafter. He had lost a great deal of weight as a result of the malaria and had come to a point where he could hardly walk. But the monk was so poor that he couldn't even consider seeking medical treatment.

One day the monk had gone to the village to beg for food as usual, but by noon had met with no success and his stomach was rumbling like crazy. The monk thought to himself, "What will happen to me when the malaria strikes again this afternoon? How can I sustain the attack without eating anything?" With this thought in his head, the monk had come to knock at yet another door. But the poor fellow who answered said, "We do not have enough food to feed ourselves, so how can we feed you? We cooked some plant roots and started eating them, but then all of us started vomiting. If you are really hungry, you can try them." Feeling that he had no choice, the monk gobbled up all the plant roots on the table and left.

Oddly enough, the monk did not vomit nor did he experience any other discomfort. After walking a short distance, he sat down on some grass to take a sunbath while waiting for the onset of the malaria. He waited and waited for many hours, until by sunset, not only had the malaria not struck, but the monk felt unusually good and comfortable.

A few days passed, but the malaria still did not attack him. The monk was quite excited by the prospect of complete recovery. But, unfortunately, a month later, the malaria recurred.

中医疗法

常山

| | |
|---|---|
| *Chinese* | *Changshan (Mount Eternity)* |
| RE | 4321 |
| COMMON NAME | antipyretic dichroa |
| FAMILY | Saxifragaceae |
| CHINESE NAME | eternal mountain |
| SCIENTIFIC NAME | Dichroa febrifuga Lour |
| PHARMACEUTICAL NAME | Radix Dichroae |
| PART USED | root |
| DOSAGE | 6 to 10g |
| FLAVOR | bitter |
| ENERGY | cold |
| CLASS | herbs to expel or destroy parasites (class 18) and herbs to induce vomiting (class 7) |
| MERIDIANS | lungs, heart and liver |
| ACTIONS | to induce vomiting of sputum, clear up heat and promote water flow. |
| INDICATIONS | sputum, malaria and amebic dysentery |
| NOTES | Experiments have shown changshan to be effective in treating various types of cancer, but it is slightly toxic and should be consumed by pregnant women with great care. Before decoction, changshan must be fried in wine in order to reduce its side effect of nausea. |

Wondering if there was any correlation between eating the roots and his temporary recovery, the monk rushed back to the poor fellow's house who had given him the roots. He asked him what the roots were and the fellow, still angry, responded, "Those were the roots my stupid son dug up on the mountain that made all of us sick for so many days." "Could you ask your son to lead me to the plants?" requested the monk.

And so, the poor fellow's son guided the monk to the mountain, where they found plenty of these plants growing on the ground. The plant turned out to be a deciduous shrub, with round stalks and branches, usu-ally found growing on wet ground in the mountains. The monk dug out the roots and brought them home to cook and eat. The next day, after eating the roots, the malaria did not attack him. After continuing to eat them for a few more days, the monk found that he was totally free of the malaria. The monk then planted some in his garden, just in case he should need them in the future.

After successfully treating his own illness, the monk became a doctor of some sort and many malaria patients began coming to him for help. The monk treated them one by one, always with the roots of the same plant and always with the same good results. As time went on, people began to ask about the name of the plant. As it had no name, the monk began to tell his patients it was called "Mount Eternity."

In Chinese herbalism, antipyretic dichroa is called Mount Eternity because the plants are so plentiful on that mountain. This plant has been used as an effective herb in treating malaria for many centuries. According to a report published in Science, antipyretic dichroa contains dichroine B, which has been proven effective for malaria. In another report, published in *Scientific Technology*, antipyretic dichroa was found to contain five different kinds of alkaloid, all of which are antimalarial agents and one of them has been found to be five times more effective than quinine in treating malaria. The leaves, stalks and roots are all effective, but the leaves have been found to be 20 times more effective than the roots, although the quantity of alkaloid contained in the leaves varies significantly from season to season.

A report published in the *Chinese Medical Journal* said that among the 24 cases of malaria treated by antipyretic dichroa, body temperature returned to normal within one day in 70 percent of the patients and malarial parasites disappeared within two days in 50 percent of the patients. The treatment takes effect more slowly when three to four dosages are used daily and takes effect more quickly when four to six dosages are used daily.

*Pugongying
(Fisherman's Herb)*

# Asian Dandelion

The 16-year-old daughter of a government official in ancient China was suffering from mastitis with a triangular lump underneath her left breast. She was in pain and was becoming very worried, but she dared not tell anybody about it, because deep down inside she felt very ashamed. But her disease was subsequently found out by her maid, who disclosed it to her father, pleading with him to hire a doctor.

On inquiry into his daughter's condition, the official became very angry, as he suspected that his daughter must have done something immoral to have caused it. He rushed to his daughter's room and began to strike her in the face. "How could you do such a shameful thing, you are a disgrace to your family," shouted the father. The maid insisted that his daughter had never gone out alone and could not have possibly done anything immoral. The father wouldn't listen and so the daughter ran away from home that night out of shame and desperation.

She went to the river bank and, thinking that no one would be around at that hour to see her, quickly jumped into the river in an attempt to commit suicide. However, a fisherman was fishing from a rowboat nearby with his 16-year-old daughter. When they heard the splash, the fisherman's daughter instantly jumped into the river to save her. Once they were both on board, the fisherman was surprised to see that the girl was just about the same age as his daughter.

The fisherman's daughter began to change the girl's clothes and in the process, discovered the swelling in the young lady's left breast. At that moment, she immediately understood the reason for her attempted suicide. After telling her father about it, the fisherman replied, "We will go dig some plants for her breast first thing in the morning."

中医疗法

蒲公英

| | |
|---|---|
| *Chinese* | *Pugongying (Fisherman's Herb)* |
| RE | 5130 |
| COMMON NAME | Asian dandelion |
| FAMILY | Compositae |
| CHINESE NAME | yellow-flowered one-leg herb (so named because its flowers are yellow and the plant looks as if it has only one leg) |
| SCIENTIFIC NAME | Taraxacum mongolicum Hand.-Mazz., Taraxacum sinicum Kitag. & Taraxacum heterolepis olepis Nakai et H. Koidz |
| PHARMACEUTICAL NAME | Herba Taraxaci |
| PART USED | entire plant |
| DOSAGE | 20g |
| FLAVOR | bitter and sweet |
| ENERGY | cold |
| CLASS | 2, herbs to reduce excessive heat inside the body |
| MERIDIANS | spleen and stomach |
| ACTIONS | to clear up heat, counteract toxic effects, disperse swelling and heal carbuncles |
| INDICATIONS | carbuncles, swelling, mastitis, urinary infections and acute tonsillitis |
| NOTES | Experts have shown that pugongying can be used for breast cancer and that it is an antibacterial herb. It contains folic acid and bacterides and it is now being widely used to treat mastitis, hepatitis, appendicitis, urinary infections, acute tonsillitis, tracheitis, laryngitis and the common cold.<br><br>In addition, pugongying can also regulate the liver and the stomach, which is why it can be used to treat mastitis and stomachache. |

The plant turned out to be a perennial herb, with white milky juice in it, yellowish flowers and straight but fleshy and thick roots. They found the plants on the roadside not far from the river. They dug out a few plants that were about 100g in weight, washed them clean and boiled them in water. Then they told the girl to drink the liquid. In the meantime, they crushed some of the plants and applied them to her breast externally.

Upon hearing of the whereabouts and the attempted suicide of their daughter, the official and his wife, feeling greatly worried and deeply regretful, rushed to see the fisherman and to take their daughter home. Their daughter, grateful and in tears, said good-bye to the fisherman and his daughter and went home with her parents, bringing a bunch of the plants with her. Before she left, the fisherman kept reminding her to continue using the herbs for her illness.

After she had recovered from her illness, she told her maid to plant the herb in their garden. So that she would always remember the fisherman, she named the plant after him without knowing his name.

Asian dandelion is now used to treat many inflammatory diseases, including mumps, tonsillitis and mastitis. Although this herb tastes bitter, the Chinese in the rural areas are in the habit of making tea out of it and then drinking it as a remedy for eye diseases, redness in the eyes, nose diseases and urination disturbances.

The Chinese use Asian dandelion to treat such symptoms by decocting 50g dandelion in two glasses of water until the water is reduced by half; then they strain it and drink the liquid once daily. In the treatment of eye disorders, they also take a cotton ball soaked in the fluid and press it over the closed eyes for about a half hour daily. Unlike most Chinese herbs, when Asian dandelion is used to treat inflammatory diseases, both internal and external methods should be applied, whether in treating mastitis, tonsillitis, or mumps.

According to a report published in *New Chinese Medicine*, Asian dandelion is effective for
1  indigestion and chronic constipation,
2  mastitis prior to pustulation by both internal and external applications simultaneously,
3  early stages of snake and insect bites prior to pustulation and
4  promoting urination in treating acute urination disturbances, by the decoction of as much as 35 to 70g of fresh dandelion, with smaller quantities producing little or no effect. The same report also indicated that when Asian dandelion is used as a tonic for the stomach, 10 to 20g should be used for a one-day dosage by decoction, but when it is used to treat inflammatory diseases and to reduce swelling, 20 to 30g should be used.

Chegian
(Plant Before-Cart)
and Chegianzi
(Seed-Before-Cart)

# Asiatic Plantain and Asiatic Plantain Seed

There was a Chinese general in the Han Dynasty (206 B.C.-A.D. 220) by the name of Ma-Wu. One summer, the country was undergoing a severe drought and the people were suffering from famine. As if things weren't bad enough for Ma-Wu, he had been defeated on the battlefield that summer and his entire army was forced to retreat to a remote region where nobody lived. Ma-Wu's soldiers couldn't find any water to drink there, nor could they find any food to eat. Many soldiers and horses died of starvation and the surviving soldiers and horses had become so weak that virtually all of them had been under the attack of one disease or another. There was one particular symptom that almost every sick soldier and horse seemed to have — and that was presence of blood in the urine.

One of the grooms under Ma-Wu was in charge of three horses and one cart. When this particular groom, who took his duties very seriously, saw that he and his three horses all showed blood in their urine, he desperately began to look for treatment.

One day, to his delight, the groom noticed that none of his three horses showed blood in their urine. Wondering what they possibly could have done, he made it a point to watch his horses very closely over the next few days and noticed that they were eating plants that were a few inches tall and crept along the ground and had oblong leaves and light-green flowers. So, he pulled out a few plants, boiled them in water and drank the liquid himself. After a few days of consuming this drink, the groom saw that the blood in his urine had completely disappeared.

The groom was so excited that he immediately told General Ma-Wu, who issued an order to all his soldiers to take this remedy themselves and to feed it to their horses. A few days later, none of the soldiers and their horses showed any sign of blood in their urine.

"Where did you find the plants?" the general asked the groom.

"I found them before the cart," replied the groom.

"What a wonderful plant before the cart!" shouted the general.

And so, the plant has been called "plant-before-cart" ever since.

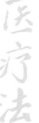

# 車前　　車前子

| Chinese | Cheqian (Plant-Before-Cart) | Cheqianzi (Seed-Before-Cart) |
|---|---|---|
| RE | 0799 | 0801 |
| COMMON NAME | Asiatic plantain | Asiatic plantain seed |
| FAMILY | Plantaginaceae | Plantaginaceae |
| CHINESE NAME | before-the-cart grass | seed-before-cart |
| SCIENTIFIC NAME | Plantago asiatica L. and Plantago depressa Willd | Plantago asiatica L. and Plantago depressa Willd |
| PHARMACEUTICAL NAME | Herba Plantaginis | Semen Plantaginis |
| PART USED | entire plant | ripe seed |
| DOSAGE | 10 to 18g | 10g |
| FLAVOR | sweet | sweet |
| ENERGY | cold | cold |
| CLASS | 5, herbs to reduce dampness in the body | 5, herbs to reduce dampness in the body |
| MERIDIANS | liver, spleen and bladder | liver, kidneys and small intestine |
| ACTIONS | to benefit water, clear heat, sharpen vision and expel sputum | to clear up heat, benefit water, relieve cough and expel sputum. |
| INDICATIONS | chronic tracheitis, urination difficulty, vaginal discharge, blood in the urine, jaundice, edema, hot dysentery and diarrhea, nosebleed, pinkeye, eye pain, sore throat, cough and skin ulcers | urination difficulty, edema, diarrhea, jaundice and cough |
| NOTES | Experiments indicate that this herb can benefit dampness and bring down blood pressure, as well as reduce blood fat and promote urination. However, this herb should be avoided by men with seminal emission due to kidney deficiency. | Experiments indicate that this herb is effective for suppression of cough and for promoting urination. Since the seeds are very small, they should be put in a cloth bag for decoction or they can be ground into powder for consumption. |

In Chinese herbalism, Asiatic plantain is called "plant before cart" because it can be found growing on the roadside along cart tracks. Both the seeds and leaves of Asiatic plantain are used as an herb and they have similar functions; however, the seeds are more commonly used than the leaves. One important use of this plant is to eliminate blood in the urine, as revealed in the legend, particularly in hot summer, when people have a tendency to develop urination disorders. Blood in the urine is frequently associated with difficulty in passing urine and this plant can promote urination, which is why it is effective for this symptom.

Cheqian and cheqianzi, which is the seeds of this herb, are similar in certain effects, but cheqian can also clear heat and detoxicate, as well as clear the lungs and transform sputum. Cheqian is also good for skin eruptions and for cough due to lung heat. In addition, fresh cheqian can be used to treat diarrhea due to damp heat.

*Lilu
(Insanity Grass)*

# Black False Hellebore

Black false hellebore is a toxic herb, which even a goat or a cow will not eat. But how did this plant become an herb for curing diseases since it's so toxic?

As the story goes, a child by the name of Lilu suffered from epilepsy and during a seizure, he would often become so violent that he would harm other children in the neighborhood. In fact, one time he hurt a child so severely that his parents were forced to pay a large sum of money in compensation.

One day Lilu's parents and his brothers were talking about the situation with Lilu and the oldest son said, "What if Lilu kills someone the next time? If that happens, the whole family would suffer terribly."

"I agree," said another brother, "so why don't we put Lilu to death?" Lilu's parents felt terrible about the thought of putting him to death, but since they couldn't figure out a better solution, they remained silent.

The following day, Lilu was undergoing another epileptic seizure. Anticipating the possibility of violence, Lilu's oldest brother pushed him to the ground and forced a cup of fresh black false hellebore juice into his mouth, in an attempt to poison him to death. Lilu began to vomit a few minutes later. His brother then forced another cup of the juice into his mouth and Lilu began to vomit again. When Lilu finally stopped vomiting, he got up and walked into the kitchen to eat a bowl of rice. From that point on, Lilu never had another seizure. This herb was appropriately named after Lilu.

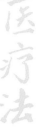

藜蘆

| Chinese | Lilu (Insanity Grass) |
|---|---|
| RE | 5652 |
| COMMON NAME | black false hellebore |
| FAMILY | Liliaceae |
| CHINESE NAME | black false hellebore |
| SCIENTIFIC NAME | Veratrum nigrum L. |
| PHARMACEUTICAL NAME | Rhizoma et Radix Veratri Nigri |
| PART USED | rhizome |
| DOSAGE | 1 to 1.5g |
| FLAVOR | bitter and pungent |
| ENERGY | cold |
| CLASS | 7, herbs to induce vomiting |
| MERIDIANS | liver, lungs and stomach |
| ACTIONS | to induce vomiting of undigested foods and sputum and destroy worms |
| INDICATIONS | epilepsy, accumulation of sputum, indigestion and scabies (by external application) |
| NOTES | Lilu is a strong emetic (vomitive) and can also drive out wind sputum in excess diseases and destroy worms; but since it is toxic, it should not be used by pregnant women and those with deficiency and loss of blood. |

# Boneset and Korean Mint

Once upon a time, a young couple and the husband's sister were living together in a small village. After the husband went off to join the army, his wife and sister remained living together. The wife was named Peilan and the sister Huoxiang and the two were very nice to each other and lived in harmony.

One summer Peilan suffered a sunstroke with a headache, dizziness, palpitations and nausea. Huoxiang put her in bed, telling her, "My brother taught me how to use two herbs to cure sunstroke. Let me go pick them in the mountains and decoct them for you to drink."

Peilan protested, saying that the mountains were too dangerous, but Huoxiang insisted on going anyway.

Peilan stayed in bed, waiting for Huoxiang to come back, but she did not return until early the next morning. No sooner had Huoxiang entered Peilan's bedroom, than she fainted and fell to the floor.

"What happened, Huoxiang?" asked Peilan, once Huoxiang had regained consciousness.

"I've been bitten by a poisonous snake," replied Huoxiang.

Realizing that snake bites could be fatal, Peilan tried to suck the poison from Huoxiang's wound. But it was all in vain; Huoxiang died an hour later. A neighbor who suspected something strange going on came knocking at the door, but nobody answered. So, the neighbor came in anyway and was astonished to see both Peilan and Huoxiang lying on the floor. Huoxiang was already dead and Peilan was on the verge of death.

Peilan explained, "Huoxiang went to the mountains to dig up two herbs for me—one for vomiting and diarrhea and one for vomiting and dizziness, particularly in the summer. Please remember these two herbs, just in case someone needs them."

No sooner had Peilan finished her last word, than she died.

Afterwards, the neighbor named the two herbs after Peilan and Huoxiang.

佩兰　　藿香

| Chinese | Peilan (Sister-in-Law's Orchid) | Huoxiang (Sister-in-Law's Mint) |
|---|---|---|
| RE | 2841 | 5685 |
| COMMON NAME | boneset | Korean mint |
| FAMILY | Compositae | Labiatae |
| CHINESE NAME | wearing orchid (so named because when it's worn, this herb smells like an orchid) | aromatic bean leaf (so named because the leaves of this herb look like those of a bean and it smells aromatic) |
| SCIENTIFIC NAME | Eupatorium fortunei Turcz. and japonicum Thunberg | Agastache rugosus (Fisch. et Mey) O. Ktze. & Pogostemon cablin Blanco Benth |
| PHARMACEUTICAL NAME | Herba Eupatorii | Herba Agastchis |
| PART USED | stalks and leaves | stalk leaves |
| DOSAGE | 8g | 8g |
| FLAVOR | pungent | pungent |
| ENERGY | neutral | slightly warm |
| CLASS | 5, herbs to reduce dampness in the body | 5, herbs to reduce dampness in the body (specifically those herbs that transform dampness by their aromatic smell) |
| MERIDIANS | lungs and spleen | spleen and stomach |
| ACTIONS | to transform dampness by aromatic flavor and relieve summer heat | to transform dampness, harmonize the stomach and relieve vomiting |
| INDICATIONS | Headache due to summer heat | Nausea and vomiting |
| NOTES | Peilan has a very strong aroma and can transform dampness and clear summer heat rather effectively. Experiments have shown that peilan can inhibit influenza | Huoxiang is pungent, warm and aromatic and it can stimulate the spleen, regulate the stomach, warm the middle region, transform dampness, relieve stomach stagnation and relieve vomiting. Experiments have shown that huoxiang is effective as a digestive and that it can inhibit influenza and also relieve vomiting. |

Huoxiang and peilan can be decocted together to harmonize the stomach and relieve vomiting. This formula is good for vomiting and abdominal swelling due to summer heat.

*Lugen
(Reed Rhizome)*

*Carrizo*

There was a small village in southern China with only one herb shop and the owner kept raising his prices. One day a child from a poor family suffered high fever, so the child's mother went to the shop to get some herbs. The owner of the shop told her that her child needed antelope's horn, which was a very expensive animal product, but the mother couldn't afford it. When she asked the shopkeeper if he would sell it to her at a cheaper price, he refused her.

So the mother went home empty-handed and her child's fever continued. Later that day a beggar knocked at her door and asked for a bowl of rice.

"We are a poor family and this is the only bowl of rice left," said the mother, as she handed it to him, with tears in her eyes.

"What is wrong, Ma'am? Why are you crying?" inquired the beggar.

The mother told him that her child had a high fever and she couldn't afford to buy antelope's horn.

"You don't need antelope's horn for high fever," said the beggar. "Those plants growing near the pond will work just as well."

On the advice of the beggar, the mother picked the plants and decocted them for her child to drink, which quickly reduced the fever and the child recovered completely a short time later. The plants she picked were lugen.

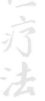

蘆根

| Chinese | Lugen (Reed Rhizome) |
|---|---|
| RE | 2191 |
| COMMON NAME | reed rhizome |
| FAMILY | Gramineae |
| CHINESE NAME | Reed rhizome |
| SCIENTIFIC NAME | Phragmites communis (L.) Trin |
| PHARMACEUTICAL NAME | Rhizoma Phragmitis |
| PART USED | rhizome |
| DOSAGE | 20g |
| FLAVOR | sweet |
| ENERGY | cold |
| CLASS | 2, herbs to reduce excessive heat inside the body |
| MERIDIANS | lungs, stomach and kidneys |
| ACTIONS | to clear up heat, produce fluids and promote urination |
| INDICATIONS | thirst, short stream of urine, vomiting due to a hot stomach, dry cough due to hot lungs and lung disease |
| NOTES | Lugen can clear heat, produce fluids and quench thirst. |

Jinyingzi
(Golden-Tassel Seed)

# Cherokee Rose

Once upon a time, there were three brothers who lived together with their wives. But only one of the couples had a child and this child grew up as the only child in this big family. After some time, all the members of the family were very anxious to see this only son in the family get married and have children. But no girl would marry him because he had a problem—bed-wetting. And so the family tried to find a cure for it.

One day an old herbalist, carrying a bag with a golden tassel, came to the village to sell some herbs. One of the brothers asked the herbalist if he had any herbs in his bag that could cure bed-wetting. The herbalist said he didn't but that he knew of one herb that could cure it that could be found in southern China. He further explained that since it would require a long journey to travel there to get the herb, they would have to pay him a huge sum of money. However, the family agreed and the old herbalist undertook the journey.

Many months passed, but the old herbalist did not return and the family had virtually given up hope, when one evening there was a knock at their door. One of the brothers opened the door and was astonished to see the old herbalist, who had fainted beside the door. He immediately carried the old herbalist into the house. Once he regained consciousness, the herbalist told the family that the herb he got in southern China was in his bag, but his voice was so low that the family could hardly hear him. The herbalist died a few days later due to physical exhaustion.

Nevertheless, the family decocted the herb, which successfully cured their son's bed-wetting. They did not know the name of the herb nor did they know the name of the old herbalist, so they decided to call the herb "golden-tassel seed," after the golden tassel attached to the old man's bag and because the seed of the plant is used as the herb.

中医疗法

# 金櫻子

| | |
|---|---|
| *Chinese* | *Jinyingzi (Golden-Tassel Seed)* |
| RE | 2898 |
| COMMON NAME | Japanese honeysuckle |
| FAMILY | Rosaceae |
| CHINESE NAME | golden-cherry seed |
| SCIENTIFIC NAME | Rosa laevigata Michx |
| PHARMACEUTICAL NAME | Fructus Rosae Laevigatae |
| PART USED | ripe fruit |
| DOSAGE | 7 to 15g |
| FLAVOR | sweet and sour |
| ENERGY | neutral |
| CLASS | 17, herbs to constrict and obstruct movements |
| MERIDIANS | kidneys, spleen and lungs |
| ACTIONS | to benefit the kidneys, constrict semen and relieve diarrhea |
| INDICATIONS | frequent urination, enuresis, chronic diarrhea, seminal emission and vaginal bleeding and discharge |
| NOTES | Experiments have shown jinyingzi to be effective as a digestive, in inhibiting gastrointestinal peristalsis and in stopping diarrhea. Jinyingzi is obstructive and should be avoided by those with constipation.<br><br>Jinyingzi can be decocted with qianshi (chicken head kernel) to solidify semen and check urination. This combination is especially beneficial for frequent urination due to kidney deficiency. |

# Chinese Clematis

At the top of a high mountain in southern China, there was a temple called "the temple of powerful spirits," which was managed by an old nun who was also a knowledgeable herbalist. She used herbs to treat the illnesses of the people who came to worship at the temple, most of whom suffered from rheumatism and arthritis.

The old nun-herbalist was a very cunning person and did not want to let people know that she was treating them with herbs. Instead, she would give a patient a cup of soup, explaining that it was the soup of Buddha, which could cure diseases because of its powerful spirits and the patient would believe her. The old nun did this in an attempt to get more people to worship at the temple and to collect more donations.

A young nun who was working under the old nun knew about her secret, because it was she who decocted the herbs for the patients. This young nun was often mistreated by the old nun and she was very unhappy about it. On top of that, she felt it was wrong for the old nun to deceive people into thinking that it was the powerful spirits of Buddha that cured their diseases and not the healing power of herbs.

One day, when the young nun was told by the old nun to decoct an herb for a patient, she deliberately decocted a different herb. The patient drank it and of course did not improve. Day after day, the same thing happened and many people even found their illnesses getting worse. After a while, people stopped coming to see the old nun and went to see the young nun instead.

One day, when the old nun found out that people were going to the young nun for treatment, she went into a frenzy and died from a heart attack. The young nun took over the temple and gave people free treatments. The herb that she used to treat their arthritis and rheumatism had no name, so the young nun named it "temple's holy root."

中医疗法

威靈仙

| | |
|---|---|
| *Chinese* | *Weilingxian (Temple's Holy Root)* |
| RE | 3372 |
| COMMON NAME | Chinese clematis |
| FAMILY | Ranunculaceae |
| CHINESE NAME | powerful soul root |
| SCIENTIFIC NAME | Clematis chinensis Osbeck, Clematis hexapetala Pall. and Clematis manshurica Rupr |
| PHARMACEUTICAL NAME | Radix Clematidis |
| PART USED | root |
| DOSAGE | 3 to 10g |
| FLAVOR | pungent |
| ENERGY | warm |
| CLASS | 3, herbs to counteract rheumatism |
| MERIDIANS | bladder |
| ACTIONS | to remove wind and dampness, facilitate passage of meridians and relieve pain |
| INDICATIONS | rheumatism, jaundice and edema |
| NOTES | Weilingxian is an effective herb for treating wind-cold rheumatism. Experiments have shown that weilingxian can benefit the gallbladder and reduce jaundice and that it is also an effective herb for relief of pain and rheumatism. |

# Chinese Ephedra

## Mahuang (Ask-For-Trouble)

A Chinese herbalist with no son decided to accept a disciple to help him with his work and to whom he could teach his trade. The disciple was an impatient person and after having studied under his master for only a few months, wanted to open a clinic of his own. However, the old herbalist was reluctant to let him go, not merely because he needed his help but because he didn't think he was ready for his own patients.

"Before you leave me to operate your own clinic, there is one thing you should remember," warned the old herbalist. "There is a plant whose leaves and roots have opposite effects: The leaves can induce perspiration, whereas the roots can reduce it. You must keep this in mind in treating your patients."

But the disciple was caught up in his own plans and barely heard what his master was saying.

On the grand-opening day of the clinic, the son of a judge fell ill and was perspiring profusely, so the judge brought his son to the clinic. The former disciple used the leaves of a plant to treat the young patient and he used the herb in huge amounts, intending to produce quick results. Rather unexpectedly, the patient began to perspire even more profusely after taking the herb. And his arms and legs became as cold as ice; in fact, his entire body was shivering with cold.

The judge was furious and rushed his son to the old herbalist, who then told the judge that his former disciple had used the wrong part of the plant; instead of using the roots of the plant, he had used the leaves, without realizing that the leaves could actually induce perspiration.

The judge later summoned the young herbalist and told him, "In treating patients without much knowledge, you are asking for trouble." Hence, the plant came to be known as "ask-for-trouble."

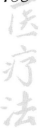

# 麻黄　　麻黄根

| Chinese | Mahuang (Ask-For-Trouble) | Mahuanggen (Root of Chinese Ephedra) |
|---|---|---|
| RE | 4615 | 4624 |
| COMMON NAME | Chinese ephedra | Chinese ephedra root |
| FAMILY | Ephedraceae | Ephedraceae |
| CHINESE NAME | numb yellow herb (so named because it produces numb sensations and is yellow) | hemp yellow root |
| SCIENTIFIC NAME | Ephedra sinica Stapf, Ephedra intermedia Schrenk et C. A. May and Ephedra equisetina Bge | Ephedra sinica Stapf and Ephedra intermedia Schrenk et C. A. Mey |
| PHARMACEUTICAL NAME | Herba Ephedrae | Radix Ephedrae |
| PART USED | dry stalks | root |
| DOSAGE | 6g | 3 to 10g |
| FLAVOR | pungent and bitter | sweet |
| ENERGY | warm | neutral |
| CLASS | 1, herbs to induce perspiration | 17, herbs to constrict and obstruct movements |
| MERIDIANS | lungs and bladder | lungs |
| ACTIONS | to induce perspiration; to disperse cold (when raw), overcome asthma (when fried) and promote urination | to check perspiration |
| INDICATIONS | asthma, edema and hypertension (if used with great care) | excessive perspiration and night sweats |
| NOTES | Mahuang can be decocted with kuxingren (bitter apricot) to reinforce the effect of calming asthma.<br><br>Experiments have shown that Mahuang is effective for asthma and can promote urination and inhibit influenza. Mahuang contains ephedrine, which accounts for its effectiveness in treating asthma.<br><br>In the treatment of asthma, mahuang should be used intermittently, particularly in chronic asthma, because a continuous, prolonged use of it can decrease its effects, as the patient may develop a resistance to it. In addition, mahuang can excite the cerebral cortex, which may lead to nervousness and insomnia. | When patients suffering from the common cold are perspiring profusely, mahuang should not be used for treatment, because mahuang is a relatively strong herb for inducing perspiration.<br><br>The following precautions should be taken in using mahuang:<br>1 Do not use excessive doses (normally between 1.5 and 10g are recommended);<br>2 when mahuang is decocted with other herbs, it should be decocted first so that the floating bubbles can be removed from the water; and<br>3 those with deficient body energy and excessive perspiration should avoid mahuang.<br><br>Mahuanggen is the root of mahuang and produces opposing effects. |

# Chinese Ginseng & Western Ginseng

*Renshen (Man's Plant) and Xiyangshen*

There was an old hunter with two sons who were just learning how to hunt. Before they left to go hunting on their own for the first time, he advised them to wait until winter was over. But the two brothers insisted on going anyway.

Within a few days, they had killed quite a few animals. Then one afternoon the weather suddenly changed and snow began to fall, virtually blocking all the passages out of the mountains. One week later, they were still unable to get out of the mountains and they had run out of food. In desperation, they searched everywhere for something to eat.

They finally spotted a plant that looked different from the others. After digging it out of the ground, the two brothers were surprised to see that the roots resembled a man standing up. They began to eat the roots, which tasted sweet and a little bitter and were very juicy. They continued eating them over the next few days and found that they were becoming very energetic. Thinking that in cold winter, they needed plenty of energy, they ate the roots in huge amounts, but then one of them began to develop a nosebleed. So, they decided to eat the roots in moderate amounts. The roots of this plant tided them over through the winter. And in spring, when the snow melted away, they headed home.

Meanwhile, the father of the two brothers was deeply worried and the people in the village all thought that the brothers had died.

The unexpected return of the two brothers shocked the entire village. Of course, the old hunter was relieved that his sons were still alive, but he did not understand how they had managed to survive under such severe conditions.

"How did you make it through the cold winter in the mountains?" asked the father.

"We ate the roots of a plant," explained one of the brothers.

"What is the name of the plant?" asked the father.

"We don't know the name of the plant," said the other brother," but its roots look like a man."

"Oh! It must be man's plant," said the father.

中医疗法

| Chinese | 人參 | 西洋參 |
|---|---|---|
| RE | *Renshen*<br>*(Man's Plant)* | *Xiyangshen*<br>*(Western ginseng)* |
| COMMON NAME | | |
| FAMILY | 0055 | 1713 |
| CHINESE NAME | ginseng | Western ginseng |
| | Araliaceae | Araliaceae |
| SCIENTIFIC NAME | man's plant (so named because the roots of this plant resemble the shape of a man) | Western ginseng |
| PHARMACEUTICAL NAME | | |
| PART USED | Panax ginseng C. A. Mey | Panax quinquefolium Linne |
| DOSAGE | Radix Ginseng | Radix Panacis Quinquefolii |
| FLAVOR | root | root |
| ENERGY | 5g | 8g |
| CLASS | sweet and slightly bitter | bitter and sweet |
| MERIDIANS | warm | cool |
| ACTIONS | 16, herbs to correct deficiencies | 16, herbs to correct deficiencies |
| | spleen and lungs | lungs and stomach |
| INDICATIONS | to tone up original energy drastically, fix prolapse, produce fluids, secure spirits and benefit brain | to tone up the lungs, benefit energy, nourish stomach, produce fluids and clear up heat. |
| NOTES | weakness after chronic illness, vaginal bleeding, diabetes, prolapse, palpitations and forgetfulness | yin deficiency with internal heat, thirst, cough and voice loss |

Experiments have shown that renshen is an effective heart tonic and anti-shock herb. It can increase red blood cells and produce adrenocortical hormones, sex hormones and excitation, as well as reduce blood sugar and blood fat.

There are three basic varieties of renshen (radix ginseng): wild ginseng, which is found in the mountains in the northeastern Chinese provinces, notably Jilin and Heilongjiang; red ginseng, which is cultivated ginseng that has been steamed to become red; and Korean ginseng, which is produced in Korea and processed with medicinal plants.

Wild ginseng tastes sweet and slightly bitter and warm. It is most frequently used as a single ingredient to drastically tonify energy, tonify the lungs and the spleen, benefit yin, produce fluids and secure the spirits; it is also used as first-aid treatment for prolapse caused by severe bleeding. Red ginseng has the same properties as wild ginseng but is weaker in its effects, while Korean ginseng is warmer and can tonify yang more effectively.

Chinese ginseng (radix ginseng) can tonify energy more effectively than Western ginseng (radix panacis quinquefolii), which is why in treating symptoms of prolapse, Chinese ginseng can be applied all by itself. Western ginseng is cool in energy and can produce fluids; it is most appropriate for patients with high fever and energy deficiency simultaneously.

# Chinese Hawthorn

A forty-year-old businessman was once married and had a son; two years after his wife died, he got married again to a cunning woman who disliked her stepchild and wanted to get rid of him.

"What is the best way to do it?" she pondered. "I can't kill him, nor can I poison him to death, because people will find out."

After her husband left on a business trip, she decided to take some action against her stepchild, who was almost ten years old. Her stepchild worked in the mountains every day and she always brought him his lunch. While her husband was gone, she intentionally prepared his lunch with half-cooked rice, with the hope that he would die from indigestion. After a few weeks, the stepchild began to complain of indigestion and was starting to lose weight. This pleased the stepmother and she continued to make him lunch with half-cooked rice.

One day the stepchild happened to find a tree growing with plenty of berries. He picked some berries out of curiosity and ate them and found them delicious. These berries seemed to quench his thirst as well. He began to feel better and continued to eat the berries every day, gradually putting on weight.

"What is happening to this child?" the stepmother asked herself. "He is not dying—on the contrary, he looks much healthier….Maybe God is protecting this child."

Being fearful of God, the stepmother stopped making his lunch with half-cooked rice. When the businessman returned home, he learned about the berries from his son and decided to market them to herbalists in town.

山楂

| Chinese | Shanzha (Mountain Hawthorn) |
|---|---|
| RE | 0323 |
| COMMON NAME | Chinese hawthorn |
| FAMILY | Rosaceae |
| CHINESE NAME | red fruits (so named because its fruits are red) |
| SCIENTIFIC NAME | Crataegus pinnatifida Bge. var. major N.E.Br. |
| PHARMACEUTICAL NAME | Fructus Crataegi |
| PART USED | fruit |
| DOSAGE | 10g |
| FLAVOR | sour |
| ENERGY | slightly warm |
| CLASS | 9, herbs to promote digestion |
| MERIDIANS | spleen, stomach and liver |
| ACTIONS | to eliminate accumulations, promote energy flow and disperse coagulations |
| INDICATIONS | indigestion, dysentery, hernia, blood coagulations & suppression of menses |
| NOTES | According to experiments, shanzha is an effective heart tonic; it can activate the blood and bring down blood pressure, it is effective as a digestive, it can treat fatty liver and it can also reduce blood fat.

Shanzha is a strong herb for transforming food and eliminating food stagnation due to indigestion; it is particularly effective for eliminating meat indigestion.

Shanzha can activate the blood and remove blood coagulations. It is often used in conjunction with danggui and yimucao to treat pain in the lower abdomen and lochiostasis. |

# Chinese Pulsatilla

A young man suffered from abdominal pain with diarrhea, which made him perspire profusely. He went to see a doctor, but the doctor wasn't in, so the young man had no choice but to return home. On his way home, his abdominal pain became so severe that he had to lie down on the wayside to rest.

An old man with grey hair all over his head walked up to him and said, "Young man, what is wrong with you? Why are you lying here?"

"I am having unbearable abdominal pain the young man replied.

"Why don't you see a doctor?" asked the old man.

"I went to see a doctor, but the doctor wasn't there," explained the young man.

Then an idea dawned on the old man. "You don't need a doctor," he said. "The plant beside you is a good remedy for abdominal pain and diarrhea. Pick some and decoct the roots. I promise it will relieve your suffering."

The young man looked at the old man in disbelief, but he picked some plants anyway and started for home after his abdominal pain had somewhat subsided.

Soon after he got home, his pain started again with severe diarrhea. Thinking that he had nothing to lose, the young man began to decoct the roots of the plant; he had the soup a few times and shortly got relief from the symptoms.

Good news travels fast and soon the whole village knew about it. People started to inquire about the plant, but all the young man could tell them was that an old man who was about the age of his grandpa with grey hair all over his head told him to use it. Thus, the herb came to be known as "grandpa's grey hair."

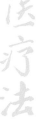

# 白头翁

| Chinese | *Baitouweng (Grandpa's Grey Hair)* |
|---|---|
| RE | 1411 |
| COMMON NAME | Chinese pulsatilla |
| FAMILY | Ranunculaceae |
| CHINESE NAME | white-headed man |
| SCIENTIFIC NAME | Pulsatilla chinensis (Bge.) Regel |
| PHARMACEUTICAL NAME | Radix Pulsatillae |
| PART USED | whole plant |
| DOSAGE | 10 to 18g |
| FLAVOR | bitter |
| ENERGY | cold |
| CLASS | 2, herbs to reduce excessive heat inside the body |
| MERIDIANS | stomach and large intestine |
| ACTIONS | to clear up heat, detoxicate cool blood and relieve dysentery |
| INDICATIONS | dysentery, nosebleed and hemorrhoids |
| NOTES | According to experiments, baitouweng is an effective heart tonic and can stop diarrhea |

*Shanyao
(Mountain Medicine)*

# Chinese Yam

Two kingdoms were at war with each other, with the stronger kingdom having won the last battle. All the soldiers in the defeated kingdom escaped to a high mountain to hide from their enemies, but they were soon surrounded by the victorious soldiers, with their lines of communication completely cut off. Thinking that the soldiers on the mountain would have no choice but to surrender sooner or later, or else starve to death, the victorious army began to enjoy themselves at the foot of the mountain. Having surrounded them for a full year, strangely enough they had not seen a single surrendering enemy soldier come down from the mountain. Then one night a strong army of soldiers suddenly appeared from the mountain to break the encirclement below and scored a decisive victory over the stronger kingdom.

What had the soldiers eaten on the mountain? After their food supply had run out, they started looking for something to eat and found plenty of plants with big roots, which they ate as food while their horses ate the vines of the plants. Since the plants were growing on the mountain and their roots were as powerful as medicine, the soldiers called the plants, "mountain medicine."

中医疗法

山藥

| Chinese | Shanyao (Mountain Medicine) |
|---|---|
| RE | 0319 |
| COMMON NAME | Chinese yam |
| FAMILY | Dioscoreaceae |
| CHINESE NAME | mountain medicine |
| SCIENTIFIC NAME | Dioscorea opposita Thunb. and Dioscorea batatas Decaisne |
| PHARMACEUTICAL NAME | Rhizoma Dioscoreae and Rhizoma Batatatis |
| PART USED | tuberous root |
| DOSAGE | 15g |
| FLAVOR | sweet |
| ENERGY | neutral |
| CLASS | 16, herbs to correct deficiencies |
| MERIDIANS | spleen, stomach, lungs and kidneys |
| ACTIONS | to strengthen the spleen and stomach, relieve diarrhea and tone up the lungs and kidneys |
| INDICATIONS | spleen deficiency with poor appetite, chronic diarrhea, seminal emission, vaginal discharge and diabetes |
| NOTES | According to experiments, shanyao can reduce blood sugar. It can also tonify the spleen and stop diarrhea, particularly diarrhea due to spleen deficiency and vaginal discharge in women. |

*Jinqiancao*

# Coin Grass

A loving couple was living happily in a small village, but since nothing lasts forever, one day the husband developed a pain below his ribs, as if he were being cut by a knife and died a few days later. The wife was so saddened and so puzzled by her husband's sudden death that she insisted on having an autopsy conducted. A stone was found in her husband's gallbladder. The wife took the stone with her, but was still perplexed by how a single stone could have killed her husband. She hung this stone in front of her neck on a string, however and kept it there day and night for many years.

One autumn, she went to the mountains to cut some plants, which she carried back home by hand. By the time she got home, she was surprised to find that the size of the stone in front of her neck had shrunk by half. She told everyone she knew about the incident, but no one seemed to believe her. Then one day an herbalist heard about it and became very curious.

"What kind of plants did you bring home that day? Could you take me to the place where you picked them?" he asked her.

The woman took the herbalist to the mountains where she picked the plants, but all the plants were gone. The two had no choice but to wait until the next year.

In the autumn of the following year, the woman and the herbalist went to the mountains once again. They cut the plants and the woman brought them home in the same manner as she had the previous year. But this time, the stone remained the same size.

In the autumn of the third year, the two went to the same place again. They cut different kinds of plants and put the stone on each of them for a period of time, finally coming upon a plant that dissolved the stone.

"This is a great discovery indeed!" exclaimed the herbalist. "We have found a cure for stones in the gallbladder."

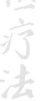

# 金錢草

| Chinese | Jinqiancao (Coin Grass) |
|---|---|
| RE | 2889 |
| COMMON NAME | herb of longtube ground ivy |
| FAMILY | Labiatae |
| CHINESE NAME | golden coin grass (so named because the leaves of the plant are as round as a coin) |
| SCIENTIFIC NAME | Glechoma longituba (Nakai) Kupr |
| PHARMACEUTICAL NAME | Herba Glechoma |
| PART USED | whole plant |
| DOSAGE | 15 to 25g |
| FLAVOR | bitter and pungent |
| ENERGY | cool |
| CLASS | 5, herbs to reduce dampness in the body |
| MERIDIANS | undetermined |
| ACTIONS | to clear up heat, promote urination, suppress cough, heal swelling and counteract toxic effects. |
| INDICATIONS | jaundice, edema, gallstones, malaria, lung disease, cough, vomiting of blood and rheumatism. |
| NOTES | Experiments have shown that jinqiancao can |

Experiments have shown that jinqiancao can
1 benefit the gallbladder and reduce jaundice,
2 promote liver bile production and bile excretion,
3 expel hepatic calculus (hepatolith),
4 expel urinary stones,
5 be used as an adjuvant herb to treat liver and gallbladder diseases and
6 promote urination.

# Danggui

A high mountain in China was full of precious herbs, but few people climbed it to pick them because the route was so treacherous.

One day a group of young men were talking among themselves and one fellow boasted, "I am the bravest of us all."

"If you're so brave," said another fellow, "I dare you to climb that mountain and bring back some herbs."

"I accept your challenge!" declared the young man.

When he told his mother of his intention to climb the Mountain, she strongly objected at first, but then later relented, saying "You are my only son and I will be completely alone after you are gone. Since you are already engaged, why don't you at least get married before you go, so that I will not be alone?"

The young man agreed and got married. Before he left, he told his wife to remarry should he fail to return home in three years, as the route through the mountain was so hazardous.

The young man did not return in one year, nor did he return in two years, nor in three years. So, the young man's mother told her daughter-in-law to remarry. She hesitated at first but then agreed, thinking that her husband must have died on the mountain.

However, a few days after her marriage, the young man suddenly returned home, which shocked everyone in the small village. All of his friends praised him for his great courage in climbing the mountain and thanked him for the many precious herbs he had picked and brought home. In the midst of the excitement, the young man was puzzled by the absence of his wife. After inquiring as to her whereabouts, he was told that she had just remarried.

Regretting his failure to return within three years, the young man asked to meet with his former wife. But on hearing of her former husband's return, the wife had burst into tears and had become seriously ill. One of the herbs the young man had picked on the mountain was a great tonic for women, so he decocted the herb and gave it to her to drink and it cured her illness in a few days.

To commemorate this incident, a Chinese poet wrote, "He ought to return a little sooner but failed to return; she ought to wait a little longer but failed to wait." The herb was thus named "ought-to-return."

中医疗法

當歸

| Chinese | Danggui (Ought-to-Return) |
|---|---|
| RE | 1763 |
| COMMON NAME | Danggui |
| FAMILY | Umbelliferae |
| CHINESE NAME | ought-to-return (so named because, according to Chinese herbalogy, by taking this herb, one's energy and blood will return without disorder) |
| SCIENTIFIC NAME | Angelica sinensis (Oliv.) Diels |
| PHARMACEUTICAL NAME | Radix Angelicae Sinensis |
| PART USED | root |
| DOSAGE | 10g |
| FLAVOR | sweet and pungent |
| ENERGY | warm |
| CLASS | 16, herbs to correct deficiencies |
| MERIDIANS | heart, liver and spleen |
| ACTIONS | to tone up blood, activate blood, regulate menstruation and produce intestinal sliding |
| INDICATIONS | blood deficiency and coagulation causing suppression of menses and abdominal pain; rheumatism and constipation |
| NOTES | Experiments have shown that danggui can protect the liver and regulate menstruation and that it contains volatile oils and folic acid.<br><br>Since danggui can tonify and activate the blood simultaneously, it is an effective herb for women. Danggui and shudihuang are two of the most important blood tonics. |

Tusizi
(Bunny's Seed)

# Dodder

A young man was hired by a farmer to look after his bunnies. Being a harsh task-master, the farmer warned the young man that the death of a bunny would cost him a quarter of his wages, which made the young man very nervous.

One day this young man accidentally dropped a bamboo stick on a bunny, which broke her spine; the bunny lay on the ground unable to move. The young man was afraid that his boss would find out, so he took the bunny from the pen and hid her in the field of soybean plants, where the poor bunny lay very still as if dying.

The farmer found one bunny missing, so the young man went to the field to bring the bunny back. To his surprise, the bunny was running around in the field. He chased after the bunny for quite a while, before finally catching her and bringing her back to the pen.

Then the young man intentionally broke another bunny's back and brought her to the soybean field. A few days later, he saw that the bunny's back had completely healed.

"How could that have happened?" he later asked his father, who suffered from a backache and had laid in bed for many years.

"Maybe it's the soybean plants," mused his father.

The next day, the young man deliberately broke the back of yet another bunny and brought her to the field. But this time, he watched closely what the bunny ate. He found that the bunny was not eating the soybean plants at all, but rather the seeds of a parasitic plant living on them. A few days later, the bunny had recovered from her back injury.

The young man started to pick the seeds of this parasitic plant and then decocted them for his father to drink; soon afterwards, his father's backache was cured! The herb has been known as "bunny's seed" ever since.

中医疗法

# 菟丝子

| Chinese | Tusizi (Bunny's Seed) |
|---|---|
| RE | 4125 |
| COMMON NAME | dodder seed |
| FAMILY | Convolvulaceae |
| CHINESE NAME | hare silk seed |
| SCIENTIFIC NAME | Cuscuta chinensis Lam. and Cuscuta japonica Choisy |
| PHARMACEUTICAL NAME | Semen Cuscutae |
| PART USED | ripe seed |
| DOSAGE | 5 to 10g |
| FLAVOR | pungent and sweet |
| ENERGY | neutral |
| CLASS | 16, herbs to correct deficiencies |
| MERIDIANS | liver and kidneys |
| ACTIONS | to tone up the liver and the kidneys, strengthen yang and relieve diarrhea |
| INDICATIONS | impotence, seminal emission, diarrhea, lumbago and insecure fetus |
| NOTES | Tusizi can tonify the liver and the kidneys to treat lumbago and weak legs due to liver and kidney deficiencies. It is an effective herb for the treatment of impotence, seminar emission and premature ejaculation and enuresis due to kidney deficiency. |

# Evergreen Artemisa

*Yinchenhao
(Evergreen Spire)*

Once a fellow suffered from jaundice, with a yellowish complexion and depressed eyes. His friends called him "Mr. Cockroach," because he had lost so much weight that he looked like a cockroach.

One day Mr. Cockroach went to see a famous doctor named Hua Duo. But Dr. Hua Duo told him that there was no cure for jaundice, so Mr. Cockroach sadly returned home.

A few months later, when Dr. Hua Duo ran into Mr. Cockroach on the street, he was surprised to see him still alive and in good health. He asked him who had treated him and what he had taken, but was told that the jaundice had disappeared all by itself. Dr. Hua Duo could not believe it, so Mr. Cockroach further explained that due to his illness, he had run out of money over the past few months and had to live on one particular plant as food. He then took Dr. Hua Duo to see the plant, which Dr. Hua Duo subsequently started using to treat his jaundice patients. But to his disappointment, the treatments didn't work, which puzzled Dr. Hua Duo a great deal.

After questioning Mr. Cockroach, Dr. Hua Duo was convinced that he had in fact identified the right plant, which he had picked in March of the previous year. Thinking that the timing of picking the plant might have something to do with its effects, Dr. Hua Duo picked the plant that March and used it to treat his patients with jaundice and this time all the patients recovered. Dr. Hua Duo then concluded that only the tender leaves and branches picked in March could be used to treat jaundice.

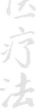

# 茵陳蒿

| Chinese | Yinchenhao (Evergreen Spire) |
|---|---|
| RE | 3305 |
| COMMON NAME | herb of virgate wormwood and herb of capillary wormwood |
| FAMILY | Compositae |
| CHINESE NAME | mattress old wormwood |
| SCIENTIFIC NAME | Artemisia capillaris Thunberg |
| PHARMACEUTICAL NAME | Herba Artemisiae Capillaris and Herba Artemisiae Scopariae |
| PART USED | seedlings and spires |
| DOSAGE | 15 to 30g |
| FLAVOR | bitter and pungent |
| ENERGY | slightly cold |
| CLASS | 5, herbs to remove dampness in the body |
| MERIDIANS | bladder |
| ACTIONS | to clear up damp heat and reduce jaundice |
| INDICATIONS | jaundice due to damp heat and acute jaundice-infectious hepatitis |
| NOTES | Experiments have shown that yinchenhao can |

NOTES (continued):

1  protect the liver,
2  reduce transaminase,
3  benefit the gallbladder and reduce jaundice,
4  promote liver bile production and bile excretion,
5  be used as a general antiviral herb and
6  be used as an adjuvant herb to treat liver and gallbladder diseases.

Yinchenhao is particularly good at clearing damp heat in the liver and gallbladder and is often used to treat damp-heat jaundice.

*Wuzhuyu
(Wu-Zhu's Fruit)*

# Evodia

In ancient China, it was customary for a smaller and weaker kingdom to pay tribute to a larger and stronger kingdom in order to avoid war between the two kingdoms. Thus, Wu Kingdom, which was small and weak, paid tribute every year to Chu Kingdom, which was much larger and stronger.

In the spring of a good year, the ambassador of Wu Kingdom brought an herb as a New Year present to the king of Chu Kingdom and told the king that it was called "Herb of Wu Kingdom" because it was the kingdom's national herb. But the king was visibly offended and declined the gift.

"How could a small and weak kingdom like Wu Kingdom have a national herb? I don't accept it as a present," said the king.

The ambassador was terribly humiliated and ready to return to his own country with the "Herb of Wu Kingdom," but a doctor in Chu Kingdom by the name of Dr. Zhu privately persuaded the ambassador to give the herb to him. Dr. Zhu planted the seeds and one year later, the "Herb of Wu Kingdom" had become readily available in Chu Kingdom.

One day the king of Chu Kingdom suffered severe abdominal pain, so Dr. Zhu decocted the "Herb of Wu Kingdom" and gave the king the soup, which cured the king's abdominal pain instantly. The king was delighted. He then asked Dr. Zhu the name of the herb and was told that it was the "Herb of Wu Kingdom." Realizing the value of the herb, the king changed the name to "Wu-Zhu's Fruit." The king gave three reasons for the new name: First, the herb was a fruit; second, it was originally the herb of Wu Kingdom; and third, it was Dr. Zhu who had planted the herb in his kingdom.

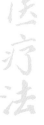

# 吴茱萸

| | |
|---|---|
| Chinese | Wuzhuyu (Wu-Zhu's Fruit) |
| RE | 2280 |
| COMMON NAME | evodia |
| FAMILY | Rutaceae |
| CHINESE NAME | evodia of Wu (so named because the herb grown in the Wu district is generally considered the best) |
| SCIENTIFIC NAME | Euodia rutaecarpa (Juss.) Benth., Euodia rutaecarpa (Juss.) Benth. var. officinalis (Dode) Huang and Euodia rutaecarpa (Juss.) Benth. var. bodinieri (Dode) Huang |
| PHARMACEUTICAL NAME | Fructus Euodiae |
| PART USED | unripe fruit |
| DOSAGE | 5g |
| FLAVOR | pungent |
| ENERGY | warm |
| CLASS | 4, herbs to reduce cold sensations inside the body |
| MERIDIANS | liver, kidneys, spleen and stomach |
| ACTIONS | to warm up the internal regions, disperse cold, relieve vomiting and relieve pain |
| INDICATIONS | cold abdominal pain, vomiting, diarrhea and headache |
| NOTES | Wuzhuyu is particularly good for warming the liver and spleen and for relieving pain; it is frequently used to treat deficiency cold of the stomach and spleen and cold liver with hernial pain in the lower abdomen, as well as menstrual pain and headache in the top of the head. |
| | Huanglian (yellow-pearl rhizome) and wuzhuyu can be decocted together to treat pain in the ribs, excessive stomach acid and belching, associated with "liver fire." |

*Cangzhu*
*(Grey Rhizome)*

# Grey Atractylodes

Once a knowledgeable old nun boasted that she could cure all sorts of illnesses with herbs. But, being cunning and greedy in nature, this nun treated only rich patients, turning away any poor patients who could not afford the herbs. The nun did not pick the herbs herself, but instead ordered a younger nun to do the chore for her.

Then one day, a poor fellow who suffered from rheumatism in the legs, with both legs swollen and painful, came to see the nun, but she turned him away because he could not pay for the herbs. The young nun, being kind in nature but knowing little or nothing about herbs, then gave the fellow an herb she had picked without knowing what it was good for.

The fellow went home and decocted the herb, which by chance cured his legs. When he came back to thank the old nun, she was naturally taken aback. The old nun remembered that she had not given any herbs to this patient, so how could he be cured? She asked the patient for details and discovered that it was the young nun who had given him the herb. She immediately expelled the young nun, who then went home and began to use that herb to treat patients with swollen and painful legs.

蒼术

| Chinese | Cangzhu (Grey Rhizome) |
|---|---|
| RE | 2174 |
| COMMON NAME | grey atractylode |
| FAMILY | Compositae |
| CHINESE NAME | grey essence (literal translation) |
| SCIENTIFIC NAME | Atractylodes lancea (Thunb.) D.C. and Atractylodes chinensis (D.C.) Koidz |
| PHARMACEUTICAL NAME | Rhizoma Atractylodis |
| PART USED | rhizome |
| DOSAGE | 10g |
| FLAVOR | pungent and bitter |
| ENERGY | warm |
| CLASS | 5, herbs to remove dampness in the body |
| MERIDIANS | spleen and stomach |
| ACTIONS | to dry up dampness, expel wind, relieve pain and sharpen vision |
| INDICATIONS | rheumatism, weak legs, night blindness and itchy skin |
| NOTES | Experiments have shown that cangzhu can reduce blood sugar and it contains volatile oils.

Cangzhu can be decocted with huang dampness. This combination is considered good for pain in the lower region associated with damp heat, such as with weakened legs and eczema. |

*Chaihu
(Who's Firewood)*

# Hare's Ear

A governor by the name of Who had hired a young fellow as his domestic servant. This servant suffered from a disease with alternating fever and chills and profuse perspiration. Since the young fellow was so ill and could not work, Governor Who dismissed him.

Having no place to go, this young servant wandered to a nearby pond. After lying by the pond for a few hours, the young servant began to feel thirsty and hungry, so he instinctively began to drink some dirty water from the pond and to eat some plants growing alongside it. The plants he ate were the ones that seemed the most edible under the circumstances.

The servant managed to survive by drinking water from the pond and eating these plants. Then strangely enough, on the seventh day, he began to regain strength and felt able to work again, so he went back to Governor Who. Surprised to see his former servant alive and well, Governor Who gave him his old job back.

One year later, Governor Who's only son suffered from a disease with alternating fever and chills and profuse perspiration — the same disease his young servant had had the year before. Governor Who ordered his young servant to go to the pond to pick the plant that he had eaten when he was ill. The servant decocted the plant and the son's disease was cured within seven days. Governor Who named the herb "Who's firewood" after himself and because the plant was normally used as firewood.

# 柴胡

| Chinese | Chaihu (Who's Firewood) |
|---------|--------------------------|
| RE | 3763 |
| COMMON NAME | hare's ear |
| FAMILY | Umbelliferae |
| CHINESE NAME | wood & vegetable (so named be-cause when the roots are young & tender, they can be eaten as a vegetable & when old, they are used as an herb) |
| SCIENTIFIC NAME | Bupleurum chinense DC. and Bupleurum Scorzonerifolium Willd |
| PHARMACEUTICAL NAME | Radix Bupleuri |
| PART USED | root |
| DOSAGE | 6g |
| FLAVOR | bitter |
| ENERGY | slightly cold |
| CLASS | 1, herbs to induce perspiration |
| MERIDIANS | liver, gallbladder, pericardium and sanjiao (including the thoracic, abdominal and pelvic cavities) |
| ACTIONS | to elevate yang, disperse heat, relieve congestion and disperse liver energy |
| INDICATIONS | malaria, rib pain, irregular menstrual flow and prolapse of the anus |
| NOTES | Experiments have shown that chaihu has six major actions: It can |

1   reinforce the resistance of capillary vessels,
2   protect the liver,
3   benefit the gallbladder and reduce jaundice,
4   promote liver bile production and bile excretion,
5   treat fatty liver and
6   soften and shrink the liver and the spleen.

Chaihu can elevate and disperse rather forcefully, which is why when used in large quantities, it may cause negative effects. Chaihu is basically a yang herb and as such, it is very flexible and can be combined with various herbs to produce different effects. For example, chaihu can be combined with gegen (radix puerariae) to induce perspiration and relax the superficial regions, with changshan (radix dichroae) to cure malaria and with huangqin (radix scutellariae) to relax the superficial regions and sedate heat.

# Japanese Honeysuckle

*Jinyinhua (Gold-Silver Flower)*

There lived a young couple in a small village with two twin girls; one was named Golden Flower and the other Silver Flower. The twin girls, who had always loved each other, grew up to be very close and had promised each other that they would never get married and would never separate from each other.

Not long after they had passed their seventeenth birthdays, Golden Flower suddenly fell ill, with a high fever and red spots all over her body.

"This is a contagious disease and there is no cure for it. Everybody should keep away from the patient," warned the doctor who made the diagnosis.

But Silver Flower insisted on staying close to her sister no matter what and nobody could convince her otherwise.

However, the doctor was right; it was indeed a contagious disease, as the twin sisters died a few days later and were buried together.

In the spring of the following year, all kinds of plants were growing all over the graveyard, but nothing grew on the graves of the twin sisters, except for one plant with an abundance of yellow and white flowers. People in the village were very curious about this strange phenomenon and some were even convinced that the twin sisters had turned into the flowers.

At the time when the plant was in full blossom, two little twin girls in the village fell ill with high fever and red spots all over their bodies—with exactly the same disease that killed Golden Flower and Silver Flower. The parents called on the same doctor to treat their little girls and the doctor gave the same diagnosis.

Although they were told that there was no cure for the disease, the parents went ahead and picked the flowers that grew on the graves of the two deceased sisters and decocted them for their daughters to drink. The two little girls soon recovered from their illness to enjoy their happiness once again.

The people in the village named the herb after the deceased twin sisters, calling it "gold-silver flower."

金銀花

| Chinese | Jinyinhua (Gold-Silver Flower) |
|---|---|
| RE | 2894 |
| COMMON NAME | Japanese honeysuckle |
| FAMILY | Caprifoliaceae |
| CHINESE NAME | gold-silver flower (so named because it has both colors) |
| SCIENTIFIC NAME | Lonicera japonica Thunb., Lonicera hypoglauca Miq., Lonicera confusa DC. and Lonicera dasystyle Rehd |
| PHARMACEUTICAL NAME | Flos Lonicerae |
| PART USED | buds |
| DOSAGE | 12g |
| FLAVOR | sweet |
| ENERGY | cold |
| CLASS | herbs to reduce excessive heat inside the body |
| MERIDIANS | lungs, stomach, heart and spleen |
| ACTIONS | to clear up heat, counteract toxic effects, cool down the blood and disperse wind and heat |
| INDICATIONS | carbuncles, dysentery and sore throat with swelling |
| NOTES | Experiments have shown that jinyinhua can produce five major effects: It can 1 protect the liver, 2 inhibit influenza, 3 inhibit mumps, 4 reduce blood fat and 5 be used as an antibacterial herb.<br><br>In addition, since this herb contains lonicerin, saponin and inositol and has been found to possess antibacterial and antiviral effects, it is now being widely used to treat the common cold, influenza, cystitis, arthritis, eye and throat infections and contagious hepatitis. |

*Gegen
(Ge's Root)*

*Kudzo Vine*

Mr. Ge was a high government official for many years, but when the government was overthrown by rebels, the members of the Ge family were all killed, except for Mr. Ge's oldest son, who had managed to escape.

An old herbalist was asleep when he heard someone screaming for help; he opened the window and saw a child about ten years old standing outside the door. The old herbalist opened the door to let him in.

"What is the matter?" asked the old herbalist.

The child explained what had happened to his family and said that he was the Ge's root, meaning that he was the only survivor in the family to carry the name of Ge to posterity.

The old herbalist was sympathetic and agreed to adopt him. The two would go to the mountain nearby to collect herbs every day, but there was one particular plant that they collected the most, whose root was especially good for neck pain and fever. Since this herb had no name, the people in the village called it "Ge's root" after the young boy and to commemorate the Ge family, who had served the government so faithfully.

中医疗法

# 葛根

| Chinese | Gegen (Ge's Root) |
|---------|---------|
| RE | 4796 |
| COMMON NAME | root of lobed kudzuvine |
| FAMILY | Leguminosae |
| CHINESE NAME | root of lobed kudzuvine |
| SCIENTIFIC NAME | Pueraria lobata (Wild.) Ohwi and Pueraria thomsanii Benth |
| PHARMACEUTICAL NAME | Radix Puerariae |
| PART USED | root |
| DOSAGE | 10 to 25g |
| FLAVOR | sweet and pungent |
| ENERGY | neutral |
| CLASS | 1, herbs to induce perspiration |
| MERIDIANS | lungs and stomach |
| ACTIONS | to induce perspiration, clear heat, facilitate measles eruption, elevate clear energy and relieve diarrhea |
| INDICATIONS | measles prior to eruptions, diarrhea (better used in roasted form), headache in forehead and stiff neck |
| NOTES | Experiments have shown that gegen can<br>1  expand coronary arteries and prevent angina pectoris,<br>2  reduce heat and bring down blood pressure and<br>3  reduce blood sugar.<br><br>In addition, from a traditional point of view, gegen is good for relaxing muscles, reducing heat, facilitating measles eruptions, producing fluids and quenching thirst. Gegen can be combined with mahuang to treat stiffness in the back of the neck. |

Gancao
(Sweet Root)

# Licorice

A popular herbalist had left home to make house calls and in over a month had still not returned. This was naturally causing anxiety among his patients who had been coming to his home for treatment. His wife was very concerned about these patients and decided to do something about it.

Since she knew little to nothing about herbs, she began to taste them all—she tasted sour herbs, bitter herbs, salty herbs, pungent herbs and sweet herbs. Thinking that most people would prefer sweet herbs, she decided to give all the patients the same sweet herb.

This sweet herb produced good results and more and more patients came back to get more of it. In fact, the business became much better in the absence of the herbalist, which puzzled him a great deal upon his return.

Wondering how this sweet herb could bring about such good results, the herbalist decided to continue giving it to all the patients who came to see him. He found that the herb was most effective for low energy, cough, pain and fatigue and he called it "sweet herb" because it tasted sweet.

甘草

| Chinese | Gancao (Sweet Root) |
|---|---|
| RE | 1187 |
| COMMON NAME | licorice |
| FAMILY | Leguminosae |
| CHINESE NAME | sweet grass (so named because it is a typical sweet herb) |
| SCIENTIFIC NAME | Glycyrrhiza uralensis Fisch., Glycyrrhiza inflata Bat. and Glycyrrhiza Glabra L |
| PHARMACEUTICAL NAME | Radix Glycyrrhizae |
| PART USED | root and tuberous root |
| DOSAGE | 5g |
| FLAVOR | sweet |
| ENERGY | neutral |
| CLASS | 16, herbs to correct deficiencies |
| MERIDIANS | twelve meridians |
| ACTIONS | to tone up the spleen, benefit energy, produce fluids, detoxicate, harmonize various herbs and slow down the advancement of symptoms |
| INDICATIONS | spleen and stomach weakness, dry cough, sore throat, acute abdominal pain, carbuncles, swelling and poisoning |
| NOTES | Experiments have shown that gancao can produce five major effects: It can<br>1  protect the liver,<br>2  produce adrenocortical hormones,<br>3  inhibit influenza,<br>4  be effective for leukemia and<br>5  reduce blood fat. |

*Xinyi
(Barbarian Bud)*

# Lily-Flowered Magnolia

A government official suffered from a nose disease, which troubled him a great deal, because the nasal discharge smelled awful and constantly blocked his nose, forcing him to breathe through his mouth. He had sought help from many herbalists, but none seemed to be able to help him. His friends advised him to retire and tour the countryside to get fresh air, which they thought might give him more relief than any herbs could.

Since he was close to retirement anyway, he decided to follow his friends' advice. He took an early retirement and soon after embarked on a tour to the frontier. There, he met a frontiersman who was an herbalist, who gave him an herbal remedy for nasal disorders. After using it for a while, it cured his condition.

The government official brought the seeds of the herb back with him to grow in his own garden. When people asked him what the herb was, he told them that it was called "barbarian bud." Why? Because the Chinese have always called frontiersmen barbarians and the bud of the plant is used as the herb.

辛夷

| Chinese | Xinyi (Barbarian Bud) |
|---|---|
| RE | 2354 |
| COMMON NAME | lily-flowered magnolia |
| FAMILY | Magnoliaceae |
| CHINESE NAME | pungent magnolia |
| SCIENTIFIC NAME | Magnolia biondii Pamp., Magnolia denudata Desr. and Magnolia liliflora Desr |
| PHARMACEUTICAL NAME | Flos Magnoliae |
| PART USED | dried buds |
| DOSAGE | 3 to 10g |
| FLAVOR | pungent |
| ENERGY | warm |
| CLASS | 1, herbs to induce perspiration |
| MERIDIANS | lungs and stomach |
| ACTIONS | to expel wind, disperse cold and open nasal passages |
| INDICATIONS | thick nasal discharge, headache and sinusitis |
| NOTES | Xinyi travels to the face and enters the nose in particular, which is why it is an effective herb for symptoms of the nose. |
| | Xinyi can be combined with huangqin and cangerzi to treat heat-predominating symptoms of the nose. |

# Mistletoe

*Sangjisheng
(Mulberry Parasite)*

The son of a wealthy man suffered from severe rheumatism. Since there was no cure, he had been bedridden for many years. The wealthy man heard about an herbalist living on a farm about five hundred miles away, so he sent his servant to buy some herbs from him.

Each time it would take the servant three weeks to get to the herbalist and back. The servant had made many trips and brought back over a hundred bags of herbs, but the wealthy man's son was still bedridden and showed not the slightest improvement.

One day when it was snowing very heavily, the servant was on his routine trip to the herbalist. He felt unusually exhausted along the way, so he stopped to rest under a white mulberry plant. He spotted a plant growing on the white mulberry that looked like the herb he brought home each time. Suddenly he thought, "Why don't I pick this plant and bring it home and tell the boss it's from the herbalist? Nothing has worked for his son's condition anyway." So the servant picked the plant and brought it home.

Since this had proven to be very convenient for the servant, he repeated it over the next two months. Strangely enough, after taking the plant picked by the servant, the wealthy man's son gradually recovered.

Seeing that the herb had cured his son, the wealthy man wanted to know its name. The servant told him that the herb was called "mulberry parasite," because it was a parasitic plant living on the white mulberry.

中医疗法

桑寄生

| Chinese | Sangjisheng (Mulberry Parasite) |
|---|---|
| RE | 4046 |
| COMMON NAME | herb of colored mistletoe |
| FAMILY | Loranthaceae |
| CHINESE NAME | mulberry parasitic herb (so named because it is parasitic on mulberry plants) |
| SCIENTIFIC NAME | Loranthus parasiticus (L.) Merr., Viscum coloratum (Kom.) Nakai & Loranthus gracilifolius Schult |
| PHARMACEUTICAL NAME | Ramulus Loranthi or Ramus Loranthi (Sangjisheng) and Herba Visci or Ramus Visci cum Folio (Hujisheng) |
| PART USED | stalks |
| DOSAGE | 10g |
| FLAVOR | bitter |
| ENERGY | neutral |
| CLASS | 16, herbs to correct deficiencies |
| MERIDIANS | liver and kidneys |
| ACTIONS | to nourish blood, expel wind, strengthen tendons and bones, secure fetus and promote milk secretion |
| INDICATIONS | blood deficiency, lumbago, weak legs, insecure fetus and shortage of milk secretion |
| NOTES | Experiments have shown that sangjisheng can produce seven major effects: It can |

NOTES (continued):

1 expand coronary arteries and prevent angina pectoris,
2 bring down blood pressure by tonification,
3 inhibit influenza,
4 reduce blood fat,
5 be generally effective in reducing blood pressure,
6 relieve pain and
7 be used as an antirheumatic herb.

*Sanqi
(Three-Seven Root)*

# Pseudo-ginseng

Two good friends promised one another that they would always help each other, like good brothers. In fact, people even started calling them brothers.

One day the younger brother suffered a severe nosebleed that wouldn't stop. So the older brother immediately rushed home to pick some herbs from his backyard and decocted them for the younger brother to drink, which stopped his nosebleed instantly. The younger brother later picked a branch to plant in his own backyard, just in case he should need it in the future.

One year later, the son of a government official suffered a severe nosebleed, so the younger brother immediately rushed to his garden to pick the herb to give it to the government official, promising that it would work. The government official decocted the herb and gave his son the soup, but it failed to stop his nosebleed. The government official was furious and the younger brother felt terribly humiliated. He went to confront his older brother, who explained that in order for the herb to be effective, the plant had to be between three and seven years old. Thus, the plant is called "three-seven root," as the root is used as the herb.

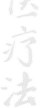

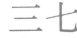

| | |
|---|---|
| *Chinese* | *Sanqi (Three-Seven Root)* |
| RE | 0096 |
| COMMON NAME | pseudoginseng |
| FAMILY | Araliaceae |
| CHINESE NAME | three-seven and mountain paint (so named because this plant has three leaves on the left and four on the right and it can heal boils like paint) |
| SCIENTIFIC NAME | Panax notoginseng (Burk.) F. H. Chen |
| PHARMACEUTICAL NAME | Radix Notoginseng |
| PART USED | root |
| DOSAGE | 8g |
| FLAVOR | sweet and slightly bitter |
| ENERGY | warm |
| CLASS | 12, herbs to regulate blood |
| MERIDIANS | liver and stomach |
| ACTIONS | to arrest bleeding of various kinds, promote blood circulation, heal swelling and relieve pain |
| INDICATIONS | bleeding of various kinds |
| NOTES | Experiments have shown that sanqi can produce four major effects: It can |

NOTES

Experiments have shown that sanqi can produce four major effects: It can
1    expand coronary arteries,
2    prevent angina pectoris,
3    increase and protect blood platelets and
4    be an effective coagulant and arrest bleeding (as a hemostatic).

Sanqi can relieve pain and reduce swelling and is often used to treat injuries. For best results, it should be applied in powder form.

*Dahuang
(Greater Yellow Root)*

# Rhubarb

There was an herbalist who was called Mr. Five Yellow because he was known to have mastered five yellow herbs—yellow bark, yellow essence, greater yellow root, yellow root and yellow pearl rhizome. This herbalist applied the five yellow herbs exclusively to treat diseases.

Mr. Five Yellow went to pick herbs every year in the country and often stayed in the house of Mr. Ma. The two had been friends for a couple of decades.

One spring when Mr. Five Yellow went to pick herbs, he found that Mr. Ma's house was gone and was told by a neighbor that it had burned down in a fire. His wife and children had died in the fire and Mr. Ma was living alone in a cave on the mountain.

Mr. Five Yellow climbed the mountain and found his friend and asked him whether he wanted to work with him. Mr. Ma agreed and from that time on, the two friends picked herbs together and lived together.

Mr. Five Yellow was an herbalist, but Mr. Ma was not; Mr. Ma wanted to become an herbalist and treat patients, but Mr. Five Yellow tried to persuade him not to.

"You are not careful enough to become an herbalist," Mr. Five Yellow told his friend, but Mr. Ma was not convinced.

One day while Mr. Five Yellow was away, Mr. Ma started treating patients on his own and obtained good results initially. One day, however, a woman came to see him for diarrhea, who looked very weak and pale. Mr. Ma remembered that his friend often used yellow root to treat diarrhea, so he decocted greater yellow root for the patient to drink. But, after drinking the soup, the patient got much worse and almost died from severe diarrhea.

Mr. Ma did not know what had gone wrong. When his friend returned, Mr. Ma told Mr. Five Yellow what had happened. Mr. Five Yellow immediately knew that Mr. Ma had used the wrong herb, because there were two yellow roots, one for diarrhea and one for constipation. Yellow root was good for diarrhea, whereas greater yellow root was good for constipation.

# 大黄

| Chinese | Dahuang (Greater Yellow Root) |
|---|---|
| RE | 0188 |
| COMMON NAME | rhubarb |
| FAMILY | Polygonacea |
| CHINESE NAME | greater yellowness (so named because it is yellow and produces a greater effect than other yellow herbs); also called "a general" |
| SCIENTIFIC NAME | Rheum palmatum L., Rheum tanguticum Maxim. ex Balf. and Rheum officinale Baill |
| PHARMACEUTICAL NAME | Radix Et Rhizoma Rhei |
| PART USED | root and rhizome |
| DOSAGE | 10g |
| FLAVOR | bitter |
| ENERGY | cold |
| CLASS | 8, herbs to induce bowel movements |
| MERIDIANS | spleen, stomach, pericardium, liver and large intestine |
| ACTIONS | to attack accumulations, sedate fire, counteract toxic effects and remove coagulations |
| INDICATIONS | excess heat in the stomach and intestine, nosebleed, coagulation, vomiting of blood and suppression of menstruation |
| NOTES | Experiments have indicated that dahuang can produce seven major effects: It can |

1  be used as an effective digestive,
2  be effective for promoting gastrointestinal peristalsis,
3  promote bowel movements,
4  benefit the gallbladder and reduce jaundice,
5  increase and protect blood platelets,
6  inhibit influenza and
7  treat bacteria.

In addition, dahuang contains anthraquinone glycosides, which accounts for its being used as a laxative; but it also contains tannin that obstructs bowel movements, which explains why, when taken in small doses, it can cause constipation.

Modern research has also revealed that dahuang contains bacterides, which is why this herb has often been used to treat acute contagious hepatitis with jaundice and constipation, dysentery and suppression of menstruation due to blood coagulations.

Aside from being a strong and forceful herb in inducing bowel movements, this herb can also activate the blood, remove blood coagulations, promote meridian energy flow and detoxicate and it is good for vomiting blood, nosebleed, suppression of menstruation and swelling.

Dahuang and huangqin (skullcap) can be decocted together to improve the effect of sedating heat. Dahuang and fanxieye (folium sennae) are both cold laxatives. But dahuang produces a more drastic action, whereas the power of fanxieye varies with the quantities consumed and the methods used in taking it. Making tea out of fanxieye will produce more drastic actions than by decocting it.

*Huangjing
(Yellow Essence)*

# Sealwort

Sometime in the third century A.D., when Dr. Hua Duo was picking herbs on a mountain, he saw two strong young men chasing after a young girl; the girl was about seventeen years old, but the two strong young men could not catch her, because they couldn't run as fast as she could. This greatly puzzled Dr. Hua Duo, who inquired about the young girl. The two young men told Dr. Hua Duo that the girl had escaped from a foster home three years before and no one had known of her whereabouts until now.

Wanting to know more about this girl, particularly about what she had been eating that had made her so energetic, Dr. Hua Duo devised a scheme to catch her. He prepared a bowl of food and placed it in a cave; then he hid in a bush to wait for the girl to come. A few hours later, the girl came to eat the food and Dr. Hua Duo immediately blocked the cave to keep her from escaping. When he questioned her, the young girl told him that she had been eating the big fleshy roots of a plant, which looked very much like a chicken.

After letting the girl go, Dr. Hua Duo found the plant and dug out the fleshy roots. He later named the plant "the yellow essence," because it was yellow and as pure as essence.

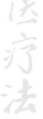

# 黄精

| Chinese | *Huangjing (Yellow Essence)* |
|---|---|
| RE | 4157 |
| COMMON NAME | sealwort |
| FAMILY | Liliaceae |
| CHINESE NAME | yellow pure substance |
| SCIENTIFIC NAME | Polygonatum kingianum Coll. et Hemsl., Polygonatum sibiricum Red & Polygonatum cyrtonema Hua |
| PHARMACEUTICAL NAME | Rhizoma Polygonati |
| PART USED | underground rhizome |
| DOSAGE | 10 to 20g |
| FLAVOR | sweet |
| ENERGY | neutral |
| CLASS | 16, herbs to correct deficiencies |
| MERIDIANS | spleen, lungs and stomach |
| ACTIONS | to water (to increase yin energy) and lubricate the heart and lungs, tone up the middle region, benefit energy and fill in semen and marrow |
| INDICATIONS | yin deficiency, blood deficiency, grey hair, dry throat, thirst and diabetes |
| NOTES | Experiments have indicated that huangjing can produce five major effects: It can |

NOTES (continued):

1 bring down blood pressure by tonification,
2 protect the liver,
3 treat fatty liver,
4 reduce blood sugar and
5 reduce blood fat.

Huangjing is an important spleen tonic. It can also lubricate the lungs and is therefore good for cough due to dry lungs, lung deficiencies, diabetes and deficiency after illness

Huangjing is sticky and for this reason, it should be decocted for a longer period of time than most other herbs in order to extract its active ingredients.

*Xiakucao
(See-Me-Not-After-
Summer)*

# Self-Heal

The mother of a mayor suffered from scrofula with a swollen neck. All the doctors said there was no cure for it. One day, however, an herbalist came along who told the mayor that he knew of an herb that could cure the disease.

The herbalist climbed a nearby mountain to pick the herb and brought it to the mayor for decoction and it indeed cured the patient.

Prior to his departure, the herbalist told the mayor that the herb grew only during the summer and that it would be gone when the summer was over.

In the winter of the following year, the governor suffered from scrofula with a swollen neck. The mayor was eager to help, so he told the governor about the herb that had cured his mother. The mayor then climbed the mountain to pick the plants, but he couldn't find any growing there and returned home empty-handed. Naturally, the governor was terribly disappointed and the mayor felt very embarrassed.

When the herbalist returned in the summer, the mayor blamed him for his failure to find the herb.

"I made it a point to tell you before I left that this herb cannot be found after the summer is over," said the herbalist. And so, the herb was named "see-me-not-after-summer" to remind herbalists that it grows only during the summer.

# 夏枯草

| Chinese | Xiakucao (See-Me-Not-After-Summer) |
|---------|------------------------------------|
| RE | 3752 |
| COMMON NAME | fruit spike of common self-heal |
| FAMILY | Labiatae |
| CHINESE NAME | summer withering grass |
| SCIENTIFIC NAME | Prunella vulgaris L |
| PHARMACEUTICAL NAME | Spica Prunellae |
| PART USED | ear of fruit (fruit spike) |
| DOSAGE | 10 to 30g |
| FLAVOR | slightly bitter |
| ENERGY | cool |
| CLASS | 2, herbs to reduce excessive heat inside the body |
| MERIDIANS | liver and gallbladder |
| ACTIONS | to calm down the liver, clear up heat, soften up hardness and disperse congestion |
| INDICATIONS | headache, pinkeye, carbuncles of the head and scrofula. |
| NOTES | Experiments have shown that this herb can produce four major effects: It can |

NOTES continued:

1  clear heat and bring down blood pressure,
2  soften and shrink the liver and the spleen,
3  treat various types of cancers and
4  treat tuberculosis.

*Yimucao
(Good-For-Mother)*

# Siberian Motherwort

A mother was living with her ten-year-old son. The mother had been ill since her child was born, with abdominal pain and irregular menstruation due to blood coagulation after childbirth. Seeing that his mother had been suffering for so long, the child tried to persuade her to see a doctor. But the mother always declined, saying that they couldn't afford it.

So the child went to see an herbalist on his own. He bought an herb from him and decocted it for his mother. After taking it, she felt a little better. The child then went back to the herbalist and asked him if he could cure his mother. The herbalist said yes but it would cost him five hundred pounds of rice. This saddened the child, as he knew that there was no way that he could come up with that much rice. Then suddenly the child had an idea and he told the herbalist that he would pay him the five hundred pounds of rice after his mother had been cured. The herbalist agreed to the child's proposal.

At midnight, the herbalist climbed the mountain to dig up the herb, with the child secretly following behind him. After the herbalist had gone home with the plants, the child stayed on to dig up some more and then brought them home to his mother.

The next day, the herbalist brought the herb to the child's house, but the child told him that he hadn't been able to come up with the five hundred pounds of rice. So the herbalist left, taking the herb with him.

The child's mother was cured by the herb her child had picked and the herb has been called "good-for-mother" ever since.

益母草

| Chinese | Yimucao (Good-for-Mother) |
|---|---|
| RE | 4016 |
| COMMON NAME | Siberian motherwort |
| FAMILY | Labiatae |
| CHINESE NAME | mother's herb (so named because this herb can benefit mothers in many ways, but in menstrual disorders in particular) |
| SCIENTIFIC NAME | Leonurus heterophyllus Sweet |
| PHARMACEUTICAL NAME | Herba Leonuri |
| PART USED | whole plant |
| DOSAGE | 10g |
| FLAVOR | bitter and pungent |
| ENERGY | neutral |
| CLASS | 12, herbs to regulate blood |
| MERIDIANS | pericardium and liver |
| ACTIONS | to activate the blood, regulate menstruation, disperse coagulations and heal edema |
| INDICATIONS | abdominal pain due to blood coagulations after childbirth, irregular menstruation and vaginal bleeding |
| NOTES | Experiments have shown that yimucao can activate the blood and bring down blood pressure, regulate menstruation and induce contraction of the uterus and labor. Yimucao contains benzoic acid. |

Xuduan
(Fracture Healer)

# Teasel

Once an herbalist was passing through a small village when he heard someone crying; he stopped to inquire about the details and was told that the child lying on the floor was dead and that the crying woman was his mother.

The herbalist took the pulse of the child and told the mother that he was still alive. He took out a bottle of herbal tablets from his briefcase and put ten tiny tablets in the child's mouth; he then washed them down with a cup of warm water. Hours later, the child regained consciousness. The herbalist told the mother that her child should fully recover within a month.

There was an herb shop in the village operated by a powerful and wealthy man who had always monopolized the herb business in the village. When this man heard about the incident, he tried to convince the herbalist to give him the tablets, but the herbalist always declined. So finally he sent two big strong fellows over to beat up the herbalist and break his legs.

Although the herbalist was hurt and had two broken legs, he still had the strength to climb the mountain to pick an herb that would heal his broken legs. A couple of months later, when the herbalist's legs had completely healed, he was able to resume treating patients.

Seeing that the herbalist could walk again and thinking that his legs had not actually been broken, the owner of the herb shop was furious. This time when he instructed the two big fellows to beat up the herbalist, he wanted them to make sure that his legs were really broken. So they beat him up once more and the herbalist became crippled again.

The herbalist could not climb the mountain to pick the herb this time; so, instead, he instructed a young man to do it for him. The young man did and once again the herbalist recovered a couple of months later.

When the owner of the herb shop learned that the herbalist had recovered from his broken legs, he instructed the two big fellows to kill him.

After the herbalist's death, the young man taught the people in the village how to heal broken bones by using the herb that the herbalist had used to heal himself; this young man named the herb "fracture healer."

續斷

| Chinese | Xuduan (Fracture Healer) |
|---|---|
| RE | 4706 |
| COMMON NAME | teazel |
| FAMILY | Dipsacaceae |
| CHINESE NAME | reconnect broken parts |
| SCIENTIFIC NAME | Dipsacus asper Wall |
| PHARMACEUTICAL NAME | Radix Dipsaci |
| PART USED | root |
| DOSAGE | 5 to 10g |
| FLAVOR | bitter and pungent |
| ENERGY | slightly warm |
| CLASS | herbs to counteract rheumatism (class 3) and herbs to correct deficiencies (class 16) |
| MERIDIANS | liver and kidneys |
| ACTIONS | to tone up the liver and kidneys, strengthen loins and knees, connect tendons and bones and secure fetus |
| INDICATIONS | lumbago, soft legs, disconnected tendons and fracture, insecure fetus and vaginal bleeding |
| NOTES | Xuduan can tonify the liver and kidneys and strengthen tendons and bones to treat lumbago. It is a particularly effective herb for promoting energy and blood circulation and for treating fractures and vaginal bleeding. |

# Chinese Magnolia-vine Fruits

Once a fellow suffered from tuberculosis and kept losing weight until he looked like a bamboo stick. The people in the small village where he lived wanted to get rid of him, because they thought that tuberculosis was highly contagious. One neighbor had suggested that they put him on a boat to die in the high seas and another had hinted that he should be burned to death or killed with a knife.

Upon hearing of the plots against their son, the parents of the patient became very worried and then finally came up with an idea.

"Son, your dad and I love you very much, but we cannot help you in any other way except to take you to the mountain where you can hide from the people in the village. If you are lucky and recover from this illness, you can return home; but if you die, we will bury you as soon as we know about it," said his mother with tears in her eyes.

And so, this fellow was taken to the mountain and put in a cave to live on his own. He had managed to survive on the dried foods he had brought with him, but when they were all used up, he didn't have the strength to look for any more food. One day he had become so weak that he was ready to give up the struggle and he started crying out loud.

Hearing his sobs, a hunter appeared at the entrance to the cave and asked him what was the matter. After the sick fellow explained his predicament, the hunter said, "I am just a hunter, not a doctor, so I am afraid I cannot help you. But I can pick some fruit for you to eat."

The fruit the hunter gave him lasted for ten days. At that point, the fellow had gradually regained enough strength to start picking the same fruit by himself.

In a few months, he had recovered from the tuberculosis and went home. When his parents saw him alive and well, at first they couldn't believe their eyes. Later when they asked him how he had managed to recover, he told them about the fruit. The whole village was in shock and this fellow lived to be over one hundred years old.

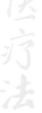

# 五味子

| Chinese | Wuweizi (Five-Flavor Seed) |
|---|---|
| RE | 0772 |
| COMMON NAME | Chinese magnoliavine fruits |
| FAMILY | Magnoliaceae |
| CHINESE NAME | five-flavored seed (so named because its bark & flesh are mixtures of sweet, sour & salty flavors & its kernel tastes pungent, bitter & salty; hence, five flavors in one herb) |
| SCIENTIFIC NAME | Schisandra chinensis (Turcz.) Baill. and Schisandra sphenanthera Rehd. et Wils |
| PHARMACEUTICAL NAME | Fructus Schisandrae |
| PART USED | ripe fruit |
| DOSAGE | 5g |
| FLAVOR | all five, but predominantly sour |
| ENERGY | warm |
| CLASS | 17, herbs to constrict and obstruct movements |
| MERIDIANS | lungs and kidneys |
| ACTIONS | to water (increase yin energy in) kidneys, constrict lungs, produce fluids, check perspiration and diarrhea and constrict semen |
| INDICATIONS | asthma and cough, excessive perspiration, night sweats, diarrhea, seminal emission and vaginal bleeding |
| NOTES | All herbs and foods have flavors; for example, grapes taste sour and sweet, ginseng tastes sweet and bitter and green onions taste pungent. But very few foods or herbs have all of the five flavors—namely, sweet, sour, bitter, pungent and salty—all at the same time Wuweizi is one of these exceptions. |

Experiments have shown that wuweizi can produce seven major effects:
1   It is effective for suppression of cough,
2   it is an effective heart tonic,
3   it is effective as a digestive,
4   it can increase acid,
5   it can reduce transaminase,
6   it can produce excitation and
7   it can be used as an adjuvant herb to treat liver and gallbladder diseases.

Wuweizi can check excessive perspiration and constrict the lungs simultaneously, which is why it is often used to treat cough and asthma due to lung deficiency. In addition, this herb is often used to produce fluids and quench thirst and in recent years it has also been used to treat insomnia, forgetfulness and hepatitis.

# *Lucid Ganoderma*

*I*n a small village a long time ago there lived a dedicated student with a great ambition to pass the empirial examinations to become a government official. This student was so ambitious that the people in the village called him Mr. Ambition.

But having failed the empirial examinations a dozen times, Mr. Ambition decided to shift his ambition and become a Taoist monk instead. Enjoying longevity as a monk, he thought, was more important than becoming a government official. And so, Mr. Ambition put the mundane world behind him and went to stay in a temple on the mountain. There, he became a dedicated Taoist monk, fasting regularly and eating nothing but vegetables.

After having been a Taoist monk for less than a year, one day Mr. Ambition looked at himself in the mirror and to his great astonishment, saw that he had lost so much weight that he looked as skinny as a stick. Mr. Ambition was so scared about his poor health that he immediately left the temple and returned to the mundane world.

Mr. Ambition had made a fortune not long after returning to the city through his construction company, but his fortune did not help him regain his good health. One day while building a large apartment building, Mr. Ambition's workers dug out a strange object from the ground. With its thick flesh and soft body, it almost looked like a huge human hand. Everyone was scared, but particularly Mr. Ambition. "Could this be a bad omen for me? Would the building collapse after its completion?" he worried. It was decided that a fortune-teller should be summoned to shed light on the situation.

"This object signals a real disaster for you, Mr. Ambition," said the fortune-teller.

靈芝草

"How can I prevent this disaster?" asked Mr. Ambition, with his face turning pale. "I would do anything."

After a long pause, the fortune-teller said, "Well, you could turn the upcoming disaster into good luck if you had the courage to eat that strange object."

Mr. Ambition was initially shocked at the suggestion, but later agreed to it and ate the big fleshy object that night at dinner. It didn't taste as bad as he had anticipated it would; in fact, he somewhat enjoyed its taste.

A few days later, Mr. Ambition began to feel dramatic changes taking place in his body: His complexion had improved considerably, he had put on weight, his grey hair had returned to its original color and he looked much younger than his age. And he really felt great!

Later that week, a Taoist monk passed by the construction site where Mr. Ambition was working. Spotting Mr. Ambition, he stopped and said to him, "Sir, you look different from other people. Did anything extraordinary happen to you recently? Have you eaten anything unusual? Let me take your pulse." Mr. Ambition sat down with the Taoist monk. After taking his pulse, the monk said, "Sir, did you possibly eat something that looks like a big human hand?" Mr. Ambition admitted that he had and told the monk the whole story. The monk said, "Sir, the strange object that you ate is an herb called 'spiritual vegetable meat,' and now that you've eaten it, you no longer belong to this mundane world. You ought to come with me to the temple on the mountain, where you can be a Taoist monk and enjoy immortality on earth."

Mr. Ambition took his advice and went with him to the temple, where he stayed for good.

| Chinese | Lingzhicao (Spiritual Vegetable Meat) |
|---|---|
| RE | 2395 |
| COMMON NAME | lucid ganoderma and glossy ganoderma |
| FAMILY | Polyporaceae |
| CHINESE NAME | lingzhi (spiritual mushroom) |
| SCIENTIFIC NAME | Ganoderma lucidum (Leyss. ex Fr.) Karst. and Ganoderma japonicum (Fr.) Lloyd |
| PHARMACEUTICAL NAME | Ganoderma Lucidum Seu Japonicum |
| PART USED | whole plant |
| DOSAGE | 2 to 4g in powder |
| FLAVOR | sweet |
| ENERGY | neutral |
| CLASS | unclassified |
| MERIDIANS | undetermined |
| ACTIONS | to benefit joints, protect the spirits, benefit pure energy, strengthen tendons & bones & improve complexion |
| INDICATIONS | deficiency fatigue, cough, asthma, insomnia, indigestion, deafness, chronic tracheitis, bronchial asthma, leukocytopenia, coronary heart disease and irregular heartbeats |
| NOTES | Experiments indicate that lingzhicao can produce nine effects: It |

Experiments indicate that lingzhicao can produce nine effects: It
1  is effective for asthma,
2  is an effective heart tonic,
3  can protect the liver,
4  can reduce transaminase,
5  can increase white blood cells,
6  can increase and protect blood platelets,
7  can sedate and inhibit,
8  can relieve pain and
9  can reduce blood fat.

*Fruit of Common Cnidium, Sche-chuangzi (Snake-Bed Seed), Chinese Cynomorium, Suoyang (Yang Locker) & Herb of Epimedium, Yinyanghuo (Sexual Plant for Goats)*

# Three Aphrodisiac Herbs

A strange skin disease had attacked many people in a small village. The people with this disease felt itchy all over and had eruptions here and there, as well as rapidly spreading boils. The disease was regarded as highly contagious.

The people in the village knew that there was an herb growing on a small island about ten miles away that could cure the disease. But they also knew that poisonous snakes were in the habit of sleeping on this herb and there were many poisonous snakes on the island. So, naturally, most herbalists were too frightened to set foot on the island.

There was one brave young man who did decide to go. He prepared himself a big bag of rice and rowed a boat to the island. This young man never returned. A few months later, another brave young man did the same thing and he, too, failed to return.

The people in the village had almost given up hope when a third brave young man said that he would go. But instead of going straight to the island, this young man went to a seaside temple, where he had heard there was a nun who was an expert at controlling snakes. The nun told the young man that poisonous snakes are afraid of realgar wine; she then gave him a bottle and he headed for the island.

Upon landing, the young man found the island to be full of poisonous snakes. He poured the realgar wine over the ground as he walked along and the snakes all remained very still. When he came to the herb he was looking for, the young man had to push them aside, as several snakes were lying on the herb.

The young man finally returned to the village with the herb, which subsequently cured the people's strange skin disease. He named the herb "snake-bed seed" because the seeds of the plant are used as the herb and snakes sleep on the plant.

蛇床子

| Chinese | Shechuangzi (Snake-Bed Seed) |
|---|---|
| RE | 4345 |
| COMMON NAME | fruit of common cnidium |
| FAMILY | Umbelliferae |
| CHINESE NAME | snake-bed seed |
| SCIENTIFIC NAME | Cnidium monnieri (L.) Cuss |
| PHARMACEUTICAL NAME | Fructus Cnidii |
| PART USED | seeds and ripe fruit |
| DOSAGE | 3 to 10g |
| FLAVOR | pungent and bitter |
| ENERGY | warm |
| CLASS | herbs to correct deficiencies (class 16) and herbs for external applications (class 20) |
| MERIDIANS | kidneys and sanjiao |
| ACTIONS | to destroy worms, dry up dampness and strengthen yang |
| INDICATIONS | chronic tinea and scabies, eczema involving scrotum, itchy genitals in women and impotence |
| NOTES | Modern experiments indicate that shechuangzi can produce sex hormones. From the traditional point of view, this herb has been found to be slightly toxic. |

Another herb that is good for improving sexual functions is suoyang. The Chinese name for this herb means "to lock the yang," with "yang" referring to a man's penis and "to lock" meaning to control. Thus, the herb is used to control the actions of the penis.

Yinyanghuo is also good for improving sexual functions. The Chinese name for this herb means "sexual plant for goats," which originated from the following story. Once there was a shepherd who wondered why his goats were so sexually active. He started watching what they were eating and noticed that they consumed a great deal of one plant in particular, which he later named "sexual plant for goats."

All three aphrodisiac herbs can warm the kidneys and strengthen the yang to treat impotence, seminal emission and premature ejaculation due to kidney yang deficiency. In terms of their differences (first) suoyang is a better herb to strengthen yang and promote bowel movements, which are essential in the treatment of constipation due to yang deficiency; (second) shechuangzi is a better herb for drying dampness and destroying worms, which is why it can be used to treat itch in the genital areas due to dampness and also scabies and sores, chronic tinea, etc.; and (third) yinyanghuo can produce sexual hormones more quickly and is also an effective herb for lumbago and arthritis and rheumatism in the legs.

# 锁阳　　淫羊霍

| Chinese | Suoyang (Yang Locker) | Yinyanghuo (Sexual Plant for Goats) |
|---|---|---|
| RE | 4976 | 4672 |
| COMMON NAME | Chinese cynomorium | herb of epimedium |
| FAMILY | Cynomoriaceae | Berberidaceae |
| CHINESE NAME | yang locker | grass for goat's sexual drive |
| SCIENTIFIC NAME | Cynomorium songaricum Rupr | Epimedium brevicornum Maxim., Epimedium koreanum Nakai and Epimedium sagittatum (Sieb. et Zucc.) Maxim |
| PHARMACEUTICAL NAME | Herba Cynomorii & Caulis Cynomorii | Herba Epimedii |
| PART USED | fleshy stems | stalk leaves or whole plant |
| DOSAGE | 2 to 4g | 4 to 15g |
| FLAVOR | sweet | pungent |
| ENERGY | warm | warm |
| CLASS | 16, herbs to correct deficiencies | 16, herbs to correct deficiencies |
| MERIDIANS | kidneys | liver and kidneys |
| ACTIONS | to tone up kidneys, strengthen yang, benefit semen and lubricate intestine. | to tone up life door and strengthen tendons and bones (Life door refers to yang energy in the kidneys that is responsible for male sexual capability.) |
| INDICATIONS | impotence, constipation due to blood deficiency and weak loins and knees | impotence, rheumatism & hypertension |
| NOTES | Suoyang can tonify and assist yang to treat impotence, seminal emission, premature ejaculation and weak loins and knees due to kidney yang deficiency on the one hand. On the other hand, it can also lubricate dryness and make the intestines smooth, which are essential in the treatment of deficiency constipation. | Experiments indicate that yinyanghuo can bring down blood pressure by tonification and can also produce sex hormones. When used to improve sexual functions in men, the leaves have stronger effects than the stalks. When used to treat hypertension, this herb can be decocted with huangbai (yellow bark), which is particularly effective for hypertension during menopause in women. Yinyanghuo is regarded as an effective herb to treat cold and damp rheumatism and hypertension due to kidney yang deficiency. |

中医疗法

# Chinese Herb's Named After Their Colors

紅花

| Chinese | Honghua |
| --- | --- |
| RE | 1999 |
| COMMON NAME | safflower |
| FAMILY | Compositae |
| CHINESE NAME | red flower (so named because of its color) |
| SCIENTIFIC NAME | Carthamus tinctorius L |
| PHARMACEUTICAL NAME | Flos Carthami |
| PART USED | corolla |
| DOSAGE | 6 g |
| FLAVOR | pungent |
| ENERGY | warm |
| CLASS | 12, herbs to regulate blood |
| MERIDIANS | heart and liver |
| ACTIONS | to activate blood, facilitate menstrual flow, disperse blood coagulations and relieve pain |
| INDICATIONS | menstrual pain, suppression of menstruation, dead fetus, swelling and lochiostasis |
| NOTES | Experiments have shown that this herb can expand coronary arteries and prevent angina pectoris, activate the blood and bring down blood pressure, treat various types of cancers and regulate menstruation. |

# 赤芍　白芷　白及

| Chinese | Chishaoyao | Baizhi | Baiji |
|---|---|---|---|
| RE | 2225 | 1380 | 1374 |
| COMMON NAME | red peony root | angelica | amethyst orchid |
| FAMILY | Ranunculaceae | Umbelliferae | Orchidaceae |
| CHINESE NAME | red peony (so named due to its color) | white rootlet (so named because the herb is white and shaped like a rootlet) | white orchid (so named due to its color) |
| SCIENTIFIC NAME | Paeonia lactiflora Pall | Angelica dahurica (Fisch. ex Hoffm.) Benth. et Hook. f., Angelica dahurica (Fisch. ex Hoffm.) Benth. et Hook. f. var. & taiwaniana (Boiss.) Shan et Yuan | Bletilla striata (Thunb.) Reichb.f |
| | Radix Paeoniae Rubra | Radix Angelicae Dahuricae | Rhizoma (Tuber) Bletillae |
| PHARMACEUTICAL NAME | root | root | underground tuberous root |
| PART USED | 5 to 10g | 5g | 10 to 20g |
| DOSAGE | sour and bitter | pungent | bitter |
| FLAVOR | cool | warm | neutral |
| ENERGY | 2, herbs to reduce excessive heat inside the body | herbs to counteract rheumatism (class 3) and herbs to induce perspiration (class 1) | 12, herbs to regulate blood |
| CLASS | liver and spleen | lungs, stomach and large intestine | lungs |
| MERIDIANS | to remove blood coagulations, relieve pain, cool the blood and reduce swelling | to induce perspiration, expel wind, heal swelling and relieve pain. | to arrest bleeding, constrict lungs, produce muscles and heal wounds |
| ACTIONS | suppression of menses due to blood coagulation, abdominal obstructions in women, abdominal pain, pain in the ribs, nosebleeds, dysentery with blood in stools, pinkeye and carbuncles | headache, toothache, pain in the bony ridge of the eye socket, sinusitis, discharge of blood from the anus & itch | vomiting of blood, coughing up blood, nosebleeds, ulcers and pulmonary tuberculosis |
| INDICATIONS | Experiments indicate that chishaoyao is effective in inhibiting gastrointestinal peristalsis and can also inhibit influenza. This herb should be avoided by those with blood deficiency.<br><br>Chishaoyao is often used to clear heat, cool the blood, activate the blood, remove coagulations, reduce swelling, relieve pain and treat sores and ulcers. | Experiments indicate that baizhi can produce excitation and is also an effective herb for relief of pain. In addition, baizhi contains volatile oils, protein, carbohydrates and fat, which make it readily eaten by insects.<br><br>Baizhi is a strong herb for relieving pain. It can also open cavities and drain off pus and is often used to treat rhinitis, sinusitis, carbuncles and burns. | Experiments indicate that baiji produce four effects:<br>1 It can increase and protect blood platelets,<br>2 it is an effective coagulant,<br>3 it is an antituberculotic herb and<br>4 it can arrest bleeding (as a hemostatic). |
| NOTES | | | |

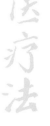

# 白薇　　白术　　青皮　　青蒿

| Baiwei | Baizhu | Qingpi | Qinghao |
|---|---|---|---|
| 1394 | 1376 | 2485 | 2491 |
| white rose | white atractylode | green orange-peel | southern wood |
| Asclepiadaceae | Compositae | Rutaceae | Compositae |
| white rose (so named due to its color) | white atractylode (so named due to its color) | green peel (so named because of its color) | green evergreen artemisia (so named because the leaves and stems of this herb remain green in autumn and it's similar to evergreen artemisia in shape) |
| Cynanchum atratum Bge. and Cynanchum versicolor Bge | Atractylodes macrocephala Koidz | Citrus reticulata Blanco, Citrus tangerina Hortorum et Tanaka, Citrus unshiu Marcovitch, Citrus sinensis (L.) Osbeckwilsonii Tanaka | Artemisia annua L. and Artemisia apiacea Hance |
| Radix Cynanchi Atrati | | | |
| root | Rhizoma Atractylodis | Pericarpium Citri Reticulate. Viride and | Herba Artemisiae Chinghao |
| 6 to 12g | rhizome | Fructus Aurantii Immaturus peel of unripe fruit and fruit | rhizome |
| bitter and salty | | | |
| cold | 5g | 5g | 6g |
| | sweet and bitter | bitter and pungent | bitter |
| 2, herbs to reduce excessive heat inside the body | warm | warm | cold |
| | 16, herbs to correct deficiencies | 11, herbs to regulate energy | 2, herbs to reduce excessive heat inside the body |
| undetermined | | | |
| to benefit yin, clear up heat and cool blood | spleen and stomach | liver and gallbladder | liver and kidneys |
| periodic fever due to yin deficiency and fever in warm-hot diseases | to tone up energy, strengthen spleen, dry up dampness, benefit water and check perspiration | to disperse energy congestion, disperse accumulations, promote energy flow and relieve pain | to relieve summer heat, clear up heat and relieve hot sensations as if coming from the bones |
| | spleen deficiency, poor appetite, edema and excessive perspiration | chest swelling and pain and hernial pain in the lower abdomen | malaria, hot sensations and scabies |
| Baiwei contains cynanchol | Experiments indicate that baizhu can protect the liver, promote urination and reduce blood sugar | This herb consists of the peel of unripe oranges. It is an effective herb for promoting energy circulation to relieve energy congestion in the liver and gallbladder, to relax the liver for the relief of pain, to break up energy and to disperse congestion. It is a strong herb in promoting energy circulation and is often used to treat pain in the chest and ribs, food stagnation and energy congestion. | Experiments indicate that this herb can inhibit influenza. It is an aromatic herb. It is good for warm diseases in their later stages, hot sensations at night and cold sensations in the morning. |

玄參

| Chinese | Xuanshen |
|---|---|
| RE | 1542 |
| COMMON NAME | figwort |
| FAMILY | Scrophulariaceae |
| CHINESE NAME | dark ginseng (so named because its stalk looks like ginseng, but it's dark) |
| SCIENTIFIC NAME | Scrophularia ningpoensis Hemsl |
| PHARMACEUTICAL NAME | Radix Scrophulariae |
| PART USED | tuberous root |
| DOSAGE | 10g |
| FLAVOR | bitter and salty |
| ENERGY | cold |
| CLASS | herbs to reduce excessive heat inside the body (class 2) and herbs for lubricating dry symptoms (class 6) |
| MERIDIANS | lungs and kidneys |
| ACTIONS | to clear up heat, water yin (increase yin energy), bring down fire, detoxicate and disperse congestion |
| INDICATIONS | hot diseases, scabies, sore throat, pain in throat, scrofula and carbuncles |
| NOTES | Experiments indicate that this herb can cool the blood and bring down blood pressure, bring down blood pressure by tonification and reduce blood sugar. |

中医疗法

Herbs can be either sweet, sour, bitter, pungent, or salty — or a combination. Some are aromatic whereas others smell offensive.

木香

# Chinese Herbs Named After Their Tastes and Aromas

| Chinese | Muxiang |
|---|---|
| RE | 0703 |
| COMMON NAME | costusroot |
| FAMILY | Compositae |
| CHINESE NAME | wood aroma (so named because it is aromatic) |
| SCIENTIFIC NAME | Aucklandia lappa Decne. and Saussurae lappa Clarke |
| PHARMACEUTICAL NAME | Radix Aucklandiae& Radix Saussureae |
| PART USED | dry root |
| DOSAGE | 6g |
| FLAVOR | pungent |
| ENERGY | warm |
| CLASS | 11, herbs to regulate energy |
| MERIDIANS | lungs, liver and spleen |
| ACTIONS | to promote energy circulation, relieve pain and eliminate accumulations |
| INDICATIONS | abdominal swelling and pain, diarrhea and dysentery |
| NOTES | Experiments indicate that this herb can be effective in promoting gastrointestinal peristalsis, can benefit the gallbladder and reduce jaundice and can promote liver bile production and bile excretion. |

Muxiang is a relatively strong herb for relieving energy stagnation in the stomach and intestine. It is often used to treat poor appetite, indigestion and abdominal swelling and pain. It can be used with huanglian to treat diarrhea and tenesmus due to damp heat.

# 小茴香 丁香　臭梧桐

| Chinese | Xiaohuixiang | Dingxiang | Chouwutong |
|---|---|---|---|
| RE | 3306 | 0026 | 3886 |
| COMMON NAME | fennel | cloves | forked clerodendron leaf |
| FAMILY | Umbelliferae | Myrtaceae | Verbenaceae |
| CHINESE NAME | fennel | T-shaped aroma (so named because its flowers are T-shaped and it's aromatic) | Stinky Chinese parasol tree (so named because of its offensive smell) |
| SCIENTIFIC NAME | Foeniculum vulgare Mill | Eugenia caryophyllata Thunberg (Caryophyllus aromaticus L.) | Clerodendron trichotomum Thunb |
| PHARMACEUTICAL NAME | Fructus Foeniculi | Flos Caryophylli | Folium Clerodendri Trichotomi |
| PART USED | ripe fruit | buds | young branches and leaves |
| DOSAGE | 2 to 5g | 2g | 10 to 20g |
| FLAVOR | pungent | pungent | bitter and sweet |
| ENERGY | warm | warm | cold |
| CLASS | 4, herbs to reduce cold sensations inside the body | herbs to regulate energy (class 11) and herbs to reduce cold sensations inside the body (class 4) | 3, herbs to counteract rheumatism |
| MERIDIANS | liver, kidneys, spleen and stomach | lungs, spleen, stomach and kidneys | undetermined |
| ACTIONS | to promote energy flow, disperse congestion, warm up internal regions and relieve pain | to bring down energy, warm up spleen and kidneys and relieve pain | to clear heat, benefit water, expel wind and dampness, relieve pain and reduce blood pressure |
| INDICATIONS | hernia, pain in the lower abdomen and intestinal rumbling | hiccups, vomiting, spleen and kidney cold deficiency and cold abdominal pain | blood in stools, suppression of urination, arthritis, lumbago and pain in legs and hypertension |
| NOTES | This herb can warm the lower abdomen. It is most frequently used to treat only acute cases of cold abdominal pain in early stages. | Experiments indicate that dingxiang is effective as a digestive and for promoting gastrointestinal peristalsis. It warms the spleen and stomach and is good for cold stomach and hiccups due to cold. | Experiments indicate that chouwutong is an effective herb for relief of pain. It is an antirheumatic herb and is also generally effective in reducing blood pressure. |

中医疗法

# 苦參　苦楝皮 酸棗仁 細辛

| Kushen | Kulianpi | Suanzaoren | Xixin |
|---|---|---|---|
| 2624 | 2658 | 5292 | 3082 |
| bitter sophora | Chinaberry tree bark | jujube | Chinese wild ginger |
| Leguminosae | Meliaceae | Rhamnaceae | Aristolochiaceae |
| bitter ginseng (so named due to its taste) | Bitter Chinaberry tree bark (so named due to its taste) | Sour date (so named because its fruits resemble dates and taste sour) | Fine & pungent (so named because its roots are very fine & taste pungent) |
| Sophora flavescens Ait | Melia toosendan Sieb. et Zucc. and Melia azedarach L | Ziziphus spinosa Hu | Asarum heterotropoides Fr. Schmidt var. mandshuricum (Maxim.) Kitag and Asarum sieboldii Miq |
| Radix Sophorae Flavescentis | Cortex Meliae | Semen Ziziphi Spinosae | Herba Asari |
| root | white root bark | kernel | root and rhizoma |
| 6 to 12g | 10 to 15g | 10g | 5g |
| bitter | bitter | sweet | pungent |
| cold | cold | neutral | warm |
| 2, herbs to reduce excessive heat inside the body | 18, herbs to expel or destroy parasites | 14, herbs to reduce anxiety | 1, herbs to induce perspiration |
| heart, spleen and kidneys | undetermined | heart, liver and gallbladder | heart, lungs, liver and kidneys |
| to clear up heat, dry up dampness, benefit water, destroy worms and relieve itch | to destroy worms | to secure the heart, calm down the spirits, check perspiration and produce fluids | to expel cold, disperse wind, promote flow of water and open up cavities |
| diarrhea, dysentery, urination difficulty, scabies and trichomonas vaginitis | roundworms and hookworms | insomnia, palpitations, forgetfulness and deficiency perspiration | headache due to wind dampness, asthma, cough and rheumatism |

Experiments indicate that kushen can produce three effects:
1   It can promote urination,
2   it can be used for various types of cancer and
3   it can be used as an antibacterial herb.

Although kushen is good for many symptoms, it is used mostly for external applications, because it is cold and bitter and can be harmful to weak patients. When kushen is used for internal consumption, it is usually combined with other herbs, such as muxiang, gancao, danggui and chishaoyao, all of which are discussed in this book.

External applications of kushen are often used to treat eczema, furuncles and carbuncles, as well as genital itch in women.

Experiments indicate that suanzaoren can sedate and inhibit. Suanzaoren can be used to treat insomnia due to anxiety by nourishing the blood and the liver.

Experiments indicate that xixin is an effective herb for relief of pain and it contains volatile oils. Since xixin is a relatively strong herb, it is particularly good at opening cavities to relieve pain. It disperses wind cold in the heart and the kidneys in particular. It is most often used to treat headache due to the common cold, body pain and nasal congestion due to external attack and yang deficiency and fever with severe fear of cold.

# Chinese Herbs Named After Their Shapes

Many herbs are named after their shapes, such as cow's knee, dog's spine and hundred parts.

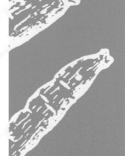

太子参

| Chinese | Taizishen |
|---|---|
| RE | 0749 |
| COMMON NAME | root of heterophylly falsestarwort |
| FAMILY | Caryophyllaceae |
| CHINESE NAME | prince ginseng (so named because its roots resemble a fat prince) |
| SCIENTIFIC NAME | Pseudostellaria heterophylla (Miq.) Pax ex Pax et Hoffm |
| PHARMACEUTICAL NAME | Radix Pseudostellariae |
| PART USED | tuberous root |
| DOSAGE | 6 to 10g |
| FLAVOR | sweet and bitter |
| ENERGY | slightly warm |
| CLASS | 16, herbs to correct deficiencies |
| MERIDIANS | spleen and lungs |
| ACTIONS | to tone up energy, benefit spleen and produce fluids |
| INDICATIONS | energy deficiency of spleen and stomach, lungs, energy deficiency, shortness of breath, asthma, cough and thirst |
| NOTES | Experiments indicate that this herb is effective in treating various types of cancer.<br><br>Taizishen can tonify energy to treat fatigue and shortness of breath. It can also tonify yin, produce fluids and quench thirst. |

# 牛膝　狗脊　鈎藤　猪苓

| *Niuxi* | *Gouji* | *Gouteng* | *Zhuling* |
|---|---|---|---|
| 0833 | 2949 | 3436 | 4545 |
| two-toothed amaranthus and root of two-toothed achyranthes | rhizome of East Asian tree fern | gambir | umbellate pore fungus |
| Amaranthaceae | Dicksoniaceae | Rubiaceae | Polyporaceae |
| cow's knee (so named because its stalks resemble the knees of a cow) | dog's spine (so named because it looks like a dog's spine) | hooky branches (so named because this herb has thorns like so many hooks) | pig's fungus (so named because it is as black as pig dung and it grows on trees like a fungus) |
| Achyranthes bidentata Bl | Cibotium barometz (L.) J. Sm | Uncaria rhynchophylla (Miq.) Jacks, Uncaria macrophylla Wall., Uncaria hirsuta Havil., Uncaria sinensis (Oliv.) Havil. and Uncaria sessilifructus Roxb | Polyporus umbellatus (Pers.) Fries |
| Radix Achyranthis Bidentatae | Rhizoma Cibotii | Ramulus Uncariae Cum Uncis and Rhynchophylla | Polyporus Umbellatus (Grifola) |
| roots | rhizome | branches | fungus nucleus |
| 10g | 5 to 25g | 10g | 10g |
| bitter and sour | bitter and sweet | sweet | sweet |
| neutral | warm | slightly cold | neutral |
| 12, herbs to regulate blood | herbs to counteract rheumatism (class 3) and herbs to correct deficiencies (class 16) | herbs to reduce anxiety (class 14) and herbs to stop involuntary movements (class 15) | 5, herbs to reduce dampness in the body |
| liver and kidneys | liver and kidneys | liver and pericardium | kidneys and bladder |
| to activate blood and facilitate menstrual flow (raw) and to tone up liver and kidneys (processed) | to tone up the liver and kidneys, strengthen the loins and legs and remove wind and dampness | to stop wind, remove heat, calm down convulsions, dizziness | to seep and benefit dampness |
| suppression of menstruation, abdominal obstructions, headache due to liver fire and pain in bones | lumbago, weak legs, enuresis, frequent urination, whitish vaginal discharge and chronic ulcers | convulsions in children, dizziness, headache, fever and twitching | diminished urination, edema, beriberi, urinary strains and vaginal discharge |
| Experiments indicate that this herb can bring down blood pressure by tonification | This herb is effective for treating pain in the spine due to an accumulation of cold and dampness | Experiments indicate that this herb can reduce anxiety and blood pressure, sedate and inhibit and counteract epilepsy and convulsions. Gouteng is an ideal herb for light cases of convulsions at the beginning stage. | Experiments indicate that this herb can promote urination |

# 川乌头　百部

| Chinese | Chuanwutou | Baibu |
|---|---|---|
| RE | 0456 | 1729 |
| COMMON NAME | monkshood | wild asparagus |
| FAMILY | Ranunculaceae | Stemonaceae |
| CHINESE NAME | crow's head from Si Chuan (so named because it looks like the head of a crow and the best quality of this herb is produced in Si Chuan) | hundred parts (so named because its roots are over one hundred in number) |
| SCIENTIFIC NAME | Aconitum chinense Paxton and Aconitum carmichaeli Debx | Stemona sessilifolia (Miq.) Miq., Stemona japonica (Bl.) Miq. and Stemona tuberosa Lour |
| PHARMACEUTICAL NAME | Radix Aconiti | Radix Stemonae |
| PART USED | tuberous root | tuberous root |
| DOSAGE | 4g | 5g |
| FLAVOR | pungent | sweet and bitter |
| ENERGY | hot | slightly warm |
| CLASS | herbs to counteract rheumatism (class 3) and herbs to reduce cold sensations inside the body (class 4) | 10, herbs to suppress cough and reduce sputum |
| MERIDIANS | spleen, kidneys and heart | lungs |
| ACTIONS | to remove wind and dampness, warm up meridians, disperse cold and relieve pain | to lubricate lungs, suppress cough, bring down energy and destroy worms |
| INDICATIONS | acute rheumatic pain, spasms of arms and legs, paralysis of limbs, twitching and numbness and cold headache | cough due to deficiency fatigue, pulmonary tuberculosis, chronic bronchitis and whooping cough |
| NOTES | Experiments indicate that this herb is effective for relief of pain. But it is extremely toxic when used in crude form and needs to be processed in order to be safe for consumption. | Experiments indicate that baibu is effective for suppression of cough and it is also an antituberculotic herb. |

中医疗法

骨碎補

Chinese
Herbs
Named
After Their
Effects

Certain Chinese herbs are named for their particular effects. For instance, some are named after eye diseases, bone diseases, or wind diseases.

| Chinese | Gusuibu |
|---|---|
| RE | 3421 |
| COMMON NAME | rhizome of fortune's drynaria |
| FAMILY | Polypodiaceae |
| CHINESE NAME | bone fracture remedy (so named due to its being effective for bone diseases) |
| SCIENTIFIC NAME | Drynaria fortunei (Kunze) J. Sm. and Drynaria baronii (Christ) Diels |
| PHARMACEUTICAL NAME | Rhizoma Drynariae |
| PART USED | rhizome |
| DOSAGE | 5 to 10g |
| FLAVOR | bitter |
| ENERGY | warm |
| CLASS | herbs to counteract rheumatism (class 3) and herbs to correct deficiencies (class 16) |
| MERIDIANS | liver and kidneys |
| ACTIONS | to tone up the kidneys, connect tendons and bones, activate the blood and relieve pain |
| INDICATIONS | fracture, lumbago and kidney deficiency with ringing in the ears |
| NOTES | This herb can tonify the kidneys to treat chronic diarrhea due to kidney deficiency. In addition, it can activate the blood and connect broken bones, which is why it can be used to treat fracture and pain in tendons and bones. |

# 遠志　　決明子　防風

| Chinese | Yuanzhi | Juemingzi, Caojueming | Fangfeng. |
|---|---|---|---|
| RE | 2087 | 1906 | 1985 |
| COMMON NAME | slender-leaved milkwort | cassia seed | Chinese fangfeng |
| FAMILY | Polygalaceae | Leguminosae | Umbelliferae |
| CHINESE NAME | Long determination (so named because it is believed that by consuming this herb, one can develop the strong determination that goes a long way) | determining brightness seed (so named because it can sharpen vision) | wind-preventing herb (so named because this herb can counteract the attack of wind to prevent wind disease and stroke) |
| SCIENTIFIC NAME | Polygala tenuifolia Willd. and Polygala sibirica L | Cassia obtusifolia L. and Cassia tora L | Ledebouriella divaricata (Turcz.) |
| PHARMACEUTICAL NAME | Radix Polygalae | Semen Cassiae | Radix Ledebouriellae |
| PART USED | root | ripe seeds | root |
| DOSAGE | 5g | | 5g |
| FLAVOR | bitter and pungent | salty | pungent |
| ENERGY | warm | neutral | slightly warm |
| CLASS | 14, herbs to reduce anxiety | 2, herbs to reduce excessive heat inside the body | 1, herbs to induce perspiration |
| MERIDIANS | heart and kidneys | liver and kidneys | bladder, liver, lungs, spleen & stomach |
| ACTIONS | to calm down the spirits, benefit intelligence, transform sputum, open cavities and disperse and eliminate | to clear up liver, benefit kidneys, expel wind, sharpen vision and lubricate intestine for constipation | to induce perspiration, disperse cold, relieve pain and overcome dampness |
| INDICATIONS | insomnia, palpitations, forgetfulness, cough with copious sputum, carbuncles and sore throat | headache due to hot liver, amaurosis, pinkeye with swelling and discharge of dry stools with constipation. | wind-dampness rheumatism |
| NOTES | Experiments indicate that this herb is effective as an expectorant and it can sedate and inhibit. It contains saponin, which accounts for its being used as an expectorant. | Experiments indicate that this herb is generally effective in reducing blood pressure | Experiments indicate that fangfeng is effective for relief of pain and it is an antirheumatic herb. Fangfeng is good for excessive perspiration due to superficial deficiency and for prevention of the common cold. |

# 大楓子

Dafengzi

0196

chaulmoogra

Flacourtiaceae

greater leprosy seed (so named
because it can treat leprosy)

Hydnocarpus anthelmintica Pierre

Semen Hydnocarpi

ripe seeds

2 to 4g

pungent

hot

20, herbs for external applications

undetermined

to expel wind, dry up dampness,
attack poisons and destroy worms

scabies, boils and leprosy

Dafengzi is toxic

# Chinese Herbs Named After Their Discoverers

徐長卿

| | |
|---|---|
| Chinese | Xuchangqing |
| RE | 3897 |
| COMMON NAME | root of paniculate swallowwort |
| FAMILY | Asclepiadaceae |
| CHINESE NAME | Mr. Xuchangqing (so named because it was discovered by him) |
| SCIENTIFIC NAME | Cynanchum paniculatum (Bge.) Kitag |
| PHARMACEUTICAL NAME | Radix Cynanchi Paniculati |
| PART USED | root and rhizome or whole plant with root |
| DOSAGE | 3 to 10g |
| FLAVOR | pungent |
| ENERGY | warm |
| CLASS | 10, herbs to suppress cough and reduce sputum |
| MERIDIANS | undetermined |
| ACTIONS | to relieve pain, suppress cough, benefit water, reduce swelling, activate blood and detoxicate |
| INDICATIONS | stomachache, toothache, rheumatic pain, abdominal pain during menstruation, chronic tracheitis and eczema |
| NOTES | Experiments indicate that Xuchangqing is effective for relief of pain and is also an antirheumatic herb. It is toxic and should be used cautiously by those with deficiency. |

# 劉寄奴　杜仲

| *Luijinu* | *Duzhong* |
|---|---|
| 1897 | 2092 |
| herb of diverse wormwood | eucommia bark |
| Compositae | Eucommiaceae |
| Mr. Liujinu (so named because it was discovered by him) | Du Zhong (so named because according to a Chinese legend, a person named Du Zhong made great intellectual achievements after taking this herb) |
| Artemisia anomala S. Moore and Siphonostegia chinensis Benth | Eucommia ulmoides Oliv |
| Scroplmlariaceae<br>Herba Artemisiae Anomalae | Cortex Eucommiae |
| whole plant | bark |
| 5 to 10g | 6g |
| bitter | sweet and bitter |
| warm | warm |
| 12, herbs to regulate blood | 16, herbs to correct deficiencies |
| heart and spleen | liver and kidneys |
| to activate the blood, relieve pain and facilitate menstruation | to tone up the liver and kidneys, strengthen tendons and bones and secure fetus |
| suppression of menstruation, pain due to blood coagulations and injuries | lumbago, fetus motion, kidney deficiency, headache and dizziness and weak legs |
| | Experiments indicate that duzhong can bring down blood pressure by tonification, reduce blood fat and be generally effective in reducing blood pressure |

Some Chinese herbs are named after the season in which they are grown, including middle summer, winter-tolerating stem and after-summer-see-me-not (which was discussed earlier).

# Chinese Herbs Named After Their Growing Seasons

半夏

| Chinese | Banxia |
|---|---|
| RE | 1550 |
| COMMON NAME | middle-summer pinellia |
| FAMILY | Araceae |
| CHINESE NAME | middle summer (so named because it grows in the middle of summer) |
| SCIENTIFIC NAME | Pinellia ternata (Thunb.) Breit |
| PHARMACEUTICAL NAME | Rhizoma Pinelliae and Tuber Pinelliae |
| PART USED | rhizome |
| DOSAGE | 8g |
| FLAVOR | pungent |
| ENERGY | warm |
| CLASS | herbs to induce vomiting (class 7) and herbs to suppress cough and reduce sputum (class 10) |
| MERIDIANS | spleen and stomach |
| ACTIONS | to dry up dampness, transform sputum, bring down upsurging energy and relieve vomiting |
| INDICATIONS | asthma, cough, vomiting and external applications for carbuncles and swelling |
| NOTES | Experiments indicate that banxia is effective as an expectorant and can relieve vomiting.<br><br>Banxia in its raw form is toxic; it can cause sore throat, swollen tongue and hoarseness, which is why it should be taken internally only after having been processed. According to a recent report, after it is decocted its toxic effects are substantially reduced. Nevertheless, pregnant women should use this herb with great care. |

# 忍冬藤 女貞子

| Rendongteng | Nuzhenzi |
|---|---|
| 2417 | 0467 |
| honeysuckle stem | wax tree |
| Caprifoliaceae | Oleaceae |
| winter-tolerating stem (so named because this plant does not wither in the severe cold of winter) | winter green or chastity seed (so named because the leaves of this plant remain green in the severe cold of winter, which is comparable to a woman remaining faithful to her lover) |
| Lonicera japonica Thunberg | Ligustrum lucidum Ait |
| Caulis Lonicerae | Fructus Ligustri Lucidi |
| leafy stems | ripe fruit |
| 11 to 33g | 10 to 15g |
| sweet | sweet and bitter |
| cold | neutral |
| 2, herbs to reduce excessive heat inside the body | 16, herbs to correct deficiencies |
| heart and lungs | liver and kidneys |
| to clear and detoxicate and open passages of meridians | to nourish yin and tone up liver and kidneys |
| fever in warm diseases, dysentery with blood in stools, contagious hepatitis, carbuncles and pain in tendons and bones | liver-kidney yin deficiency, dizziness, seminal emission and palpitations |
| Experiments indicate that this herb is effective for various types of cancer. | Experiments indicate that this herb is an effective heart tonic. In addition, nuzhenzi can tonify the kidneys and sharpen vision and it is an effective herb for dizziness, ringing in the ears and premature grey hair due to liver and kidney deficiency. |

# Chinese Flowering Herbs

Once upon a time, a goddess threw a party for her seven daughters. In the food she cooked, she used seven flowers, with one flower for each daughter. As a result, all her seven daughters grew up to be beautiful women and remained beautiful and youthful forever. The seven daughters were so happy about the wonderful effects of the flowers that they begged their mother to do the same for women in the mundane world so that they too would remain beautiful forever. And so, the goddess ordered her seven daughters to plant flowers on earth for the women in the mundane world, which is why most flowers in Chinese medicine are good for women's disorders.

合欢花

| Chinese | Hehuanhua |
|---|---|
| RE | 1880 |
| COMMON NAME | silk-tree flower |
| FAMILY | Leguminosae |
| CHINESE NAME | meeting-happiness flower |
| SCIENTIFIC NAME | Albizzia julibrissin Durazz |
| PHARMACEUTICAL NAME | flos Albiziae |
| PART USED | flower or bud |
| DOSAGE | 3 to 10g |
| FLAVOR | sweet |
| ENERGY | neutral |
| CLASS | 14, herbs to reduce anxiety |
| MERIDIANS | heart and spleen |
| ACTIONS | to relax liver, regulate energy and secure spirits |
| INDICATIONS | congested chest, insomnia, forgetfulness, wind-fire eye diseases, blurred vision, sore throat, carbuncles and injuries from falls |
| NOTES | |

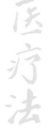

# 蓮花　　蒲黃　　菊花　　玫瑰花

| *Lianhua* | *Puhuang* | *Juhua* | *Meiguihua* |
|---|---|---|---|
| 3693 | 5126 | 4127 | 2483 |
| lotus flower | cattail pollen | mulberry-leaved chrysanthemum | rose |
| Nymphaceae | Typhaceae | Compositae | Rosaceae |
| lotus flower | cattail pollen | peak flower of September (so named because the flower of this plant reaches its peak in September and should be picked at that time) | rose |
| Nelumbo nucifera Gaertn | Typha angustifolia L. and Typha orientalis Presl | Chrysanthemum morifolium Ramat | Rosa rugosa Thunb |
| Flos Nelumbinis | Pollen Typhae | Flos Chyrsanthemi | Flos Rosae Rugosae |
| flower | pollen | dry inflorescence | flower |
| 5 to 10g | 3 to 10g | 8g | 3 to 6g |
| bitter and sweet | sweet | sweet and bitter | sweet and slightly bitter |
| warm | neutral | cool | warm |
| 12, herbs to regulate blood | 12, herbs to regulate blood | 1, herbs to induce perspiration | 11, herbs to regulate energy |
| heart and liver | liver, spleen and pericardium | lungs, liver and kidneys | liver and spleen |
| to activate the blood, arrest bleeding and remove dampness and wind | to disperse coagulation when used fresh and arrest bleeding when fried | to induce perspiration, clear heat, clear liver and detoxicate | to regulate energy, relieve energy congestion, harmonize the blood and disperse blood coagulation |
| vomiting of blood due to injuries from falls, eczema and carbuncles | menstrual pain due to blood coagulation, pain due to injuries causing blood coagulation, sore throat and bleeding | eye diseases, pain in ears, dizziness, carbuncles, swelling and headache due to wind heat | energy pain in the liver and stomach, wind rheumatism, vomiting blood, discharge of blood from the mouth, irregular menstruation, vaginal discharge, dysentery, mastitis and swelling. |
| | Experiments indicate that puhuang is an effective coagulant and can arrest bleeding (as a hemostatic). In addition, puhuang is good for irregular menstruation, acute pain in the lower abdomen and dizziness. | Juhua is good for dispersing wind heat in the liver and gallbladder meridians and also in the ears and eyes; it is often used to treat pinkeye, pain in the ears and vertigo, due to wind heat. | |
| | | It is estimated that in China, there are several hundred varieties of this herb. However, only the four that follow are commonly used. Sweet juhua, which is yellowish and is used to disperse wind and reduce fever; white juhua, which is drunk as tea and is used to clear the liver and sharpen vision; aromatic juhua, which is white and aromatic and is used to treat dizziness and twitching in warm-hot diseases; and wild juhua, which is used to clear heat and to detoxicate. | |

鶏冠花 射干　丹參

| Chinese | Jiguanhua | Shegan | Danshen |
|---|---|---|---|
| RE | 2451 | 3875 | 0977 |
| COMMON NAME | cockscomb | blackberry lily | purple sage |
| FAMILY | Amaranthaceae | Iridaceae | Labiatae |
| CHINESE NAME | cockscomb | shooting dryness | red ginseng (so named because it is red and is shaped like ginseng) |
| SCIENTIFIC NAME | Celosia cristata L | Belamcanda chinensis (L.) DC | Salvia miltiorrhiza Bge |
| PHARMACEUTICAL NAME | Flos Celosiae Cristatae | Rhizoma Belamcandae | Radix Salviae Miltiorrhizae |
| PART USED | inflorescence | rhizome | root |
| DOSAGE | 5 to 10g | 3 to 10g | 10g |
| FLAVOR | sweet | bitter | bitter |
| ENERGY | cool | cold | slightly cold |
| CLASS | herbs to induce perspiration (class 1) and herbs to regulate blood (class 12) | 2, herbs to reduce excessive heat inside the body | 12, herbs to regulate blood |
| MERIDIANS | liver and kidneys | lungs and liver | heart and liver |
| ACTIONS | to cool blood and arrest bleeding | to clear up heat, counteract toxic effects, bring down energy, expel sputum, disperse blood and heal swelling | to activate the blood, regulate menstruation, clear up heat and cool the blood |
| INDICATIONS | hemorrhoids with discharge of blood, vomiting blood, coughing up blood, blood in urine and vaginal bleeding and discharge | sore throat with swelling, cough and carbuncles | irregular menstruation, suppression of menstruation, vaginal bleeding, abdominal obstructions and insomnia |
| NOTES | | Experiments indicate that this herb is effective as an expectorant and can inhibit influenza. This herb is slightly toxic. | Experiments indicate that this herb can produce seven effects. It can: 1 expand coronary arteries and prevent angina pectoris, 2 activate the blood and bring down blood pressure, 3 protect the liver, 4 soften and shrink the liver and the spleen, 5 increase red blood cells, 6 increase white blood cells and 7 sedate and inhibit. |

# 垂盆草 槐花 　密蒙花 桔梗

| Chuipencao | Huaihua | Mimenghua | Jiegeng |
|---|---|---|---|
| 1245 | 5078 | 4700 | 3642 |
| weeping-plate plant | Japanese pagoda tree | butterfly bush | kikio root |
| Crassulaceae | Leguminosae | Loganiaceae | Campanulaceae |
| stone nail (so named because it grows on cliffs with its leaves all over stones and is shaped like a nail) | Japanese pagoda flower | dense-covered flower | Solid and straight root (so named because the roots are straight and solid) |
| Sedum sarmentosum Bge | Sophora japonica L | Buddleja officinalis Maxim | Platycodon grandiflorum (Jacq.) A.DC |
| Herba Sedi Sarmentosi | Flos Sophorae | Flos Buddlejae | Radix Platycodi |
| whole plant | buds | dried flowers or buds | root |
| 50g | 6 to 15g | 3 to 10g | 6g |
| light, sweet and slightly sour | bitter | sweet | pungent and bitter |
| cool | slightly cold | cool | slightly warm |
| 19, herbs for ulcers and tumors | 12, herbs to regulate blood | 2, herbs to reduce excessive heat inside the body | 10, herbs to suppress cough and reduce sputum |
| undetermined | liver and large intestine | liver | lungs |
| to clear up heat, counteract toxic effects, heal swelling and benefit water | to sedate heat, cool the blood and arrest bleeding | to expel wind, cool blood, lubricate liver and sharpen vision | to expand lung energy, expel sputum, suppress cough and drain off pus |
| burns, carbuncles, snakebite and cancerous swelling, particularly in liver cancer | hemorrhoids, discharge of blood from the anus, discharge of urine containing blood, nosebleeds and dysentery | pinkeye with swelling, watering of eyes and amaurosis (optic atrophy) | sore throat, hoarseness, cough and copious sputum, abscess of the lungs, suppurative pneumonia and pulmonary gangrene |
| | Experiments indicate that this herb can produce four effects:<br>1　It can cool the blood and bring down blood pressure,<br>2　it can reinforce the resistance of capillary vessels,<br>3　it is an effective coagulant and<br>4　it is generally effective in reducing blood pressure. | Mimenghua is effective for nourishing the blood and sharpening the vision. It is good for those with liver-kidney yin deficiency and heat. | Experiments indicate that this herb is effective as an expectorant, as it contains saponin |

# 旋復花　千日紅　紫菀

| Chinese | Xuanfuhua | Qianrihong | Ziwan |
|---|---|---|---|
| RE | 4608 | 0439 | 4866 |
| COMMON NAME | innula flower | flower of Globeamaranth | purple aster |
| FAMILY | Compositae | Amaranthaceae | Compositae |
| CHINESE NAME | innula flower | thousand-day red flower | purple-soft roots (so named because the roots are purple and soft) |
| SCIENTIFIC NAME | Inula japonica Thunb | Gomphrena globosa L | Aster tataricus L.f. |
| PHARMACEUTICAL NAME | Flos Inulae | Flos Gomphrenae | Radix Asteris |
| PART USED | flower head | inflorescence or whole plant | root |
| DOSAGE | 3 to 10g | 3 to 10g (flower), 15 to 30g (whole plant) | 8g |
| FLAVOR | salty | sweet | bitter |
| ENERGY | warm | neutral | warm |
| CLASS | 10, herbs to suppress cough and reduce sputum | 12, herbs to regulate blood | 10, herbs to suppress cough and reduce sputum |
| MERIDIANS | lungs and large intestine | undetermined | lungs |
| ACTIONS | to expel sputum, suppress cough, bring down energy and calm down asthma | to clear liver, disperse congestion, relieve cough, treat asthma and cool blood | to warm up the lungs, expel sputum, suppress cough and relieve asthma |
| INDICATIONS | cough, asthma and hiccups | headache, cough, dysentery, whooping cough, scrofula, boils, eye pain due to hot liver, headache from hypertension and chronic tracheitis | cough due to wind cold, asthma and vomiting of blood in cough due to deficiency fatigue |
| NOTES | Xuanfuhua is slightly toxic. It is good for internal obstruction of thick sputum with uprising energy | | Experiments indicate that this herb is effective as an expectorant. It contains flavonone, which can act on the cardiovascular system, on the one hand and arrest bleeding, suppress cough and expel sputum, on the other. |

**F**or each of the treatment

formulas listed in this

book, information is included here

in the following two categories: the

formula name and the ingredients.

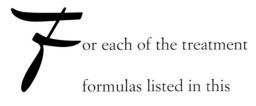

# Herbal Formulas

### Formula

This is the Romanization of the name of the formula; it is also the Chinese pronunciation of the name. The number within the brackets after the name of the formula is the reference number of the formula as shown in *An Encyclopedic Dictionary of Chinese Herbal Formulas*, which I compiled and which contains more than 4,000 formulas. Take the first formula as an example. Ai-Fu-Nuan-Gong-Wan is the Romanization of the name of this formula and 0196i is its reference number. Following the reference number are the Chinese characters for the formula.

### Ingredients

Each ingredient is written in the Romanization of the name of that herb, followed by its pharmaceutical name and standard dosage and then by its dosage used in the particular formula. Take the first formula as an example. Ai-ye is the name of an herb used in this formula, its pharmaceutical name is Folium Artemisiae Argyi, 4-11 g is the standard daily dosage when this herb is decocted by itself for consumption and 90 g is the amount of this herb used in this particular formula.

### Instructions

For some of the formulas, special instructions are presented. If no special instructions are presented, the formula is to be used by decoction for single-day consumption. It is always wise to ask your herbalist for instructions to meet your needs.

Since each herbal formula is accompanied by its Chinese characters, any knowledgeable Chinese herbalist should be able to make the formula for you. If there are no Chinese herb shops in your area, write to Natural Chinese Herbs Information Resources, Box 236, 1857 West 4th Avenue, Vancouver, BC V6J 1M4, Canada.

*Formula*

## AI-FU-NUAN-GONG-WAN
(01961)

*Ingredients*
Ai-Ye-(Folium Artemisiae Argi, 4 to 11g), 90g • Bai-shao-yao (Radix Paeoniae Alba, 5 to 11g), 90g • Chuan-xiong (Rhizoma Ligustici Chuanxiong, 2 to 6g), 90g • Dang-gui (Radix Angelicae Sinensis, 5 to 11g), 90g • Huang-qi (Radix Astragali Seu Hedysari, 5-40g), 90g • Rou-gui (Cortex Cinnamomi, 1 to 5g), 15g • Shui-di-huang (Radix Rehmanniae Praeparatae, 11 to 18g), 30g • Wu-zhu-yu (Fructus Euodiae, 2 to 7g), 90g • Xiang-fu (Rhizoma Cyperi, 5 to 11g), 180g • Xu-Duan (Radix Dipsaci, 5 to 11g), 45g

*Instructions*
Grind into powder to make tablets and take 9g of tablets twice daily.

*Formula*

## AN-GONG-NIU-HUANG WAN
(0286)

*Ingredients*
Bing-pian (Borneol, 0.2 to 0.3g), 8g • Huang-lian (Rhizoma Coptidis, 2 to 12g), 30g • Huang-qin (Radix Scutellariae, 4 to 15g), 30g • Niu-huang (Calculus Bovis, 0.2 to 0.5g), 30g • She-xiang (Moschus, 0.01 to 0.03g), 8.30g • Xi-jiao (Cornu Rhinoceri, 1 to 2g), 30g • Xiong-huang (Realgar, 0.3 to 1.5g), 30g • Yu-jin (Radix Curcumae, 4 to 11g), 30g • Zhen-Zhu (Margarita, 0.3 to 0.7g), 15g • Zhi-zi (Fructus gardeniae, 7 to 16g), 30g • Zhu-sha (Cinnabaris, 0.3 to 1g), 30g

*Formula*

## AN-SHEN-DING-ZHI-WAN
(0324)

*Ingredients*
Chang-pu (Rhizoma Calami, 4 to 7g), 3g • Fu-Ling (Poria, 7 to 14g), 12g • Fu-shen (Buyury, with pine root, 11 to 15g), 9g • Long-chi (Dens Draconis, 11 to 18g), 15g • Ren-shen (Radix Ginseng, 1 to 35g), 9g • Yuan-zhi (Radix Polygalae, 4 to 11g), 6g

*Instructions*
Grind into powder and take 2g of powder each time, twice daily.

*Formula*

## BA-ZHEN-TANG
(0182)

*Ingredients*
Bai-shao-yao (Radix Paeoniae Alba, 5 to 11g), 12g • Bai-zhu (Rhizoma Atractylodis Macrocephalae, 5 to 11g), 10g • Chuan-xiong (Rhizoma Ligustici Chuanxiong, 2 to 6g), 6g • Dang-gui (Radix Angelicae Sinensis, 5 to 11g), 12g • Dang-shen (Radix Codonopsis Pilosulae, 11 to 15g), 10g • Fu-ling (Poria, 7 to 14g), 12g • Gan-cao (Radix Glycyrrhizae, 2 to 11g), 3g • Shu-di-huang (Radix Rehmanniae Praeparatae, 11 to 18g), 15g

*Formula*

## BA-ZHEN-YI-MU-TANG
(0872)

*Ingredients*
(Use equal quantities of all ingredients.) Bai-shao-yao (Radix Paeoniae Alba, 5 to 11g)• Bai-zhu (Rhizoma Atractylodis Macrocephalae, 5 to 11g) • Chuan-xiong (Rhizoma Ligustici Chuanxiong 2 to 6) • Dang-gui (Radix Angelicae Sinensis, 5 to 11g) • Dang Shen (Radix Codonopsis Pilosulae, 11 to 15g) • Fu-ling (Poria, 7 to 14g) • Gan-cao (Radix Glycyrrhizae, 2 to 11g) • Shu-di-huang (Radix Rehmanniae Praeparatae, 11 to 18g) • Yi-mu-cao (Herba Leonuri, 11 to 36g)

*Formula*

## BA-ZHENG-SAN
(0349)

*Ingredients*
(Use equal quantities of all ingredients.) Bian-xu (Herba Polygoni Avicularis, 5 to 11g) • Che-qian-zi (Semen Plantaginis, 4 to 11g) • Da-huang (Radix Et Rhizoma Rhei, 4 to 15g) • Gan-cao-shao (Fine Root Glycyrrhizae, 2 to 5g) • Hua-shi (Talcum, 11 to 15g) • Mu-tong (Caulis Aristolochiae, 4 to 8g) • Qu-mai (Herba Dianthi, 5 to 11g) • Zhi-zi (Fructus Garderniae, 7 to 16g)

*Instructions*
Grind into powder and take 6 to 8g of powder each time.

*Formula*

## BAI-HE-GU-JIN-TANG
(0360)

*Ingredients*
Bai-he (Bulbus Lilii, 5 to 11g), 15g •Chi-shao-yao (Radix Paeoniae Rubra, 5 to 11g), 9g •

Chuan-bei-mu (Bulbus Fritillariae Cirrhosae, 4 to 14g), 6g •Dang-gui (Radix Angelicae Sinensis, 5 to 11g), 9g • Gan-cao (Radix Glycyrrhizae, 2 to 11g), 3g • Jie-geng (Radix Platycodi, 2 to 5g), 6g • Mai-men-dong (Radix Ophiopogonis, 5 to 11g), 6g • Sheng-di (Radix Rehamanniae, 14 to 35g), 12g • Shu-di-huang (Radix Rehmanniae Praeparatae, 11 to 18g), 9g • Xuan-shen (Radix Scrophulariae, 7 to 35g), 9g

*Formula*

## BAI-HU-JIA-GUI-ZHI-TANG
(0065A)

*Ingredients*

Gan-cao (Radix Glycyrrhizae, 2 to 11g), 6g • Gui-zhi (Ramulus Cinnamomi, 2 to 10g), 6g • Jing-mi (polished rice, flexible quantity), 9g • Shi-gao (Gypsum Fibrosum, 10 to 70g), 15-60g • Zhi-mu (Rhizoma Anemarrhenae, 4 to 15g), 12g

*Formula*

## BAN-XIA-BAI-ZHU-TIAN-MA-TANG
(0122)

*Ingredients*

Bai-zhu (Rhizoma Atracylodis Macrocephalae, 5 to 11g), 12g • Ban-xia, zhi-ban-xia (Rhizoma Pinelliae, 4 to 12g), 12g • Chen-pi (Pericarpium Papaveris, 4 to 11g), 10g • Fu-ling (Poria, 7 to 14g), 15g • Gan-cao (Radix Glycyrrhizae, 2 to 11g), 3g • Tian-ma (Rhizoma Gastrodiae, 4 to 11g), 10g

*Formula*

## BAN-XIA-HOU-PU-TANG
(0099)

*Ingredients*

Ban-xia (Rhizoma Pinelliae, 4 to 12g), 12g • Fu-ling (Poria, 7 to 14g), 12g • Hou-po (Cortex Magnoliae Officinalis, 4 to 11g), 12g • Sheng-jiang (Rhizoma Zingiberis Recens, 4 to 10g), 9g • Zi-su-ye (Folium Perillae, 5 to 10g), 12g

*Formula*

## BAN-XIA-XIE-XIN-TANG
(0105)

*Ingredients*

Ban-xia (Rhizoma Pinelliae, 4 to 12g), 15g • Da-zao (Fructus Ziziphi Jujubae, 7 to 18g), 9g • Gan-cao, zhi-gan-cao (Radix Glycyrrhizae, 2 to 11g), 3g • Gan-jiang (Rhizoma Zingiberis, 3 to 7g), 9g • Huang-lian (Rhizoma Coptidis, 2 to 12g), 6g • Huang-qin (Radix Scutellariae, 4 to 15g), 9g • Ren-shen (Radix Ginseng, 1 to 35g), 9g

*Formula*

## BAO-HE-WAN
(0074)

*Ingredients*

Ban-xia (Rhizoma Pinelliae, 4 to 12g), 10g • Chen-pi (Pericarpium Papaveris, 4 to 11g), 10g • Fu-ling (Poria, 7 to 14g), 10g • Lai-fu-zi (Semen Raphani, 5 to 11g), 10g • Lian qiao (Fructus Forsythiae, 5 to 11g), 10g • Shan-zha (Fructus Crataegi, 7 to 14g), 10g • Shen-qu (Massa Medicata Fermentata, 7 to 15g), 12g

*Formula*

## BEI-XIE-FEN-QING-YIN
(0358)

*Ingredients*

Bai-zhu (Rhizoma Atractylodis Macrocephalae, 5 to 11g), 6g • Bei-xie (Rhizoma Dioscoreae Bishie, 11 to 18g), 24g • Che-qian-Zi (Semen Plantaginis, 4 to 11g), 12g • Dan-shen (Radix Salviae Miltiorrhizae, 5 to 10g), 6g • Fu-ling (Poria, 7 to 14g), 6g • Huang-bai (Cortex Phellodendri, 4 to 15g), 6g • Lian-zi-xin (Plumula Nelumbinis, 2 to 4g), 6g • Shi-chang-pu (Rhizoma Acori Graminei, 2 to 5g), 3g

*Formula*

## BU-FEI-TANG
(0043)

*Ingredients*

Huang-qi (Radix Astragali Seu Hedysari, 5 to 40g), 24g • Ren-shen (Radix Ginseng, 1 to 35g), 9g • Sang-bai-pi (Cortex Mori Radicis, 5 to 11g), 12g • Shu-di-huang (Radix Rehmanniae Praepar-atae, 11 to 18g), 24g • Wu-wei-zi (Fructus Schisandrae, 2 to 4g), 6g • Zi-wan (Radix Asteris, 5 to 11g), 9g

*Formula*

## BU-HUAN-JIN-ZHENG-QI-SAN
(0117D)

*Ingredients*
Ban-xia (Rhizoma Pinelliae, 4 to 12g), 10g • Cang-zhu (Rhizoma Atractylodis Macrocephalae, 4 to 11g), 10g • Chen-pi (Pericarpium Papaveris, 4 to 11g), 10g • Gan-cao (Radix Glycyrrhizae, 2 to 11g), 3g • Hou-po (Cortex Magnoliae Officinalis, 4 to 11g), 10g • Huo-xiang (Herba Agastachis, 5 to 11g), 10g

*Formula*

## BU-XIN-DAN
(0297)

*Ingredients*
Bai-zi-ren (Semen Biotae, 4 to 11g), 30g • Dan-shen (Radix Salviae Miltiorrhizae, 5 to 10g), 15g • Dang-gui (Radix Angelicae Sinensis, 5 to 11g), 21g • Fu-ling (Poria, 7 to 14g), 12g • Jie-geng (Radix Platycodi, 2 to 5g), 9g • Mai-men-Dong (Radix Ophiopogonis, 5 to 11g), 9g • Ren-shen (Radix Ginseng, 1 to 35g), 9g • Sheng-di (Radix Rehmanniae, 14 to 35g), 30g • Suan-zao-Ren (Semen Ziziphi Spinosae, 7 to 18g), 30g • Tian-dong (Radix Asparagi, 7 to 14g), 9g • Wu-wei-zi (Fructus Schisandrae, 2 to 4g) 9g • Xuan-shen (Radix Scrophulariae, 7 to 35g), 12g • Yuan-zhi (Radix Polygalae, 4 to 11g), 9g

*Instructions*
Grind into powder to make tablets and take 9 to 15g of tablets each time.

*Formula*

## BU-YANG-HUAN-WU-TANG
(0212)

*Ingredients*
Chi-shao-yao (Radix Paeoniae Rubra, 5 to 11g), 6g • Chuan-xiong (Rhizoma Ligustici Chuanxiong, 2 to 6g), 3g • Dang-gui (Radix Angelicae Sinensis, 5 to 11g), 6g • Di-long (Lumbricus, 5 to 11g), 3g • Hong-hua (Flos Carthami, 4 to 7g), 3g • Huang-qi (Radix Astragali Seu Hedysari, 5 to 40g), 120g • Tao-ren (Semen Persicae, 5 to 11g), 3g

*Formula*

## BU-ZHONG-YI-QI-TANG
(0084)

*Ingredients*
Bai-zhu (Rhizoma Atractylodis Macrocephalae, 5 to 11g), 10g • Chai-hu (Radix Bupleuri, 4 to 16g), 6g • Chen-pi (Pericarpium Papaveris, 4 to 11g), 9g • Dang-gui (Radix Angelicae Sinensis, 5 to 11g), 10g • Dang-shen (Radix Codonopsis Pilosulae, 11 to 15g), 15g • Gan-cao (Radix Glycyrrhizae, 2 to 11g), 6g • Huang-qi (Radix Astragali Seu Hedysari, 5 to 40g), 24g • Sheng-ma (Thizoma Cimicifugae, 3 to 10g), 6g

*Formula*

## CANG-ER-ZI-SAN
(0563)

*Ingredients*
Bai-zhi (Radix Angelicae Dahuricae, 4 to 10g), 3g • Bo-he (Herba Menthae, 3 to 10g), 6g • Cang-er-zi (Fructus Xanthii, 4 to 11g), 9g • Xin-yi (Flos Magnoliae, 4 to 10g), 6g

*Formula*

## CHAI-HU-SHU-GAN-SAN
(0230A)

*Ingredients*
Bai-shao-yao (Radix Paeoniae Alba, 5 to 11g), 24g • Chai-hu (Radix Bupleuri, 4 to 16g), 9g • Chuan-xiong (Rhizoma Ligustici Chuanxiong, 2 to 6g), 6g • Gan-cao (Radix Glycyrrhizae, 2 to 11g), 6g • Gan-jiang (Rhizoma Zingiberis, 3 to 7g),g • Xiang-fu (Rhizoma Cyperi, 5 to 11g), 12g • Zhi-qiao (Fructus Auranth, 4 to 11g), 9g • Zhi-zi (Fructus Gardeniae, 7 to 16g),g

*Formula*

## CHEN-SHI-YI-SHUAN-DAI-DAN
(3358)

*Ingredients*
Bai-shao-yao (Radix Paeoniae Alba, 5 to 11g), 8g • Ban-xia (Rhizoma Pinelliae, 4 to 12g), 6g • Chai-hu (Radix Bupleuri, 4 to 16g), 7g • Chen-pi (Pericarpium Citri Reticulatae, 4 to 11g), 6g • Dan-shen (Radix Salviae Miltiorrhizae, 5 to 10g), 6g • Dang-gui (Radix Angelicae Sinensis, 5 to 11g), 7g • Dang-shen (Radix Codonopsis Pilosulae, 11 to 15g), 6g • Fu-shen (Buyury with pine root, 11 to 15g), 6g • Gan-cao (Radix Glycyrrhizae, 2 to 11g), 5g • Mai-men-Dong (Radix Ophiopogonis, 5 to 11g), 6g • Shen-qu (Massa Medicata Fermentata, 7 to 15g), 8g • Shi-chang-pu (Rhizoma Acori Graminei, 2 to 5g), 5g • Suan-

zao-ren (Semen Ziziphi Spinosae, 7 to 18g), 8g • Tao-ren (Semen Persicae, 5 to 11g), 6g • Tian hua-fen (Radix Trichosanithis, 10 to 14g), 10g • Xiang-fu (Rhizoma Cyperi, 5 to 11g), 6g

## Formula

### CHI XIAO-DOU-DANG-GUI-SAN
(0571)

### Ingredients
Chi-xioa-dou (Semen Phaseoli, 11 to 18g) 30g • Dang-gui (Radix Angelicae Sinensis 5 to 11g), 15g

## Formula

### CHUAN-XIONG-CHA-TIAO-SAN
(0011)

### Ingredients:
Bai-zhi (Radix Angelicae Dahuricae, 4 to 10g), 6g • Bo-he (Herba Menthae, 3 to 10g), 3g • Chuan-xiong (Rhizoma Ligustici Chuanxiong, 2 to 6g), 12g • Fang-feng (Radix Ledebouriellae, 5 to 10g), 6g • Gan-cao (Radix Glycyrrhizae, 2 to 11g), 6g • Jing-jie (Herba Schizonepetae, 5 to 10g), 12g • Qiang-huo (Rhizoma Seu Radix Notopterygii Notopterygii, 4 to 10g), 6g • Xi-xin (Herba Asari, 1 to 4g), 3g

## Formula

### DA-BU-YIN-WAN
(0273)

### Ingredients
Gui-ban (Plastrum Testudinis, 11 to 30g), 180g • Huang-bai (Cortex Phellodendri, 4 to 15g), 120g • Shu-di-huang (Radix Rehmanniae Praeparatae, 11 to 18g), 180g • Zhi-mu (Rhizoma Anemarrhenae, 4 to 15g), 120g

### Instructions
Grind into powder and make tablets. Take six to nine tablets twice daily; if decoction is done, reduce dosages.

## Formula

### DA-BU-YUAN-JIAN
(0399)

### Ingredients
Dang-gui (Radix Angelicae Sinensis, 5 to 11g), 9g • Du-zhong (Cortex Eucommiae 7 to 11g), 9g • Gan-cao (Radix Glycyrrhizae, 2 to 11g), 6g • Gou-qi-zi (Fructus Lych, 5 to 11g), 9g • Ren-shen (Radix Ginseng, 1 to 35g), 9g • Shan-yao (Rhizoma Dioscoreae, 10 to 20g), 9g • Shan-zhu-yu (Fructus Corni, 5 to 11g), 9g • Shu-di-huang (Radix Rehmanniae Praeparatae, 11 to 18g), 15g

## Formula

### DA-CHAI-HU-TANG
(0256)

### Ingredients
Bai-shao-Yao (Radix Paeoniae Alba, 5 to 11g), 30g • Ban-xia (Rhizoma Pinelliae, 4 to 12g), 15g • Chai-hu (Radix Bupleuri, 4 to 16g), 21g • Da-huang (Radix Et Rhizoma Rhei, 4 to 15g), 15g • Da-zao (Fructus Ziziphi Jujubae, 7 to 18g), four dates • Huang-qin (Radix Scutellariae, 4 to 15g), 15g • Sheng-jiang (Rhizoma Zingiberis Recens, 4 to 10g), 9g • Zhi-shi (Fructus Aurantii Immaturus, 4 to 7g), 6g

## Formula

### DA-CHENG-QI-TANG
(0146)

### Ingredients
Da-huang (Radix Et Rhizoma Rhei, 4 to 15g), 12g • Hou-po (Cortex Magnoliae Officinalis, 4 to 11g), 15g • Pu-xiao (Mirabilitum Depuratum, 5 to 11g), 12g • Zhi-shi (Fructus Aurantii Immaturus, 4 to 7g), 10g

## Formula

### DA-DING-FENG-ZHU
(0247)

### Ingredients
Bai-shao-yao (Radix Paeoniae Alba, 5 to 11g), 18g • Bie-jia (Carapax Trionycis, 11 to 18g), 12g • E-jiao (Colla Corii Asini, 5 to 11g), 9g • Gan-cao (Radix Glycyrrhizae, 2 to 11g), 12g • Gui-ban (Plastrum Testudinis, 11 to 30g), 12g • Huo-ma-Ren (Fructus Cannabis, 11 to 17g), 6g • Ji-zi-huang (Chicken egg yolk, flexibleg), two eggs • Mai-men-dong (Radix Ophiopogonis, 5 to 11g), 18g • Mu-li (Concha Ostrae, 11 to 35g), 12g • Sheng-di (Radix Rehmanniae, 14 to 35g), 18g • Wu-wei-zi (Fructus Schisandrae, 2 to 4g), 6g

nalis, 4 to 11g), 9g • Huang-qin (Radix Scutellariae, 4 to 15g), 12g • Zhi-mu (Rhizoma Anemarrhenae, 4 to 15g), 12g

*Formula*

## DA-QIN-JIAO-TANG
(0279)

*Ingredients*
Bai-shao-yao (Radix Paeoniae Alba, 5 to 11g), 18g • Bai-zhi (Radix Angelicae Dahuricae, 4 to 10g), 9g • Bai-zhu (Rhizoma Atractylodis Macrocephalae, 5 to 11g), 12g • Chuan-xiong (Rhizoma Ligustici Chuanxiong, 2 to 6), 9g • Dang-gui (Radix Angelicae Sinensis, 5 to 11g), 9g • Du-huo (Radix Angelicae Pubescentis, 2 to 5g), 12g • Fang-feng (Radix Ledebouriellae, 5 to 10g), 9g • Fu-ling (Poria, 7 to 14g), 12g • Gan-cao (Radix Glycyrrhizae, 2 to 11g), 6g •Huang-qin (Radix Scutellariae, 4 to 15g), 9g • Qiang-Huo (Rhizoma Seu Radix Notopterygii Notopterygh, 4 to 10g), 9g •Qin-jiao (Radix Gentianae Macrophyllae, 4 to 11g), 15g • Sheng-di (Radix Rehmanniae, 14 to 35g), 12g • Shi-gao (Gypsum Fibrosum, 10 to 70g), 18g • Shu-di-huang (Radix Rehmannice Praeparatae, 11 to 18g), 12g • Xi-xin (Herba Asari, 1 to 4g), 6g

*Formula*

## DA-YUAN-YIN
(0257)

*Ingredients*
Bai-shao-Yao (Radix Paeoniae Alba, 5 to 11g), 9g • Bing-lang (Semen Areca, 4 to 11g), 12g • Cao-guo (Fructus Tsaoko, 2 to 5g), 3g • Gan-cao (Radix Glycyrrhizae, 2 to 11g), 3g • Houpo (Cortex Magnoliae Offici-

*Formula*

## DAI-DI-DANG-WAN
(0982)

*Ingredients*
Chuan-shan-jia (Squama Manitis, 5 to 11g), 30g • Da-huang (Radix Et Rhizoma Rhei, 4 to 15g), 120g • Dang-gui (Radix Angelicae Sinensis, 5 to 11g), 30g • Mang-xiao (Natrii Sulfas, 4 to 11g), 30g • Rou-gui (Cortex Cinnamomi, 1 to 5g), 15g • Sheng-di (Radix Rehmanniae, 14 to 35g), 30g • Tao-ren (Semen Persicae, 5 to 11g), 30g

*Instructions*
Grind into powder to make tablets and take 9g of tablets twice daily.

*Formula*

## DAN-TIAN-JIANG-ZHI-WAN
(3359)

*Ingredients*
Chuan-xiong (Rhizoma Ligustici Chuanxiong, 2 to 6g), 6g • Dan-shen (Radix Salviae Miltiorrhizae, 5 to 10g), 10g • Dang-gui (Radix Angelicae Sinensis, 5 to 11g), 11g • He-shou-Wu (Radix Polygoni Multiflori, 11 to 15g), 15g • Huang-jing (Rhizoma Polygonati, 11 to 15g), 15g • Ren-shen (Radix Ginseng, 1 to 35g), 35g • San-qi (Radix Notoginseng, 2 to 10g), 10g • Ze-xie (Rhizoma Alismatis, 7 to 14g), 14g

*Formula*

## DAN-ZHI-XIAO-YAO-SAN
(0229A)

*Ingredients*
Bai-shao-yao (Radix Paeoniae Alba, 5 to 11g), 30g • Bai-zhu (Rhizoma Atractylodis Macrocephalae, 5 to 11g), 9g • Chai-hu (Radix Bupleuri, 4 to 16g), 9g • Dang-gui (Radix Angelicae Sinensis, 5 to 11g), 9g • Fu-ling (Poria, 7 to 14g), 15g • Gan-cao (Radix Glycyrrhizae, 2 to 11g), 6g • Mu-dan-pi (Cortex Moutan Radicis, 5 to 11g),g • Zhi-zi (Fructus Gardeniae, 7 to 16g), 8g

*Formula*

## DANG-GUI-JIAN-ZHONG-TANG
(0064C)

*Ingredients*
Chi-shao-yao (Radix Paeoniae Rubra, 5 to 11g), 30g • Da-zao (Fructus Ziziphi Jujubae, 7 to 18g), 10g • Dang-gui (Radix Angelicae Sinensis, 5 to 11g), 20g • Gan-cao (Radix Glycyrrhizae, 2 to 11g), 10g • Gui-zhi (Ramulus Cinnamomi, 2 to 10g), 15g • Sheng-jiang (Rhizoma Zingiberis Recens, 4 to 10g), 15g • Yi-tang (Saccharum Granorum, 30 to 60g), 60g

*Formula*

## DANG-GUI-LONG-HUI-WAN
(0189)

*Ingredients*

Da-huang (Radix Et Rhizorna Rhei, 4 to 15g), 15g • Dang-gui (Radix Angelicae Sinensis, 5 to 11g), 30g • Huang-bai (Cortex Phellodendri, 4 to 15g), 30g • Huang-lian (Rhizoma Coptidis, 2 to 12g), 30g • Huang-qin (Radix Scutellariae, 4 to 15g), 30g • Long-dan (Radix Gentianae, 7 to 10g), 30g • Lu-hui (Aloe, 2 to 5g), 15g • Mu-xiang (Radix Aucklandiae/Radix Saussureae, 2 to 6g), 6g • Qing-dai (Indigo Naturalis, 2 to 4g), 15g • She-xiang (Moschus, 0.01 to 0.03g), 1.5g • Zhi-zi (Fructus Gardeniae, 7 to 16g), 30g

*Instructions*

Grind into powder and take 5g of powder each time, twice daily.

*Formula*

### DAO-CHI-CHENG-QI-TANG
(1049)

*Ingredients*

(Use equal quantities of all ingredients.) Chi-shao-yao (Radix Paroniae Rubra, 5 to 11g) • Da-huang (Radix Et Rhizoma Rhei, 4 to 15g) • Huang-bai (Cortex Phellodendri, 4 to 15g) • Huang-lian (Rhizoma Coptidis, 2 to 12g) • Mang-xiao (Natrii Sulfas/Mirabilitum Depuratum, 4 to 11g) • Sheng-di (Radix Rehmanniae, 14 to 35g)

*Instructions*

Grind into powder and take 6g of powder each time, twice daily.

*Formula*

### DAO CHI SAN
(0357)

*Ingredients*

Gan-cao shao (Fine Root Glycyrrhizae, 2 to 5g), 6g • Mutong (Caulis Aristolochiae, 4 to 8g), 12g • Sheng-di (Radix Rehmanniae, 14 to 35g), 24g • Zhu-ye (Foliuim Bambusae, 4 to 20g), 6g

*Instructions*

Decoct the herbs by adding Deng-Xin-Cao (Medulla Junci, 2 to 3g), 6g

*Formula*

### DAO-TAN-TANG
(0123)

*Ingredients*

Ban-xia (Rhizoma Pinelliae, 4 to 12g), 15g • Chen-pi Pericarpium Papaveris, 4 to 11g), 10g • Fu-ling (Poria, 7 to 14g), 12g • Gan-cao (Radix Glycyrrhizae, 2 to 11g), 3g • Sheng-jiang (Rhizoma Zingiberis Recens, 4 to 10g), 10g • Tian-nan-xing (Rhizoma Arisaematis, 2.5 to 5g), 12g • Zhi-qiao (Fructus Aurantii, 4 to 11g), 10g

*Formula*

### DE-SHENG-DAN
(1841)

*Ingredients*

Bai-shao-yao (Radix Paeoniae Alba, 5 to 11g), 80g • Chai-hu (Radix Bupleuri, 4 to 16g), 30g • Dang-gui (Radix Angelicae Sinesis, 5 to 11g), 80g • Mu-xiang (Radix Aucklandiae, 6g), 30g • Qiang-huo (Rhizoma Seu Radix Notopterygii, 4 to 10g), 30g • Yi-mu-cao (Herba Leonuri, 11 to 36g), 320g

*Instructions*

Grind into powder to make tablets with honey and take 10g of tablets twice daily.

*Formula*

### DI-HUANG-YIN-ZI
(0532)

*Ingredients*

Gan-cao (Radix Glycrrhizae, 2 to 11g), 5g • Huang-qi (Radix Astragati seu Hedysari, 5 to 40g), 20g • Mai-men-dong (Radix Ophiopogonis, 5 to 11g), 5g • Pi-pa-ye (Folium Eriobotryae, 5 to 11g), 5g • Ren-shen (Radix Ginseng, 1 to 35g), 20g • Sheng-di (Radix Rehmanniae, 14 to 35g), 25g • Shi-hu (Herba Dendrobii, 7 to 14g), 10g • Shu-di-huang (Radix Rehmanniae Praeparatae, 11 to 18g), 15g • Tian-dong (Radix Asparagi, 7 to 14g), 10g • Ze-xie (Rhizoma Alismatis, 7 to 14g), 10g • Zhi-qiao (Fructus Aurantii, 4 to 11g), 5g

*Formula*

### DI-TAN-TANG
(0293)

*Ingredients*

Ban xia (Rhizoma Pinelliae, 4 to 12g), 15g • Chang-pu (Rhizoma Calami, 4 to 7g), 6g • Chen-pi (Pericarpium Papaveris, 4 to 11g), 9g • Dan-nan-xing (Arisaema Cum Bile, 4 to 8g), 12g • Fu-ling (Poria, 7 to 14g),

12g • Gan-cao (Radix Gly-cyrrhizae, 2 to 11g), 3g • Ren-shen (Radix Ginseng, 1 to 35g), 9g • Zhi-shi (Fructus Aurantii Immaturus, 4 to 7g), 9g • Zhu-ru (Caulis Bambusae in Taeniam, 5 to 11g), 15g

## Formula
### DING-XIAN-WAN
(0592)

*Ingredients*
Ban-xia (Rhizoma Pinelliae, 4 to 12g), 30g • Chang-pu (Rhizoma Calami, 4 to 7g), 15g • Chen-pi (Pericarpium Citri Reticulatae Viride, 4 to 11g), 21g • Chuan-bei-mu (Bulbus Fritillariae Thunbergii Cirrhosae, 4 to 14g), 21g • Dan-nan-xing (Arisaema Cum Bile, 4 to 8g), 15g • Dan-shen (Radix Salviae Miltiorrhizae, 5 to 10g), 60g • Fu-ling (Poria, 7 to 14g), 30g • Fu-shen (Buyury with pine root, 11 to 15g), 30g • Gan-cao (Radix Glycyrrhizae, 2 to 11g), 21g • Hu-po (Suc-cinum, 1 to 2g), 15g • Jiang-can (Bombyx Batryticatus, 5 to 11g), 15g • Mai-men-dong (Radix Ophiopogonis, 5 to 11g), 60g • Quan-xie (Scorpio, 2 to 5g) 15g • Sheng-jiang (Rhizoma Zin-giberis Recens, 4 to 10g), 10g • Tian-ma (Rhizoma Gastrodiae, 4 to 11g), 30g •Yuan-zhi (Radix Polygalae, 4 to 11g), 21 • Zhu-li (Bamboo Liquid, 30 to 60g), 10g • Zhu-sha (Cinnabaris, 0.3 to 1g), 15g

*Instructions*
Grind into powder and take 9g of powder twice daily.

## Formula
### DING-XIANG-SHI-DI-TAN
(0092)

*Ingredients*
Ding-xiang (Flos Caryophylli, 1 to 4g), 10g • Ren-shen (Radix Ginseng, 1 to 35g), 10g • Sheng-jiang (Rhizoma Zingiberis Recens, 4 to 10g), 12g • Shi-di (Calyx Kaki, 5 to 11g), 10g

## Formula
### DING-ZHI-WAN
(0306)

*Ingredients*
Fu-ling (Poria, 7 to 14g), 30g • Ren-shen (Radix Ginseng, 1 to 35g), 30g • Shi-chang-pu (Rhizoma Acori Graminei, 2 to 5g), 60g • Yuan-zhi (Radix Poly-galae, 4 to 11g), 60g

*Instructions*
Grind into powder and take 6g of powder each time; you may also decoct.

## Formula
### DU-HUO-JI-SHENG-TANG
(0278)

*Ingredients*
Chi-shao-yao (Radix Paeoniae Rubra, 5 to 11g), 30g • Chuan-xiong (Rhizoma Ligustici Chuanxiong, 2 to 6g), 9g • Dang-gui (Radix Angelicae Sinensis, 5 to 11g), 9g • Du-huo (Radix Angelicae Pubescentis, 2 to 5g), 15g • Du-zhong (Cortex Eucommiae, 7 to 11g), 15g • Fang-feng (Radix Ledebouriel-lae, 5 to 10g), 9g • Fu-ling

(Poria, 7 to 14g), 12g • Gan-cao (Radix Glycyrrhizae, 2 to 11g), 3g • Gan-di (Dried Radix Rehmanniae, 11 to 18g), 18g • Niu-xi (Radix Achyranthis Bidentatae, 5 to 11g), 15g • Qin-jiao (Radix Gentianae Macrophyllae, 4 to 11g), 10g • Ren-shen (Radix Ginseng, 1 to 35g), 12g • Rou-gui (Cortex Cinnamomi, 1 to 5g), 9g • Sang-ji-sheng (Ramulus Loran-thi, 11 to 18g), 24g • Xi-xin (Herba Asari, 1 to 4g), 6g

## Formula
### ER-CHEN-TANG
(0121)

*Ingredients*
Ban-xia (Rhizoma Pinelliae, 4 to 12g), 15g • Chen-pi (Pericarpi-um Papaveris, 4 to 11g), 10g • Fu-ling (Poria, 7 to 14g), 15g • Gan-cao (Radix Glycyrrhizae, 2 to 11g), 3g

## Formula
### ER-LONG-ZUO-ZI-WA
(0327D)

*Ingredients*
Ci-shi (Magnetitum, 11 to 35g), 90g • Fu-ling (Poria, 7 to 14g), 90g • Mu-dan-pi (Cortex Moutan Radicis, 5 to 11g), 90g • Shan-yao (Rhizoma Dioscoreae, 10 to 20g), 120g • Shan-zhu-yu (Fructus Corni, 5 to 11g), 120g • Shi-chang-pu (Rhizoma Acori Graminei, 2 to 5g), 90g • Shu-di-huang (Radix Rehmanniae Praeparatae, 11 to 18g), 240g • Wu-wei-zi (Fructus Schisandrae, 2 to 4g), 90g • Ze-Xie (Rhizoma Alismatis, 7 to 14g), 90g

*Instructions*

Grind into powder to make tablets and take three tablets or 9g two to three times daily.

*Formula*

## ER-MU-SAN
(0366)

*Ingredients*

(Use equal quantities of ingredients.) Zhe-bei-mu (Bulbus Fritillariae Thunbergii, 5 to 11g) • Zhi-mu (Rhizoma Anemarrhenae, 4 to 15g)

*Instructions*

Grind into powder and take 6g of powder twice daily.

*Formula*

## ER-YIN-JIAN
(0860)

*Ingredients*

Deng-xin-cao (Medulla Junci, 2 to 3g), 30g • Fu-ling (Poria, 7 to 14g), 12g • Gan-cao (Radix Glycyrrhizae, 2 to 11g), 10g • Huang-lian (Rhizoma Coptidis, 2 to 12g), 9g • Mai-men dong (Radix Ophiopogonis, 5 to 11g), 12g • Mu-tong (Caulis Aristolochiae, 4 to 8g), 9g • Sheng-di (Radix Rehmanniae, 14 to 35g), 12g • Suan-zao-ren (Semen Ziziphi Spinosae, 7 to 18g), 18g • Xuan-shen (Radix Scrophulariae, 7 to 35g), 10g • Zhu-ye (Folium Bambusae, 4 to 20g), 6g

*Formula*

## FANG-FENG-TANG
(0535)

*Ingredients*

Dang-gui (Radix Angelicae Sinensis, 5 to 11g), 6g • Fang-feng (Radix Ledebouriellae, 5 to 10g), 6g • Fu-ling (Poria, 7 to 14g), 6g • Gan-cao (Radix Glycyrrhizae, 2 to 11g), 3g • Ge-gen (Radix Puerariae, 4 to 20g), 9g • Gui-zhi (Ramulus Cinnamomi, 2 to 10g), 3g • Huang-qin (Radix Scutellariae, 4 to 15g), 9g • Qiang-huo (Rhizoma Seu Radix Notopterygii, 4 to 10g), 3g • Qin-Jiao (Radix Gentianae Macrophyllae, 4 to 11g), 9g • Xing-Ren (Semen Armeniacae Arnarae, 5 to 11g), 6g

*Formula*

## FANG-FENG-TONG-SHENG-SAN
(0536)

*Ingredients*

Bai-shao-yao (Radix Paeoniae Alba, 5 to 11g), 15g • Bai-zhu (Rhizoma Atractylodis Macrocephalae, 5 to 11g), 15g • Bo-he (Herba Menthae, 3 to 10g) 15g • Chuan-xiong (Rhizoma Ligustici Chuanxiong, 2 to 6g), 15g • Da-huang (Raidix Et Rhizoma Rhei, 4 to 15g), 15g • Dang-gui (Radix Angelicae Sinensis, 5 to 11g), 15g • Fang-feng (Radix Ledebouriellae, 5 to 10g), 15g • Gan-cao (Radix Glycyrrhizae, 2 to 11g), 60g • Hua-shi (Talcum, 11 to 15g), 90g • Huang-qin (Radix Scutellariae, 4 to 15g), 30g • Jie-geng (Radix Platycodi, 2 to 5g), 30g • Jing-Jie (Herba Schizonepetae, 5 to 10g), 15g • Lian-qiao (Fructus Forsythiae, 5 to 11g), 15g • Ma-huang (Herba Ephedrae, 5 to 10g), 15g • Mang-xiao (Natrii Sulfas, 4 to 11g), 15g • Shi-gao (Gypsum Fibrosum,

10 to 70g), 30g • Zhi-zi (Fructus Gardeniae, 7 to 16g), 15g

*Instructions*

Grind into powder and take 9g of powder twice daily.

*Formula*

## FANG-JI-HUANG-QI-TANG
(0131)

*Ingredients*

Bai-zhu (Rhizoma Atractylodis Macrocephalae, 5 to 11g), 10g • Fang-ji (Radix Stephaniae Tetrandrae, 5 to 11g), 15g • Gan-cao (Radix Glycyrrhizae, 2 to 11g), 6g • Huang-qi (Radix Astragali Seu Hedysari, 5 to 40g), 30g

*Formula*

## FENG-SUI-DAN
(0666)

*Ingredients*

Gan-Cao (Radix Glycyrrhizae, 2 to 11g), 21g • Huang-bai (Cortex Phellodendri, 4 to 15g), 90g • Sha-ren (Fructus Amomi, 2 to 7g), 30g

*Formula*

## FU-YUAN-HUO-XUE-TANG
(0209)

*Ingredients*

Chai-hu (Radix Bupleuri, 4 to 16g), 15g • Chuan-shan-jia (Squama Manitis, 5 to 11g), 9g • Da-huang (Radix Et Rhizoma Rhei, 4 to 15g), 30g • Dang-gui (Radix

Angelicae Sinensis, 5 to 11g), 9g • Gan-cao (Radix Glycyrrhizae, 2 to 11g), 9g • Hong-hua (Flos Carthami, 4 to 7g), 9g • Tao-ren (Semen Persicae, 5 to 11g), 50 kernels • Tian-hua-jen (Radix Trichosanthis, 10 to 14g), 12g

## Formula

### FU-ZI-LI-ZHONG-TANG
(0062A)

### Ingredients
(Use 90g of each ingredient)
Bai-zhu (Rhizoma Atractylodis Macrocephalae, 5 to 11g) • Fu-zi (Radix Aconiti Praeparata, 4 to 11g) • Gan-cao, zhi-gan-cao (Radix Glycyrrhizae, 2 to 11g) • Gan-jiang (Rhizoma Zingiberis, 3 to 7g) • Ren-shen (Radix Ginseng, 1 to 35g)

### Instructions
Take 10g in tablet form each time; reduce the quantity in decoction.

## Formula

### GAN-MAI-DA-ZAO-TANG
(0489)

### Ingredients
Da-zao (Fructus Ziziphi Jujubae, 7 to 18g), 10 red dates • Gan-cao (Radix Glycyrrhizae, 2 to 11g), 9g • Xiao-mai (wheat 20 to 50g), 30g

## Formula

### GE-GEN-QIN-LIAN-TANG
(1509)

### Ingredients
Gan-cao (Radix Glycyrrhizae, 2 to 11g), 60g • Ge-gen (Radix Puerariae, 4 to 20g), 240g • Huang-lian (Rhizoma Coptidis, 2 to 12g), 90g • Huang-qin (Radix Scutellariae, 4 to 15g), 90g

### Instructions
Grind into powder and take 6g of powder twice daily.

## Formula

### GE-XIA-ZHU-YU-TANG
(0119)

### Ingredients
Chi-shao-yao (Radix Paeoniae Rubra, 5 to 11g), 9g • Chuan-xiong (Rhizoma Ligustici Chuanxiong, 2 to 6g), 9g • Dang-gui (Radix Angelicae Sinensis, 5 to 11g), 9g • Gan-cao (Radix Glycyrrhizae, 2 to 11g), 3g • Hong-hua (Flos Carthami, 4 to 7g), 6g • Mu-dan-pi (Cortex Moutan Radicis, 5 to 11g), 6g • Tao-ren (Semen Persicae, 5 to 11g), 9g • Wu-ling-zhi (Faeces Trogopterorum, 5 to 11g), 9g • Wu-yao (Radix Linderae, 5 to 10g), 12g • Xiang-fu (Rhizoma Cyperi, 5 to 11g), 12g • Yan-hu-suo (Rhizoma Corydalis, 4 to 11g), 9g • Zhi-qiao (Fructus Aurautii, 4 to 11g), 9g

## Formula

### GUA-LOU-XIE-BAI-BAI-JIU-TANG
(0215A)

### Ingredients
Gua-lou (Fructus Trichosanthis, 11 to 15g), 24g • Xie-bai (Bulbus Allii Macrostemi, 5 to 11g), 30g

### Instructions
Add wine to decoct in water, or grind into powder and take 6g of powder with a half glass of wine.

## Formula

### GUA-LOU-XIE-BAI-BAN-XIA-TANG
(0215B)

### Ingredients
Ban-xia (Rhizoma Pinelliae, 4 to 12g), 15g • Gua-lou (Fructus Trichosanthis, 11 to 15g), 24g • Xie-bai (Bulbus Allii Macrostemi, 5 to 11g), 20g

### Instructions
Add wine to decoct in water, or grind into powder and take 6g of powder with a half glass of wine.

## Formula

### GUAN-XIN-ER-HAO-FANG
(0198A)

### Ingredients
Chi-shao-yao (Radix Paeoniae Rubra, 5 to 11g), 15g • Chuan-xiong (Rhizoma Ligustici Chuanxiong, 2 to 6g), 15g • Dan-shen (Radix Salviae Miltiorrhizae, 5 to 10g), 30g • Hong-hua (Flos Carthami, 4 to 7g), 15g • Jiang-xiang (Lignum Acronychiae, 15 to 30g), 10g

## Formula

### GUI-PI-TANG
(0173)

*Ingredients*
Bai-zhu (Rhizoma Atractylodis Macrocephalae, 5 to 11g), 10g • Dang-gui (Radix Angelicae Sinensis, 5 to 11g), 12g • Dang-shen (Radix Codonopsis Pilosulae, 11 to 15g), 12g • Fu-shen (Buyury with pine root, 11 to 15g), 12g • Gan-cao (Radix Glycyrrhizae, 2 to 11g), 6g • Huang-qi (Radix Astragali Seu Hedysari, 5 to 40g), 20g • Long-yan-rou (Arillus Longan, 4 to 11g), 15g • Mu-xiang (Radix Aucklandiae/Radix Saussureae, 2 to 6g), 3g • Suan-zao-ren (Semen Ziziphi Spinosae, 7 to 18g), 15g • Yuan-zhi (Radix Polygalae, 4 to 11g), 6g

*Formula*

## GUI-SHAO-DI-HUANG-TANG
(0996)

*Ingredients*
Bai-shao-yao (Radix Paeoniae Alba, 5 to 11g), 120g • Dang-gui (Radix Angelicae Sinensis, 5 to 11g), 120g • Fu-ling (Poria, 7 to 14g), 90g • Mu-dan-pi (Cortex Moutan Radicis, 5 to 11g), 90g • Shan-yao (Rhizoma Dioscoreae Bulbiferae, 10 to 20g), 120g • Shan-zhu-yu (Fructus Corni, 5 to 11g), 120g • Sheng-di (Radix Rehmanniae, 14 to 35g), 240g • Ze-xie (Rhizoma Alismatis, 7 to 14g), 90g

*Instructions*
Grind into powder to make tablets and take 9g of tablets twice daily.

*Formula*

## GUI-ZHI-FU-LING-WAN
(0204)

*Ingredients*
(Use equal quantities of all ingredients.) Chi-shao-yao (Radix Paeoniae Rubra, 5 to 11g) • Fu-ling (Poria, 7 to 14g) • Gui-zhi (Ramulus Cinnamomi, 2 to 10g) • Mu-dan-pi (Cortex Moutan Radicis, 5 to 11g) • Tao-ren (Semen Persicae, 5 to 11g)

*Instructions*
Grind into powder to make tablets with honey and take 10g of tablets each time.

*Formula*

## GUI-ZHI-GAN-CAO-TANG
(0309)

*Ingredients*
Gan-cao (Radix Glycyrrhizae, 2 to 11g), 6g • Gui-zhi (Ramulus Cinnamomi, 2 to 10g), 12g

*Formula*

## GUI-ZHI-SHAO-YAO-ZHI-MU-TANG
(0003K)

*Ingredients*
Bai-shao-yao (Radix Paeoniae Alba, 5 to 11g), 10g • Bai-zhu (Rhizoma Atractylodis Macrocephalae, 5 to 11g), 15g • Fang-feng (Radix Ledebouriellae, 5 to 10g), 10g • Fu-zi (Radix Aconiti Praeparata, 4 to 11g), 6g • Gan-cao (Radix Glycyrrhizae, 2 to 11g), 6g • Gui-zhi (Ramulus Cinnamomi, 2 to 10g), 10g • Ma-Huang (Herba Ephedrae, 5 to 10g), 6g • Sheng-jiang (Rhizoma Zingiberis Recens, 4 to 10g), 10g • Zhi-mu (Rhizoma Anemarrhenae, 4 to 15g), 10g

*Formula*

## HE-CHE-WAN
(1153)

*Ingredients*
Dan-shen (Radix Salviae Miltiorrhizae, 5 to 10g), 18g • Fu-ling (Poria, 7 to 14g), 30g • Fu-shen (Buyury with pine root, 11 to 15g), 30g • Ren-shen (Radix Ginseng, 1 to 35g), 15g • Yuan-zhi (Radix Polygalae, 4 to 11g), 30g • Zi-he-che (Placenta Hominis, 2 to 5g), 25g

*Instructions*
Grind into powder to make tablets and take 9g of tablets twice daily.

*Formula*

## HOU-PU-SAN-WU-TANG
(0670)

*Ingredients*
Da-huang (Radix Et Rhizoma Rhei, 4 to 15g), 15g • Hou-po (Cortex Magnoliae Officinalis, 4 to 11g), 18g • Zhi-shi (Fructus Aurantii Immaturus, 4 to 7g), 15g

*Formula*

## HUAI-HUA-SAN
(0223)

*Ingredients*
Ce-bai-ye (Caumen Biotae, 7 to 14g), 15g • Huai-hua (Flos Sophorae, 5 to 11g), 30g • Jing-

jie (Herba Schizonepetae, 5 to
10g), 9g • Zhi-qiao (Fructus
Aurantii 4 to 11g), 9g

4 to 15g), 3g • Zhi-zi (Fructus
Gardeniae, 7 to 16g), 3g

*Formula*

## HUANG-LIAN-E-JIAO-TANG
(0302)

*Ingredients:*
Bai-shao yao (Radix Paeoniae
Alba, 5 to 11g), 15g • E-jiao
(Colla Corii Asini, 5 to 11g),
12g • Huang-lian (Rhizoma
Coptidis, 2 to 12g), 6g • Huang-
qin (Radix Scutellariae, 4 to
15g), 12g • Ji-zi-huang (Chicken
egg yolk, 10 to 20g), one egg

*Formula*

## HUANG-TU-TANG
(0144)

*Ingredients*
Bai-zhu (Rhizoma Atractylodis
Macrocephalae, 5 to 11g), 10g •
E-jiao (Colla Corii Asini, 5 to
11g), 12g • Fu-long-gan (Terra
Flava Usta, 17 to 35g), 30g • Fu-
zi (Radix Aconiti Praeparata, 4 to
11g), 10g • Gan-cao (Radix Gly-
cyrrhizae, 2 to 11g), 3g • Gan-di
(Dried Radix Rehmanniae, 11 to
18g), 15g • Huang-qin (Radix
Scutellariae, 4 to 15g), 12g

*Formula*

## HUO-XIANG-ZHENG-QI-SAN
(0101)

*Ingredients*
Bai-zhi (Radix Angelicae Dahuricae, 4 to 10g), 9g • Bai-zhu (Rhizoma Atractylodis Macrocephalae, 5 to 11g), 9g • Ban-xia (Rhizoma Pinelliae, 4 to 12g), 12g •
Chen-pi (Pericarpium Papaveris,
4 to 11g), 9g • Da-fu-pi (Pericarpium Papaveris/Fructus Papaveris Arecae, 5 to 18g), 15g • Fu-
ling (Poria, 7 to 14g), 12g • Gan-
cao (Radix Glycyrrhizae, 2 to
11g), 3g • Hou-po (Cortex Magnoliae Officinalis, 4 to 11g), 12g
• Huo-xiang (Herba Agastachis,
5 to 11g), 9g • Jie-geng (Radix
Platycodi, 2 to 5g), 6g • Zi-su-ye
(Folium Perillae, 5 to 10g), 9g

*Formula*

## HUANG-LIAN-TANG
(0105E)

*Ingredients*
Ban-xia (Rhizoma Pinelliae, 4
to 12g), 15g • Da-zao (Fructus
Ziziphi Jujubae, 7 to 18g), 9g •
Gan-cao, Zhi-Gan-Cao (Radix
Glycyrrhizae, 2 to 11g), 3g •
Gan-jiang (Rhizoma Zingiberis,
3 to 7g), 9g • Gui-zhi (Ramulus
Cinnamomi, 2 to 10g), 9g •
Huang-lian (Rhizoma Coptidis,
2 to 12g), 6g • Ren-shen (Radix
Ginseng, 1 to 35g), 9g

*Formula*

## HUO-PU-XIA-LING-TANG
(0118)

*Ingredients*
Bai-dou-kou (Fructus Amomi
Cardamomi, 2 to 7g), 3g • Ban-
xia (Rhizoma Pinelliae, 4 to 12g),
10g • Dan-dou-chi (Semen Sojae
Praeparatum, 7 to 14g), 10g •
Fu-ling (Poria, 7 to 14g), 10g •
Hou-po (Cortex Magnoliae
Officinalis, 4 to 11g), 6g • Huoxiang (Herba Agastachis, 5 to
11g), 10g • Xing-ren (Semen
Armeniacae Amarae, 5 to 11g),
6g • Yi-yi-ren (Semen Coicis,
11 to 22g), 20g • Ze-xie (Rhizoma Alismatis, 7 to 14g), 6g •
Zhu-ling (Polyporus Umbellatus, 7 to 14g), 6g

*Formula*

## JI-CHUAN-JIAN
(1203)

*Ingredients*
Dang-gui (Radix Angelicae
Sinensis, 5 to 11g), 10g • Niu-
xi (Radix Achyranthis bideni-
tatae 5 to 11g), 6g • Rou-cong-
rong (Herba Cistanchis, 7 to
11g), 9g • Sheng-ma (Rhizoma
Cimicifugae, 3 to 10g), 2g • Ze-
xie (Rhizoma Alismatis, 7 to
14g), 4g • Zhi-qiao (Fructus
Aurantii, 4 to 11g), 3g

*Formula*

## HUANG-QIN-QING-FEI-YIN
(0786)

*Ingredients*
Huang-qin (Radix Scutellariae,

*Formula*

## JI-SHENG-SHEN-QI-WAN
(0331A)

*Ingredients*
Che-qian-zi (Semen Plantaginis,

4 to 11g), 80g • Fu-ling (Poria, 7 to 14g), 90g • Fu-zi (Radix Aconiti Praeparata, 4 to 11g), 30g • Gan-di (dried Radix Rehmanniae, 11 to 18g), 240g • Gui-zhi (Ramulus Cinnamomi, 2 to 10g), 30g • Mu-dan-pi (Cortex Moutan Radicis, 5 to 11g), 90g • Niu-xi (Radix Achyranthis Bidentatae, 5 to 11g), 80g • Shan-yao (Rhizoma Dioscoreae, 10 to 20g), 120g • Shan-zhu-yu (Fructus Corni, 5 to 11g), 120g • Ze-xie (Rhizoma Alismatis, 7 to 14g), 90g

*Instructions*

Grind into powder to make tablets with honey. Take 9g of tablets one to two times daily, with warm or lightly salted water. Use reduced quantities of ingredients if decoction is done.

*Formula*

## JIA-WEI-ER-CHEN-TANG
(0121M)

*Ingredients*

Bai-guo (Semen Ginkgo, 5 to 11g), 9g • Ban-xia (Rhizoma Pinelliae, 4 to 12g), 15g • Che-qian-zi (Semen Plantaginis, 4 to 11g), 9g • Chen-pi (Pericarpium Citri Reticulatae, 4 to 11g), 10g • Chun-bai-pi (Cortex Toona, 7 to 14g), 9g • Fu-ling (Poria, 7 to 14g), 15g • Gan-cao (Radix Glycyrrhizae, 2 to 11g), 3g • Huang-bai (Cortex Phellodendri, 4 to 15g), 9g • Tiani-nan-xing (Rhizoma Arisaematis, 2.5 to 5g), 9g

*Formula*

## JIA-WEI-SHI-XIAO-SAN
(0201A)

*Ingredients*

(Use equal amounts of all ingredients.) Mu-dan-pi (Cortex Moutan Radicis, 5 to 11g)• Pu-huang (Pollen Typhae, 5 to 11g) • Tao-ren (Semen Persicae, 5 to 11g) • Wu-ling-zhi (Faeces Trogopterorum, 5 to 11g) • Wu-yao (Radix Linderae, 5 to 10g) • Xiang-fu (Rhizoma Cyperi, 5 to 11g) Xuan-ming-Fen (Mirabilitum Dehydratum, 4 to 11g)

*Instructions*

Grind into powder and take 9g of powder two times daily.

*Formula*

## JIA-WEI-SI-LING-SAN
(0348F)

*Ingredients*

Bai-zhu (Rhizoma Atractylodis Macrocephalae, 5 to 11g), 9g • Chen-pi (Pericarpium Papaveris, 4 to 11g), 9g • Fu-ling (Poria, 7 to 14g), 12g • Hou-po (Cortex Magnoliae Officinalis, 4 to 11g), 12g • Ze-xie (Rhizoma Alismatis, 7 to 14g), 15g • Zhu-ling (Polyporus Umbellatus, 7 to 14g), 12g

*Formula*

## JIAN-LING-TANG
(0242B)

*Ingredients*

Bai-shao-yao (Radix Paeoniae Alba, 5 to 11g), 12g • Bai-zi-ren (Semen Biotae, 4 to 11g), 12g • Dai-zhe-shi (Ocherum Rubrum, 1 to 35g), 24g • Long-gu (Os Draconis, 11 to 18g), 18g • Mu-li (Concha Ostrae, 11 to 35g), 18g • Niu-xi (Radix Achyranthis

Bidentatae, 5 to 11g), 30g • Shan-yao (Rhizoma Dioscoreae, 10 to 20g), 30g • Sheng-di (Radix Rehmanniae, 14 to 35g), 18g

*Formula*

## JIANG-TANG ER-HAO-FANG
(3362)

*Ingredients*

Bai-Zhu (Rhizoma Atractylodis Macrocephalae, 5 to 11g), 30g • He-shou-Wu (Radix Polygoni Multiflori, 11 to 15g), 30g • Huang-qi (Radix Astragali Seu Hedysari, 5 to 40g), 30g • Shan-yao (Rhizoma Dioscoreae, 10 to 20g), 30g • Sheng-di (Radix Rehmanniae, 14 to 35g), 24g • Shi-gao (Gypsum Fibrosum, 10 to 70g), 30g • Shu-di-huang (Radix Rehmanniae Praeparatae, 11 to 18g), 30g • Tian-dong (Radix Asparagi, 7 to 14g), 15g • Tian-hua-Fen (Radix Trichosanthis, 10 to 14g), 90g • Xuan-shen (Radix Scrophulariae, 7 to 35g), 24g • Yu-zhu (Rhizoma Polygonati Odorati, 5 to 11g), 20g • Zhi-mu (Rhizoma Anemarrhenae, 4 to 15g), 15g

*Formula*

## JIANG-TANG-SAN-HAO-FANG
(3363)

*Ingredients*

Bai-zhu (Rhizoma Atractylodis Macrocephalae 5 to 11g), 30g • Gou-qi-zi (Fructus Lych, 5 to 11g), 30g • He-shou-wu (Radix Polygoni Multiflori, 11 to 15g), 30g • Huang-bai (Cortex Phellodendri, 4 to 15g), 12g • Huang-qi (Radix Astragali Seu Hedysari, 5 to 40g), 30g • Sang-piao-xiao

(Ootheca Mantidis, 5 to 11g), 12g • Shan-yao (Rhizoma Dioscoreae, 10 to 20g), 40g • Shan-zhu-yu (Fructus Corni, 5 to 11g), 18g • Sheng-di (Radix Rehmanniae, 14 to 35g), 20g • Shu-di-huang (Radix Rehmanniae Praeparatae, 11 to 18g), 20g • Tian-hua-fen (Radix Trichosanthis, 10 to 14g), 12g • Xuan-shen (Radix Scrophulariae, 7 to 35g), 20g

## Formula

### JIANG-TANG-SI-HAO-FANG
(3364)

#### Ingredients
Bai-zhu (Rhizoma Atractylodis Macrocephalae, 5 to 11g), 30g • Cang-zhu (Rhizoma Atractylodis, 4 to 11g), 15g • Ge-gen (Radix Puerariae, 4 to 20g), 12g • Gou-qi-zi (Fructus Lych, 5 to 11g), 30g • He-shou-wu (Radix Polygoni Multiflori, 11 to 15g), 30g • Huang-jing (Rhizoma Polygonati, 11 to 15g), 30g • Huang-qi (Radix Astragali Seu Hedysari, 5 to 40g), 20g • Shan-yao (Rhizoma Dioscoreae, 10 to 20g), 30g • Sheng-di (Radix Rehmanniae, 14 to 35g), 20g • Tian-hua-fen (Radix Trichosanthis, 10 to 14g), 30g • Xuan-Shen (Radix Scrophulariae, 7 to 35g), 30g

## Formula

### JIANG-TANG-YI-HAO-FANG
(3361)

#### Ingredients
Bei-sha-shen (Radix Glehniae, 5 to 11g), 24g • Shan-yao (Rhizoma Dioscoreae, 10 to 20g), 45g • Sheng-di (Radix Rehmanniae, 14 to 35g), 30g • Shi-gao (Gypsum Fibrosum, 10 to 70g), 60g • Tian-Dong (Radix Asparagi, 7 to 14g), 20g • Tian-hua-fen (Radix Trichosanthis, 10 to 14g), 120g • Xuan-shen (Radix Scrophulariae, 7 to 35g), 30g • Yu-zhu (Rhizoma Polygonati Odorati, 5 to 11g), 20g • Zhi-mu (Rhizoma Anemarrhenae, 4 to 15g), 18g

## Formula

### JIN-SUO-GU-JING-WAN
(0342)

#### Ingredients
Lian-xu (Stamen Nelumbinis, 3 to 7g), 60g • Long-gu, duan-long-gu (OS Draconis, 11 to 18g), 30g • Mu-li duan-mu-li (Concha Ostrae, 11 to 35g), 30g • Qian-shi (Semen Euryales, 7 to 11g), 60g • Sha-wan-zi (Semen Astragalus, 7 to 11g), 60g

#### Instructions
Grind into powder to make tablets with cooked lotus powder and take 9g of tablets twice daily.

## Formula

### JING-FANG-BAI-DU-SAN
(0004B)

#### Ingredients
Chai-hu (Radix Bupleuri, 4 to 16g), 10g • Chuan-xiong (Rhizoma Ligustici Chuanxiong, 2 to 6g), 10g • Du-huo (Radix Angelicae Pubescentis, 2 to 5g), 10g • Fang-feng (Radix Ledebouriellae, 5 to 10g), 10g • Fu-ling (Poria, 7 to 14g), 10g • Gan-cao (Radix Glycyrrhizae, 2 to 11g), 3g • Jing-jie (Herba Schizonepetae, 5 to 10g), 10g • Jie-geng (Radix Platycodi, 2 to 5g), 10g

• Qian-hu (Radix Peucedani, 5 to 11g), 10g • Qiang-huo (Rhizoma Seu Radix Notopterygii, 4 to 10g), 10g • Zhi-qiao (Fructus Auranth, 4 to 11g), 10g

## Formula

### JU-FANG-ZHI-BAO-DAN
(1823)

#### Ingredients
An-xi-xiang (Benzoinum, 0.3 to 2g), 45g • Bing-pian (Borneol, 0.2 to 0.3g), 7.5g • Dai-mao (Carapax Eretmochelydis Erethmochelyos, 4 to 7g), 30g • Hu-po (Succinum, 1 to 2g), 30g • Jin-bo (Native Gold Slice flexibleg), 50g • Niu-huang (Calculus Bovis, 0.2 to 0.5g), 15g • She-xiang (Moschus, 0.01 to 0.03g), 7.5g • Xi-jiao (Cornu Rhinoceri, 1 to 2g), 30g • Xiong-huang (Realgar, 03. to 1.5g), 30g • Yin-bo (Native Silver Slice flexibleg), 50g • Zhu-sha (Cinnabaris, 0.3 to 1g), 30g

#### Instructions
Grind into powder to make tablets and take 3g of tablets twice daily.

## Formula

### JUAN-BI-TANG
(1485)

#### Ingredients
Chuan-xiong (Rhizoma Ligustici Chuanxiong 2 to 6g), 2g • Dang-gui (Radix Angelicae Sinensis, 5 to 11g), 9g • Du-huo (Radix Angelicae Pubescentis, 2 to 5g), 3g • Gan-cao (Radix Glycyrrhizae, 2 to 11g), 1.5g • Hai-feng-teng (Caulis Piperis Futokadsurae, 7 to 18g), 6g • Jiang-

huang (Rhizoma Curcumae Longae, 4 to 11g), 6g • Mu-xiang (Radix Aucklandiae/Radix Saussureae, 2 to 6g), 2g • Qiang-huo (Rhizoma Seu Radix Notopterygii, 4 to 10g), 3g • Qin-jiao (Radix Gentianae Macrophyllae, 4 to 11g), 3g • Rou-gui (Cortex Cinnamomi, 1 to 5g), 1.5g • Ru-xiang (Mastix/resina, 4 to 11g), 2g • Sang-zhi (Ramulus Mori, 11 to 18g), 9g

*Formula*

## KAI-GUAN-SAN
(0438)

*Ingredients*
Bai-zhi (Radix Angelicae Dahuricae, 4 to 10g), 2g • Chuan-xiong (Rhizoma Ligustici Chuanxiong, 2 to 6g), 3g

*Instructions*
Grind into powder for consumption as one dose and take two doses daily.

*Formula*

## KE-XUE-TANG
(0280)

*Ingredients*
Gua-lou-ren (Semen Trichosanthis, 11 to 15g), 9g • Hai-fu-shi (Pumex, 10 to 18g), 9g • He-zi (Fructus Chebulae, 2 to 5g), 9g • Qing-dai (Indigo Naturalis, 2 to 4g), 9g • Zhi-zi (Fructus Gardeniae, 7 to 16g), 9g

*Formula*

## LI-ZHONG-WAN
(0062)

*Ingredients*
(Use 90g of each ingredient.) Bai-zhu (Rhizoma Atractylodis Macrocephalae, 5 to 11g) • Gan-cao, zhi-gan-cao (Radix Glycyrrhizae, 2 to 11g) • Gan-jiang (Rhizoma Zingiberis, 3 to 7g) • Ren-shen (Radix Ginseng, 1 to 35g)

*Instructions*
Take 10g in tablet form each time; reduce the quantity if decoction is done

*Formula*

## LING-GUI-ZHU-GAN-TANG
(0119)

*Ingredients*
Bai-zhu (Rhizoma Atractylodis Macrocephalae, 5 to 11g), 15g • Fu-ling (Poria, 7 to 14g), 20g • Gan-cao (Radix Glycyrrhizae, 2 to 11g), 6g • Gui-zhi (Ramulus Cinnamomi, 2 to 10g), 15g

*Formula*

## LING-YANG-GOU-TENG-TANG
(0243)

*Ingredients*
Bai-shao-yao (Radix Paeoniae Alba, 5 to 11g), 30 to 60g • Chuan-bei-mu (Bulbus Fritillariae Cirrhosae, 4 to 14g), 6g • Fu-shen (Buyury with pine root, 11 to 15g), 15g • Gan-cao (Radix Glycerrhizae, 2 to 11g), 6g • Gou-teng (Ramulus Uncariae Cum Uncis, 5 to 11g), 12g • Ju-hua (Flos Chrysanthemi, 4 to 20g), 12g

• Ling yang-Jiao (Cornu Antelopis, 1 to 1.5g), 9g • Sang-ye (Folium Mori, 5 to 10g), 9g • Sheng-di (Radix Rehmanniae, 14 to 35g), 24g • Zhu-ru (Caulis Bambusae in Taeniam, 5 to 11g), 12g

*Formula*

## LIU-JUN-ZI TANG
(0080C)

*Ingredients*
Bai-zhu (Rhizoma Atractylodis Macrocephalae, 5 to 11g), 10g • Ban-xia (Rhizoma Pinelliae, 4 to 12g), 10g • Cheng-pi (Pericarpium Papaveris, 4 to 11g), 10g • Fu-ling (Poria, 7 to 14g), 12g • Gan-cao (Radix Glycyrrhizae, 2 to 11g), 3g • Ren-shen (Radix Ginseng, 1 to 35g), 15g

*Formula*

## LIU-MO-YIN
(0419)

*Ingredients*
Bing-lang (Semen Areca, 4 to 11g), 6g • Chen-xiang (Lignum Aquilariae Resinatum, 1 to 4g), 3g • Da-huang (Radix Et Rhizoma Rhei, 4 to 15g), 8g • Mu-xiang (Radix Aucklandiae/Radix Saussureae, 2 to 6g), 4g • Wu-yao (Radix Linderae, 5 to 10g), 7g • Zhi-shi (Fructus Aurantii Immaturus, 4 to 7g), 5g

*Formula*

## LIU-WEI-DI-HUANG-WAN
(0307)

Fu-ling (Poria, 7 to 14g), 90g • Mu-dan-pi (Cortex Moutan Radicis, 5 to 11g), 90g • Shan-yao (Rhizoma Dioscoreae, 10 to 20g), 120g • Shan-zhu-yu (Fructus Corni, 5 to 11g), 120g • Shu-di-huang (Radix Rehmanniae Praeparatae, 11 to 18g), 240g • Ze-xie (Rhizoma Alismatis, 7 to 14g), 90g

*Instructions*

Grind into powder to make tablets and take three tablets or 9g two to three times daily.

*Formula*

### LONG-DAN-XIE-GAN-TANG
(0188)

*Ingredients*

Chai-hu (Radix Bupleuri, 4 to 16g), 9g • Che-qian-zi (Semen Plantaginis, 4 to 11g), 12g • Dang-gui (Radix Angelicae Sinensis, 5 to 11g), 9g • Gan-cao (Radix Glycyrrhizae, 2 to 11g), 3g • Huang-qin (Radix Scutellariae, 4 to 15g), 12g • Long-dan (Radix Gentianae, 7 to 10g), 9g • Mu-tong (Caulis Aristologhiae, 4 to 8g), 12g • Sheng-di (Radix Rehmanniae, 14 to 35g), 15g • Ze-xie (Rhizoma Alismatis, 7 to 14g), 9g • Zhi-zi (Fructus Gardeniae, 7 to 16g), 9g

*Formula*

### MA-HUANG-LIAN-QIAO-CHI-XIAO DOU-TANG
(0059)

*Ingredients*

Chi-xiao-dou (Semen Phaseoli, 11 to 18g), 15g • Da-zao (Fructus Ziziphi Jujabae, 7 to 18g), 4 dates • Gan-cao (Radix Glycyrrhizae, 2 to 11g), 6g • Lian-qiao (Fructus Forsythiae, 5 to 11g), 15g • Ma-huang (Herba Ephedrae, 5 to 10g), 9g • Sheng-jiang (Rhizoma Zingiberis Recens, 4 to 10g), 9g • Xing-ren (Semen Armeniacae Amarae, 5 to 11g), 9g • Zi-bai-pi (Cortex Catalpa 5 to 15g), 15g

*Formula*

### MA-XING-SHI-GAN-TANG
(0028)

*Ingredients*

Gan-cao (Radix Glycyrrhizae, 2 to 11g), 3g • Ma-huang (Herba Ephedrae, 5 to 10g), 9g • Shi-gao (Gypsum Fibrosum, 10 to 70g), 30g • Xing-ren (Semen Armeniacae Amarae, 5 to 11g), 9g

*Formula*

### MA-ZI-REN-WAN
(0161)

*Ingredients*

Chi-shao-yao (Radix Paeoniae Rubra, 5 to 11g), 15g • Da-Huang (Radix Et Rhizoma Rhei, 4 to 15g), 20g • Hou-po (Cortex Magnioliae Officinalis, 4 to 11g), 15g • Huo-ma-ren (Fructus Cannabis, 11 to 17g), 30g • Xing-ren (Semen Armeniacae Amarae, 5 to 11g), 15g • Zhi-shi (Fructus Aurantii Immaturus, 4 to 7g), 10g

*Formula*

### MAI-MEN-DONG-TANG
(0140)

*Ingredients*

Ban-xia (Rhizoma Pinelliae, 4 to 12g), 10g • Da-zao (Fructus Ziziphi Jujubae, 7 to 18g), 10g • Gan-cao (Radix Glycyrrhizae, 2 to 11g), 6g • Jing-Mi (Polished rice, flexible quantity), 10g • Mai-men-dong (Radix Ophiopogonis, 5 to 11g), 30g • Ren-shen (Radix Ginseng, 1 to 35g), 6g

*Formula*

### MAI-WEI-DI-HUANG-WAN
(0327C)

*Ingredients*

Fu-ling (Poria, 7 to 14g), 90g • Mai-men-dong (Radix Ophiopogonis, 5 to 11g), 90g • Mu-dan-pi (Cortex Moutan Radicis, 5 to 11g), 90g • Shan-yao (Rhizoma Dioscoreae, 10 to 20g), 120g • Shan-zhu-yu (Fructus Corni, 5 to 11g), 120g • Shu-di-huang (Radix Rehmanniae Praeparatae, 11 to 18g), 240g • Wu-wei-zi (Fructus Schisandrae, 2 to 4g), 90g • Ze-xie (Rhizoma Alismatis, 7 to 14g), 90g

*Instructions*

Grind into powder to make tablets and take three tablets or 9g two to three times daily.

*Formula*

### MI-NIAO-XI-TONG-GAN-RAN-HE-JI
(1903)

*Ingredients*

Chai-hu (Radix Bupleuri, 4 to

16g), 25g • Che-qian-Zi (Semen Plantaginis, 4 to 11g), 15g • Huang-bai (Cortex Phellodendri, 4 to 15g), 15g • Huang-qin (Radix Scutellariae, 4 to 15g), 15g • Wu-wei-zi (Fructus Schisandrae, 2 to 4g), 15g

## Formula
### MU-XIANG-BING-LANG-WAN
(0076)

**Ingredients**
Bing-lang (Semen Areca, 4 to 11g), 15g • Chen-pi (Pericarpium Papaveris, 4 to 11g) 15g • Da-huang (Radix Et Rhizoma Rhei, 4 to 15g), 30g • E-zhu (Rhizoma Zedoariae, 5 to 11g), 15g • Huang-bai (Cortex Phellodendri, 4 to 15g), 15g • Huang-lian (Rhizoma Coptidis, 2 to 12g), 15g • Mu-xiang (Radix Aucklandiae /Radix Saussureae, 2 to 6g), 15g • Qian-niu-zi (Semen Pharbitidis, 4 to 7g), 60g • Qing-pi (Pericarpium Papaveris, 4 to 11g), 15g • Xiang-fu (Rhizoma Cyperi, 5 to 11g), 60g

## Formula
### MU-XIANG-SHUN-QI-WAN
(0442)

**Ingredients**
Bing-lang (Semen Areca, 4 to 11g), 30g • Cang-zhu (Rhizoma Atractylodis Macrocephalae, 4 to 11g), 30g • Chen-pi (Pericarpium Citri Reticulatae Viride, 4 to 11g), 30g • Gan-cao (Radix Glycyrrhizae, 2 to 11g), 15g • Hou-po (Cortex Magnoliae Officinalis, 4 to 11g), 30g • Mu-xiang (Radix Aucklandiae/Radix Saussureae, 2 to 6g),

30g • Qing-pi (Pericarpium Citri Reticulatae Viride, 4 to 11g), 30g • Sha-ren (Fructus Amomi, 2 to 7g), 30g • Xiang-fu (Rhizoma Cyperi, 5 to 11g), 30g • Zhi-Qiao (Fructus Aurantii, 4 to 11g), 30g

**Instructions**
Grind into powder and take 9g of powder twice daily.

## Formula
### PING-WEI-SAN
(0117)

**Ingredients**
Cang-zhu (Rhizoma Atractylodis Macrocephalae, 4 to 11g), 10g • Chen-pi (Pericarpium Papaveris, 4 to 11g), 10g • Gan-cao (Radix Glycyrrhizae, 2 to 11g), 3g • Hou-po (Cortex Magnoliae Officinalis, 4 to 11g), 10g

## Formula
### QI-GONG-WAN
(0559)

**Ingredients**
Ban-xia (Rhizoma Pinelliae, 4 to 12g), 45g • Cang-zhu (Rhizoma Atractylodis Macrocephalae, 4 to 11g), 60g • Chen-pi (Pericarpium Citri Reticulatae Viride, 4 to 11g), 45g • Chuan-xiong (Rhizoma Ligustici Chuanxiong, 2 to 6g), 45g • Fu-ling (Poria, 7 to 14g) 45g • Shen-qu (Massa Medicata Fermentata, 7 to 15g), 45g • Xiang-fu (Rhizoma Cyperi, 5 to 11g), 60g

## Formula
### QIAN-JIN-XI-JIAO-TANG
(0411)

**Ingredients**
Da-huang (Radix Et Rhizoma Rhei, 4 to 15g), 5g • Dou-chi (Semen sojae Praeparatum, 10 to 15g), 8g • Huang-qin (Radix Scutellariae, 4 to 15g), 5g • Ling-yang-Jiao (Cornu Antelopis, 1 to 1.5g), 1g • Qian-hu (Radix Peucedani, 5 to 11g), 5g • She-gan (Rhizoma Belamcandae, 2 to 5g), 3g • Sheng-ma (Rhizoma Cimicifugae, 3 to 10g), 6g • Xi-jiao (Cornu Rhinoceri, 1 to 2g), 1g • Zhi-Zi (Fructus Gardeniae, 7 to 16g), 8g

## Formula
### QIAN-ZHENG-SAN
(0253)

**Ingredients**
(Use equal quantities of all ingredients.) Du-jiao-lian (Rhizoma Typhonii, external uses) • Jiang-can (Bombyx Batryticatus, 5 to 11g) • Quan-xie (Scorpio, 2 to 5g)

**Instructions**
Grind into powder and take 3g of powder each time with hot wine.

## Formula
### QIANG-HUO-SHENG-SHI-TANG
(0010)

**Ingredients**
Chuan-xiong (Rhizoma Ligusticti Chuanxiong, 2 to 6g), 6g • Du-huo (Raidix Angelicae Pubescentis, 2 to 5g), 9g • Gan-

cao (Radix Glycyrrhizae, 2 to 11g), 3g • Gao-ben (Rhizoma Et Radix Ligustici, 4 to 10g), 6g • Man-jing-Zi (Fructus Viticis, 4 to 15g), 6g • Qiang-huo (Rhizoma Seu Radix Notopterygii Notopterygii, 4 to 10g), 9g

## Formula
### QIN-JIAO-BIE-JIA-SAN
(0275)

### Ingredients
Bie-jia (Carapax Trionycis, 11 to 18g), 30g • Chai-hu (Radix Bupleuri, 4 to 16g) 30g • Dang-gui (Radix Angelicae Sinensis, 5 to 11g), 15g • Di-gu-pi (Cortex Lych Radicis, 5 to 11g), 30g • Qin-jiao (Radix Genitianae Macrophyllae, 4 to 11g), 15g • Zhi-mu (Rhizoma Anemarrhenae, 4 to 15g), 15g

## Formula
### QING-GAN-TANG
(0756)

### Ingredients
Bai-shao-yao (Radix Paeoniae Alba, 5 to 11g), 5g • Chai-hu (Radix Bapleuri, 4 to 16g), 2g • Chuan-xiong (Rhizoma Ligustici Chuanxiong, 2 to 6g), 3g • Dang-gui (Radix Angelicae Sinensis, 5 to 11g), 3g • Mu-dan-pi (Cortex Moutan Radicis, 5 to 11g), 1.5g • Zhi-zi (Fructus Gardeniae, 7 to 16g), 1.5g

## Formula
### QING-GONG-TANG
(0281A)

### Ingredients
Lian-Qiao (Fructus Forsythiae, 5 to 11g), 6g • Lian-zi-xin (Plumula Nelumbinis, 2 to 4g), 3g • Mai-men-dong (Radix Ophiopogonis, 5 to 11g), 9g • Xi-jiao (Cornu Rhinoceri, 1 to 2g), 2 to 3g • Xuan-shen (Radix Scrophulariae, 7 to 35g), 12g • Zhu-juan-xin (young bamboo leaf, 3 to 5g), 6g

## Formula
### QING-GU-ZI-SHEN-TANG
(0755)

### Ingredients
Bai-zhu (Rhizoma Atractylodis Mactocephalae, 5 to 11g), 10g • Bei-sha-shen (Radix Glehniae, 5 to 11g), 15g • Di-gu-pi (Cortex Lych Radicis, 5 to 11g), 30g • Mai-men-dong (Radix Ophiopogonis, 5 to 11g), 15g • Mu-dan-pi (Cortex Moutan Radicis, 5 to 11g), 15g • Shi-hu (Herba Dendrobii, 7 to 14g), 6g • Wu-wei-zi (Fructus Schisandrae, 2 to 4g), 1.5g • Xuan-shen (Radix Scrophulariae, 7 to 35g), 15g

## Formula
### QING-HAO-BIE-JIA-TANG
(0277)

### Ingredients
Bie-jia (Carapax Trionycis, 11 to 18g), 15g • Mu-dan-pi (Cortex Moutan Radicis, 5 to 11g), 9g • Qing-hao (Herba Artemisiae Chinghao, 5 to 11g), 15g • Sheng-di (Radix Rehmanniae, 14 to 35g), 12g • Zhi-mu (Rhizoma Anemarrhenae, 4 to 15g), 9g

## Formula
### QING-JING-TANG
(0272A)

### Ingredients
Bai-shao-yao (Radix Paeoniae Alba, 5 to 11g), 12g • Di gu-pi (Cortex Lych Radicis, 5 to 11g), 12g • Fu-ling (Poria, 7 to 14g), 9g • Huang-bai (Cortex Phellodendri, 4 to 15g), 9g • Mu-dan-pi (Cortex Moutan Radicis, 5 to 11g), 9g • Qing-hao (Herba Artemisiae Chinghao, 5 to 11g), 12g • Shu-di-huang (Radix Rehmanniae Praeparatae, 11 to 18g), 15g

## Formula
### QING-XUE-YANG-YIN-TANG
(0754)

### Ingredients
Bai-shao-yao (Radix Paeoniae Alba, 5 to 11g), 8g • Huang-bai (Cortex Phellodendri, 4 to 15g), 9g • Mo-han-lian (Herba Ecliptae, 5 to 11g), 7g • Mu-dan-pi (Cortex Moutan Radicis, 5 to 11g), 8g • Noncontributory and unchanged-zhen-zi (Fructus Ligustri Lucidi, 5 to 11g), 7g • Sheng-di (Radix Rehmanniae, 14 to 35g), 25g • Xuan-shen (Radix Scrophulariae, 7 to 35g), 20g

## Formula
### QING-YING-TANG
(0281)

*Ingredients*
Dang-shen (Radix Salviae Miltiorrhizae, 5 to 10g), 6g • Huang-
lian (Rhizoma Coptidis, 2 to 12g),
5g • Jin-yin-hua (Flos Lonicerae, 7 to 18g), 15g • Lian-qiao
(Fructus Forsythiae, 5 to 11g),
6g • Mai-men-dong (Radix
Ophiopogonis, 5 to 11g), 9g •
Sheng-di (Radix Rehmanniae,
14 to 35g), 15g • Xi-jiao (Cornu
Rhinoceri, 1 to 2g), 9g • Xuan-
shen (Radix Scrophulariae, 7 to
35g), 9g • Zhu-juan-xin (young
bamboo leaf, 3 to 5g), 3g

*Formula*

**QING-ZAO-JIU-FEI-TANG**
(0049)

*Ingredients*
E-jiao (Colla Corii Asini, 5 to
11g), 6g • Gan-cao (Radix Gly-
cyrrhizae, 2 to 11g), 3g • Hu-
ma (Semen Sesami, 3 to 10g),
3g • Mai-men-Dong (Radix
Ophiopogonis, 5 to 11g), 6g •
Pi-pa-ye (Folium Eriobotryae, 5
to 11g), three leaves • Ren-shen
(Radix Ginseng, 1 to 35g), 10g
• Sang-ye (Folium Mori, 5 to
10g), 10g • Shi-gao (Gypsum
Fibrosum, 10 to 70g), 15g •
Xing-ren (Semen Armeniacae
Amarae, 5 to 11g), 10g

*Formula*

**QING-ZHI-TANG**
(3365)

*Ingredients*
He-shou-wu (Radix Polygoni
Multiflori, 11 to 15g), 12g • Hei-
zhi-ma (Semen Sesami, 4 to 11g),
12g • Nu-zhen-zi (Fructus Ligustri Lucidi, 5 to 11g), 12g • Sheng-

di (Radix Rehmanniae, 14 to
35g), 12g • Tu-si-zi (Semen
Cuscutae, 5 to 11g), 15g • Yin-
yang-huo (Herba Epimedii, 4 to
11g), 10g • Ze-xie (Rhizoma
Alismatis, 7 to 14g), 15g

*Formula*

**REN-SHEN-YANG-YING-TANG**
(0182B)

*Ingredients*
Bai-shao-yao (Radix Paeoniae
Alba, 5 to 11g), 12g • Bai-zhu
(Rhizoma Atractylodis Macrocephalae, 5 to 11g), 10g • Chen-
pi (Pericarpium Papaveris, 4 to
11g), 6g • Dang-gui (Radix
Angelicae Sinensis, 5 to 11g),
12g • Dang-shen (Radix Codonopsis Pilosulae, 11 to 15g), 10g
• Fu-ling (Poria, 7 to 14g), 12g
• Gan-cao (Radix Glycyrrhizae,
2 to 11g), 3g • Huang-qi (Radix
Astragali Seu Hedysari, 5 to 40g),
12g • Rou-gui (Cortex Cinnamomi, 1 to 5g), 6g • Shu-di-huang
(Radix Rehmanniae Praeparatae,
11 to 18g), 15g • Wu-wei-zi
(Fructus Schisandrae, 2 to 4g),
6g • Yuan-zhi (Radix Polygalae,
4 to 11g), 6g

*Formula*

**RUN-CHANG-WAN**
(0159)

*Ingredients*
Dang-gui (Radix Angelicae
Sinensis, 5 to 11g), 10g • Huo-
ma-ren (Fructus Cannabis, 11
to 17g), 15g • Sheng-di (Radix
Rehmanniae, 14 to 35g), 30g •
Tao-ren (Sernen Persicae, 5 to
11g), 10g • Zhi-qiao (Fructus
Aurantii, 4 to 11g), 10g

*Formula*

**SAN-MIAO-WAN**
(0392)

*Ingredients*
Cang-zhu (Rhizoma Atractylodis Macrocephaiae, 4 to 11g),
60g • Huang-bai (Cortex Phellodendri, 4 to 15g), 40g • Niu-
xi (Radix Achyranthis Bidentatae, 5 to 11g), 20g

*Formula*

**SAN-QI-HONG-TENG-ER-HAO-FANG**
(3367)

*Ingredients*
Chi-shao yao (Radix Paeoniae
Rubra, 5 to 11g), 15g • Chuan
shan-jia (Squama Manitis, 5 to
11g), 12g • Da-xue-teng (Caulis
Sargentodoxae, 10 to 15g), 15g
• Dan-shen (Radix Salviae Miltiorrhizae, 5 to 10g), 15g • Dang-
gui (Radix Angelicae Sinensis, 5
to 11g), 15g • E-zhu (Rhizoma
Zedoariae, 5 to 11g), 15g • Pu-
gong-ying (Herba Taraxaci, 7 to
15g), 15g • San-qi (Radix Notoginseng, 2 to 10g), 3g • Shui-zhi
(Hirudo, 2 to 4g), 6g • Wu-ling-
zhi (Faeces Trogopterorum, 5 to
11g), 12g • Xuan-shen (Radix
Scrophulariae, 7 to 35g), 15g

*Formula*

**SAN-QI-HONG-TENG-SAN-HAO-FANG**
(3368)

*Ingredients*

Bai-jiang (Herba Patriniae, 10 to 18g), 30g • Chuan-lian-zi (Fructus Meliae Toosendan, 5 to 11g), 10g • Da-qing-ye (Folium Isatidis, 11 to 18g), 15g • Ji-xue-teng (Caulis Spatholobi, 11 to 35g), 30g • Jin-yin-hua (Flos Lonicerae, 7 to 18g), 15g • Jin-ying-zi (Fructus Rosae Laevigatae, 5 to 11g), 30g • Qian-cao (Radix Rubiae, 7 to 11g), 10g • San-qi (Radix Notoginseng, 2 to 10g), 3g •Xiang-fu (Rhizoma Cyperi, 5 to 11g), 10g • Yan-hu-suo (Rhizoma Corydalis, 4 to 11g), 15g • Yi-mu-cao (Herba Leonuri, 11 to 36g), 30g

*Formula*

### SAN-QI-HONG-TENG-YI-HAO-FANG
(3366)

*Ingredients*

Chuan-xiong (Rhizoma Ligustici Chuanxiong, 2 to 6g), 6g • Da-xue-teng (Caulis Sargentodoxae 10 to 15g), 30g • Dang-gui (Radix Angelicae Sinensis, 5 to 11g), 15g • Jin-yin-hua (Flos Lonicerae, 7 to 18g), 15g • Mai-men-dong (Radix Ophiopogonis, 5 to 11g), 10g • Mu-dan-pi (Cortex Moutan Radicis, 5 to 11g), 10g • San-qi (Radix Notoginseng, 2 to 10g), 30g • Tao-ren (Semen Persicae, 5 to 11g), 12g • Xiang-fu (Rhizoma Cyperi, 5 to 11g), 12g • Yi-yi-ren (Semen Coicis, 11 to 22g), 30g

*Formula*

### SAN-REN-TANG
(0107)

*Ingredients*

Bai-dou-kou (Fructus Amomi Cardamomi, 2 to 7g), 10g • Ban-xia (Rhizoma Pinelliae, 4 to 12g), 12g • Hou-po (Cortex Magnoliae Officinais, 4 to 11g), 12g • Hua-shi (Talcum, 11 to 15g), 18g • Tong-cao (Medulla Tetrapanacis, 2 to 5g), 6g • Xing-ren (Semen Armeniacae Amarae, 5 to 11g), 10g • Yi-yi-ren (Semen Coicis, 11 to 22g), 24g • Zhu-ye (Folium Bambusae, 4 to 20g), 6g

*Formula*

### SAN-ZI-TANG
(1885)

*Ingredients*

Bai-jie-zi (Semen Sinapis Albae, 4 to 11g), 6g • Lai-fu-zi (Semen Raphani, 5 to 11g), 9g • Zi-su-zi (Fructus Perillae, 5 to 11g), 9g

*Formula*

### SANG-JU-YIN
(0016)

*Ingredients*

Bo-he (Herba Menthae, 3 to 10g), 3g • Gan-cao (Radix Glycyrrhizae, 2 to 11g), 3g • Jie-geng (Radix Platycodi, 2 to 5g), 9g • Ju-hua (Flos Chrysanthemi, 4 to 20g), 12g • Lian-qiao (Fructus Forsythiae, 5 to 11g), 9g • Lu-gen (Rhizoma Phragmitis, 15 to 65g), 15g • Sang-ye (Folium Mori, 5 to 10g), 9g • Xing-ren (Semen Armeniacae Amarae, 5 to 11g), 9g

*Formula*

### SANG-NU-SAN-JIA-TANG
(3369)

*Ingredients*

Bai-shao-yao (Radix Paeoniae Alba, 5 to 11g), 15g • Gui-ban (Plastrum Testudinis, 11 to 30g), 30g • Long-gu (Os Draconis, 11 to 18g), 30g • Mu-li (Concha Ostrae, 11 to 35g), 30g • Nu-zhen-zi (Fructus Ligustri Lucidi, 5 to 11g), 20g • Sang-ji-sheng (Ramulus Loranthi, 11 to 18g), 20g • Sheng-di (Radix Rehmanniae, 14 to 35g), 15g • Tian-dong (Radix Asparagi, 7 to 14g), 15g

*Formula*

### SANG-PIAO-XIAO-SAN
(0326)

*Ingredients*

(Use 30g of each ingredient.) Chang-pu (Rhizoma Calami, 4 to 7g) • Dang-gui (Radix Angelicae Sinensis, 5 to 11g) • Fu-shen (Buyury with pine root, 11 to 15g) • Gui-ban (Plastrum Testudinis, 11 to 30g) Long-gu (Os Draconis, 11 to 18g) • Ren-shen (Radix Ginseng, 1 to 35g) • Sang-piao-xiao (Ootheca Mantidis, 5 to 11g) • Yuan-zhi (Radix Polygalae, 4 to 11g)

*Formula*

### SANG-XING-TANG
(0047)

*Ingredients*

Dan-dou-chi (Semen Sojae Praeparatum, 7 to 14g), 10g • Li-pi (Pericarpium Papaveris/ Fructus Papaveris Pyrus, 11 to

18g), 30g • Nan-sha-shen (Radix Adenophorae, 5 to 11g), 15g • Sang-ye (Folium Mori, 5 to 10g), 15g • Xing-ren (Semen Armeniacae Amarae, 5 to 11g), 10g • Zhe-bei-mu (Bulbus Fritillariae Thunbergh, 5 to 11g), 10g • Zhi-zi-pi (Pericarpium Papaveris/ Fructus Papaveris Gardenia, for external use), 12g

*Formula*

## SHA-SHEN-MAI-DONG-TANG
(0048)

*Ingredients*

Bian-dou (Semen Lalab, 11 to 22g), 5g • Gan-cao (Radix Glycyrrhizae, 2 to 11g), 3g • Mai-men-dong (Radix Ophiopogonis, 5 to 11g), 10g • Nan-sha-shen (Radix Adenophorae, 5 to 11g), 10g • Sang-ye (Folium Mori, 5 to 10g), 6g • Tian-Hua-fen (Radix Trichosanthis, 10 to 14g), 6g • Yu-zhu (Rhizoma Polygonati Odorati, 5 to 11g), 6g

*Formula*

## SHAO-FU-ZHU-YU-TANG
(0205)

*Ingredients*

Chi-shao-yao (Radix Paeoniae Rubra, 5 to 11g), 9g • Chuan-xiong (Rhizoma Ligustici Chuanxiong, 2 to 6g), 6g • Dang-gui (Radix Angelicae Sinensis, 5 to 11g), 9g • Gan-jiang, pao-jiang, or baked ginger (Rhizoma Zingiberis, 3 to 7g), 6g • Mo-yao (Myrrha, 4 to 11g), 6g • Pu-huang (Pollen Typhae, 5 to 11g), 9g • Rou-gui (Cortex Cinnamomi, 1 to 5g), 6g • Wu-ling-zhi (Faeces Trogopterorum, 5 to

11g), 9g • Xiao-Hui-Xiang (Fructus Foeniculi, 4 to 11g), 9g • Yan-Hu-Suo (Rhizoma Corydalis, 4 to 11g), 6g

*Formula*

## SHAO-YAO-TANG
(0165)

*Ingredients*

Bing lang (Semen Areca, 4 to 11g), 15g • Chi-shao-yao (Radix Paeoniae Rubra, 5 to 11g), 15g • Da-huang (Radix Et Rhizoma Rhei, 4 to 15g), 12g • Dang-gui (Radix Angelicae Sinensis, 5 to 11g), 6g • Gan-cao (Radix Glycyrrhizae, 2 to 11g), 3g • Huang-lian (Rhizoma Coptidis, 2 to 12g), 10g • Huang-qin (Radix Scutellariae, 4 to 15g), 12g • Mu-xiang (Radix Aucklandiae/ Radix Saussureae, 2 to 6g), 10g • Rou-gui (Cortex Cinnamomi, 1 to 5g), 6g

*Formula*

## SHE-GAN-MA-HUANG-TANG
(0026)

*Ingredients*

Ban-xia (Rhizoma Pinelliae, 4 to 12g), 12g • Da-Zao (Fructus Ziziphi Jujubae, 7 to 18g), 9g • Kuan-dong-hua (Flos Farfarae, 5 to 11g), 12g • Ma-huang (Herba Ephedrae, 5 to 10g), 9g • She-gan (Rhizoma Belamcandae, 2 to 5g), 9g • Sheng-jiang (Rhizoma Zingiberis Recens, 4 to 10g), 9g • Wu-wei-zi (Fructus Schisandrae, 2 to 4g), 6g • Xi-xin (Herba Asari, 1 to 4g), 6g • Zi-wan (Radix Asteris, 5 to 11g), 9g

*Formula*

## SHEN-FU-LONG-MU-JIU-NI-TANG
(1898)

*Ingredients*

Fu-zi (Radix Aconiti Praeparata, 4 to 11g), 11g • Long-gu (Os Draconis, 11 to 18g), 18g • Mu-li (Concha Ostrae, 11 to 35g), 35g • Ren-shen (Radix Ginseng, 1 to 35g), 35g

*Formula*

## SHEN-FU-TANG
(0318)

*Ingredients*

Fu-zi (Radix Aconiti Praeparata, 4 to 11g), 15 to 60g • Ren-shen (Radix Ginseng, 1 to 35g), 15g

*Formula*

## SHEN-HUANG-GAN-QI-TANG
(3370)

*Ingredients*

Dang-shen (Radix Codonopsis Pilosulae, 11 to 15g), 15g • Gan-cao (Radix Glycyrrhizae, 2 to 11g), 11g • Gou-qi-zi (Fructus Lych, 5 to 11g), 11g • Huang-jing (Rhizoma Polygonati, 11 to 15g), 15g

*Formula*

## SHEN-LING-BAI-ZHU-SAN
(0081)

*Ingredients*

Bai-zhu (Rhizoma Atractylodis

Macrocephalae, 5 to 11g), 10g • Bian-dou (Semen Lalab, 11 to 22g), 12g • Chen-pi (Pericarpium Papaveris, 4 to 11g), 12g • Dang-shen (Radix Codonopsis Pilosulae, 11 to 15g), 15g • Fu-ling Poria, 7 to 14g), 15g • Gan-cao (Radix Glycyrrhizae, 2 to 11g), 3g • Jie-geng (Radix Platycodi, 2 to 5g), 6g • Lian-zi (Semen Nelumbinis, 7 to 18g), 15g • Sha-ren (Fructus Amomi, 2 to 7g), 9g • Shan-yao (Rhizoma Dioscoreae, 10 to 20g), 15g • Yi-yi-ren (Semen Coicis, 11 to 22g), 24g

## Formula

### SHEN-QI-SI-WU-TANG
(3371)

#### Ingredients
Bai-shao-yao (Radix Paeoniae Alba, 5 to 11g), 10g • Bai-zhu (Rhizoma Atractylodis Macrocephalae, 5 to 11g), 10g • Chuan-xiong (Rhizoma Ligustici Chuanxiong, 2 to 6g), 6g • Dang-gui (Radix Angelicae Sinensis, 5 to 11g), 10g • Dang-shen (Radix Codonopsis Pilosulae, 11 to 15g), 10g • Gan-cao (Radix Glycyrrhizae, 2 to 11g), 6g • Huang-qi (Radix Astragali Seu Hedysari, 5 to 40g), 30g • Shu-di-huang (Radix Rehmanniae Praeparatae, 11 to 18g), 12g • Suan-zao-ren (Semen Ziziphi Spinosae, 7 to 18g), 12g • Wu-wei-zi (Fructus Schisandrae, 2 to 4g), 10g

## Formula

### SHEN-QI-WAN
(0331)

#### Ingredients
Fu-ling (Poria, 7 to 14g), 90g •

Fu-zi (Radix Aconiti Praeparata, 4 to 11g), 30g • Gan-di (Dried Radix Rehmanniae, 11 to 18g), 240g • Gui-zhi (Ramulus Cinnamomi, 2 to 10g), 30g • Mu-dan-pi (Cortex Mouton Radicis, 5 to 11g), 90g • Shan-yao (Rhizoma Dioscoreae, 10 to 20g), 120g • Shan-zhu-yu (Fructus Corni, 5 to 11g), 120g • Ze-xie (Rhizoma Alismatis, 7 to 14g), 90g

#### Instructions
Grind into powder to make tablets with honey. Take 9g of tablets one to two times daily, with warm or lightly salted water. Use reduced quantities of ingredients if decoction is done.

## Formula

### SHEN-TONG-ZHU-YU-TANG
(1084)

#### Ingredients
Chuan-xiong (Rhizoma Ligustici Chuanxiong, 2 to 6g), 6g • Dang-gui (Radix Angelicae Sinensis, 5 to 11g), 9g • Di-long (Lumbricus, 5 to 11g), 6g • Gan-cao (Radix Glycyrrhizae, 2 to 11g), 6g • Hong-hua (Flos Carthami, 4 to 7g), 9g • Mo-yao (Myrrha, 4 to 11g), 6g • Niu-xi (Radix Achyranthis Bidentatae, 5 to 11g), 9g • Qiang-huo (Rhizoma Seu Radix Noto-pterygii, 4 to 10g), 3g • Qin-jiao (Radix Gentianae Macrophyllae 4 to 11g), 3g • Tao-ren (Semen Persicae, 5 to 11g), 9g • Wu-ling-zhi (Faeces Trogopterorum, 5 to 11g), 6g • Xiang-fu (Rhizoma Cyperi, 5 to 11g), 3g

## Formula

### SHEN-ZHE-ZHEN-QI-TANG
(1839)

#### Ingredients
Bai-shao-yao (Radix Paeoniae Alba, 5 to 11g), 12g • Dai-zhe-shi (Ocherum Rubrum, 1 to 35g), 18g • Dang-shen (Radix Codonopsis Pilosulae, 11 to 15g), 12g • Long-gu (Os Draconis, 11 to 18g), 18g • Mu-li (Concha Ostrae, 11 to 35g), 18g • Qian-shi (Semen Euryales, 7 to 11g), 15g • Shan-yao (Rhizoma Dio-scoreae, 10 to 20g), 15g • Shan-zhu-yu (Fructus Corni, 5 to 11g), 18g • Zi-su-zi Fructus Perillae, 5 to 11g), 6g

## Formula

### SHEN-ZHUO-TANG
(0617)

#### Ingredients
Bai-zhu (Rhizoma Atractylodis Macrocephalae, 5 to 11g), 6g • Fu-ling (Poria, 7 to 14g), 9g • Gan-cao (Radix Glycyrrhizae, 2 to 11g), 3g • Gan-Jiang (Rhizoma Zingiberis, 3 to 7g), 6g

## Formula

### SHENG-MAI-SAN
(0315)

#### Ingredients
Mai-men-dong (Radix Ophio-pogonis, 5 to 11g), 9g • Ren-shen (Radix Ginseng, 1 to 35g), 15g • Wu-wei-zi (Fructus Schisandrae, 2 to 4g), 6g

中医疗法

## Formula

### SHI-GAO-ZHI-MU-JIA-REN-SHEN-TANG
(0065G)

### Ingredients
Gan-cao (Radix Glycyrrhizae, 2 to 11g), 6g • Jing-mi (polished rice, flexible quantity), 9g • Ren-shen (Radix Ginseng, 1 to 35g), 10g • Shi-gao (Gypsum Fibrosum, 10 to 70g), 15 to 60g • Zhi-mu (Rhizoma Anemarrhenae, 4 to 15g), 12g

## Formula

### SHI-PI-YIN
(0132)

### Ingredients
Bai-zhu (Rhizoma Atractylodis Macrocephalae, 5 to 11g), 10g • Bing-lang (Semen Areca, 4 to 11g), 15g •Cao-Guo (Fructus Tsaoko, 2 to 5g), 10g • Fu-ling (Poria, 7 to 14g), 15g • Fu-zi (Radix Aconiti Praeparata, 4 to 11g), 15g • Gan-cao (Radix Glycyrrhizae, 2 to 11g), 3g • Gan-Jiang (Rhizoma Zingiberis, 3 to 7g), 10g • Hou-po (Cortex Magnoliae Officinalis, 4 to 11g), 12g • Mu-gua (Fructus Chaenomelis, 5 to 11g), 12g • Mu-xiang (Radix Aucklaridiae/Radix Saussureae, 2 to 6g), 6g

## Formula

### SHI-QUAN-DA-BU-WAN
(0182A)

### Ingredients
Bai-shao-yao (Radix Paeoniae Alba, 5 to 11g), 12g • Bai-zhu (Rhizoma Atractylodis Macrocephalae, 5 to 11g), 10g • Chuanxiong (Rhizoma Ligustici Chuanxiong, 2 to 6g), 6g • Dang-gui (Radix Angelicae Sinensis, 5 to 11g), 12g • Dang-shen (Radix Codonopsis Pilosulae, 11 to 15g), 10g • Fu-ling (Poria, 7 to 14g), 12g • Gan-cao (Radix Glycyrrhizae, 2 to 11g), 3g • Huang-qi (Radix Astragali Seu Hedysari, 5 to 40g), 12g • Rougui (Cortex Cinnamomi, 1 to 5g), 4g • Shu-di-huang (Radix Rehmanniae Praeparatae, 11 to 18g), 15g

## Formula

### SHI-XIAO-SAN
(0201)

### Ingredients
(Use equal quantities of both ingredients.) Pu-huang (Polien Typhae, 5 to 11g) • Wu-ling-zhi (Faeces Trogopterorum, 5 to 11g)

### Instructions
Grind into powder and take 6g of powder twice daily.

## Formula

### SHU-ZAO-YIN-ZI
(0134C)

### Ingredients
(Use 8g of each ingredient.) Bing-lang (Semen Areca, 4 to 11g) • Chi-xiao-dou (Semen Phaseoli, 11 to 18g) • Da-fu-pi (Pericarpium Arecae, 5 to 18g) • Fu-ling-pi (Poria, outer skin, 10 to 18g) • Jiang-pi (Exocarpium Zingiberis (Recens, 15 to 45g) • Jiao-mu (Semen Zanthoxyli, 8g) • Mu-tong (Caulis Aristolochiae, 4 to 8g) • Qiang-huo (Rhizoma Seu Radix Notopterygii, 4 to 10g) • Qin-jiao (Radix Gentianae Macrophyllae, 4 to 11g) • Shang-lu (Radix Phytolaccae, 2 to 5g) • Ze-xie (Rhizoma Alismatis, 7 to 14g)

## Formula

### SI-HAI-SHU-YU-WAN
(0993)

### Ingredients
Chen-pi (Pericarpium Citri Reticulatae Viride, 4 to 11g), 9g • Ge-li-fen (Clam-Shell Powder, 3 to 10g), 9g • Hai-dai (Seaweed, 5 to 10g), 60g • Hai-piao-xiao (Os Sepiellae Seu Sepiae, 5 to 11g), 60g • Hai-zao (Sargassum 5 to 11g), 60g • Kun-bu (Thallus Laminariae Seu Eckloniae, 5 to 11g), 60g • Qing-mu-xiang (Radix Aristolochiae, 4 to 11g), 15g

### Instructions
Grind into powder and take 6g of powder twice daily.

## Formula

### SI-JUN-ZI TANG
(0080)

### Ingredients
Bai-zhu (Rhizoma Atractylodis Macrocephalae, 5 to 11g), 10g • Fu-ling (Poria, 7 to 14g), 12g • Gan-cao (Radix Glycrrhizae, 2 to 11g), 3g • Ren-shen (Radix Ginseng, 1 to 35g), 15g

## Formula

### SI-NI-JIA-REN-SHEN-TANG
(0317C)

*Ingredients*
Fu-zi (Radix Aconiti Praeparata, 4 to 11g), 15 to 30g • Gan-cao, zhi-gan-cao (Radix Glycyrrhizae, 2 to 11g), 12g • Gan-jiang (Rhizoma Zingiberis, 3 to 7g), 9g • Ren-shen (Radix Ginseng, 1 to 35g), flexible quantity

## Formula

### SI-NI-SAN
(0178)

*Ingredients*
Chai-hu (Radix Bupleuri, 4 to 16g), 12g • Chi-shao-yao (Radix Paeoniae Rubra, 5 to 11g), 30 to 100g • Gan-cao (Radix Glycyrrhizae, 2 to 11g), 6g • Zhi-shi (Fructus Auranth Immaturus, 4 to 7g), 12g

*Instructions*
Grind into powder and take 6g of powder twice daily.

## Formula

### SI-NI-TANG
(0317)

*Ingredients*
Fu-zi (Radix Aconiti Praeparata, 4 to 11g), 15 to 30g • Gan-cao, zhi-gan-cao (Radix Glycyrrhizae, 2 to 11g), 12g •Gan-jiang (Rhizoma Zingiberis, 3 to 7g), 9g

## Formula

### SI-SHEN-WAN
(0169)

*Ingredients*
Bu-gu-zhi (Fructus Psoraleae, 4 to 11g), 120g • Rou-dou-kou (Semen Myristicae, 2 to 8g), 60g • Wu-wei-zi (Fructus Schisandrae, 2 to 4g), 60g • Wu-zhu-yu (Fructus Euodiae, 2 to 7g), 30g

*Instructions*
Grind into powder to make tablets and take 6g of tablets each time.

## Formula

### SI-SHENG-WAN
(0984)

*Ingredients*
Ai-ye (Folium Artemisiae Argyi, 4 to 11g), 60g • Ce-bai-ye (Caumen Biotae, 7 to 14g), 60g • He-ye (Folium Nelumbinis, 4 to 11g), 60g • Sheng-di (Radix Rehmanniae, 14 to 35g), 60g

*Instructions*
Grind into powder and take 6g of powder twice daily.

## Formula

### SI-WU-TANG
(0196)

*Ingredients*
Bai-shao-yao (Radix Paeoniae Alba, 5 to 11g), 24g • Chuan-xiong (Rhizoma Ligustici Chuanxiong, 2 to 6g), 3g • Dang-gui (Radix Angelicae Sinensis, 5 to 11g), 12g • Shu-di-huang (Radix Rehmanniae Praeparatae, 11 to 18g), 20g

## Formula

### SU-HE-XIANG-WAN
(0292)

*Ingredients*
An-xi-xiang (Benzoinum, 0.3 to 2g), 60g • Bai-zhu (Rhizoma Atractylodis Macrocephalae, 5 to 11g), 60g • Bi-bo (Fructus, Piperis Longi, 2 to 4g), 60g • Bing-pian (Borneol, 0.2 to 0.3g), 60g • Chen-xiang (Lignum Aquilariae Resinatum, 1 to 4g), 60g • Ding-xiang (Flos Caryo-phylli, 1 to 4g), 60g • He-zi (Fructus Chebulae, 2 to 5g), 60g • Qing-mu-xiang (Radix Aristolochiae, 4 to 11g), 60g • Ru-xiang (Mastix/Resina, 4 to 11g), 30g • She-xiang (Moschus, 0.01 to 0.03g), 60g • Su-he-xiang (Styrax Liquidus oil, 0.5g), 30g • Tan-xiang (Lignum Santali Album, 2 to 4g), 60g • Xi-jiao (Cornu Rhinoceri, 1 to 2g), 60g • Xiang-fu (Rhizoma Cyperi, 5 to 11g), 60g • Zhu-sha (Cinna-baris, 0.3 to 1g), 60g

*Instructions*
Grind into powder to make tablets and take half to one tablet or 3geach time.

## Formula

### SUO-NIAO-WAN
(0334)

*Ingredients*
(Use equal quantities of both ingredients.) Wu-yao (Radix Linderae, 5 to 10g) • Yi-zhi-ren (Fructus Zigiberis Nigri, 4 to 11g)

*Instructions*
Decoct Shan-Yao powder in

wine and grind the ingredients into powder. Use the decoction to make tablets, with each one the size of a Chinese parasol seed, called wu-tong-zi. Take 6g of tablets each time.

## Formula

### TAI-WU-SHEN-ZHU-SAN
(2164)

### Ingredients
Cang-zhu (Rhizoma Atractylodis, 4 to 11g), 30g • Chen-pi (Pericarpium Citri Reticulatae, 4 to 11g), 30g • Da-zao (Fructus Ziziphi Jujubae, 7 to 18g), 40g • Hou-po (Cortex Magnoliae Officinalis, 4 to 11g), 30g • Huo-xiang (Herba Agastachis, 5 to 11g), 30g • Sheng-jiang (Rhizoma Zingiberis Recens, 4 to 10g), 35g • Shi-chang-pu (Rhizoma Acori Graminei, 2 to 5g), 20g

### Instructions
Grind into powder and take 9g of powder twice daily.

## Formula

### TAO-HONG-SI-WU-TANG
(0196G)

### Ingredients
Bai-shao-yao (Radix Paeoniae Alba, 5 to 11g), 24g • Chuan-xiong (Rhizoma Ligustici Chuanxiong, 2 to 6g), 3g • Dang-gui (Radix Angelicae Sinensis, 5 to 11g), 12g • Hong-hua (Flos Carthami, 4 to 7g), 3g • Shu-di-huang (Radix Rehmanniae Praeparatae, 11 to 18g), 20g • Tao-ren (Semen Persicae, 5 to 11g), 3g

## Formula

### TAO-REN-FU-SU-FANG
(3373)

### Ingredients
Da-huang (Radix Et Rhizoma Rhei, 4 to 15g), 10g • Gan-cao (Radix Glycyrrhizae, 2 to 11g), 6g • Gui-zhi (Ramulus Cinnamomi, 2 to 10g), 10g • Mu-li (Concha Ostrae, 11 to 35g), 30g • Shi-chang-pu (Rhizoma Acori Graminei, 2 to 5g), 10g • Tao-ren (Semen Persicae, 5 to 11g), 10g • Wu-gong (Scolopendra, 0.1 to 0.2g), 10g • Xuan-ming-fen (Mirabilitum Dehydratum, 4 to 11g), 10g • Yuan-zhi (Radix Polygalae, 4 to 11g), 10g • Zhu-sha (Cinnabaris, 0.3 to 1g), 15g

## Formula

### TIAN WANG-BU-XIN-DAN
(0920)

### Ingredients
Bai-zi-ren (Semen Biotae, 4 to 11g), 30g • Dan-shen (Radix Salviae Miltiorrhizae, 5 to 10g), 15g • Dang-gui (Radix Angelicae Sinensis, 5 to 11g), 30g • Fu-ling (Poria, 7 to 14g), 15g • Jie-geng (Radix Platycodi, 2 to 5g), 15g • Mai-men-dong (Radix Ophiopogonis, 5 to 11g), 30g • Ren-shen (Radix Ginseng, 1 to 35g), 15g • Sheng-di (Radix Rehmanniae, 14 to 35g), 120g • Suan-zao-ren (Semen Ziziphi Spinosae, 7 to 18g), 30g • Tian-dong (Radix Asparagi, 7 to 14g), 30g • Wu-wei-zi (Fructus Schis-andrae, 2 to 4g), 30g • Xuan-shen (Radix Scrophulariae, 7 to 35g), 15g • Yuan-zhi (Radix Polygalae, 4 to 11g),

15g • Zhu-sha (Cinnabaris, 0.3 to 1g), 1.5g

### Instructions
Grind into powder to make tablets with honey and take 9g of tablets twice daily.

## Formula

### TONG-GUAN-WAN
(0732)

### Ingredients
Huang-bai (Cortex Phellodendri, 4 to 15g), 30g • Rou-gui (Cortex Cinnamomi, 1 to 5g), 1.5g • Zhi-mu (Rhizoma Anemarrhenae, 4 to 15g), 30g

## Formula

### TONG-QIAO-HUO-XUE-TANG
(0214)

### Ingredients
Chi-shao-yao (Radix Paeoniae Rubra, 5 to 11g), 9g • Chuan-xiong (Rhizoma Ligustici Chuanxiong, 2 to 6g), 9g • Da-zao (Fructus Ziziphi Jujubae, 7 to 18g), 9g • Hong-hua (Flos Carthami, 4 to 7g), 9g • She-xiang (Moschus, 0.01 to 0.03g), 0.3g • Sheng-jiang (Rhizoma Zingiberis Recens, 4 to 10g), 9g • Tao-ren (Semen Persicae, 5 to 11g), 9g, Old green onion, three roots

## Formula

### TONG-XIE-YAO-FANG

*Ingredients*
Bai-shao-yao (Radix Paeoniae Alba, 5 to 11g), 20g • Bai-zhu (Rhizoma Atractylodis Macrocephalae, 5 to 11g), 12g • Chen-pi (Pericarpium Papaveris, 4 to 11g), 9g • Fang-feng (Radix Ledebouriellae, 5 to 10g), 6g

*Formula*

## WEI-JING-TANG
(0037)

*Ingredients*
Dong-gua-ren (Semen Benincasae, 3 to 14g), 24g • Lu-jing (Caulis Phragmitis, 15gto 35g) 60 to 120g • Tao-ren (Semen Persicae, 5 to 11g), 9g • Yi-yi-ren (Semen Coicis, 11 to 22g), 30g

*Formula*

## WEI-LING-TANG
(0117F)

*Ingredients*
Bai zhu (Rhizoma Atractylodis Macrocephalae, 5 to 11g), 9g • Cang-zhu (Rhizoma Atractylodis Macrocephalae, 4 to 11g), 10g • Chen-pi (Pericarpium Papaveris, 4 to 11g), 10g • Fu-ling (Poria, 7 to 14g), 12g • Gan-cao (Radix Glycyrrhizae, 2 to 11g), 3g • Gui-zhi (Ramulus Cinnamomi, 2 to 10g), 9g • Hou-po (Cortex Magnoliae Officinalis, 4 to 11g), 10g • Ze-xie (Rhiozoma Alismatis, 7 to 14g), 15g • Zhu-ling (Polyporus Umbellatus, 7 to 14g), 12g

*Formula*

## WEN DAN TANG
(0124)

*Ingredients*
Ban-xia (Rhizoma Pinelliae, 4 to 12g), 12g • Chen-pi (Pericarpium Papaveris, 4 to 11g), 10g • Fu-ling (Poria, 7 to 14g), 12g • Gan-cao (Radix Glycyrrhizae, 2 to 11g), 3g • Zhi-shi (Fructus Aurantii Immaturus, 4 to 7g), 6g • Zhu-ru (Caulis Bambusae in Taeniam, 5 to 11g), 10g

*Formula*

## WEN-FEI-ZHI-LIU-DAN
(0807)

*Ingredients*
Gan-cao (Radix Glycyrrhizae, 2 to 11g), 4g • He-zi (Fructus Chebulae, 2 to 5g), 4g • Jie-geng (Radix Platycodi, 2 to 5g), 12g • Jing-jie (Herba Schizonepetae, 5 to 10g), 2g • Ren-shen (Radix Ginseng, 1 to 35g), 2g • Xi-xin (Herba Asari, 1 to 4g), 2g

*Formula*

## WEN-PI-TANG
(0158)

*Ingredients*
Da-Huang (Radix Et Rhizoma Rhei, 4 to 15g), 12g • Fu-zi (Radix Aconiti Praeparata, 4 to 11g), 15g • Gan-cao (Radix Glycyrrhizae, 2 to 11g), 6g • Gan-jiang (Rhizoma Zingiberis, 3 to 7g), 10g • Ren-shen (Radix Ginseng, 1 to 35g), 6g

*Formula*

## WU-HU-ZHUI-FENG-SAN
(0250)

*Ingredients*
Chan-tui (Periostracum Cicadae, 2 to 5g), 30g • Jiang-can (Bombyx Batryticatus, 5 to 11g), seven pieces • Quan-xie (Scorpio, 2 to 5g), seven insects • Tian-ma (Rhizoma Gastrodiae, 4 to 11g), 6g • Tian-nan-xing (Rhizoma Arisaematis, 2.5 to 5g), 6g • Zhu-sha (Cinnabaris, 0.3 to 1g), 1.5g

*Instructions*
Decoct the herbs; then strain and mix with 60g of yellow wine. Drink 1.5g of Zhu-Sha first, before drinking the decoction. Take once daily for three days.

*Formula*

## WU-LING-SAN
(0348)

*Ingredients*
Bai-zhu (Rhizoma Atractylodis Macrocephalae, 5 to 11g), 9g • Fu-ling (Poria, 7 to 14g), 12g • Gui-zhi (Ramulus Cinnamomi, 2 to 10g), 9g • Ze-xie (Rhizoma Alismatis, 7 to 14g), 15g • Zhu-ling (Polyporus Umbellatus, 7 to 14g), 12g

*Formula*

## WU-MO-YIN-ZI
(0433)

## Ingredients

(Use equal quantities of all ingredients.) Bing-lang (Semen Areca, 4 to 11g) • Chen-xiang (Lignum Aquilariae Resinatum, 1 to 4g) • Wu-Yao (Radix Linderae, 5 to 10g) • Zhi-shi (Fructus Aurantii Immaturus, 4 to 7g)

## Instructions

Grind into powder and take 6g of powder twice daily.

## Formula

### WU-PI-YIN
(0130)

## Ingredients

(Use equal quantities of all ingredients.) Chen-pi (Pericarpium Papaveris, 4 to 11g) • Da-fu-pi (Pericarpium Papaveris/Fructus Papaveris Arecae, 5 to 18g) • Fu-ling-pi (Poria, outer skin, 10 to 18g) • Sang-bai-pi (Cortex Mori Radicis, 5 to 11g) • Sheng-jiang (Rhizoma Zingiberis Recens, 4 to 10g)

## Formula

### WU-TOU-TANG
(0465)

## Ingredients

Bai-shao-yao (Radix Paeoniae Alba, 5 to 11g), 9g • Chuan-wu (Radix Aconiti, 1.5 to 5g), 15g • Gan-cao (Radix Glycyrrhizae, 2 to 11g), 9g • Huang-qi (Radix Astragali Seu Hedysari 5 to 40g), 15g • Ma-Huang (Herba Ephedrae, 5 to 10g), 8g

## Formula

### WU-WEI-DI-HUANG-TANG
(2157)

## Ingredients

Gou-qi-zi (Fructus Lych, 5 to 11g), 10g • Ren-shen (Radix Ginseng, 1 to 35g), 24g • Shan-zhu-yu (Fructus Corni, 5 to 11g), 10g • Shu-di-huang (Radix Rehmanniae Praeparatae, 11 to 18g), 15g • Tian-dong (Radix Asparagi, 7 to 14g), 10g

## Formula

### WU-ZHU-YU-TANG
(0185)

## Ingredients

Da-zao (Fructus Ziziphi Jujubae, 7 to 18g), 9g • Ren-shen (Radix Ginseng, 1 to 35g), 9g • Sheng-jiang (Rhizoma Zingiberis Recens, 4 to 10g), 9g • Wu-zhu-yu (Fructus Euodiae, 2 to 7g), 9g

## Formula

### WU-ZI-YAN-ZONG-WAN
(0915)

## Ingredients

Che-qian-zi (Semen Plantaginis, 4 to 11g), 60g • Fu-pen-zi (Fructus Rubi, 5 to 11g), 120g • Gou-qi-zi (Fructus Lych, 5 to 11g), 240g • Tu-si-zi (Semen Cuscutae, 5 to 11g), 240g • Wu-wei-zi (Fructus Schisandrae, 2 to 4g), 30g

## Instructions

Grind into powder to make tablets with honey and take 9g of tablets twice daily.

## Formula

### XI-GAN-SAN
(3376)

## Ingredients

(Use equal quantities of all ingredients.) Da-huang (Radix Et Rhizoma Rhei, 4 to 15g), 50g • Dang-gui (Radix Angelicae Sinensis, 5 to 11g), 50g • Fang-feng (Radix Ledebouriellae, 5 to 10g), 50g • Huang-qin (Radix Scutellariae, 4 to 15g), 50g • Qiang-huo (Rhizoma Seu Radix Notopterygii, 4 to 10g), 50g • Xuan-shen (Radix Scrophulariae, 7 to 35g), 50g

## Instructions

Grind into powder and take 9g of powder twice daily.

## Formula

### XI-JIAO-DI-HUANG-TANG
(0285)

## Ingredients

Chi-shao-yao (Radix Paeoniae Rubra, 5 to 11g), 12g • Mu-dan-pi (Cortex Moutan Radicis, 5 to 11g), 9g • Sheng-di (Radix Rehmanniae, 14 to 35g), 30g • Xi-jiao (Cornu Rhinoceri, 1 to 2g), 9g

## Formula

### XI-XIN-TANG
(1147)

## Ingredients

Chong-wei-zi (Fructus Leonuri,

5 to 11g), 60g • Da-huang (Radix
Et Rhizoma Rhei, 4 to 15g), 30g
• Fang-feng (Radix Ledebouriel-
lae, 5 to 10g), 60g • Jie-geng
(Radix Platycodi, 2 to 5g), 60g
• Ling-yang-jiao (Cornu Antelop-
is, 1 to 1.5g), 10g • Xi-xin (Herba
Asari, 1 to 4g), 60g • Xuan-shen
(Radix Scrophulariae, 7 to 35g),
60g • Zhi-mu (Rhizoma Ane-
marrhenae, 4 to 15g), 60g

*Instructions*
Grind into powder and take 6g
of powder twice daily.

*Formula*

## XIANG-SHA-LIU-JUN-ZI-TANG
(0080D)

*Ingredients*
Bai-zhu (Rhizoma Atractylodis
Macrocephalae, 5 to 11g), 10g •
Ban-xia (Rhizoma Pinelliae, 4 to
12g), 7g • Chen-pi (Pericarpium
Papaveris, 4 to 11g), 7g • Fu-ling
(Poria, 7 to 14g), 12g • Gan-cao
(Radix Glycyrrhizae, 2 to 11g),
3g • Mu-xiang (Radix Aucklan-
diae/Radix Saussureae, 2 to 6g),
7g • Ren-shen (Radix Ginseng,
1 to 35g), 15g • Sha-ren (Fructus Amomi, 2 to 7g), 5g

*Formula*

## XIAO-BAN-XIA-JIA-FU-LING-TANG
(0093A)

*Ingredients*
Ban-xia (Rhizoma Pinelliae, 4 to
12g), 15g • Fu-ling (Poria, 7 to
14g), 9g • Sheng-jiang (Rhizoma
Zingiberis Recens, 4 to 10g), 9g

*Formula*

## XIAO-BAN-XIA-TANG
(0093)

*Ingredients*
Ban-xia (Rhizoma Pinelliae, 4 to
12g), 15g • Sheng-jiang (Rhizoma
Zingiberis Recens, 4 to 10g), 9g

*Formula*

## XIAO-CHAI-HU-TANG
(0255)

*Ingredients*
Ban-xia (Rhizoma Pinelliae, 4
to 12g), 9g • Chai-hu (Radix
Bupleuri, 4 to 16g), 15g • Da-
Zao (Fructus Ziziphi Jujubae,
7 to 18g), four dates • Gan-cao
(Radix Glycyrrhizae, 2 to 11g),
3g • Huang-qin (Radix Scutel-
lariae, 4 to 15g), 12g • Ren-shen
(Radix Ginseng, 1 to 35g), 9g
• Sheng-Jiang (Rhizoma Zin-
giberis Recens, 4 to 10g), 9g

*Formula*

## XIAO-FENG-SAN
(0014)

*Ingredients*
Bo-he (Herba Menthae, 3 to
10g), 9g • Chan-tui (Perios-
tracum Cicadae, 2 to 5g), 9g
• Chen-pi (Pericarpium Citri
Reticulatae, 4 to 11g), 6g •
Chuan-xiong (Rhizoma Ligusti-
ci Chuanxiong, 2 to 6g), 9g •
Dang-shen (Radix Codonopsis
Pilosulae, 11 to 15g), 20g • Fang-

feng (Radix Ledebouriellae, 5
to 10g), 9g • Fu-ling (Poria, 7
to 14g), 9g • Hou-po (Cortex
Magnolia Officinalis, 4 to 11g),
6g • Jiang-can (Bombyx Batryticatus, 5 to 11g), 9g • Jing-jie
(Herba Schizonepetae, 5 to 10g),
9g • Qiang-huo (Rhizoma Seu
Radix Notopterygii, 4 to 10g), 9g

*Formula*

## XIAO-JI-YIN-ZI
(0353)

*Ingredients*
Dan-zhu-ye (Herba Lophatheri,
4 to 11g), 9g • Dang-gui (Radix
Angelicae Sinesis, 5 to 11g), 6g
• Gan-cao (Radix Glycyrrhizae,
2 to 11g), 3g • Hua-shi (Talcum,
11 to 15g), 15g • Mu-tong (Caulis
Aristolochiae, 4 to 8g), 12g • Ou-
jie (Nodus Nelumbinis Rhizoma-
tis, 5 to 11g), 15g • Pu-huang
(Pollen Typhae, 5 to 11g), 9g •
Sheng-di (Radix Rehmanniae,
14 to 35g), 15g • Xiao-ji (Herba
Cephalanoploris, 6 to 11g), 15g
• Zhi-zi (Fructus Gardeniae, 7
to 16g), 9g

*Formula*

## XIAO-KE-FANG
(0704)

*Ingredients*
Huang-lian (Rhizoma Coptidis,
2 to 12g), 8g • Sheng-di (Radix
Rehmanniae, 14 to 35g), 30g •
Tian-hua fen (Radix Trichosan-
this, 10 to 14g), 12g

*Instructions*
Grind into powder and take 9g of
powder with honey twice daily.

## Formula

### XIAO-YAO-SAN
(0229)

*Ingredients*
Bai-shao-yao (Radix Paeoniae Alba, 5 to 11g), 30g • Bai-zhu (Rhizoma Atractylodis Macrocephalae, 5 to 11g), 9g • Chai-hu (Radix Bupleuri, 4 to 16g), 9g • Dang-Gui (Radix Angelicae Sinensis, 5 to 11g), 9g • Fu-ling (Poria, 7 to 14g), 15g • Gan cao (Radix Glycyrrhizae, 2 to 11g), 6g

## Formula

### XIAO-ZHI-TANG
(3377)

*Ingredients*
Fu-ling (Poria, 7 to 14g), 15g • He-ye (Folium Nelumbinis, 4 to 11g), 12g • Ju-hua (Flos Chrysanthemi, 4 to 20g), 12g • Jue-ming-zi (Semen Cassiae, 7 to 18g), 15g • Ren-dong-teng (Caulis Lonicerae, 11 to 35g), 15g • Yi-yi-ren (Semen Coicis, 11 to 22g), 15g • Yu-mi-xu (Stigma Maydis, 30 to 60g), 10g • Ze-xie (Rhizoma Alismatis, 7 to 14g), 12g

## Formula

### XIE-GAN-AN-SHEN-WAN
(3372)

*Ingredients*
Bai-zi-ren (Semen Biotae, 4 to 11g), 10g • Che-qian-zi (Semen Plantaginis, 4 to 11g), 10g • Ci-ji-li (Fructus Tribli, 7 to 10g), 10g • Dang-gui (Radix Angelicae Sinesis, 5 to 11g), 10g • Fu-shen (Buyury with pine root, 11 to 15g), 10g • Gan-cao (Radix Glycyrrhizae, 2 to 11g), 3g • Huang-qin (Radix Scutellariae, 4 to 15g), 10g • Long-dan (Radix Gentianae, 7 to 10g), 10g • Long-gu (Os Draconis, 11 to 18g), 10g • Mai-men-dong (Radix Ophiopogonis, 5 to 11g), 10g • Mu-li (Concha Ostrae, 11 to 35g), 10g • Sheng-di (Radix Rehmanniae, 14 to 35g), 30g • Shi-jue-ming (Concha Haliotids, 11 to 35g), 30g • Suan-zao-ren (Semen Ziziphi Sinosae, 7 to 18g), 10g • Yuan-zhi (Radix Polygalae, 4 to 11g), 10g • Ze-xie (Rhizoma Alismatis, 7 to 14g), 10g • Zhen-zhu-mu (Concha Margaritifera Usta, 10 to 30g), 30g • Zhi-zi (Fructus Gardeniae, 7 to 16g), 10g

## Formula

### XIE-XIN-TANG
(0367)

*Ingredients*
Da-haung (Radix Et Rhizoma Rhei, 4 to 15g), 9g • Huang-lian (Rhizoma Coptidis, 2 to 12g), 6g • Huang-qin (Radix Scutellariae, 4 to 15g), 6g

## Formula

### XIN-JIA-XIANG-RU-YIN
(0012 C)

*Ingredients*
Bian-dou-hua (Flos Dolichoris, 5 to 11g), 12g • Hou-po (Cortex Magnoliae Officinalis, 4 to 11g), 9g • Jin-yin-hua (Flos Lonicerae, 7 to 18g), 12g • Lian-qiao (Fructus Forsythiae, 5 to 11g), 9g • Xiang-ru (Herba Elsholtziae Seu Moslae, 4 to 10g), 9g

## Formula

### XING-SU-SAN
(0046)

*Ingredients*
Ban-xia (Rhizoma Pinelliae, 4 to 12g), 10g • Da-zao (Fructus Ziziphi Jujubae, 7 to 18g), three dates • Fu-ling (Poria, 7 to 14g), 12g • Gan-cao (Radix Glycyrrhizae, 2 to 11g), 2g • Jie-geng (Radix Platycodi, 2 to 5g), 6g • Ju-pi (Tangerine peel, 3 to 17g), 6g • Qian-hu (Radix Peucedani, 5 to 11g), 6g • Sheng-jiang (Rhizoma Zingiberis Recens, 4 to 10g), 6g • Xing-ren (Semen Armeniacae Amarae, 5 to 11g), 9g • Zhi-qiao (Fructus Aurantii, 4 to 11g), 6g • Zi-su-ye (Folium Perillae, 5 to 10g), 6g

## Formula

### XUAN-FU-DAI-ZHE-TANG
(0096)

*Ingredients*
Ban-xia (Rhizoma Pinelliae, 4 to 12g), 12g • Da-zao (Fructus Ziziphi Jujubae, 7 to 18g), four dates • Dai-zhe-shi (Ocherum Rubrum, 1 to 35g), 30g • Gan-cao (Radix Glycyrrhizae, 2 to 11g), 6g • Ren-shen (Radix Ginseng, 1 to 35g), 9g • Sheng-jiang (Rhizoma Zingiberis Recens, 4 to 10g), 9g • Xuan-fu-hua (Flos Inulae, 4 to 11g), 15g

## XUE-FU-ZHU-YU-TANG
(0198)

Chai-hu (Radix Bupleuri, 4 to 16g), 9g • Chi-shao-yao (Radix Paeoniae Rubra, 5 to 11g), 9g • Chuan-xiong (Rhizoma Ligustici Chuanxiong, 2 to 6g), 6g • Dang-gui (Radix Angelicae Sinensis, 5 to 11g), 12g • Gan-cao (Radix Glycyrrhizae, 2 to 11g), 3g • Hong-hua (Flos Carthami, 4 to 7g), 9g • Jie-geng (Radix Platy-codi, 2 to 5g), 6g • Niu-xi (Radix Achyranthis Bidentatae, 5 to 11g), 12g • Sheng-di (Radix Rehmanniae, 14 to 35g), 12g • Tao-ren (Semen Persicae, 5 to 11g), 9g • Zhi-qiao (Fructus Aurantii, 4 to 11g), 9g

## YANG-JING-ZHONG-YU-TANG
(0652)

Bai-shao-yao (Radix Paeoniae Alba, 5 to 11g), 15g • Dang-gui (Radix Angelicae Sinensis, 5 to 11g), 15g • Shan-zhu-yu (Fructus Corni, 5 to 11g), 15g • Shu-di-huang (Radix Rehmanniae Praeparatae, 11 to 18g), 15g

## YANG-XIN-TANG
(1212)

Bai-zi-ren (Semen Biotae, 4 to 11g), 8g • Ban-xia-qu (Pinelliae mixture, 7 to 10g), 15g • Chuan-xiong (Rhizoma Ligustici Chuan-xiong, 2 to 6g), 15g • Dang-gui (Radix Angelicae Sinensis, 5 to 11g), 15g • Fu-ling (Poria, 7 to 14g), 15g • Fu-shen (Buyury with pine root, 11 to 15g), 15g • Gan-cao (Radix Glycyrrhizae, 2 to 11g), 12g • Huang-qi (Radix Astragali Seu Hedysari, 5 to 40g), 15g • Ren-shen (Radix Ginseng, 1 to 35g), 8g • Rou-gui (Cortex Cinnamomi, 1 to 5g), 8g • Suan-zao-ren (Semen Ziziphi Spin-osae, 7 to 18g), 8g • Wu-wei-zi (Fructus Schisandrae, 2 to 4g), 8g • Yuan-zhi (Radix Polygalae, 4 to 11g), 8g

## YANG-YIN-QING-FEI-TANG
(0050)

Bai-shao-yao (Radix Paeoniae Alba, 5 to 11g), 12g • Bo-he (Herba Menthae, 3 to 10g), 6g • Chuan-bei-mu (Bulbus Fritil-lariae Cirrhosae, 4 to 14g), 10g • Gan-cao (Radix Glycyrrhizae, 2 to 11g), 6g • Mai-men-dong (Radix Ophiopogonis, 5 to 11g), 20g • Mu-dan-pi (Cortex Moutan Radicis, 5 to 11g), 12g • Sheng-di (Radix Rehmanniae, 14 to 35g), 30g • Xuan-shen (Radix Scrophulariae, 7 to 35g), 24g

## YANG-YIN-TONG-BI-TANG
(2930)

Dang-shen (Radix Codonopsis Pilosulae, 11 to 15g), 12g • Gua-lou (Fructus Trichosanthis, 11 to 15g), 18g • Hong-hua (Flos Carthami, 4 to 7g), 6g • Mai-men-dong (Radix Ophio-pogonis, 5 to 11g), 12g • Nu-zhen-zi (Fructus Ligustri Luci-di, 5 to 11g), 15g • Sheng-di (Radix Rehmanniae, 14 to 35g), 18g • Tao-ren (Semen Persicae, 5 to 11g), 10g • Wu-wei-Zi (Fructus Schisandrae, 2 to 4g), 10g • Yan-hu-suo (Rhizoma Corydalis, 4 to 11g), 10g

## YI-GONG-SAN
(0533)

Bai-zhu (Rhizoma Atractylodis Macrocephalae, 5 to 11g), 10g • Chen-pi (Pericarpium Citri Reticulatae Viride, 4 to 11g), 10g • Fu-ling (Poria, 7 to 14g), 12g • Gan-cao (Radix Glycyrrhizae, 2 to 11g), 3g • Ren-shen (Radix Ginseng, 1 to 35g), 15g

## YI-GONG-SAN
(0240)

Chuan-lian-zi (Fructus Meliae Toosendan, 5 to 11g), 6g • Dang-gui (Radix Angelicae Sinensis, 5 to 11g), 9g • Gou-qi-zi (Fructus Lycii, 5 to 11g), 9g • Mai-men-dong (Radix Ophiopogonis, 5 to 11g), 9g • Nan-sha-shen (Radix Adenophorae, 5 to 11g), 9g • Sheng-di (Radix Rehmanniae, 14 to 35g), 18g

## Formula

### YI-WEI-TANG
(0136)

#### Ingredients
Bing-tang (Rock Sugar, flexible g), flexible quantity • Mai-men-dong (Radix Ophiopogonis, 5 to 11g), 15g • Nan-sha-shen (Radix Adenophorae, 5 to 11g), 10g • Sheng-di (Radix Rehmanniae, 14 to 35g), 30g • Yu-zhu (Rhizoma Polygonati Odorath, 5 to 11g), 10g

## Formula

### YI-YI-REN-TANG
(1477)

#### Ingredients
Cang-zhu (Rhizoma Atractylodis Macrocephalae, 4 to 11g), 11g • Cao-wu (Radix Aconiti/ Radix Aconiti Kusnezoffi, 2 to 5g), 5g • Chuan-xiong (Rhizoma Ligustici Chuanxiong, 2 to 6g), 6g • Dang-gui (Radix Angelicae Sinensis, 5 to 11g), 11g • Du-huo (Radix Angelicae Pubescentis, 2 to 5g), 5g • Fang-feng (Radix Ledbouriellae, 5 to 10g), 10g • Gan-cao (Radix Glycyrrhizae, 2 to 11g), 11g • Gui-zhi (Ramulus Cinnamomi, 2 to 10g), 10g • Ma-huang (Herba Ephedrae, 5 to 10g), 10g • Qiang-huo (Rhizoma Seu Radix Notopterygii, 4 to 10g), 10g • Sheng-jiang (Rhizoma Zingiberis Recens, 4 to 10g), 10g • Yi-yi-ren (Semen Coicis, 11 to 22g), 22g

#### Instructions
Grind into powder and take 6g of powder twice daily.

## Formula

### YIN-CHEN-HAO-TANG
(0261)

#### Ingredients
Da-huang (Radix Et Rhizoma Rhei, 4 to 15g), 9g • Yin-chen (Herba Artemisiae Scopariae, 7 to 21g), 60g • (Fructus Gardeniae, 7 to 16g), 9g

## Formula

### YIN-CHEN-WU-LING SAN
(0348B)

#### Ingredients
Bai-zhu (Rhizoma Atractylodis Macrocephalae, 5 to 11g), 9g • Fu-ling (Poria, 7 to 14g), 12g • Gui-zhi (Ramulus Cinnamomi, 2 to 10g), 9g • Yin-chen-hao (Herba Artemisiae Capillaris, 10 to 18g), 9g • Ze-xie (Rhizoma Alismatis, 7 to 14g), 15g • Zhu-ling (Polyporus Umbellatus, 7 to 14g), 12g

## Formula

### YIN-CHEN-ZHU-FU-TANG
(0656)

#### Ingredients
Bai-zhu (Rhizoma Atractylodis Macrocephalae, 5 to 11g), 6g • Fu-zi (Radix Aconiti Praeparata, 4 to 11g), 2g • Gan-cao (Radix Glycyrrhizae, 2 to 11g), 3g • Gan-jiang (Rhizoma Zingiberis, 3 to 7g), 2g • Rou-gui (Cortex Cinnamomi, 1 to 5g), 1g • Yin-chen (Herba Artemisiae Capillaris/Herba Artemisiae Scopariae Scopariae, 7 to 21g), 3g

## Formula

### YIN-QIAO-SAN
(0015)

#### Ingredients
Bo-he (Herba Menthae, 3 to 10g), 18g • Dou-chi (Semen Sojae Praeparatum, 10 to 15g), 15g • Gan-cao (Radix Glycyrrhizae, 2 to 11g), 9g • Jie-geng (Radix Platycodi, 2 to 5g), 6g • Jin-yin-hua (Flos Lonicerae, 7 to 18g), 30g • Jing-jie (Herba Schizonepetae, 5 to 10g), 18g • Lian-qiao (Fructus Forsythiae, 5 to 11g), 30g • Lu-gen (Rhizoma Phragmitis, 15 to 65g), 30g • Niu-bang-zi (Fructus Arctii, 6 to 10g), 18g • Zhu-ye (Folium Bambusae, 4 to 20g), 12g

## Formula

### YOU-GUI-WAN
(0963)

#### Ingredients
Dang-gui (Radix Angelicae Sinensis, 5 to 11g), 90g • Du-zhong (Cortex Eucommiae, 7 to 11g), 120g • Fu-zi (Radix Aconiti Praeparata, 4 to 11g), 60g • Gou-qi-zi (Fructus Lych, 5 to 11g), 120g • Lu jiao-jiao (Colla Cornus Cervi, Xg), 120g • Rou-gui (Cortex Cinnamomi, 1 to 5g), 60g • Shan-yao (Rhizoma Dioscoreae Bulbiferae, 10 to 20g), 120g • Shan-zhu-yu (Fructus Corni, 5 to 11g), 90g • Shu-di-huang (Radix Rehmanniae Praeparatae, 11 to 18g), 240g • Tu-si-zi (Semen Cuscutae, 5 to 11g), 120g

#### Instructions
Grind into powder to make

tablets and take 15g of tablets twice daily.

*Formula*

## YOU-GUI-YIN
(0331D)

*Ingredients*
Du-zhong (Cortex Eucommiae, 7 to 11g), 120g • Fu-zi (Radix Aconiti Praeparata, 4 to 11g), 30g • Gan-cao (Radix Glycyrrhizae, 2 to 11g), 15g • Gan-di (Dried Radix Rehmanniae, 11 to 18g), 240g • Gou-qi-zi (Fructus Lych, 5 to 11g), 120g • Rou-gui (Cortex Cinnamomi, 1 to 5g), 30g • Shan-yao (Rhizoma Dioscoreae, 10 to 20g), 120g • Shan-zhu-yu (Fructus Corni, 5 to 11g), 120g

*Instructions*
Grind into powder to make tablets with honey. Take 9g of tablets one to two times daily, with warm or lightly salted water. Use reduced quantities of ingredients if decoction is done.

*Formula*

## YU-NU-JIAN
(0476)

*Ingredients*
Mai-men-dong (Radix Ophiopogonis, 5 to 11g), 6g • Nu-xi (Radix Achyranthis Bidentatae, 5 to 11g), 5g • Shi-gao (Gypsum Fibrosum, 10 to 70g), 30g • Shu-di-huang (Radix Rehmanniae Praeparatae, 11 to 18g), 15g • Zhi-mu (Rhizoma Anemarrhenae, 4 to 15g), 5g

*Formula*

## YU-PING-FENG-SAN
(0022)

*Ingredients*
Bai-zhu (Rhizoma Atractylodis Macrocephalae, 5 to 11g), 9g • Fang-feng (Radix Ledebouriellae, 5 to 10g), 9g • Huang-qi (Radix Astragali Seu Hedysari, 5 to 40g), 24g

*Formula*

## YUE-BI-JIA-ZHU-TANG
(0053)

*Ingredients*
Bai-zhu (Rhizoma Atractylodis Macrocephalae, 5 to 11g), 10g • Da-zao (Fructus Ziziphi Jujubae, 7 to 18g), 12g • Gan-cao (Radix Glycyrrhizae, 2 to 11g), 3g • Ma-huang (Herba Ephedrae, 5 to 10g), 10g • Sheng-jiang (Rhizoma Zingiberis Recens, 4 to 10g), 10g • Shi-gao (Gypsum Fibrosum, 10 to 70g), 40g

*Formula*

## YUE-BI-TANG
(0051)

*Ingredients*
Da-Zao (Fructus Ziziphi Jujubae, 7 to 18g), 10g • Gan-cao (Radix Glycyrrhizae, 2 to 11g), 6g • Ma-huang (Herba Ephedrae, 5 to 10g), 15g • Sheng-jiang (Rhizoma Zingiberis Recens, 4 to 10g), 9g • Shi-gao (Gypsum Fibrosum, 10 to 70g), 50g

*Formula*

## YUE-HUA-WAN
(0468)

*Ingredients*
Bai-bu (Radix Stemonae, 4 to 7g), 60g • Bei-sha-shen (Radix Glehniae, 5 to 11g), 60g • Chuan-bei-mu (Bulbus Fritillariae Thunbergii Cirrhosae, 4 to 14g), 21g • E-jiao (Colla Corii Asini, 5 to 11g), 21g • Fu-ling (Poria, 7 to 14g), 60g • Ju-hua (Flos Chrysanthemi, 4 to 20g), 60g • Mai-men-dong (Radix Ophiopogonis, 5 to 11g), 30g • San-qi (Radix Notoginseng, 2 to 10g), 15g • Sang-ye (Folium Mori, 5 to 10g), 60g • Shan-yao (Rhizoma Dioscoreae, 10 to 20g), 60g • Sheng-di (Radix Rehmanniae, 14 to 35g), 60g • Shu-di-huang (Radix Rehmanniae Praeparatae, 11 to 18g), 60g • Tian-Dong (Radix Asparagi, 7 to 14g), 30g

*Instructions*
Grind into powder and take 9g of powder twice daily.

*Formula*

## ZENG-YI-CHENG-QI-TANG
(0155)

*Ingredients*
Da-huang (Radix Et Rhizoma Rhei, 4 to 15g), 6g • Mai-men-dong (Radix Ophiopogonis, 5 to 11g), 12g • Pu-xiao Mirabilitum Depuratum, 5 to 11g), 5g • Sheng-di (Radix Rehmanniae, 14 to 35g), 24g • Xuan-shen (Radix Scrophulariae, 7 to 35g), 24g

中医疗法

## Formula

### ZENG-YI-TANG
(0138)

#### Ingredients

Mai-men-dong (Radix Ophio-pogonis, 5 to 11g), 24g • Sheng-di (Radix Rehmanniae (fresh), 14 to 35g), 24g • Xuan-shen (Radix Scrophulariae, 7 to 35g), 30g

## Formula

### ZHEN-GAN-XI-FENG-TANG
(0242)

#### Ingredients

Bai-shao-yao (Radix Paeoniae Alba, 5 to 11g), 15g • Chuan-lian-zi (Fructus Meliae Toosen-dan, 5 to 11g), 6g • Dai-zhe-shi (Ocherum Rubrum, 1 to 35g), 15g • Gan-cao (Radix Gly-cyrrhizae, 2 to 11g), 4g • Gui-ban (Plastrum Testudinis, 11 to 30g), 15g • Long-gu (Os Draco-nis, 11 to 18g), 15g • Mai-ya (Fructus Hordei Germinatus, 11 to 13g), 6g • Mu-li (Concha Ostrae, 11 to 35g), 15g • Niu-xi (Radix Achyranthis Bidentatae, 5 to 11g), 30g • Tian-dong (Radix Asparagi, 7 to 14g), 15g • Xuan-shen (Radix Scrophu-lariae, 7 to 35g), 15g • Yin-chen (Herba Artemisiae Scopariae, 7 to 21g), 15g

## Formula

### ZHEN-WU-TANG
(0347)

#### Ingredients

Bai-zhu (Rhizoma Atractylodis Macrocephalae, 5 to 11g), 9 to 15g • Chi-Shao-yao (Radix Paeo-niae Rubra, 5 to 11g), 9 to 18g • Fu-ling (Poria, 7 to 14g), 15 to 24g • Fu-zi (Radix Aconiti Prae-parata, 4 to 11g), 15 to 60g • Sheng-jiang (Rhizoma Zingiberis Recens, 4 to 10g), 9 to 18g

#### Instructions

Decoct fu-zi over low heat for half an hour, add the remaining ingredients to the decoction and divide into three doses for one-day consumption; drink it warm.

## Formula

### ZHI-BAI-DI-HUANG-WAN
(0327E)

#### Ingredients

Fu-ling (Poria, 7 to 14g), 90g • Huang-bai (Cortex Phelloden-dri, 4 to 15g), 90g • Mu-dan-pi (Cortex Moutan Radicis, 5 to 11g), 90g • Shan-yao (Rhizoma Dioscoreae, 10 to 20g), 120g • Shan-zhu-yu (Fructus Corni, 5 to 11g), 120g • Shu-di-huang (Radix Rehmanniae Praeparatae, 11 to 18g), 240g • Ze-xie (Rhi-zoma Alismatis, 7 to 14g), 90g • Zhi-mu (Rhizoma Anemar-rhenae, 4 to 15g), 90g

#### Instructions

Grind into powder to make tablets and take three tablets or 9gtwo to three times daily.

## Formula

### ZHI-BAO-DAN
(0288)

#### Ingredients

An-xi-xiang (Benzoinum, 0.3 to 2g), 45g • Bing-pian (Borneol, 0.2 to 0.3g), 3g • Dai-mao (Cara-pax Eretmochelydis, 4 to 7g), 30g • Hu-po (Succinum, 1 to 2g), 30g • Niu-huang (Calculus bovis, 0.2 to 0.5g), 15g • She-xiang (Moschus, 0.01 to 0.03g), 3g • Xi-jiao (Cornu Rhinoceri, 1 to 2g), 30g • Xiong-huang (Realgar, 0.3 to 1.5g), 30g • Zhu-sha (Cinnabaris, 0.3 to 1g), 30g

#### Instructions

Grind into powder to make tablets and take one tablet or 3geach time. (Patent medicine also available.)

## Formula

### ZHI-GAN-CAO-TANG
(0311)

#### Ingredients

Da-zao (Fructus Ziziphi Jujubae, 7 to 18g), 12g • E-jiao (Colla Corii Asini, 5 to 11g), 12g • Gan-cao, zhi-gan-cao (Radix Gly-cyrrhizae, 2 to 11g), 15g • Gui-zhi (Ramulus Cinnamomi, 2 to 10g), 9g • Huo-ma-ren (Fructus Cannabis, 11 to 17g), 15g • Mai-men-dong (Radix Ophiopogonis, 5 to 11g), 9g • Ren-shen (Radix Ginseng, 1 to 35g), 9g • Sheng-jiang (Rhizoma Zingiberis Recens, 4 to 10g), 9g • Shu-di-huang (Radix Rehmanniae Praeparatae, 11 to 18g), 30g

## Formula

### ZHI-SHI-DAO-ZHI-WAN
(0075)

#### Ingredients

Bai-zhu (Rhizoma Atractylodis Macrocephalae, 5 to 11g), 10g • Da-Huang (Radix Et Rhizoma Rhei, 4 to 15g), 10g • Fu-ling

(Poria, 7 to 14g), 10g • Huang-lian (Rhizoma Coptidis, 2 to 12g), 10g • Huang-qin (Radix Scutellariae, 4 to 15g), 10g • Shen-qu (Massa Medicata Fermentata, 7 to 15g), 12g • Ze-xie (Rhizoma Alismatis, 7 to 14g), 6g • Zhi-shi (Fructus Aurantii Immaturus, 4 to 7g), 10g

*Formula*

## ZHI-SHI-XIE-BAI-GUI-ZHI-TANG
(0215C)

*Ingredients*
Gua-lou (Fructus Trichosanthis, 11 to 15g), 24g • Gui-zhi (Ramulus Cinnamomi, 2 to 10g), 10g • Hou-po (Cortex Magnoliae Officinalis, 4 to 11g), 12g • Xie-bai (Bulbus Allii Macrostemi, 5 to 11g), 30g • Zhi-shi (Fructus Aurantii Immaturus, 4 to 7g), 12g

*Formula*

## ZHU-YE-SHI-GAO-TANG
(0545)

*Ingredients*
Ban-xia (Rhizoma Pinelliae, 4 to 12g), 12g • Gan-cao (Radix Glycyrrhizae, 2 to 11g), 6g • Jing-mi (polished rice, flexible quantity), 10g • Mai-men-dong (Radix Ophiopogonis, 5 to 11g) 30g • Ren-shen (Radix Ginseng, 1 to 35g), 6g • Shi-gao (Gypsum Fibrosum, 10 to 70g), 30g • Zhu-ye (Folium Bambusae, 4 to 20g), 10g

*Formula*

## ZI-SHEN-YANG-XUE-JIAN-BU-TANG
(3378)

*Ingredients*
Bai-shao-yao (Radix Paeoniae Alba, 5 to 11g), 12g • Dang-gui (Radix Angelicae Sinensis, 5 to 11g), 12g • Du-zhong (Cortex Eucommiae, 7 to 11g), 12g • Gou-qi-zi (Fructus Lycii, 5 to 11g), 12g • Gou-teng (Ramulus Uncariae Cum Uncis, 5 to 11g), 30g • Gui-ban (Plastrum Testudinis, 11 to 30g), 30g • Huang-qi (Radix Astragali Seu Hedysari, 5 to 40g), 30g • Jiang-can (Bombyx Batryticatus, 5 to 11g), 15g • Niu-xi (Radix Achyranthis Bidentatae, 5 to 11g), 15g • Rou-gui (Cortex Cinnamomi, 1 to 5g), 6g • Sha-wan-zi (Semen Astragalus, 7 to 11g), 12g • Shu-di-huang (Radix Rehmanniae Praeparatae, 11 to 18g), 30g • Tu-si-zi (Semen Cuscutae, 5 to 11g), 12g

*Formula*

## ZUO-GUI-WAN
(0962)

*Ingredients*
Gou-qi-zi (Fructus Lycii, 5 to 11g), 120g • Gui-ban-jiao (Colla Plastri Testudinis, 3 to 10g), 120g • Lu-jiao-jiao (Colla cornus Cervi, 6 to 12g), 120g • Niu-xi (Radix Achyranthis Bidentatae, 5 to 11g), 90g • Shan-yao (Rhizoma Dioscoreae Bulbiferae, 10 to 20g), 120g • Shan-zhu-yu (Fructus Corni, 5 to 11g), 120g • Shu-di-huang (Radix Rehmanniae Praeparatae, 11 to 18g), 240g • Tu-si-zi (Semen Cuscutae, 5 to 11g), 120g

*Instructions*
Grind into powder to make

tablets and take 9g of tablets twice daily.

*Formula*

## ZUO-GUI-YIN
(0328)

*Ingredients*
Fu-ling (Poria, 7 to 14g), 6g • Gan-cao, zhi-gan-cao (Radix Glycyrrhizae, 2 to 11g), 3g • Gou-qi-zi (Fructus Lycii, 5 to 11g), 6g • Shan-yao (Rhizoma Dioscoreae, 10 to 20g), 6g • Shan-zhu-yu (Fructus Corni, 5 to 11g), 3 to 6g(reduce in case of fear of cold) • Shu-di-huang (Radix Rehmanniae Praeparatae, 11 to 18g), 6 to 10g(or as much as 30 to 60g)

中医疗法

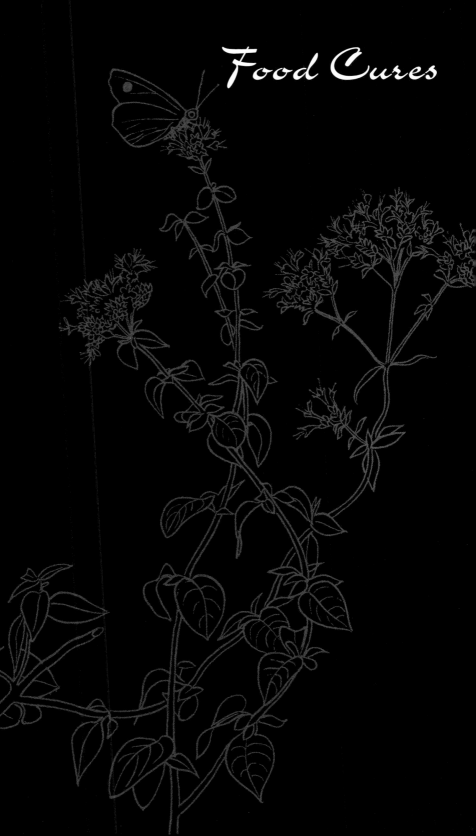

# Food Cures

## THE CHINESE DIET: DIFFERENCES FROM WESTERN DIET

There are two basic differences between Chinese and Western diets. First of all, Western diet focuses almost exclusively on diet for weight loss. Chinese diet is designed not only to help you lose weight but also to treat many other ailments, including hypertension, diabetes, common cold, gastritis, diarrhea, constipation, cough, hepatitis, psoriasis, common acne, eczema and so on.

# *Energies and Flavors of Foods*

In Chinese diet, for example, it is considered bad for someone with constipation to drink tea; it is good for someone with a cough to eat apple with honey. When I have a headache, I want to know which foods I should eat to cure my headache and which I should avoid to prevent my headache from becoming worse. When I have diarrhea or am suffering from diabetes, I want to know which foods I should eat to treat my symptoms and which to avoid to prevent my problems from becoming worse. When I am overweight, I want to know which foods I should eat to reduce my weight and which not to eat to avoid gaining more weight.

To lose weight, no doubt, is part of Chinese diet, but there are many other considerations as important as weight loss in the minds of Chinese dietitians. Recently, I read a diet book written by a well-known Western physician and to my great amazement, I found no information on dietary treatment of such symptoms as sore throat, hemorrhoids, hiccupping, vomiting, fever, toothache, psoriasis, stomachache and other ailments—all important treatments when using the Chinese diet.

The second difference between Chinese and Western diets: In Western diet, foods are considered for their protein, calorie, carbohydrate, vitamin and other nutrient content, but in Chinese diet, foods are considered for their flavors, energies, movements and common and organic actions. It works like this: If I feel cold in my body and limbs, naturally I like to eat something that will warm me; if I feel hot, something to cool me. If I have a weak stomach, naturally I like to eat something that will make my stomach stronger; if I feel my kidneys are weakening, something that will make my kidneys stronger. Ginger will warm me, because it has a warm energy; mung beans will cool me, because they have a cool energy; sugar can make my stomach stronger, because it tastes sweet and acts on the stomach; yam will make my kidneys stronger, because it acts on the kidneys in a special way.

To be sure, we can find nutritional information on foods in Western diet. For example, we know that red pepper contains vitamins A and C, but it does not tell us that it can warm us; we know mung beans contain some protein and carbohydrates, but not that mung beans can cool us; we know that black pepper contains some protein, but not that it can make our stomachs stronger; we know that yam contains protein, carbohydrate, calcium and many vitamins, but not that it can make our kidneys stronger. Thus, it is easy to see how Chinese diet differs from Western diet.

The essential aspects of Chinese diet in regard to foods are: the five flavors of foods, the five energies of foods, the movements of foods and the common and organic actions of foods.

## THE FIVE FLAVORS OF FOODS

The five flavors of foods include pungent (acrid), sweet, sour, bitter and salty.

Pungent foods include green onion, chive, clove, parsley and coriander.

Sweet foods include sugar, cherry, chestnut and banana.

Sour foods include lemon, pear, plum and mango.

Bitter foods include hops, lettuce, radish leaf and vinegar (I list vinegar as bitter because the Chinese call vinegar "bitter wine." Vinegar tastes both sour and bitter; it is common for some foods to have two simultaneous flavors).

Salty foods include salt, kelp and seaweed.

The flavors of foods are important in Chinese diet, because different flavors have their respective important effects upon the internal organs. Foods that have a pungent flavor can act on the lungs and large intestine; foods with a sweet flavor on the stomach and spleen; with sour flavor on the liver and gall bladder; with a bitter flavor on the heart and small intestine; foods that have a salty flavor can act on the kidneys and bladder.

Let's take the sweet flavor as an example, that acts on the stomach and spleen. It is common knowledge among Chinese and Western dietitians, that eating sweet foods will put on weight, but Chinese and Western dietitians give different explanations. According to Western dietitians, eating sweet foods puts on weight because sweet foods contain a large number of calories; according to Chinese dietitians, eating sweet foods will put on weight because sweet foods can act on the stomach and spleen, which are in charge of digestive functions. In other words, in Chinese diet, sweet foods are considered capable of improving the digestive functions, which is why they are good for people with a weak digestive system. In talking to a Western audience about Chinese diet, one question frequently comes up: How do we determine the flavors of such foods as beef, pork and celery that have no distinct tastes? In Chinese diet, beef has a sweet flavor, pork has a sweet and salty flavor and celery a sweet flavor. Some foods have one flavor, but others may have two or three. Undoubtedly, the flavors of many foods are very difficult to determine precisely, but the Chinese have done it through many centuries of experience.

The process may look like this: At the beginning, some foods with obvious flavors are found to act on some internal organs and perform specific actions in the human body. The basic relationships between flavors and internal organs and the actions are studied and analyzed by a process in science called the inductive method. As time goes on, other foods whose flavors are more difficult to determine may be found capable of acting upon some internal organs and performing some specific actions. The flavors of such foods are determined on the basis of their organic effects and specific actions. This process in science is called the deductive method.

In general, the common actions of foods in regard to their flavors are as follows:

Pungent foods (ginger, green onion and peppermint) can induce perspiration and promote energy circulation.

Sweet foods (honey, sugar and watermelon) can slow down the acute symptoms and neutralize the toxic effects of other foods.

Sour foods (lemon and plum) can obstruct the movements and are useful, therefore, in checking diarrhea and excessive perspiration.

Bitter foods, such as animals' gall bladder and hops, can reduce body heat, dry body fluids and induce diarrhea (which is why many Chinese herbs recommended to reduce fever and induce diarrhea taste bitter).

Salty foods (kelp and seaweed) can soften hardness, which explains their usefulness in treating tuberculosis of the lymph nodes and other symptoms involving the hardening of muscles or glands.

In addition, some foods have a light flavor or little taste. These foods normally have two flavor classifications. Cucumber, for example, has sweet and light flavors. Foods with a light flavor promote urination and may be used as diuretics. Job's tears is one of the outstanding examples.

The following are foods arranged by different flavors:

- BITTER: apricot seed, asparagus, bitter gourd, wild cucumber, celery, cherry seed, coffee, grapefruit peel, hops, kohlrabi, lettuce, lotus plumule, radish leaf, sea grass, vinegar, wine.
- SLIGHTLY BITTER: ginseng, pumpkin.
- LIGHT: Job's tears, kidney bean, sunflower seed, white fungus, Chinese wax gourd.
- PUNGENT: black pepper, castor bean, cherry seed, chive, chive root, chive seed, cinnamon bark, cinnamon twig, clove, Chinese parsley, cottonseed, dillseeds, fennel, garlic, ginger, dried or fresh, grapefruit peel, green onion, leaf and white head, green pepper, kohlrabi, kumquat, leaf mustard, leek, marjoram, nutmeg, peppermint, radish and radish leaf, red pepper, rice bran, rosemary, soybean oil, spearmint, star anise, sweet basil, taro, tobacco, white pepper, wine.
- SLIGHTLY PUNGENT: asparagus, caraway.
- SALTY: abalone, barley, chive seeds, clam (sea, fresh water, river clamshell, sea clam-shell), crab, cuttlebone, cuttlefish, duck, eel blood, ham, kelp, milk (human), oyster, oyster shell, pork, salt, seagrass, seaweed. (All recommended shells are crushed into powder before using them.)
- SOUR: apple, apricot, crab apple, grape, grapefruit, hawthorn fruits, kumquat, litchi, loquat, mandarin orange, mango, olive, peach, pineapple, plum, raspberry, small red or adzuki bean, star fruit or carambola, strawberry, tangerine, tomato, vinegar.
- EXTREMELY SOUR: lemon, pear, sour plum.
- SWEET: abalone, apple, apricot, apricot seeds (sweet), bamboo shoots, banana, barley, bean curd, beef, beetroots, black fungus, black sesame seeds, black soybean, brown sugar, cabbage (Chinese), carp (common carp, gold carp, grass carp), carrot, castor bean, celery, cherry, chestnut, chicken, chicken egg, yolk and white, Chinese wax gourd, cinnamon bark, cinnamon twig, clam (fresh water), coconut, coffee, common button mushroom, corn, corn silk, crab apple, cucumber, red and black date, dry mandarin orange peel, duck, eel, eel blood, eggplant, fig, ginseng, grape, grapefruit, grapefruit peel, guava, guava leaf, hawthorn fruits, honey, horse bean, hyacinth bean, Job's tears, kidney bean, kohl-rabi, kumquat, lettuce, licorice, lily flower, litchi, longan, longevity fruit, loquat, lotus (fruit and seed), malt, maltose, mandarin orange, mango, milk (cow's and human), mung bean, muskmelon, mutton, olive, oyster, papaya, peach, peanuts, pear, persimmon, pineapple, plum, pork, potato, pumpkin, radish, raspberry, red small bean or adzuki bean, rice bran, rice (polished), saffron, sesame oil, shiitake mushroom, shrimp, soybean oil, spearmint, spinach, squash, star anise, star fruit, strawberry, string bean, sugar cane, sunflower seed, sweet rice, sweet potato, sword bean, tangerine-orange, taro, tomato, walnut, water chestnut, watermelon, wheat, wheat bran, white fungus, white sugar, wine, yellow soybean.

## THE FIVE ENERGIES OF FOODS

The energies of foods refer to their capacity to generate sensations—either hot or cold—in the human body. As an example, eating foods with a hot energy will make us experience hot sensations in the body and foods with a cold energy, cold sensations. In daily life, each of us knows that eating ice makes us feel cold and drinking hot water makes us feel warm. This is because ice has a cold energy and hot water, a hot energy. But ice or hot water produce only temporary effects. To produce long-lasting effects, herbs are used as substitutes for foods that provide only temporary relief. In other words, to produce cold or hot sensations, herbs are more effective than foods and foods are more effective than ice or hot water.

The five energies of foods are cold, hot, warm, cool and neutral. But the adjectives, "cold," "hot," "warm," "cool," "neutral," do not refer to the present state of foods. For example, tea has a cold energy, so even though you may drink hot tea, you are actually drinking a cold beverage. Shortly after the tea enters your body, its heat (a temporary phenomenon) will be lost and as it begins to generate cold energy, your body begins to cool off. Another example, red pepper, has a hot energy. Even though you may eat cold red pepper from the refrigerator, you still consume a hot food. Shortly after it enters your body, its temporary coldness is lost and your body begins to feel hot.

When I discuss the energies of foods, therefore, I refer to what the foods do in our bodies —whether they generate hot or cold, warm or cool, or neutral sensations. Hot is opposed to cold; warm is opposed to cool; neutral is somewhere between warm and cool. Cold and cool foods differ from each other, as do warm and hot foods. Bamboo shoots have a cold energy, black pepper a hot energy; cucumber has a cool energy, chicken a warm and corn a neutral energy.

It is important for us to know the energies of foods, because different energies act upon the human body in different ways. This has important effects on good health. As an example, when a person suffers from cold rheumatism and the pain is particularly severe on cold winter days, then it is good for him or her to eat foods with a warm or hot energy, which should considerably relieve the pain. Or if you suffer from skin eruptions that worsen when exposed to heat, it is good to eat foods with a cold or cool energy to relieve your symptoms.

While the energies of foods play an important role in Chinese diet, the Chinese also classify the human body into cold and hot types. One person may have a hot physical constitution, another a cold one. The person with a hot physical constitution should consume more foods with a cold or cool energy; the person with a cold physical constitution, more foods with a hot or warm energy—a plan the Chinese call "a balanced diet." Such a diet is always related to each individual's physical constitution and may differ from one person to another.

During my lectures and in my clinical practice, people often ask me: Is tea good? Is coffee better than tea? Is liquor good for you? There are no absolute answers. In fact, these are the wrong questions. It would make more sense to ask: Is tea good for me? Which is better for me, coffee or tea? Is it good for me to drink liquor? Those questions can be answered correctly. Tea is good for you if you have a hot physical constitution, because tea has a cold energy; if you have a cold physical constitution, coffee is better for you than tea, because coffee has a warm energy. If you have a cold physical constitution, liquor can warm you, but if you have a hot physical constitution, it may create many symptoms of certain hot diseases, such as skin problems. For this reason, in the Chinese diet, foods with a cold energy are used to counteract intoxication and alcoholism.

The process of learning the energies of foods is basically the same as that of finding the flavors of foods. At first, the foods that obviously make us feel hot may be considered as having a hot energy; the foods that make us cold, a cold energy. For example, obviously ice makes us feel cold, so it is believed to have a cold energy; and since red pepper makes us feel hot, it is thought to have a hot energy. As time goes on, any food that can make us hot is regarded as having a hot energy; any food that can make us cold, a cold energy.

It's interesting to see how important and relevant the energies of foods in Chinese diet can be. Suppose on a cold rainy day, on your way home from work, your car breaks down. You walk to a service station to hire a tow truck and by the time you get home, you're soaked to the skin and shivering with cold. You suspect that you caught cold. If you have some knowledge of the Chinese diet, you prepare a bowl of fresh old ginger soup and drink it hot. You feel much better, because fresh old ginger has a warm energy that warms you and a pungent flavor that makes you perspire.

Let's use another example. Suppose you develop hives with severe itching. You cannot cook your meals, because the heat in the kitchen makes your itching intolerable. If you have a fair knowledge about Chinese diet, you cook a bowl of mung bean soup and stir in some sugar. After drinking the soup a few times, your symptoms disappear, because the cold energy in both mung beans and sugar heal your hot symptoms. Of course, many other factors need to be considered as well, but the energy of foods is important.

Suppose you suffer from hemorrhoids and know about Chinese diet. You eat two cooked (underdone) whole bananas (with the peels) every day. The bananas should improve the symptoms, because banana has a cold energy.

On the negative side, let's suppose you have no knowledge about Chinese diet and you happen to make a mistake. In the first example, when you had the cold, instead of drinking hot ginger soup, you drank a bowl of mung bean soup. That would have made your symptoms worse. With the hives, had you taken hot sauce at dinner instead of mung bean soup, your itching would probably have become much worse. With the hemorrhoids, if instead of eating bananas, you drank whiskey every day, that too could make your symptoms deteriorate.

The following foods arranged by their different energies:

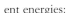 COLD: bamboo shoot, banana, bitter gourd, clam (sea and freshwater), clamshell, crab, grapefruit, kelp, lettuce, lotus plumule, muskmelon, persimmon, salt, sea grass, seaweed, star fruit, sugar cane, water chestnut, watermelon.

SLIGHTLY COLD: hops, tomato.

COOL: apple, barley, bean curd, chicken egg white, Chinese wax gourd, common button mushroom, cucumber, eggplant, Job's tears, lettuce, lily flower, longevity fruit, loquat, mandarin orange, mango, marjoram, mung bean, oyster shell, pear, peppermint, radish, sesame oil, spinach, strawberry; tangerine, wheat, wheat bran.

HOT: black pepper, cinnamon bark, cottonseed, ginger (dried ginger), green pepper, red pepper, soybean oil, white pepper.

NEUTRAL: abalone, apricot, beef, beetroot, black fungus, black sesame seed, black soybean, cabbage (Chinese), carp (common carp, gold carp), carrot, castor bean, celery, cherry seed, chicken egg, chicken egg yolk, corn, corn silk, crab apple, cuttlefish, dry mandarin orange peel, duck, eel blood, fig, grape, guava leaf, honey, horse bean, hyacinth bean, kidney bean, kohlrabi, licorice, lotus fruit and seed, milk (cow's and human), olive, oyster, papaya, peanuts, pineapple, plum, polished rice, pork, potato, pumpkin, radish leaf, small red or adzuki bean, rice bran, saffron, shiitake mushroom, sour plum, string bean, sunflower seed, sweet, ice, sweet potato, taro, taro flower, white fungus, white sugar, yellow soybean.

WARM: apricot seed (bitter and sweet apricot), brown sugar, caraway, carp (grass carp), cherry, chestnut, chicken, chive, chive seeds, chive roots, cinnamon twig, clove, coconut, coffee, coriander (Chinese parsley), date (both red and black), dillseeds, eel, fennel, garlic, ginger (fresh ginger), ginseng, grapefruit peel, green onion leaf, green onion white head, guava, ham, kumquat, leaf mustard, leek, litchi, longan, maltose, mutton, nutmeg, peach, raspberry, rosemary, shrimp, spearmint, squash, star anise, sunflower seed, sweet basil, sword bean, tobacco, vinegar, walnut, wine.

SLIGHTLY WARM: asparagus, cuttlebone, hawthorn fruits, malt.

## THE MOVEMENTS OF FOODS

Foods have a tendency to move in different directions in the body. Some foods move outward, some inward; some foods have a tendency to move upwards; some downwards. To see how this works, think of the human body as divided into four regions: inside (internal region); outside (skin and body surface); upper (above the waist); lower (below the waist).

To move outward means to move from inside towards outside; so foods with outward move-

ments can induce perspiration and reduce fever.

To move inward means to move from outside towards inside; so foods with inward movements can ease bowel movements and abdominal swelling.

To move upwards means to move from the lower region towards the upper region; so foods with upward movements can relieve diarrhea, prolapse of anus, prolapse of uterus and falling of stomach.

To move downwards means to move from the upper region towards the lower region; so foods with downward movements can relieve vomiting, hiccupping and asthma.

In general, leaves and flowers have a tendency to move upwards. Roots and seeds and fruits have a tendency to move downwards. But this is just a general principle. There are many exceptions.

Among the foods we eat every day, peppermint has a tendency to move outward; banana has a tendency to move inward; wine has a tendency to move upwards; salt has a tendency to move downwards. Some foods can move in two directions.

Two additional characteristics of food are associated with the movements, namely, glossy (sliding) and obstructive. Glossy foods, such as honey and spinach, facilitate the movements. Obstructive foods, such as guava and olive, slow down the movements. Glossy foods are good for constipation and internal dryness, but bad for diarrhea and seminal emission. Conversely, obstructive foods are good for diarrhea and seminal emission, but bad for constipation and internal dryness. The movements of foods are important in Chinese diet, because foods moving in different directions have different applications in coping with human health problems.

The symptoms treated by the different movements of foods are classified into four categories: First, upward symptoms, such as vomiting, hiccupping, coughing, etc., should be treated by foods that can move downwards. Second, downward symptoms, such as diarrhea, falling of the stomach and prolapse of uterus and anus, should be treated by foods that can move upwards. Third, the outward symptoms, such as excessive perspiration, premature ejaculation, seminal emission, frequent urination, should be treated by foods that can obstruct. The inward symptoms, such as constipation and abdominal swelling, should be treated by foods that can move outward in combination with other foods that cleanse the internal regions.

The movements of foods change after they are prepared in a certain way. Foods prepared with wine develop a tendency to move upwards. That is the reason, in treating falling symptoms like prolapse of uterus and anus, herbs are very often processed along with the wine. Foods prepared with ginger juice develop a tendency to move outward. When foods are prepared with vinegar, they have a tendency to become obstructive. Foods processed with salt (as in frying) develop a tendency to move downwards.

In clinical practice, we often see patients with

falling of the stomach, which is called gastroptosis in Western medicine. When a patient with this symptom consults a physician, he or she is often told to stay upside down so that the stomach is restored to its original position. This sounds like a sensible treatment, because when the person is upside down, the stomach will surely fall in the opposite direction—but it's impractical. A person is born to stand on his feet and not on his head. And it is also ineffective, because when the person stands upright, the stomach will fall again.

From the Chinese point of view, a far more effective treatment of this downward symptom is to eat foods that can move upwards, so they will push up the energy. Although none of the common foods we eat every day push upwards forcefully, plenty of herbs do the job very effectively. For example, *rhizoma cimicifugae* is called the "elevating herb" because of its power to push upwards. *Radix bupleuri* is also used for the same purpose.

The movements of foods are also related to the flavors and energies of foods. Generally, warm and hot foods that have a pungent and sweet flavor tend to move upwards or outward; cold and cool foods that have a sour or salty or bitter flavor tend to move downwards or inward. In addition, the movements of foods also relate to the four seasons: Foods that move upwards are good to consume in spring, the time when living things begin to grow; growth means to move upwards. Foods that move outward are good in summer, when everything is outgoing (as in perspiration and expansion). Foods that move downwards are good in autumn, when things begin to fall (such as leaves). Foods that move inward are good in winter, when things move inward (and stay indoors). The following foods are arranged by their combinations of energies and flavors suitable for the four seasons.

- Foods with an *upward movement* are good to eat in spring. Such foods have a neutral energy and three flavors—pungent or sweet or bitter. These include abalone, apricot, beef, beetroots, black fungus, black sesame seed, black soybean, cabbage (Chinese), carp (common and gold carp), carrot, celery, cherry seed, chicken egg, chicken egg yolk, corn silk, crab apple, dry mandarin orange peel, duck, eel blood, fig, grape, guava leaf, honey, horse bean, hyacinth bean, kidney bean, kohlrabi, licorice, lotus fruit and seed, milk (cow's and human milk), olive, oyster, peanuts, pineapple, plum, pork, potato, pumpkin, radish leaf, small red bean or adzuki bean, rice bran, saffron, shiitake mushroom, string bean, sunflower seed, sweet rice, sweet potato, taro, white fungus, white sugar, yellow soybean.

- Foods with an *outward movement* are good in summer. These foods have a hot energy and two different flavors—pungent or sweet. Among these are black pepper, cinnamon bark, cottonseed, ginger (dried), green pepper; red pepper; soybean oil; white pepper.

- Foods with a *downward movement*, good in autumn. Such foods have three energies—cold or cool or warm—and two flavors—sweet or sour. This list includes apple, bamboo shoots, banana, barley, bean curd, chicken egg white, Chinese wax gourd, clam (freshwater), common button mushroom, cucumber, eggplant, grapefruits, hawthorn fruits, kumquat, Job's tears, lettuce, lily flower, litchi, longevity fruit, loquat, mango, mung bean, muskmelon, peach, persimmon, spinach, star fruit, strawberry, sugar cane juice, tangerine, water chestnut, watermelon, wheat, wheat bran.

- Foods with an *inward movement*, good in winter. They have a cold energy and two different flavors—bitter or salty. Bitter gourd, clam (salt and freshwater), crab, hops, kelp, lettuce, lotus plumule, salt, sea grass and seaweed are among these foods.

## THE ORGANIC ACTIONS OF FOODS

*O*rganic actions of foods refer to specific internal organs on which the foods can act. The Chinese people focus on ten internal organs for dietary treatment: lungs, large intestine, small intestine, gall bladder, bladder, liver, kidneys, spleen, heart and stomach. Each food acts on one or more internal organs the organic actions of that particular food. For example, celery acts on the stomach and liver, carrot on the

the nose may be traced to the lungs. Mouth and lips are associated with the spleen; mouth and lip diseases may be traced to the spleen. And since the tongue is associated with the heart, diseases of the tongue may be traced to the heart.

After the associations between internal organs and body surface are established, some foods may be found very effective when treating symptoms on the body surface. Gradually, these foods are used to establish the associations between foods and internal organs. This is arrived at by the deductive method. Chicken liver, for example, is

# Actions of Foods and The Balanced Diet

lungs and spleen, eggplant on the spleen, stomach and large intestine, wheat on the heart, spleen and kidneys.

Flavors and energies of foods are important factors in determining the organic actions of foods. Generally, when the energy and flavor of a specific food are relatively simple, that food may only act on one organ. For example, almond is neutral and sweet, so it only acts on the lungs; wheat bran is cool and sweet, so it only acts on the stomach; kelp is cold and salty, so it only acts on the stomach. But when a food has more than one energy or one flavor, it may act on two or more organs at the same time. For example, tea is cool (or slightly cold) and bittersweet; it acts upon three internal organs—the heart, lungs and stomach; barley is cool and sweet and salty; it acts on the spleen and stomach. But this is just a general principle, because many foods that have one energy and one flavor still act upon two or more internal organs simultaneously; and conversely, many foods that have two or more energies and flavors act only on one organ.

The organic actions of foods, like the flavors and energies of foods, have been discovered by the inductive and deductive methods throughout Chinese history. At first, certain foods may be effective in the treatment of some organic diseases. Consequently, such foods are considered good for specific actions on the diseased organs. This is arrived at by the inductive method. After many isolated instances have been observed, gradually, the results are used to establish the associations between foods and internal organs. Chinese physicians have always put great emphasis on the relationships between internal organs and body surface, including the skin, the five senses and visible symptoms. The diseases on body surface are then traced back to the related internal organs.

In Chinese belief, the eyes are associated with the liver; eye diseases may be traced to the liver. Ears are associated with the kidneys; deafness and hearing loss may be traced to the kidneys. The nose is associated with the lungs; disease of

effective for blurred vision; since the eyes are associated with the liver, it follows that the relationship between chicken liver and our liver may be established. Another example, honey is effective for relief of constipation—a symptom related to the large intestine—so that the association between honey and the large intestine is established. The following foods of different organic actions are listed with the organ on which they act.

- BLADDER: Chinese wax gourd, cinnamon bark, cinnamon twig, fennel, grapefruit peel, watermelon.
- GALL BLADDER: chicory, corn silk.
- HEART: bitter gourd, chicken egg yolk, cinnamon twig, crab apple, green pepper, longan, lotus fruit and seed, lotus plumule, milk (cow's and human), mung bean, muskmelon, persimmon, red pepper, small red or adzuki bean, saffron, watermelon, wheat, wine.
- KIDNEYS: black sesame seed, black soybean, caraway, carp (common), chestnut, chicken egg yolk, chive, chive seeds, cinnamon bark, clam (freshwater), clove, cuttlebone, cuttlefish, dillseed, duck, eel, eel blood, fennel, grape, grapefruit peel, Job's tears, lotus fruit and seed, lotus plumule, mutton, oyster shell, plum, pork, salt, star anise, string bean, tangerine, walnut, wheat.
- LARGE INTESTINE: bean curd, black fungus, black pepper, cabbage (Chinese), carp (gold carp), castor bean, Chinese wax gourd, corn, cucumber, eggplant, fig, honey, lettuce, nutmeg, persimmon, rice bran, salt, spinach, sweet basil, sword bean, taro, white pepper, yellow soybean.
- LIVER: black sesame seed, brown sugar, celery, chicory, chive, chive seed, clam (freshwater), clarnshell (river), corn silk, crab, crab apple, cuttlefish, eel, eel blood, hawthorn fruits, leek, litchi, loquat, oyster shell, peppermint, plum, saffron, sour plum, star anise, vinegar, wine.
- LUNGS: carrot, castor bean, Chinese wax gourd, cinnamon twig, clarnshell (river), common button mushroom, coriander, crab apple,

duck, garlic, ginger (fresh and dried), ginseng, grape, green onion white head, honey, Job's tears, leaf mustard, leek, licorice, lily flower, loquat, lotus plumule, maltose, milk (cow's and human), olive, peanut, pear, peppermint, persimmon, radish, sugar cane, sweet basil, tangerine, walnut, water chestnut, wine.

- SMALL INTESTINE: Chinese wax gourd, small red or adzuki bean, salt, spinach.
- SPLEEN: barley, bean curd, beef, bitter gourd, black soybean, brown sugar, carp (common, gold and grass), carrot, chestnut, chicken, cinnamon bark, clove, coriander, cucumber, date (red and black), dillseed, eel, eggplant, fig, garlic, ginger (fresh and dried), ginseng, grape, grapefruit peel, green pepper, hawthorn fruit, honey, horse bean, hyacinth bean, job's tears, licorice, litchi, longan, loquat, lotus fruit and seed, malt, maltose, mutton, nutmeg, peanuts, pork, radish leaf, red pepper, rice (polished), squash, star anise, string bean, sweet basil sweet rice, wheat, white sugar, yellow soybean.
- STOMACH: barley, bean curd, beef, bitter gourd, black fungus, black pepper, brown sugar, cabbage (Chinese), caraway, carp (gold and grass), celery, chestnut, chicken, chive, clam (saltwater and freshwater), clamshell (river and sea), clove, common button mushroom, corn, crab, cucumber, date (red and black), eggplant, fennel, garlic, ginger (fresh and dried), green onion white head, hawthorn fruit, horse bean, hyacinth bean, kelp, lettuce, licorice, malt, maltose, milk (cow's and human), mung bean, muskmelon, olive, pear, pork, radish, radish leaf, rice bran, rice (polished), salt, shiitake mushroom, squash, sugar cane, sweet basil, sweet rice, sword bean, tangerine, taro, vinegar, water chestnut, watermelon, wheat bran, white pepper, wine.

## THE COMMON ACTIONS OF FOODS

The common actions of foods refer to the general actions of foods without referring to any specific internal organ. Many actions are familiar to the Western reader. As an example, the action called "to relieve asthma" means that it is beneficial to asthma patients; the action called "to check perspiration" means that it can reduce perspiration.

Other familiar actions include: to arrest bleeding, to promote blood circulation, to induce bowel movements, to check urination and so on.

There are also a few actions that are totally unfamiliar to Western readers who do not have backgrounds in Chinese medicine. For instance, what is meant by the terms, "to cool blood" or "to tone up yang"? After reading this book, however, you should have a clear understanding of such actions. Of the large number of actions known in Chinese medicine, less than 100 are commonly used in Chinese diet. Here are actions and effective foods:

- ARREST BLEEDING black fungus, chestnut, chicken eggshell, cottonseed, cuttlebone, guava, lotus plumule, spinach, vinegar.
- CALM DOWN THE SPIRITS licorice, lily flower.
- CHECK ACID chicken eggshell, cuttlebone.
- CHECK PERSPIRATION oyster shell, peach.
- CHECK URINATION raspberry.
- CHECK SEMINAL EJACULATION lotus plumule, oyster shell, walnut, black fungus.
- COUNTERACT TOXIC EFFECTS abalone, banana, bean curd, black soybean, castor bean, cherry seed, chicken egg white, Chinese wax gourd, clam (freshwater), cucumber, date (red and black), fig, honey, Job's tears, kohlrabi, radish, salt, sesame oil, small red bean, star fruit, vinegar.
- DISPERSE BLOOD COAGULATIONS brown sugar, chive, chive root, crab, hawthorn fruit, saffron, vinegar.
- DISPERSE COLD ginger (fresh), wine.
- ELIMINATE SPUTUM Chinese wax gourd, clam (saltwater), longevity fruit, pear, radish, sea grass, seaweed.
- FACILITATE MEASLES ERUPTION cherry seed, coriander, sunflower seed.
- IMPROVE APPETITE green pepper, ham, red pepper.
- INDUCE BOWEL MOVEMENT castor bean, sesame oil.
- INDUCE PERSPIRATION cinnamon twig, coriander, ginger (fresh), green onion leaf, green onion white head, marjoram, rosemary.
- LUBRICATE DRYNESS bean curd, chicken egg, chicken egg yolk, honey, maltose, milk (human), pear, pork, sesame oil, spinach, sugar cane juice, yellow soybean.
- LUBRICATE INTESTINES apricot seed (bitter and sweet), banana, milk (cow's), peach, soybean oil, walnut, watermelon.
- LUBRICATE LUNGS apple, apricot, chicken egg white, ginseng, lily flower, longevity fruit, loquat, mandarin orange, peanuts, persimmon, strawberry, white fungus, white sugar.
- PRODUCE FLUIDS apple, apricot, bean curd, coconut, date (red and black), ham, lemon, licorice, litchi, maltose, milk (cow's), peach, pear, plum, sour plum, star fruit, strawberry, sugar cane juice, tomato, white fungus, white sugar.
- PROMOTE BLOOD CIRCULATION black soybean, brown sugar, chestnut, eel blood, peach, saffron, sweet basil, wine.
- PROMOTE DIGESTION apple, coriander, ginseng, green pepper, hops, malt, nutmeg, papaya, pineapple, plum, radish, radish leaf, red pepper, sweet basil, tomato.
- PROMOTE ENERGY CIRCULATION caraway, chive, chive roots, dillseeds, dry mandarin orange peel, fennel, garlic, kumquat, litchi, marjoram, radish leaf, spearmint, star anise, sweet basil, tangerine, tobacco.
- PROMOTE MILK SECRETION common carp, lettuce.
- PROMOTE URINATION asparagus, barley, Chinese cabbage, carrot, Chinese wax gourd, coconut, coffee, corn, corn silk, cucumber, grape, hops, Job's tears, kidney bean, lettuce, mandarin orange, mango, mung bean, muskmelon, onion, pineapple, plum, star fruit, sugar cane juice, water chestnut, watermelon.

- QUENCH THIRST crab apple, cucumber, loquat, mango, muskmelon, persimmon, pineapple.
- REDUCE FEVER muskmelon, star fruit, water chestnut. Relieve asthma: apricot seed (bitter).
- RELIEVE COUGH apricot seed (sweet and bitter), kumquat, longevity fruit, mandarin orange, tangerine, thyme.
- RELIEVE DIARRHEA guava, sunflower seed.
- RELIEVE HOT SENSATIONS IN THE BODY chicken egg white, crab, mung bean, sea grass.
- RELIEVE PAIN honey, litchi, spearmint, squash, tobacco.
- SHARPEN VISION abalone, bitter gourd, wild cucumber, freshwater clam, cuttlefish.
- SOFTEN HARDNESS clam (saltwater), kelp, oyster shell, sea grass, seaweed.
- TONE UP BLOOD DEFICIENCY beef, chicken egg, chicken egg yolk, cuttlefish, milk (human), oyster, spinach.
- TONE UP ENERGY DEFICIENCY apricot seed (sweet), bean curd, beef, brown sugar, chicken, eel, licorice, maltose, mutton, polished rice, potato, sweet rice, sweet potato.
- TONE UP THE HEART coffee, wheat.
- TONE UP THE KIDNEYS black sesame seed, string bean, sword bean, wheat, kidneys.
- TONE UP THE LIVER black sesame seed, liver.
- TONE UP THE LUNGS Job's tears, milk (cow's).
- TONE UP THE SPLEEN beef, carp (gold), ham, horse bean, hyacinth bean, Job's tears, polished rice, potato, string bean, sweet potato, yellow soybean.
- TONE UP THE STOMACH beef, hops, milk (cow's), rosemary.
- RELIEVE DRUNKENNESS apple, ginseng, strawberry.
- WARM UP THE INTERNAL REGIONS black pepper, chicken, chive roots, clove, fennel, ginger (dried), green pepper, mutton, nutmeg, red pepper, sword bean, white pepper.

## THE BALANCED DIET IN CHINESE THEORY

Basically, a balanced diet means two different things: First, it means that you should eat foods of various flavors, energies and organic actions rather than concentrate on a single flavor or energy or organic action. Second, a balanced diet also means that foods are selected according to your needs and physical constitution. The balanced diet in the first sense may be called the common balanced diet and in the second, the individual's balanced diet.

It is not easy to eat foods of various energies, flavors and organic actions, because we are inclined to eat what we like. The foods we like are determined by our taste, which is judged by our mouth and tongue. The mouth and tongue represent only the internal organs of the digestive system. This implies that the foods we like most are pleasing to the organs of the digestive system without considering the internal organs of other body systems (the bladder, liver, kidneys, heart and others). According to the Chinese theory, sweet foods are pleasing to the stomach and the spleen, pungent foods to the lungs and large intestine, salty foods to the kidneys and bladder, bitter foods to the heart and small intestine, sour foods to the liver and gallbladder.

The foods we enjoy most and eat most frequently are sweet foods, followed by salty foods; therefore, to have a balanced diet, we need to eat more pungent, sour and bitter foods. This sense of balanced diet is very different from the balanced diet in the Western sense. I have compiled a balanced diet in the Western sense to point out the differences between Chinese and Western balanced diets. The following list of foods represents essential nutrients in Western diet and a comparison from the Chinese point of view.

Western foods: beef for phosphorus; seaweed for iodine; banana for potassium; corn for protein and fat; sweet rice for carbohydrate; celery for calcium; spinach for iron; tomato for vitamin A; potato and chicken liver for vitamin B; lemon for vitamin C; butter for vitamin D; lettuce for vitamin E; honey for vitamin K.

According to Chinese diet, beef is neutral in energy, sweet in flavor and acts on the spleen and stomach.

Seaweed is cold in energy and salty in flavor, with undetermined organic actions.

Banana is cold in energy and sweet in flavor, with undetermined organic actions.

Corn is neutral in energy and sweet in flavor and acts on the stomach and large intestine.

Sweet rice is warm in energy and sweet in flavor and acts on the spleen, the stomach and lungs.

Celery is neutral in energy and sweet in flavor and acts on the stomach and liver.

Spinach is cool in energy and sweet in flavor and acts on the stomach and large intestine.

Tomato is slightly cold in energy and sweet and sour in flavor, with undetermined organic actions.

Potato is neutral in energy and sweet in flavor, with undetermined organic actions.

Chicken liver is slightly warm in energy and sweet in flavor and acts upon the liver and kidneys.

Lemon is extremely sour in flavor, with undetermined energy and organic actions.

Butter is warm in energy and sweet in flavor with undetermined organic actions.

Lettuce is cool in energy and bitter and sweet in flavor and acts on the stomach and large intestine.

Honey is neutral in energy and sweet in flavor and acts on the lungs, the spleen and large intestine.

We can classify all the above foods into groups according to their energies, flavors and organic actions by ignoring all undetermined items.

- COLD ENERGY seaweed, banana, tomato.
- HOT ENERGY none.
- COOL ENERGY spinach, lettuce.
- WARM ENERGY sweet rice, chicken liver, butter.
- NEUTRAL ENERGY beef, corn, celery, potato, honey.
- PUNGENT FLAVOR none.
- SWEET FLAVOR beef, banana, corn, sweet rice, celery, spinach, tomato, potato, chicken liver, butter, lettuce, honey.

- SOUR FLAVOR tomato, lemon.
- SALTY FLAVOR seaweed.
- BITTER FLAVOR lettuce.
- ACTS ON THE SPLEEN beef, sweet rice, honey.
- ACTS ON THE STOMACH beef, corn, sweet rice, celery, spinach, lettuce.
- ACTS ON THE LARGE INTESTINE corn, spinach, lettuce, honey.
- ACTS ON THE SMALL INTESTINE none.
- ACTS ON THE LIVER celery, chicken liver.
- ACTS ON THE GALL BLADDER none.
- ACTS ON THE BLADDER none.
- ACTS ON THE KIDNEYS chicken liver.
- ACTS ON THE HEART none.
- ACTS ON THE LUNGS sweet rice, honey.

You can see that in the above, there is no food with a hot energy or with a pungent flavor and no food to act on the small intestine, gall bladder, bladder, or the heart. Especially, the majority of foods are sweet and act on the spleen, stomach and large intestine, which are related to the digestive system. Although the foods listed above are selected at random with only Western nutritional balance in mind, they reflect how the Western people eat. Specifically, Westerners eat more sweet foods, which taste good and act predominantly on organs of the digestive system. Small wonder that there are more overweight people in the West than in the East!

## THE INDIVIDUAL'S BALANCED DIET

The individual's balanced diet must consider each person's physical constitution. In Chinese diet, there are six different types of physical constitution: hot, cold, dry, damp, deficient and excessive. Individuals with different types of physical constitution should follow a different balanced diet. This means that if you have a hot physical constitution, you should eat more cold and cool foods; if you have a cold physical constitution, you should eat more hot and warm foods in order to strike a balance in your body. It is very important, therefore, to know what type of physical constitution you have in order to design a balanced diet for yourself.

A person's physical constitution may be determined in terms of a number of key factors, including subjective sensations, urine, stools, the tongue and other factors. If you often feel hot, thirsty and if you normally prefer cold drink and have a reddish complexion, you probably have a hot physical constitution.

A person with a hot physical constitution may discharge scanty urine (reddish yellow in color) and hard stools. The tongue may appear red with a yellowish coating, but sometimes, the tongue may also appear red with no coating at all.

If you often feel cold and not thirsty and you normally prefer hot or warm drink and have a pale or whitish complexion, you probably have a cold physical constitution. A person with a cold physical constitution may discharge clear urine (that looks white) and soft stools. The tongue of a person with a cold physical constitution normally appears light in color with a thin whitish coating.

If you easily feel thirsty and your lips, nose, throat and skin are all dry and when you cough (when you have a cold) it is mostly dry cough without mucus, then you probably have a dry physical constitution. A person with a dry physical constitution may easily have an itch in the skin or nose or eyes. And he may also display symptoms of constipation, due to the dry conditions of his intestines. A person with a dry physical constitution is normally skinny and cannot gain weight easily.

If you feel heavy in the body and very often tired and if your tongue appears glossy and greasy, then you probably have a damp physical constitution. A person with a damp physical constitution easily becomes overweight due to water retention, called edema. This type of person may look fat but is rather weak in energy. The Chinese believe that to remove water from the body, it is necessary for this type of person to promote urination and induce perspiration and to eat aromatic foods, which are believed to have the effects of drying the internal region.

Another type of physical constitution is called deficient. A person with a deficient physical constitution is weak in energy and normally in low spirits. This type of person may have a pale complexion, feet tired very often, perspire excessively, have palpitations or shortness of breath. The tongue may appear clean and light without a coating. A person with a deficient physical constitution is underweight or skinny and often suffers from falling symptoms (falling of the stomach, prolapse of the uterus, prolapse of the anus), which are caused by energy deficiency. The body does not have sufficient energy to support the internal organs, so the organs begin to fall.

The last type of physical constitution is called excessive. A person with an excessive physical constitution is strong and energetic and often in high spirits and speaks in a high-pitched voice. This type of person normally has a reddish complexion and may suffer from constipation, hypertension, or heart disease. Because the body has accumulated too much energy, traffic jams are created leading to blockages of various kinds. It must be emphasized here, however, people usually have a mixed physical constitution—cold and dry, damp and hot, cold and deficient, or another combination.

The individual's balanced diet, therefore, is always a mixture of foods with different flavors and energies suited to the needs of the individual's physical constitution. To design a balanced diet for yourself, there are some general principles you can follow: If you have a cold physical constitution, eat more foods with a hot or warm energy and fewer foods with a cold or cool energy. As for the flavors of foods, eat more sweet and pungent foods and decrease bitter foods.

If you have a hot physical constitution, eat more foods with a cool or cold energy; consider-

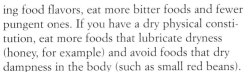

ing food flavors, eat more bitter foods and fewer pungent ones. If you have a dry physical constitution, eat more foods that lubricate dryness (honey, for example) and avoid foods that dry dampness in the body (such as small red beans).

If you have a damp physical constitution, eat more foods that dry dampness and promote water passage; avoid foods that can produce fluids. If you have a deficient physical constitution, you should eat more foods that can move you towards the excessive side in energy. Such foods are called tonics (yam and red date, for example); eat fewer foods that can make you deficient (these normally taste bitter). If you have an excessive physical constitution, choose more foods that can promote energy and blood circulation; avoid foods that can decrease your energy.

I have discussed how the individual's balanced diet may be designed according to six types of individual physical constitution. In addition, each person should also pay attention to a diet that maintains the balance of internal organs. This is called the organic balanced diet.

## THE ORGANIC BALANCED DIET

The organic balanced diet refers to a diet that maintains the balance of internal organs. Since each person has different organic conditions, the organic balanced diet also varies with these conditions. Each individual has organic strengths and organic weaknesses. For example, a person may be strong in the digestive functions but weak in the reproductive functions. The fact that a person has an excellent appetite does not necessarily mean that his heart is also in good shape or his sexual capacities measure up to the standard.

Ideally, the diet for organic balance guarantees that all internal organs are kept in good condition. This is important, not only because all internal organs should be in good shape, but also because when one organ is excessively strong, it tends to weaken another organ, creating an organic imbalance. Here is a simple example: When a person gains twenty or thirty pounds within two or three months, he may become sexually weak or even impotent. Why? Because the excessive strength of his stomach is putting pressure on his kidneys, which, according to Chinese medical theory, are responsible for sexual capacities.

It is rather difficult for a layman to determine personal organic strengths and weaknesses that require expert knowledge about Chinese medicine. Suppose as an example, a person suffering from heartburn consults his doctor and is advised to have a physical check-up that may turn up nothing no gastritis, gastric ulcers, or excessive gastric acid. His stomach may also look normal, so the doctor tells him that he is in good health. But then the person suffering with heartburn begins to wonder whether he really is in good health. A question emerges in his mind, "If I am in good health, why do I have heartburn?"

Let's assume this person is quite curious and one day decides to consult a Chinese herbalist. The Chinese herbalist asks him how his stomach feels and he answers that he feels burning sensations in his stomach. The Chinese herbalist asks him whether he enjoys drinking liquor and he replies that drinking whiskey produces even more severe hot sensations in his stomach. The Chinese herbalist asks him whether spicy foods agree with him and he answers that spicy foods make his hot sensations worse. The Chinese herbalist then diagnoses that the patient's stomach is too hot. But the patient insists that his doctor checked his stomach very thoroughly and found nothing wrong with his stomach.

How does the Chinese herbalist know that this person's stomach is too hot? In fact, the answer is not as difficult as it appears. The fact that the patient feels burning sensations in the stomach indicates that this is a hot disease which gets worse when consuming liquor and spicy foods. Both liquor and spicy foods are either very warm or hot—bad for a hot stomach. A hot stomach should be cooled down by eating foods that have a cold or cool energy. If such foods cannot heal the symptoms, then cold herbs should be used; herbs are stronger than foods. This brings out another important aspect of balanced diet, namely, the diet for restoring the balance of the body.

## RESTORING THE BODY BALANCE

When a person becomes ill, the balance of his or her body is lost—at least temporarily. If you have a headache, for example, it means your body balance is lost; it is necessary to create a diet to restore the balance, or in other words, to relieve your symptoms. Normally, the symptoms you develop are consistent with your physical constitution: If you have a hot physical constitution, you will probably develop hot symptoms (such as skin eruptions and hot rheumatism), a cold physical constitution, cold symptoms (such as cold vomiting and cold rheumatism). For this reason, it is important to know your own physical constitution to deal with occasional symptoms. Conversely, it is also easy for you to identify your physical constitution through the symptoms. If you have a tendency to suffer from constipation, you most probably have a hot or dry physical constitution; if you suffer from rheumatic pain that gets worse on cold days or on exposure to cold environments, then you most probably have a cold physical constitution. People who suffer rheumatic pain in the same joints—with increasing pain on rainy days—have damp rheumatism. These people probably have a damp physical constitution.

The symptoms may sometimes run counter to one's physical constitution, however, which means that a person with a hot physical constitution may develop cold symptoms from time to time and a person with a cold physical constitution may develop hot symptoms as well. As an example, even though you have a hot physical constitution, you may still suffer though you have a cold physical constitution, sometimes you may still have fever (a hot symptom). For this reason, treatment of symptoms may involve foods that are normally not good for the person who develops the temporary symptoms. When a person with a cold physical constitution develops fever (a hot symptom), he or she may have to eat foods with a cold energy, although such foods may normally be bad for that person.

The more you learn about Chinese diet, the more you will be able to apply it with flexibility. Even with a fair knowledge of the Chinese beliefs, you will benefit from it. How would you feel if you recovered from eczema simply by drinking mung bean soup for a few weeks? How would you feel if you recovered from neuralgic pain simply by drinking hot ginger soup? How would you feel if you recovered from migraine headache simply by drinking peppermint tea?

I had runny nose yesterday and my eyes were itchy. I knew I had caught cold—but I did not have cold sensations nor did I have fever. The only symptoms were runny nose and itchy eyes. So, I boiled hot water, cut up a lemon, squeezed juice into the hot water and added one spoonful of sugar. I drank the warm lemon juice. At this writing I feel fine. Why did I drink lemon juice? Everybody knows that lemon has lots of vitamin C. But yesterday, I was not interested in vitamin C, I only wanted to stop my nasal discharge. I know that lemon is extremely sour and the foods that have a sour flavor are obstructive. This is why I used lemon juice—its obstructive nature can stop my runny nose. Moreover, lemon can produce fluids that are good for me, not only because my eyes were itchy (due to dryness) but also because I have a dry physical constitution. Why did I add sugar? There are two reasons: One, lemon juice is so sour that it is not very pleasing to me; two, sugar can also produce fluids that are good for my dry symptom. I could have made a mistake by adding honey instead of sugar; honey is very glossy, which could make my nasal discharge worse and cancel out the obstructive nature of lemon. Why did I drink very warm lemon juice instead of chilling it in the refrigerator and drinking it cold? Because my runny nose was caused by coldness and I knew the warm lemon juice would make me warm.

In the previous chapters, I discussed energies and flavors of foods. Now you can put this knowledge to use. But before you begin to apply my suggestions to benefit your health, there is one important concept you should know about — yin and yang. The theory of yin and yang is fundamental in Chinese medicine and should be regarded as such when discussing food cures. In fact, everything in the universe can be classified into yin and yang: man is yang, woman is yin; the sun is yang, the moon is yin; day is yang, night is yin; functions of the human body are yang, its

food should be calculated separately; then add them and divide by 2 to arrive at the y-score. As an example, garlic has a warm energy and a pungent flavor. It has a y-score of +4 in energy and +8 in flavor with a total score of +12 (4+8), which means garlic has a y-score of +6. Take watermelon as another example; it has a cold energy and a sweet flavor. This means that watermelon has a y-score of -8 in energy and +4 in flavor with the total score of -4, which means watermelon has a y-score of -2.

If a given food has two or more flavors or

# Body Types and The Yin-Yang Principles

shape is yin; heaven is yang, earth is yin; skin and muscles are yang, internal organs are yin; the back is yang, the abdomen is yin.

The energies and flavors of foods are also classified into yin and yang. Hot and warm energies are yang; cool and cold energies are yin. Pungent and sweet flavors are yang; sour, bitter and salty flavors are yin. When we try to classify foods into yin and yang, we must consider both their energies and flavors. Sometimes, the energy of a food may be yang and its flavor yin, which seems contradictory but is not.

## Y-SCORES

I have designed a comprehensive chart of y-scores (Table 1) by which food and body types, diseases, moods and four seasons may be classified into yin and yang. Y-scores stand for the yin or yang scores of a given item. This table is not only simple in design but also accurate to apply. After you have learned how to use the table by reading this chapter, you will find it very convenient to use in deciding what foods to eat and under what circumstances to eat them.

Y-scores can be used to determine to what extent a given food or disease or body type or season is yin or yang because it is a quantification of yin and yang. If a given item is preceded by +, it is yang; if preceded by -, it is yin.

Yin and yang may be better understood as two adjectives, instead of nouns, because as adjectives, we can say one thing is more yang or more yin than another. For example, if the energy of a food is hot, it has a y-score of +8 and if the energy of another food is warm, it has a y-score of +4, which means that the first food is more yang than the second one. Again, if the energy of one food is cool, it has a y-score of -4 and if the energy of another food is cold, it has a y-score of -8, which means the second food is more yin than the first one.

In determining the y-score of a given food, both the y-score of its energy and that of its flavor should be taken into account. To compute it, the y-scores of flavor and those of energy of a given

energies, their y-scores should average out to the mean score. As an example, kumquat has three flavors, namely, pungent (+8), sweet (+4) and sour (-4), with a total score of +8, which averages out to +3 as its flavor; and since kumquat is warm (+4), you add it to +3 (flavor average) and divide by 2. The y-score of kumquat is +3 or +4.

After determining the y-score of a given food, you can know its movements simply by reading Table 3.

If a food has a y-score of +8, it can move outward; if it has a y-score of +4, it can move upwards; if it has a y-score of -4, it can move downwards; if it has a y-score of -8, it can move inward; if it has a y-score of 0, it is neutral. What if a food has a y-score of +6? Does it move upwards or outward? To answer this question, it is important to remember that there is a continuity between yin and yang which, in turn, means there is also a continuity between upward and outward movements. If a food has a y-score of +6, it may move upwards and outward simultaneously, or it may move more upwards then outward or vice versa. As we have just seen, garlic has a y-score of +6 and watermelon has a y-score of -2. With this information, we know that garlic moves upwards or outward but that watermelon moves downwards. This is the general principle governing the relationships between energy and flavor of foods on the one hand and the movements of foods on the other. There are exceptions to this general principle, which are usually stated in this book under each food involved. One such exception is sword bean. According to the general principle, sword bean should move upwards since it is warm and sweet. Nevertheless, sword bean moves downwards instead of upwards according to the established theory.

As already discussed in the previous chapter, many health problems are classified into outward, upward, downward, inward diseases, symptoms, or ailments. Vomiting, panting and hiccupping are upward ailments; prolapse of anus and falling of the stomach are downward problems; fever, excessive perspiration and night sweat are outward symptoms; diarrhea and abdominal swelling are inward ailments. Certainly exceptions exist, but as a general rule, foods that have a y-score of +4 (upward movement) may be used to treat downward diseases; foods that have a y-score of -4 (downward movement) may be used to treat upward diseases; foods that have a y-score of +8 (outward movement) may be used to treat inward diseases; and foods that have a y-score of -8 (inward movement) may be used to treat outward diseases.

Suppose you are hiccupping at this moment and try to decide whether to eat garlic or watermelon to stop the hiccupping. It is obvious that watermelon should be your logical choice: It has a y-score of -2, which means that it can move downwards; that is good for hiccupping. Let's further assume that you have a mild cold and try to decide whether to eat garlic or watermelon in order to speed up your recovery. It is obvious that garlic should be your logical choice, because it has a y-score of +6, which means that it can move upwards and outward to induce perspiration; thus it is good for a common cold.

The movements of foods may also be applied to treat the diseases that are not in motion, namely, they are not moving upwards or downwards or outward or inward, but stay in the same region. For example, if you have a headache, the pain may stay in your head without moving in any direction; if you have a stomachache, the pain may stay in the stomach without moving in any direction; if you suffer from arthritis, the pain may stay in the knee joint without moving in any direction. Such symptoms are called symptoms in the fixed regions and they may be treated by foods with different y-scores: When a disease occurs in the upper region, like headache or stomachache, it should be treated by foods with a y-score of +4 (upward movement) so that the effects of foods can reach the head; when a disease occurs in the lower region, like arthritis involving the knee joints, it should be treated by foods with a y-score of -4 (downward movement) so that the foods can reach the knee joints; when a disease occurs in the outer region, like pain in the muscles, it should be treated by foods with a y-score of +8 (outward movement) so that the foods can reach the muscles; when a disease occurs in the inner region, like constipation or abdominal swelling, it should be treated by foods with y-score of -8 (inward movement) so that the foods can reach the affected regions.

## YOUR BODY TYPE

What if you are not suffering from any disease? What foods should you eat? To choose foods wisely, it is necessary to have an adequate knowledge of your body type. Body types, like foods, may also be classified into yin and yang to be determined by the concept of y-scores. If your body type has a y-score of, say, +8, it is wise for you to eat more foods with a y-score of -8 to strike a balance; if you have a y-score of -8, for example,

it is wise to eat more foods with a y-score of +8 to strike a balance. In other words, a yin person wisely should eat more yang foods and a yang person more yin foods to create a balance between yin and yang in the body.

But how can you determine your body type, whether it is yin or yang? There are four basic factors that should be taken into consideration: hot/cold, dry/damp, dispositions and sex life.

The hot/cold dichotomy may be determined by the answers to the following four questions:

First, do you normally have cold hands or cold feet? If your answer is yes, then your y-score is -8.

Second, do you normally have warm hands or warm feet? If your answer is yes, then your y-score is +8.

Third, do you generally prefer cold winter to hot summer? If your answer is yes, then your y-score is -4.

Fourth, do you generally prefer hot summer to cold winter? If your answer is yes, then your y-score is +4.

If you cannot decide on the answer to any of the above questions, then your y-score is 0 (neutral). Let's assume that your answers to the first and third questions are positive, then your y-score, the addition of -8 and -4 divided by 2, is -6.

The dry/damp dichotomy may be determined by your body weight, with each 5 overweight or underweight pounds to be counted as +1 or -1, making a maximum score of either +8 or -8. Here's how it works: If you are 5 pounds overweight, your y-score is -1; if you are 5 pounds underweight, your y-score is +1; if you are 10 pounds overweight, your y-score is -2; if you are 40 pounds (or more) overweight, your y-score is -8. As you can see, overweight is yin, underweight is yang. Men are yang and women are yin (small wonder there are more overweight women than men); a rooster is a very yang creature (small wonder that each rooster is underweight); a hen is a very yin creature (small wonder that each hen is overweight). One man may be more underweight than another, because the former is more yang than the latter; by the same token, a woman may be more overweight than another, because the former is more yin than the latter.

The dichotomy of excess and deficiency may be determined by the conditions of body energy. If you normally feel energetic, your y-score is +8; if you seldom feel tired, but only once in a while, your y-score is +4; if you normally feel lazy but not tired, your y-score is -4; if you normally feel tired, your y-score is -8; if you do not know the answer, your y-score is 0. If both +8 and +4 are applicable to you, pick +8 as your y-score; if both -8 and -4 are applicable to you, pick -8 as your y-score; if more than two scores are applicable to you, average them out to arrive at a y-score.

The dichotomy of dispositions may be determined by the nature of your answer to this question: Do you fall to sleep while you are on board a plane or sitting in a chair or in the car as a passenger? If your answer is "very often or easily," your y-score is -8; if your answer is "never or only when extremely tired," your y-score is +8; if your answer is "easily when a little tired," your y-score is +4; if your answer is "occasionally even though not tired," your y-score is -4. If both +4 and +8 are applicable to you, pick +8; if both -4 and -8 are applicable to you, pick -8.

The dichotomy of sex life is self-evident, requiring no further explanations with the exception of the greater than symbol (>), which is used here to denote preference. Sex > foods denotes enjoyment of sex more than foods, which has a y-score of +4; and foods > sex denotes enjoyment of foods more than sex, which has a y-score of -4. In case two scores are equally applicable to you, pick the higher score as your y-score. As an example, if both +4 and +8 are applicable to you, your y-score should be +8; if both -4 and -8 are applicable to you, your y-score should be -8. If you cannot decide on which category you belong to, your y-score is 0, which means neutral or indecisive.

After you have arrived at a y-score in each of the above five dichotomies, add the five y-scores and then divide by 5 to arrive at your y-score — a description of your body type. For example, if your y-score in the hot/cold dichotomy +4, in the dry/damp dichotomy +8, in the excessive/deficient dichotomy +8, in the dispositions dichotomy 0 and in the sex life dichotomy +4, then your y-scores should average out to +5. This is the y-score of your body type.

You are ready to choose foods for your needs on this basic principle: A person with a yang body type should eat more yin foods and a person with a yin body type should eat more yang foods in order to create a yin-yang balance in the body.

## ALLERGIES AND BODY TYPES

All of us have heard about the word "allergy" in modern medicine, but what does it mean? Some people cannot stand certain foods and they are often told by their doctors that they cannot stand such foods because they are allergic to them. Thus the word allergy, in fact, is nothing but a vicious circle in disguise, neither better nor worse than no explanation at all.

The concept of allergies in modern medicine may be explained better in terms of the interaction between foods and body types, however. An individual with a body type y-score of -8 for example, may not tolerate foods with a y-score of -8, because they will drive him towards the yin limit; an individual with a y-score of +8 in body type may not tolerate foods with a y-score of +8, because they will drive him towards the yang limit, particularly when such foods are consumed for a prolonged period of time. If your body type has a y-score of +8, it is better for you to eat more seaweed, for example, which has a y-score of -6 than fresh ginger, which has a y-score of +6; fresh ginger adds +6 to your body and makes a total y-score of +14; by eating seaweed, -6 is added to your body, which makes only a total of +2. Thus, the choice of eating seaweed and fresh ginger equals the difference between +14 and +2, indeed, a very significant difference. It is important, therefore, to select foods according to your body type so that a balance between yin and yang may be created in the body to maintain good health and to prevent disease.

## DISEASES AND Y-SCORES

The hot/cold dichotomy concept may be applied to disease as well, because some diseases are hot, while others are cold diseases. Here are the criteria to help you distinguish between the two: If the disease gets worse on exposure to cold surroundings or if it gets better on exposure to warm or hot surrounding, then it is a cold disease and should be assigned a y-score of -8; if the disease deteriorates on exposure to warm or hot surroundings or if it gets better on exposure to cool or cold surroundings, then it is a hot disease and should be assigned a y-score of +8. If the patient prefers cool or cold surroundings, it is a warm disease, which should be assigned a y-score of +4; if the patient prefers warm or hot surroundings, it is a cool disease and should be assigned a y-score of -4. In case both +4 and +8 are applicable to a patient, +8 should be chosen as its y-score; in case both -4 and -8 are applicable to a patient, -8 should be chosen as its y-score. In case a patient cannot decide on the right answer, the y-score is 0.

The y-scores of diseases may be applied to choose foods for patients the same way the y-scores of body types are applied to choose foods for different people. When a person has a high fever (obviously a hot disease), it is only logical for him to eat more yin foods; conversely, if a person is shivering with cold, it is only logical for him to eat more yang foods. Some arthritis patients get worse in winter, which means that it is a cold disease; therefore, they should eat more yang foods. If some people have a skin disease that gets worse in summer, on exposure to sunlight or heat in the kitchen, it is a hot disease; they should eat more yin foods to improve the conditions. In my clinical practice, I have seen patients with skin itch (like urticaria) which starts as soon as they come close to the kitchen as if they were allergic to the kitchen. In fact, they are not allergic to the kitchen; it is the kitchen heat that triggers their itch. Conversely, some patients with itchy skin feel much better when they are in the kitchen; but as soon as they are exposed to cold air, their itching starts, because they are suffering from a cold disease.

## MOODS AND Y-SCORES

Moreover, our knowledge of food y-scores also enables us to control our moods—or create moods we desire. As you can see from the chart, cheerful and joyful moods have a y-score of +8, hopeful and comfortable a y-score of +4, thinking and reasoning a y-score of 0, depressed and sad moods have a y-score of -4, scary and fearful moods a y-score of -8. Assume that you feel depressed and sad, for one reason or another and begin to wonder, "Which food will change my depressed or sad moods—garlic or watermelon?" The answer seems clear from the chart: Garlic should be your logical choice, because it can increase your yang scores and shift your moods towards the yang side.

There is another example demonstrating how to create the moods by eating suitable foods. People often say, "I can't think straight." To think straight, the y-score of moods should be 0, as indicated in the chart; foods with a neutral energy and light flavor are the most suitable foods to eat.

It is important to remember, however, that the above examples are given merely from the point of view of y-scores of foods. In actual practice, we must also consider y-scores of our body types. For example, if your body type has a y-score of +8 and you eat the foods with a y-score of +8, your body conditions will stay in the same position, namely, a y-score of +8 that creates cheerful and joyful moods instead of thinking and reasoning ones. On the other hand, if you eat the foods with a y-score of -8, it will shift your body conditions from +8 towards 0 to create thinking and reasoning moods.

The formula that creates the desired moods may be stated as follows: Y-score of moods equals the addition of y-score of body type and y-score of foods divided by 2. By using this formula, a person with a body type y-score of +4 should eat foods with a y-score of +4 to create hopeful and comfortable moods; a person with body type y-score of -4 should eat foods with a y-score of +4 to create the moods conducive to thinking and reasoning.

According to the y-scores of Table 5, it seems impossible for a person with a body type y-score of -8 to have cheerful and joyful moods no matter which foods he or she eats. This conclusion is wrong. "Body type" refers only to a relatively constant state of physical conditions that may change occasionally to create a different mood. When we say, "He is a cheerful person," we are talking about the constant mood consistent with his body type; but when we say, "He is cheerful," we mean the temporary mood (that may not be consistent with his body type) created by a combination of body type and foods or a temporary change in body conditions due to other environmental factors.

## Y-SCORES AND THE FOUR SEASONS

Is it true that a person with a body type y-score of +4, for example, always or frequently remains hopeful and comfortable and that a person with a y-score of -4 is always or frequently in a depressed or sad mood? The answer depends mostly on what he eats as well as on other environmental factors. We have to eat and live in some environment. Our body begins to interact with the foods and surroundings, which combine to create different moods.

The four seasons are environmental factors that can significantly affect our moods. Like foods, the four seasons are also classified into yin and yang with different y-scores assigned to them: summer, +8; spring, +4; autumn, -4; winter, -8.

In summer, people of all body types move towards the yang side, in winter, towards the yin side, hence creating seasonal moods. So in summer it is easier to create cheerful and joyful moods and in winter to become depressed and sad or even scared and fearful.

It is important to remember, whichever your body type, you should eat more hot and pungent foods in summer, more warm and sweet foods in spring, more neutral and light foods in between summer and autumn, more cool and sour foods in autumn and more cold and bitter foods in winter. This may seem to contradict the principle stated earlier that to create the yin-yang balance people with a hot body type should eat more cold foods and people with a cold body type more hot foods, which implies that one should eat more cold foods in summer, more hot in winter to create a yin-yang balance. Nevertheless, the two seemingly contradictory principles are resolved by the fact that foods and seasons have a difference in their impact on the human body: Foods, when eaten, become part of the human body; the four seasons (as environmental factors) are external to the human body. When a person with a hot body type eats cold foods, for example, the cold energy of foods is absorbed to become part of his body so that the heat of the body is reduced and the yin-yang balance within the body is achieved; on the other hand, summer heat is always external to the body and in summer, the body surface is constantly under the impact of summer heat that creates an imbalance between the internal body region and the body surface; for this reason, in summer, it is necessary to eat more hot and warm foods to increase internal body heat so that a yin-yang balance between the internal region and body surface can be achieved. By the same token, in winter, the body surface is constantly under the impact of winter cold that creates an imbalance between the internal region and the body surface and it is necessary to eat more cold and cool foods to cool the internal region to achieve a yin-yang balance between the internal body region and the surface.

Chinese herbalists believe that in spring, one should eat more foods that move upwards (warm and sweet foods) to stay in harmony with the growing season (living things begin to grow, an upward movement); in summer, eat more foods that move outward (hot and pungent foods) to remain harmonious with the season (living things begin to expand, an outward movement); in autumn, eat more foods that move downwards (cool and sour foods) (living things begin to fall, a downward movement); in winter, eat more foods that move inward (cold, salty and bitter foods) (living things begin to shrink, an inward movement). This theory is consistent with the common practice of applying fertilizers to plants in spring when living things begin to grow, but futile to do in winter when plants are ready to move downwards.

I take this principle of harmony between foods and the four seasons very seriously, not only because I practice Chinese medicine, but also because of a painful personal experience. I used to develop swelling and pain in my foot every winter. Each recurrence brought severe pain and the swelling lasted for a month or longer, virtually preventing me from walking and working. At first, I kept asking myself why this happened only in winter, not in summer. I figured that it must have something to do with the winter cold. So I started warming my foot in hot water every day, which seemed to help a little bit but not enough to cure the pain or heal the swelling to any significant degree. This problem lasted for three years. One day, this principle of harmony between the internal region and body surface suddenly dawned on me. I began to suspect the swelling and pain could have developed from the disparity between my internal region and body surface since the body surface was constantly exposed to severe winter cold whereas my internal region remained hot. When a disparity between the internal region and

body surface developed, the heat in the internal region erupted like a volcano, the cause of the pain and swelling. When I tried to warm my foot in hot water, I tried to counteract the cold impact of winter on my body surface instead of staying in harmony with the winter by cooling down my internal region. So I began to eat yin foods and yin herbs and finally bade farewell to those annual miseries, thanks to the master Chinese herbalist Shi-Chen Li (1518-1593). He stated, in his most celebrated book in Chinese herbal therapy, *An Outline of Materia Medica*, published in 1578: "In spring, one should eat more pungent and warm foods to stay in harmony with the upward movement of the season; in summer, one should eat more pungent and hot foods to stay in harmony with the outward movement of the season; in autumn, one should eat more sour and warm foods to stay in harmony with the downward movement of the season; in winter, one should eat more bitter and cold foods to stay in harmony with the inward movement of the season."

In China today, diseases are treated either by Western medicine or traditional Chinese medicine or both, depending on the nature of the diseases and the patient's choice. When I visited China in 1983, our bus driver told me of his plans to see a doctor the following day and I asked him which doctor he wanted to see, a doctor of Western medicine or a doctor of Chinese medicine. He had made an appointment to see the latter, he said. I asked him how he made that choice. Normally, he replied, a Chinese patient relies on the advice of a friend or acquaintance,

and a pungent flavor (foods with a warm or hot energy will relieve shivering and foods with a pungent flavor will induce perspiration). When the patient with a common cold begins to develop fever, the foods consumed should have a cold or cool energy to reduce the fever (the disease has changed from a cold disease into a hot one); therefore, to reduce the fever the patient should eat foods with a cold or cool energy instead of foods with a warm or hot energy. But the foods with a pungent flavor should still be used to induce

# Preventing and Curing Ailments

for that matter, someone who had suffered from a similar disease and had been cured.

## COMMON COLD

- Cook noodles according to the patient's taste and add 25g fresh onion white heads and 25g fresh ginger; mix thoroughly. The patient may begin to perspire afterwards and should stay in bed after eating it.
- Peel and crush 15g garlic; add 15ml rice vinegar. Use this mixture the same as the noodles (above).
- Slice 30g old or fresh ginger and boil in 300ml water until the water is reduced to 100ml; add some brown sugar and boil again until the sugar dissolves. Drink the whole thing and stay in bed to perspire.
- Boil 30g hyacinth beans in water until they break; add 30g sugar and boil again until the sugar dissolves. After eating, stay in bed to perspire.
- Boil 10g peppermint and 10g crushed green onion white heads in water to make tea to relieve headache due to common cold.
- Other foods considered beneficial to common cold are orange peel, peppermint, green onion bulb and radish.
- Crush 100g fresh ginger and squeeze out the juice; mix the juice with rice wine and warm in a small pan. Drink the beverage to induce perspiration.
- Fry a few garlic cloves and grind into powder; mix 2 teaspoonfuls of the garlic powder with a little sugar and eat it to relieve cough due to common cold.
- Break an egg into a glass of rice wine and mix with a spoon; warm it over low heat until the egg is half cooked; add some sugar. Drink it as soup to relieve headache and shivering due to common cold.
- Like any other disease, treatment of common cold varies with different symptoms. At the beginning stage, the patient may shiver with cold but without fever, which should be relieved by foods with a warm or hot energy

perspiration. On the other hand, common cold with a sore throat or any other inflammation should be treated as a hot symptom.

## Internal Conditions

### INFLUENZA

- Boil 10g yellow soybeans in water for 15 minutes; add 30g parsley and boil it again for 15 minutes. Drink the soup and stay in bed to perspire.
- Slice 250g fresh radish and soak it in a suitable quantity of vinegar for a few hours. Eat it as salad.
- Put a few slices green onion white heads or garlic in a respiratory mask; inhale for prevention of and recovery from influenza.
- Grate 150g fresh radish and mix it with honey in a jar. Seal the jar for 1 week. Eat a small cupful each time, 3 times a day.

### DIABETES

Sugar in the urine as one of the most important symptoms of diabetes was included in the Chinese medical classic, *A Collection of Diseases*, by Wang Shou, published in 752. For the first time in Chinese medical history, diabetes was listed among the eleven hundred diseases in the book. The author recommended pork pancreas as treatment for the disease and had also used a special method of testing sugar in the urine: The patient passed urine on a wide, flat brick to see if ants gathered to collect the sugar. This method of testing urine was more than ten centuries ahead of Richard Thomas Williamson (1862-1937), who invented a test for the same purpose. The Chinese author's treatment using pork pancreas was similar to modern treatment by insulin, a hormone secreted by the beta cells of the islets of Langerhans of the pancreas.

In Chinese medicine, however, thirst, weight

loss, fatigue and sugar in the urine are considered the key symptoms of diabetes. When a patient recovers from any of these symptoms, the diabetes treatment is considered successful.

Twenty-five diabetes patients were treated at the Canton College of Traditional Chinese Medicine by dried bitter melon slices; each dosage per day consisted of 250g dried bitter melon slices boiled in water. The levels of their blood sugar taken 2.5 hours after meals and of their urine sugar taken 24 hours after meals, were both statistically very significant; the same method has subsequently been applied on diabetic rats, which also resulted in a significant decrease in the level of blood sugar; the same report concludes that the effects of dried bitter melon are comparable to those of insulin. It is also suggested that when 100g fresh clams are boiled in water with the dried bitter melon slices, the results should be better.

A clinic in the Province of Jiangxi in China reports the treatment of a diabetic patient with good results in which a total of 100g fresh corn are boiled each time as one dosage. The patient had suffered from diabetes for over 2 years with sugar in the urine, puffiness in the body, frequent urination and had been treated by Western medicine with no results. Under the treatment by corn the patient had recovered after taking only 4 dosages. Subsequently, another Chinese physician, on reading this report from a medical journal, had used the same remedy to treat a 63-year-old diabetic patient and found it to be equally effective —the patient showed a very significant decrease in the level of blood sugar after undergoing less than 10 treatments. Another clinic in the same province had developed a food cure for diabetes which consists of 60 percent wheat bran and 40 percent wheat powder, mixed with chicken eggs to make a cake remedy (without sugar). At the beginning, the patients were treated with 500g of this cake remedy each day, with the proportion of wheat bran gradually decreased as symptoms improved. Among the 15 cases treated by this method, the level of blood sugar was tested in 10 cases, among them, blood sugar was reduced to lower than 140mg per 100ml blood in 3 cases and reduced to the level lower than 180mg per 100ml blood in 7 cases. All 13 cases showed a general improvement in all other symptoms.

At the International Symposium on the Effects of Ginseng held in the Soviet Union in 1954, a report indicates that ginseng is capable of lowering the level of blood sugar; and a Chinese physician also points out that according to his experiments, ginseng is capable of reducing the level of blood sugar by as much as 40 to 50mg per 100ml blood; such effects can continue for more than 2 weeks after the patient stops taking ginseng. Moreover, in some cases, insulin intake can be reduced while the patient is taking ginseng.

- Chop 50g fresh potato leaves and 100g wax gourd; steam over water as a dosage for daily consumption.
- Soak 100g fresh onion in boiling water for 1 minute; season with a little salt. Eat twice a day.
- Boil 1 cup mare's milk as a daily dosage. Drink the milk twice a day. Mare's milk has a cool energy and sweet flavor; it can lubricate dryness, reduce heat and quench thirst; it is used for fatigue and diabetes. A Chinese diet classic says, "Mare's milk has the same function as cow's milk, but it is not as fatty as cow's milk; it is effective for reducing the heat of the gall bladder and the stomach, considered beneficial to sore throat, good for the head and the eyes and also effective for the relief of diabetes."
- According to Chinese herb remedies, pork pancreas has a neutral energy and a sweet flavor; it is used to treat chronic tracheitis, cough, shortage of milk secretion and emphysema. Boil a pork, beef, or lamb pancreas in water with 200g yam; season with some salt. Divide into 4 parts. Eat each part once a day for 4 days. Or cut up a pork pancreas and bake until dry over low heat; grind into powder. Take 3 to 5g in warm water each time, 3 times a day. Or wash the pork pancreas, remove and discard all the white fat and cut into thin pieces; boil over low heat in water with 20g corn silk; season with some salt. Eat daily. The use of pork pancreas as an ingredient in a dietary formula to treat diabetes in China was originally published in 1846 in a Chinese diet classic, *New Collected Works of Proven Dietary Recipes*.
- Mix 50g yam powder with 10g ginseng powder (readily available in shops). Take 3 times a day, 15g each time, dissolved in warm water.
- Boil 30g fresh watermelon peel in 2 glasses water. Drink 1 glass each time, twice a day.
- Soak 100g mung beans overnight; boil in 3 glasses water over low heat until beans break. Eat as soup in a day.
- Boil 250 to 300g fresh radish in water with 20 to 25g abalone. Drink as soup, once every other day. Repeat 6 to 7 times as a treatment program (this is a time-honored recipe in Chinese folk medicine for diabetes).
- Boil 150g chive (or chive shoots) with 200g clams and suitable seasoning. Eat in a day. This remedy is also good for excessive perspiration and pulmonary tuberculosis.

## HYPERTENSION

- In the Ping-Yang Seaweed Culture Unit in the Province of Zhejiang, China, 110 cases of hypertension were treated by seaweed root powder; in 19 cases (17.3 percent), diastolic blood pressure was reduced by over 20mm of mercury and in 65 cases (59.1 percent), diastolic blood pressure was reduced by 10 to 19mm or to lower than 90mm of mercury and systolic blood pressure reduced by more than 20mm of mercury. The report concluded that the total effective rate of 76.4 percent was achieved and that seaweed roots are waste materials, readily available without any side effects, thus making the therapy both effective and economical.

- In a clinical report, 30 to 40g dried peanut plants were boiled to make tea as a daily dosage for 2 weeks; patients were instructed to drink the tea from peanut plants on an irregular basis after blood pressure returned to normal. Twenty cases of hypertension were treated by this method; the majority showed improvements within 3 days with a significant decrease in blood pressure (the mean value-systolic pressure was reduced by 29mm and diastolic pressure by 30mm of mercury).
- A patient of hypertension in Tianjin, China, wrote to an editor to say that he had been suffering from hypertension with dizziness and constipation for many years but had been unable to find a cure; subsequently, he began to eat 5 bananas every day, which eventually cured his disease.
- A Chinese physician reported a 49-year-old female patient suffered from hypertension with occasional constipation, headache and dizziness; she had taken honey for 2 months, which reduced her blood pressure to normal and cured her constipation as well.
- There are basically 3 ways to cope with hypertension, according to the Chinese diet system. First, eat more foods that can soften the blood vessels, such as kelp, sea grass, mung bean sprouts, fruits and others, to prevent arteriosclerosis. Second, use vegetable oils such as sesame, peanut and corn oil, instead of animal fats and oils to reduce the level of cholesterol; and avoid foods with a high cholesterol level, such as egg yolk, liver and kidneys. Third, eat more foods that can reduce blood pressure, such as celery, hawthorn fruit, banana and persimmon.
- Wash 500g fresh celery and squeeze out the juice; mix the juice with 50ml honey and warm it in a small pan. Divide and drink twice a day.
- Soak mung beans in water overnight; the next day, boil with an equal amount of seaweed and some rice (for long-term consumption).
- Eat 1 to 2 fresh tomatoes on an empty stomach first thing in the morning for 15 days. Repeat from time to time as a treatment program. This is also good for constipation.
- Cook tomatoes with celery as soup; season with a little salt.
- Chop 750g water chestnuts and 750g radishes; squeeze out the juice; mix with a few teaspoonfuls honey. Drink the juice twice a day, half of the portion each time.
- Fry 20g kelp with 20 black soybeans; boil kelp and soybeans in 3 cups water until water is reduced by half. Eat as soup.
- Regularly eat seaweed, mung beans, hawthorn fruit, clams and mung bean sprouts.

## KIDNEY DISEASE

- Wash and peel 300g old ginger; crush it to squeeze out the juice; soak 50g red dates in water for half an hour until soft; crush them after peeling and removing the seeds. Combine ginger juice and crushed dates in container; add 100g brown sugar and steam until they become like a pudding. Eat 3 times a day for 5 days.
- Chinese people in small villages have the habit of eating "watermelon sugar" as a food to treat kidney disease. Slice watermelon (red part only) into thin pieces and cook over low heat; then add a little sugar and strain; after 4 or 5 days, the juice will thicken like honey, which is called watermelon sugar. Eat 1 tablespoonful each time, twice a day.

## NEPHRITIS

- Using a sharp knife, make a triangular hole in a 1.5kg watermelon to remove some flesh; place 70g peeled garlic cloves inside the watermelon; cover the hole with cut piece of the rind; steam the watermelon with the garlic; and eat the whole thing while hot.
- Boil 30g dried watermelon peel in water. Drink as tea. Or boil 2 corncobs in water and drink it as tea.
- Eat 1 or 2 fresh cucumbers; or crush the cucumbers to squeeze out the juice. Drink as tea; or boil dried cucumbers in water as soup.
- Prepare a large carp by removing the internal organs; do not scrape off the scales; use a cloth to dry the fish. Boil the carp in water with 1 cup small red beans without salt. Drink the soup, which is also good for edema due to nephritis during pregnancy in women.
- For difficulty when urinating, eat more foods that can promote urination, such as eggplant roots, cucumber, wax melon seeds and peel, corncob, watermelon peel, small red beans, sea grass, lily flowers, radish, black soybeans. Avoid fresh garlic, green onion, chive, red pepper, nicotine, alcohol.

## BRONCHITIS

- Crush 500g unpeeled radish or pear and soak in 2 teaspoonfuls honey for a few hours before eating it.
- In case of hoarseness due to bronchitis, boil some licorice in water over low heat. Eat as soup.
- Clean out a chicken and peel a grapefruit; stuff the grapefruit into the chicken cavity, place in a pan and add a little water; steam the chicken with the grapefruit inside. Eat the chicken and drink the broth. Repeat this remedy 3 times, once every other week.
- Older patients suffering with chronic bronchitis should be more energetic by eating fish, seafoods and yam.

## BRONCHIAL ASTHMA

- Wash and boil a pumpkin with 2 teaspoonfuls honey in water until the pumpkin becomes extremely soft; use the condensed pumpkin soup to mix with 10g fresh ginger juice. Boil the new mixture for a few minutes. Drink 1 cupful each time with warm water, 3 times a day.
- Boil together 200g bean curd, 60g maltose or honey and 30g fresh radish. Eat in 1 day to relieve the symptoms.
- Boil 2g fennel seed or anise seed, 10g apricot seed, 5g dry orange peel and 8g seaweed in 3 cups water until the water is reduced to 1 cup. Drink 1 cup as tea each time, 3 times a day.

## TUBERCULOSIS OF THE LYMPH NODE

- Boil together 50g dried litchi, 15g seaweed, 15g kelp and 1 teaspoonful wine in water. Eat the mixture in 1 day.
- Boil some noodles in water until half cooked; add 50g fresh oyster meats and 15g fresh garlic, crushed; boil again for a few minutes and season with some salt. Eat the entire stew in 1 day.
- Peel 90g garlic cloves; boil them in water with 2 unshelled duck eggs; when the eggs are hard-cooked, peel them and cook again for a while. Drink the soup and eat the eggs and garlic. (Duck eggs should be used instead of chicken eggs, for duck eggs can tone up yin energy and cool down the lungs.)
- Boil 120g fresh kelp or 60g dried kelp with an adequate amount of rice vinegar. Eat it as soup. This is not recommended for people with gastric and duodenal ulcers or excessive stomach acid.

## MUMPS

- Boil 50g fresh lily flowers or 20g dried lily flowers; add some salt. Drink it as soup.
- Crush 10g peeled garlic cloves in 10ml rice vinegar for external application to the affected region; or soak 50g small red beans in water for 30 minutes and crush them for external application to the affected region; or soak 50g small red beans overnight; boil until tender the next day. Eat it as soup in 1 day.

## CONTAGIOUS HEPATITIS

- Boil together 4 cups rice vinegar, 500g pork spareribs, 125g brown sugar and 125g white sugar for 30 minutes or less without adding water. Strain and drink each time as follows: 10 to 15ml for 5- to 10-year-old children; 20 to 30ml for 11- to 15-year-olds; 30 to 40ml for adults; 3 times a day after meals for 1 month as a treatment program; and 2 to 3 treatment programs for chronic patients.
- Wash 100 to 150g fresh celery and squeeze out the juice; steam the juice with honey. Eat it warm once a day.

## GASTROENTERITIS

- Bake 100g tea leaves and 50g fresh ginger; when dry, grind into powder. Take 3g of the powder each time, 3 times a day, with warm water. This is a good remedy for acute gastroenteritis.
- Boil 50g hyacinth beans in water as a day's dosage; divide and eat it twice a day. Or bake hyacinth beans until dry and grind into powder. Take 15g of the powder in warm water each time, twice a day. Another good remedy for acute gastroenteritis.
- Wine made from grapes is considered good for chronic gastroenteritis.
- Mix large pinches of ground nutmeg, ground cinnamon and a small pinch of ground cloves; divide into 3 equal portions. Take 1 portion in warm water each time, 3 times a day: Good for chronic gastroenteritis and cold stomach.

## GASTRIC AND DUODENAL ULCERS

- A well-known Japanese physician reported that a German professor at Berlin University used licorice powder to treat patients of gastric ulcers with remarkable results. According to this report in a German medical journal, 38 patients were treated with 20 to 25g licorice every day for 6 weeks; the gastric ulcers were completely gone in 32 cases, verified by x-ray examination; subjective sensations of stomach discomfort were eliminated in 3 cases. The remaining 3 cases showed no effects, but when subsequently treated by surgery were found to have stomach cancers.
- During the treatment, salt intake should be controlled and patients should be on high-protein and -vitamin diets. The professor pointed out that if a patient of gastric ulcer does not respond to treatment of licorice powder, the possibility of stomach cancer may be indicated. Subsequently, a professor and 2 assistants at Kyushu University in Japan also reported their treatment of licorice powder for 6 Japanese patients of gastric ulcers; the results indicated that abdominal pain and heartburn were completely gone within a week, gastric juices returned to normal and stools were free of blood within 2 weeks. X-ray examinations a month later verified the patients were completely cured. This dramatic cure of gastric ulcers, they pointed out, has never occurred in the past except by surgery.
- Soak 50g fresh peanuts in water for 30 minutes, drain and crush them; bring 200ml fresh milk to a boil and add the peanuts; again bring to a boil; remove from the heat to cool; add 30ml honey. Eat it once a day, an hour before bedtime.
- Cut up and crush 50g unpeeled fresh potatoes; squeeze out the juice and add a suitable quantity of honey to the juice. Drink the juice on an empty stomach first thing in the morning for 20 days. The potato's sour flavor will

be neutralized by the honey.

- Avoid irritating foods (liquor, coffee, red and black pepper, ginger), foods with a cold energy (crab, clam, seaweed, mung beans, wax gourd) and foods with a sour flavor (vinegar, lemon, plum, hawthorn fruits).
- Boil 3 bean curds with 60g brown sugar in a glass of water for 10 minutes. Drink it as soup. This remedy is recommended for bleeding or vomiting of blood or discharge of black stools caused by gastric and duodenal ulcers.
- Boil 50g Job's tears and 10g licorice in 2 cups water. Drink it as soup.
- Boil fresh lotus roots in water over low heat to make a concentrated juice. Drink 1 cup a day for 2 weeks as a treatment program.

### GASTROXIA (HYPERCHLORHYDRIA)

- Take 5g abalone bone powder with warm water each time, half an hour before meals, 3 times a day. Avoid getting too hungry, too full, or too tired. To make abalone bone powder, wash the bones and bake until dry; scrape the outer layer and grind into powder. Store the powder in a jar.
- Eat some fresh ginger or sweet fruits or strong tea or a few slices of garlic 2 or 3 hours after meals to relieve pain or heartburn.
- Roast oyster shells and grind into powder. Take 2g of the powder in warm water each time, 3 times a day.

### STOMACHACHE

- A Chinese physician reported that he treated 34 cases of cold diseases with remarkable results; these included cold stomachache, vomiting of acid, abdominal swelling, intestinal rumbling, diarrhea, chest pain, cough and abdominal pain during menstruation in women. The above diseases are classified as cold diseases, because all the patients show 3 basic cold symptoms: dislike of cold as it makes their symptoms get worse, absence of fever and no sensations of thirst. The remedy consists of 10 to 15g licorice and dried ginger mixed together as a dosage for one day.
- A Chinese physician reported his successful treatment of 20 cases of cold stomachache. To make his remedy: combine 10 raw black peppercorns, 3 red seeded dates, 5 apricot seeds (from sweet or bitter apricots) and immerse in warm water for 2 days (change water 5 times during that period); drain and crush the 3 ingredients, mix them with a small amount of warm water to make a thick soup. Drink the soup with water for a dosage (reduce for children). A 75-year-old patient treated in this program who had a 10-year history of stomachache, came to the clinic because his chronic stomachache was triggered by a cold meal the previous evening. His stomachache was gone only 30 minutes after drinking the soup. The Chinese doctor visited him

a month later and found the patient in good health.

- Warm ¾ cup fresh milk with 1 teaspoonful fresh ginger juice and a little sugar; drink the whole thing. It's also good for vomiting, belching and difficulty when swallowing.
- Dissolve 4g ground cinnamon in a cup of warm water; cover it for 15 minutes. Drink it as tea.

### ABDOMINAL PAIN

- Boil a few garlic cloves in water with black sugar over low heat. Drink a cupful each time, 3 times a day, after meals.
- Chew a few dried sour plums slowly like chewing gum.
- Consume a large quantity of cooked chives.

### BACILLARY DYSENTERY

- In a Chinese clinic, 24 patients of bacillary dysentery were cured by tomato plants. To make the remedy: wash tomato stalks, branches and leaves of 2 to 3 tomato plants (about 1 kg); boil them in water for 3 hours and make juice by straining through a clean cloth and squeezing. Drink 1 to 2 cupfuls each time, 6 to 10 times a day.
- Two Chinese hospitals in the Province of Sandong reported that 91 patients, 34 with bacillary dysentery and 57 with enteritis, were treated by a simple remedy with remarkable results. The remedy: charred hawthorn fruits and hyacinth bean flowers; the patients, divided into 3 groups, were treated separately by 3 remedies— charred hawthorn fruits, hyacinth bean flowers and a combination of the 2 ingredients; 24 cases of bacillary dysentery (83.33 percent) were cured by charred hawthorn fruits alone, 35 cases of acute enteritis (71.43 percent) by hyacinth bean flowers alone. It is also pointed out raw and charred hawthorn fruits do not have significant differences in treatment results, which means that either may be used for the treatment.
- Cut up peeled fresh radishes; add some rice vinegar and sugar. Eat twice a day.
- Eat steamed potatoes with honey, 3 times a day.
- Place 100g green tea leaves in 700ml water; bring to a boil and cook for 20 minutes or until reduced to 75ml water; remove from heat to cool; add 25ml white wine. Drink 2ml each time, 3 times a day.

### CHRONIC AMOEBIC DYSENTERY

- Chew 1 garlic clove each time, 3 times a day for 7 days, along with other foods.
- Boil 50g fresh guava peel in water as a day's dosage.
- The above 2 remedies are not suitable for acute amoebic dysentery.

## ROUNDWORMS ON THE BILIARY TRACT

A 27-year-old female patient of biliary ascariasis was cured by a formula of 3 ingredients: 15g licorice, 12g honey and 10g nonglutinous ground rice. To make the remedy, boil licorice in water; then pour the hot licorice juice into the mixture of honey and rice powder. Drink it hot.

When the patient with 10 roundworms was admitted to the clinic, she was in severe pain in the right upper abdomen and vomiting frequently. She was treated by both Western and Chinese medicines for 3 days without results but with severe pain (the doctors refrained from using strong pain killer due to her pregnancy). By taking this remedy, the patient's pain was gone within a day and she recovered completely within 6 days when some Chinese herbs comparable to piperazine were also administered; she gave birth to a boy a few months later.

- Mix 40ml rice vinegar with an equal amount of warm water for 1 dosage. Drink 3 times a day for 3 days.
- Drink 10ml fresh ginger juice with warm water each time, once every hour for 4 times; repeat 3 times a day for 2 days.
- Grind 10 black peppercorns; add 100ml water and boil for 30 minutes. Strain and drink all the liquid each time, twice a day.
- The above 3 recipes may be used alternately; after symptoms are eliminated, piperazine should be used to prevent a recurrence.

## IRON-DEFICIENCY ANEMIA

- Boil 50g mung beans and 50g dried red dates in water until the beans break; add some brown sugar. Drink once a day for 15 days as a treatment program.
- Put 100g sweet or brown rice and 30g black soybeans in boiling water; simmer until half cooked; add 30g red dates and continue cooking until well done; add brown sugar as seasoning. Eat once a day.

## MACROCYTIC ANEMIA

- Wash 150g spinach; cut up 50g pork liver. Bring water to a boil; add the spinach and pork liver and boil for a few more minutes; season with salt. Eat once a day until recovery.
- Prepare a pork kidney as you would normally; soak it in warm water for 30 minutes; cut it up in thin pieces and boil the pieces in water. Add salt as seasoning. Eat it once a day or every other day until recovery. (Beef, veal, or lamb kidneys may be used as substitute).

## APLASTIC ANEMIA

- Soak 30g black fungus in water for 30 minutes; drain. Boil the fungus with 30 red dates and some brown sugar. Eat once a day until recovery.

## GRANULOPENIA

- Boil 50g fresh mushrooms; add salt as seasoning. Eat daily until recovery.

## HEMOPHILIA

- Eat 50g unshelled fresh peanuts, including the peanut and skin, 3 times a day for 2 weeks as a treatment program.

## ANAPHYLACTOID PURPURA (ALLERGIC PURPURA)

Two Chinese physicians reported they cured 6 cases of athrombopenic purpura, including purpura simplex and allergic purpura, by using red dates. For the remedy, wash fresh red dates (or dried ones). Eat 10 dates each time, 3 times daily, until purpura is completely gone.

No other remedies are used except in one case, which is also given vitamins C and K and benadryl. Purpura disappeared within 2 days in 1 case, 3 days in 3 cases, 7 days in 2 cases, with an average of 4 days. A follow-up visit indicated no recurrence in 5 cases and recurrence in 1 case, possibly caused by premature termination of the treatment. The physician indicated treatment should continue for a few days after purpura is gone, to prevent a recurrence.

- Boil 100g barley with 15g red dates in 500ml water until reduced to 150ml water. Eat the whole thing as a day's dosage.
- Put 250g red dates in 1,500ml water and bring to a boil; crush the dates as soon as they swell; continue to boil for 40 minutes, then drain over a bowl and save the juice. Add 300ml water to the dates and boil over low heat for 20 minutes; drain it again and save the juice. Boil the reserved juice until reduced to 750ml. Drink 1 cup of the juice each time, 3 times a day.
- Prepare 30g peanut shells and 30g red dates. Boil the 2 ingredients; drain and save the soup. Drink the soup all at once as a day's dosage; repeat for 5 days as a treatment program.

## CORONARY ARTHEROSCLEROTIC HEART DISEASE

- Boil 50g yellow soybeans in water; add salt as seasoning. Eat in 1 day; repeat as often as necessary.
- Boil 30 hawthorn fruits in water; season with sugar and eat this amount each day of the treatment; repeat as often as necessary.

## SIMPLE GOITER

- Bake 500g seaweed and 500g sea grass until dry; grind into powder. Take 10g of the powder in warm water each time, once a day.
- Boil 10g seaweed and 10g kelp in water. Drink the soup as tea.

### SUNSTROKE

- Boil 50g hyacinth beans in 500ml water until reduced to 300ml; add salt as seasoning. Drink half the cooled juice each time, twice a day and eat the beans.
- Peel a wax gourd weighing about 500g; crush it to squeeze out the juice; season with salt. Drink it slowly.
- Wash and peel a radish; grate it to squeeze out the juice. Drink it with cold water.
- Slice a bitter melon in small pieces; cook in water as soup or as an ingredient in a recipe.

### ALCOHOLISM

- Pour boiling water into a teapot containing 15g tea leaves; wait for 10 minutes. Drink it all at once.
- Boil 60g black soybeans in water. Drink it as soup.
- Put 15g sugar in 30ml rice vinegar; add a little hot water to dissolve the sugar. Drink it all at once.
- Boil 30g hyacinth beans in water. Drink it as soup.
- Cut finely 2g dried orange peel; add 2 sliced seeded plums; boil the peel and plums in 2 glasses water over low heat for 30 minutes; drain over a bowl; add fresh ginger juice and strong tea to the liquid. Drink it as tea.
- Wash 20g black soybeans; cut open a coconut (saving the liquid) and place the black soybeans in the coconut and close it again; steam the coconut in a bowl for 4 hours; add salt to the coconut liquid.
- Use American or Western ginseng (not Korean or Chinese ginseng, which have altogether different actions) either in soup or in powder form, once a day.

### SMOKING

- Grate a fresh radish and mix with 2 teaspoonfuls honey. Drink as juice.
- Prepare 100g fresh bean curd and 50g black sugar; make a few holes in the bean curds and put black sugar into the holes; steam bean curds. Whenever a person has an urge to smoke, eat a few spoonfuls of bean curds with black sugar inside to quit smoking. This will make the habitual smoker want to vomit on exposure to the smell of tobacco.

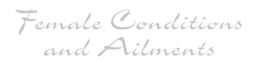

*Female Conditions and Ailments*

### MENSTRUAL DISORDERS

- Prepare 120g lamb liver, 90g chives, 1 tablespoon peanut oil and some light soy sauce. Cut chives and liver as you would in normal cooking. Heat a wok or fry pan over high heat and pour the oil into the pan; add the chives and stir-fry for a short while; drop the liver into the wok and stir-fry again for a short while; season with light soy sauce and cook for a few more seconds. Good for irregular menstruation and vaginal bleeding; also good for vaginal discharge.
- Fry 30g black fungus over low heat, add a bowl of water and continue cooking; add 15g sugar as seasoning. Good for excessive menstrual flow that belongs to a hot symptom only. This remedy is not recommended for treatment of excessive menstrual flow due to blood deficiency.
- Scrape and slice 120g fresh celery and 120g lotus roots as you would in normal cooking; place a wok or fry pan over high heat and pour 1 tablespoon peanut oil into the pan; when hot, add the celery and lotus roots and stir-fry for 5 minutes before adding salt as seasoning. Good for irregular menstruation and vaginal bleeding of a hot nature.
- Boil 30g dried ginger in water along with 30g brown sugar and 30g seeded red dates. Good for menstrual pain of a cold nature.
- Prepare 24g fresh ginger, 30g red dates and 9g red pepper. Cut the ginger and pepper as you would in normal cooking; boil the 3 ingredients in 3 glasses water until the water is reduced by half. Drink it hot to relieve cold menstrual pain.
- Cook 60g black soybeans, 2 unshelled eggs and 120g rice wine over low heat; peel eggs after cooking and then cook eggs again; add rice wine. Eat the eggs and drink the hot soup to relieve menstrual pain due to energy and blood deficiency.
- Boil 5g cinnamon twigs, 15g hawthorn fruits and 30g brown sugar in 3 glasses water until water is reduced by half; add brown sugar and continue to boil for a few seconds. Drink it hot to relieve menstrual pain due to coldness and blood coagulations.
- Boil 50g fresh parsley in 3 cups water until the water is reduced to 1 cup; crack 1 egg into the boiling water (the egg coagulates to look like flowers); add some seasoning. Eat it to relieve menstrual pain. This recipe is also good for stomachache and nervous headache.
- Fry a 250g cuttlefish in vegetable oil with 40g thinly sliced fresh ginger; season with salt. This is a remedy for relief of suppression of menstruation.

### LEUKORRHEA

- Boil 15g hyacinth beans, 30g yam, 60g sweet rice in 500ml water over low heat. Drink as soup to relieve whitish vaginal discharge. Or boil 60g hyacinth beans in water; add some sugar as seasoning. Drink as tea for relief of whitish vaginal discharge. Or, fry an equal amount of hyacinth beans and yam and make tea to stop whitish vaginal discharge.

Boil 30g Job's tears in 750ml water with 30g seeded red dates and 60g sweet rice over low heat. Drink as soup to relieve whitish vaginal discharge due to weakness.

Boil 2 cuttlefish with 250g lean pork in water; season with salt. Eat it once a day for 5 days as a treatment program to relieve whitish vaginal discharge.

Boil 10 dried radish leaves in 3 glasses water; add a little salt. Drink the hot soup to induce perspiration, twice a day, for 1 to 2 months to relieve whitish vaginal discharge.

## SYMPTOMS ASSOCIATED WITH PREGNANCY

Clean a 250g gold carp as you would in normal cooking; steam it along with 90g small red beans until the beans are soft. In general, edema during pregnancy should be cured after eating this 5 or 7 times.

Boil 50g wax gourd peel and 50g small red beans in water without adding salt. Drink as tea to relieve edema during pregnancy.

Prepare 125g fresh peanuts, 10 red dates, 30 garlic cloves, thinly sliced and 15g peanut oil. Heat a wok or fry pan over high heat; pour peanut oil into the wok and stirfry the garlic; then add peanuts and dates with 1,000ml water; boil until peanuts are very soft. This dish should produce effects for edema during pregnancy after eating it for 7 to 10 times.

Steam 9g grapefruit peel and 12g Chinese salted brown olives in 600 to 700ml water until olives are fully cooked. In general, this remedy should relieve morning sickness after eating it 5 to 7 times.

Boil 15 to 20g grapefruit peel in water. Drink it as tea to relieve morning sickness.

Bring 1,000ml water to a boil over high heat; add 100g black soybeans and 30g sliced garlic cloves and 30g brown sugar; boil over low heat until the soybeans are fully cooked. In general, edema during pregnancy should be cured after eating this 5 or 7 times.

Fry 250g sweet rice with 30ml of fresh ginger juice until the rice breaks; grind into powder. Take 10 to 20g in warm water each time, twice a day, to cure morning sickness.

Bring 60ml rice vinegar to a boil; add 30g sugar and stir until dissolved; break the egg into the boiling vinegar. When the egg is cooked, drink the whole thing to relieve morning sickness.

Fry 1 cup rice bran; then wrap it in a cloth bag or cheesecloth; add water and simmer over low heat, add some sugar, if desired. Drink it as tea to cure beriberi during pregnancy.

Soak 100g small red beans overnight; next day, boil in 3 glasses water until beans begin to break. Drink as soup to cure edema and water retention during pregnancy.

## SYMPTOMS AFTER CHILDBIRTH

Boil 150g bean curd with 50g brown sugar in 3 cups water; add 50ml rice wine when sugar dissolves. Drink all at once, once a day for 5 days to increase milk supply after childbirth.

Crush a river crab; boil it with 60ml rice wine. Eat in 1 day. In general, this dish should produce results in increasing the milk supply following childbirth after eating it 3 to 5 times.

Prepare 30g lily flowers and 60g lean pork as you would in normal cooking; steam the 2 ingredients over high heat until the pork is well done. Eat the whole thing to increase the milk supply after childbirth and also to relieve mastitis.

Simmer 500g papaya along with 500ml rice vinegar and 30g fresh ginger over low heat for 40 minutes. Drink as tea, twice a day, 1 small glass each time, to increase the milk supply after childbirth and also to relieve lochiostasis.

Fry 120g malt over low heat for a few seconds; add 750ml water and bring it to a boil and cook until the malt is fully cooked; add 30g brown sugar. Drink it as soup once a day for 5 to 7 days to stop milk secretion.

Boil 30g hawthorn fruits in water until very soft; add 30g brown sugar. Drink as tea to relieve lochiostasis and blood coagulations after childbirth.

Fry 500g black soybeans over low heat until they become half burned, add 350ml rice wine and marinate overnight. Next day, strain it and drink half a glass of wine each time, 3 times a day, to relieve rheumatic pain after childbirth.

Eat cracked wheat and brown rice on a regular basis to promote milk secretion.

Boil 10g anise seed in water to make soup; add some wine. Drink it to promote milk secretion.

## OTHER WOMEN'S DISEASES

Put 1kg fresh litchis with seeds (or dry litchis in a reduced quantity) in 1 L rice wine; seal the container and put away for 1 week. Drink twice a day, depending on your appetite, to cure prolapse of the uterus.

Wash and steam a few crabs; when they are fully cooked, add 2 teaspoonfuls rice wine and steam for 1 more minute. Drink the soup and eat the crab with soy sauce to relieve abdominal pain after childbirth.

Put a grapefruit or its peel in the bathtub while taking a bath; this will give off an aromatic smell, considered good to warm cold sensations in women.

Steam black soybeans and dry them in the sun; grind into powder; add an equal amount of ground sesame seeds and some honey; drink the 3 ingredients with warm water to cure frigidity in women.

# *Other Health Problems*

## PROLAPSE OF THE ANUS

- Boil 200g fresh parsley in water. Wash the anus with the liquid once a day. Boil fig leaves in water. Use the liquid to wash the affected region or sit in the liquid while taking a bath.

## HEMORRHOID

- Fry 250g clams in some peanut oil; add 10g sliced fresh ginger and some water and cook until the clams are very soft; add some salt. Eat it on an empty stomach, once every other day, 7 times as a treatment program.
- Eat 1 to 2 bananas with the peel on an empty stomach first thing in the morning.
- Eat 1 to 2 figs on an empty stomach first thing in the morning. Or boil fig leaves in water; use the liquid to wash the affected region or sit in the liquid in the bathtub.
- Steam 60g dried figs in an adequate amount of water with 100g lean pork; season to your taste. Eat for as long as a month as a treatment program.
- A Chinese army physician writes a report on his successful treatment of 27 cases of hemorrhoids by a simple remedy of figs. To use his remedy, prepare 10 fresh or dried figs and simmer in 1L water over low heat for 30 minutes after the water begins to boil; the water should be reduced to about .7L. Eat 5 figs each time, twice a day; also, repeatedly wash the affected region with the hot cooking water of the figs for 20 minutes. During the treatment, the patient should refrain from eating pungent or hot foods. The history of hemorrhoids among the 27 cured cases is as follows: 3 cases more than 10 years; 7 cases between 6 and 10 years; 17 cases between 1 and 5 years; patients recovered within 12 treatments in 4 cases, within 5 treatments in 9 cases and within 6 to 11 treatments in 14 cases, with the average being 7.6 treatments.
- Boil 30g black fungus with 30 red dates over low heat. Eat once a day for 10 days as a treatment program.
- Boil 60g lily flowers in water with an adequate amount brown sugar. Eat before breakfast for 1 week as a treatment program.
- Peel 2 bananas and steam them with an adequate amount of rock sugar. Eat them twice a day for 1 week.

## MASTITIS

- See Symptoms after Childbirth.
- Boil 150g green onion white heads and 60g malt in 500ml water for 20 minutes; wrap the onion heads and malt in a clean white cloth.

Use hot to rub repeatedly along the breast towards the nipple, particularly in the hard area, until the breast becomes red and soft. This treatment is applicable only in the early stage of acute mastitis prior to suppuration.

## CARBUNCLE

- See the bean remedy under Erysipelas.
- Bake some small red beans and grind them into powder; mix with honey to make an ointment. Apply externally to the affected region until healed; change the dressing as soon as it dries.

## ERYSIPELAS

- Soak 1kg whole wheat in 1,500ml water for 3 days; crush the wheat to squeeze out the juice; store juice in a container until it settles, discard the clear liquid; dry the sediment in the sun. Fry the dry sediment over low heat until yellowish; grind into powder. Mix the powder with some rice vinegar. Apply externally to the affected region and its surrounding areas prior to eruption; after the eruption, apply only to the surrounding area, leaving the middle open for drainage of the pus.
- Grind 50g small red beans into powder; add 3 egg whites to make an ointment. Apply externally to the affected region, one to two times a day. This treatment may also be applied to the swelling of carbuncle and burns.

## BURN

- A Chinese physician reported, "In the past 20 years, I have applied fresh ginger juice to treat 400 or 500 cases of burns by hot water or fire and I have not failed a single case." To use his treatment method, crush fresh ginger and squeeze out juice. Apply it to burns with a cotton ball, which should stop pain instantly; and it can also heal inflammation, reduce swelling and eliminate blisters after the burns have pustulated.
- Apply fresh aloe juice to the burn.
- Crush fresh pumpkin pulp and apply externally to the burn.
- Crush the pulp of fresh wax gourd and apply externally to the burn.

## FROSTBITE

- Chop and crush 5 red chilies; boiling in 100ml water. Wash the frostbite twice a day.
- Mix 70ml honey with 30ml lard to make an ointment. Apply externally to the frostbite.
- Heat chilies in sesame oil. Apply the cold oil to the frostbite.
- Soak red chilies in alcohol. Use a cotton ball to apply to the affected region, 3 times a day, both for a cure and to prevent future attacks.

## VITILIGO

- Slice a piece of fresh ginger or garlic clove. Rub the affected region until the juice is gone; repeat the same procedure with a new slice of ginger or garlic until hot sensations are generated in the skin, 3 to 4 times a day, until the skin returns to normal. This treatment may also be applied to alopecia areata and alopecia premature.

## ALOPECIA AREATA AND ALOPECIA PREMATURA

- Cook sesame seeds until half burned; grind into powder and mix with cold lard to make an ointment. Apply externally to the affected region, a few times daily, until hair starts growing again.
- Cut up and crush 10g red chilies; soak in 50ml white wine (60 percent alcohol) for 10 days; strain and apply the wine to the affected region, a few times daily.
- Treat the same way as vitiligo.

## FUNGUS INFECTION, SCALD, TINEA CORPORIS AND PSORIASIS

- Cut up and crush 250g fresh ginger and soak it in 500ml white wine for 2 days. Use a cotton ball to apply externally to the affected region, several times a day.
- Crush peeled garlic cloves; mix with sesame oil or lard to make an ointment. Cut the hair in the affected area before application, once a day and apply externally to the affected region.
- Mix 20g whole cloves with 70 percent alcohol to make 100ml. Apply externally to the affected region.
- Apply vinegar to the affected region, 3 times a day. Or fill a plastic bag with vinegar and tie the bag around the hand overnight to heal greyish nails.
- Boil a few eggs and remove the egg white; fry the yolks until dried and burned; mix yolks with boiling water so that yolk oil will float on the surface. Cool it and use to rub the affected region.

## INSOMNIA

- Crush an onion and put it in a jar. Inhale the vapor through the nose while in bed. Normally you fall asleep within 15 minutes.
- Wrap 30g wheat bran in a clean cloth as a tea bag; make tea with the bran. Drink it all at once before bedtime.
- Prepare 50g fresh lily flowers (reduced by half if dried lily flowers are used) and 15g rock sugar; boil in water for 30 minutes; remove the lily flowers; add 15g rock sugar to the liquid and boil for 2 minutes. Drink 1 hour before bedtime, once a day for 1 week.
- Eat cooked egg yolk every day for a few weeks.

- Fry 20g wheat until yellowish; add 5g licorice and 10 red dates; boil the 3 ingredients in water over low heat until water is reduced by half. Drink as soup.

## NEURASTHENIA

- See the last remedy under Insomnia.
- Regular consumption of honey with milk at breakfast is a good remedy.
- Regularly eat garlic.
- Regularly eat walnuts.

## HICCUPPING

- A Chinese physician in the Hebei Provincial Hospital in China reports he has cured more than 30 cases of hiccupping with fresh ginger slices. But he cautions that when the patient under treatment is also suffering from acute mouth infections or laryngitis, this method should be applied with great care. The method is as follows: Select juicy fresh ginger and cut it in slices; when hiccupping occurs, put 1 ginger slice in the mouth and chew it slowly and swallow the juice; in general, 1 to 3 slices should stop the hiccupping.
- Boil 15g sword beans in water. Drink it as soup.
- Bake fresh litchis with shells until half charred; grind into powder. Drink with warm water.
- Prepare 30g fresh ginger and squeeze out the juice; mix with 30ml honey. Slowly drink it all.
- Mix 20ml rice vinegar with an equal amount of cold water. Slowly drink it all.

## CHRONIC CONSTIPATION

- Peel and chop 500g sweet potatoes as you would in normal cooking: boil the potatoes in water; add salt or sugar as seasoning. Eat before bedtime.
- Cut up 100g white radish and squeeze out the juice; mix with some honey. Eat every day.
- Mix 2 teaspoonfuls honey with a glass warm water. Drink it on an empty stomach first thing in the morning.
- Cut up and crush fresh unpeeled potatoes and squeeze out the juice. Drink 2 teaspoonfuls of the juice with honey on an empty stomach first thing in the morning for 2 to 3 weeks. This remedy also applies to gastric and duodenal ulcers.
- Crush 7 star anise, 20g hemp and 7 green onion white heads; boil in water. Eat it twice a day. This also applies to difficulty when urinating.
- Eat a few very ripe bananas or dry figs on an empty stomach first thing in the morning (hard bananas could produce negative results).
- Regularly drink milk first thing in the morning on an empty stomach.
- Soak 1 glass rice in water overnight. Next day, boil 10 walnuts for 5 minutes; grind them in a blender; pour the rice and soaking water into

the blender and grind them again; add more water and a little sugar and continue boiling the walnuts and rice over low heat until they become sticky. Eat this dish regularly.

- Drink a glass of grapefruit juice first thing in the morning on an empty stomach.

## ENURESIS AND FREQUENT URINATION

- Chew a few fresh chestnuts (uncooked) in the morning and in the evening to reduce frequent urination, particularly in older persons.
- Mix half a spoonful of ground cinnamon twig with maltose and a little licorice powder. Drink twice a day to stop bed-wetting in children.
- Soak 30 dried mushrooms in water until they are soft; cook with a few green onion white heads, add soy sauce as seasoning, for normal consumption at meals.
- Steam 2 chicken livers with 3g ground cinnamon and a little water. Eat the livers to relieve frequent urination and enuresis in children. This cannot be taken by pregnant women, for cinnamon is very pungent and hot, which could cause damage to the energy of the fetus.
- Boil 150g string beans in water; add a little salt as seasoning when the beans become very soft. Drink as soup on an empty stomach to stop frequent urination.

## DIARRHEA

- A Chinese hospital in Shanghai presents this simple remedy effective for the treatment of diarrhea: Peel 2 cloves garlic (about 15 g) and crush them; add 2 teaspoonfuls brown sugar and boil the 2 ingredients in half a glass water. Drink the hot soup each time, 2 to 3 times daily.
- Eat 1 peeled crabapple first thing in the morning on an empty stomach; eat a crabapple after lunch and another after dinner.
- Fry fresh ginger without oil until it becomes dry and burned on the outside; grind into powder. Take 8g ground ginger each time, 3 times a day, with warm water.
- Crush a few fresh radishes to squeeze out the juice. Drink a cup of juice each time, twice a day.
- Boil in water 60g fried hyacinth beans with 60g yam and 50g white long grain rice (not brown rice). Drink it as soup.
- Boil a chicken egg until hard cooked; peel the shell and save the egg white for another dish; place the yolk in a fry pan to fry over low heat to extract the oil. The oil of 1 egg may be used as a one-day dosage for infants under a year old, divided into 3 dosages; children over one year may take the oil of 2 eggs in 1 day; each treatment program lasts 4 to 5 days. This recipe is particularly designed for diarrhea or vomiting in infants due to simple indigestion; it is not good for chronic indigestion or diarrhea. In general, improvement in stools should appear in 2 to 3 days; otherwise, stop the treatment.

- Fry 3 bean curds in peanut oil over low heat; add a little salt and 60ml rice vinegar and boil for a short while. Eat it for relief of diarrhea.
- Bring a glass of water to a boil; crack a duck egg into the boiling water and stir it; add 1 teaspoonful fresh ginger juice and a little salt as seasoning. Eat the bean curds and drink the soup.

## HOARSENESS

- Crush a few pears and squeeze out the juice. Drink it slowly.
- Boil 50 fresh peanuts in water. Eat every day.
- Mix a teaspoonful of honey with a glass of warm water. Drink it 3 hours after meals, 3 times a day for 1 week. This is beneficial to sudden loss of voice or hoarseness due to excessive fatigue, but not beneficial to loss of voice in common cold.

## COUGHING

- Slice 2 snow pears into small pieces; add 3 bowls water and boil until the water is reduced to 2 bowls; strain and discard the pears; add 30g white rice to the liquid and boil again until cooked. Drink the rice soup.
- Peel 200g fresh radishes and cut into small pieces; prepare 1 or 2 gold carps by removing the internal organs without scraping off the scales; simmer the radishes and carps and add some seasoning. Drink the soup.
- Peel 50g fresh ginger and cut into small slices; boil the ginger slices with 100g maltose in 2 glasses water for 30 minutes. Drink it hot, twice a day, in 1 day.
- Boil 20 red dates with 60g maltose in an adequate amount of water. Eat once a day.
- Mix 150ml fresh lotus juice with 30g honey. Drink as juice, once a day, for a few days.
- Make a hole on the side of a pear or an apple; pour some honey into the hole; steam the pear or the apple. Crush it and eat.

## EDEMA

- Use 15g of the shells of dried broad beans and 6g red tea leaves to make tea or to simmer over low heat. Drink the juice regularly.
- Remove and discard the internal organs of a chicken; squeeze 60g small red beans into the chicken cavity; simmer in water and season the chicken. Eat the chicken and beans and drink the broth.
- Boil 60g mung beans in water with 100g pork liver and an adequate amount of white rice. Season and eat the stew.
- Boil 60g Job's tears in water with an adequate amount of white rice. Season the soup before eating it.

## VOMITING

Three Chinese physicians report they jointly treated 20 cases of vomiting with remarkable results. To use their remedy, first, fry 20 to 30g long-grain rice until yellowish; second, cut up some fresh ginger, add a little salt, then wrap them in a wet paper towel and heat in a pan; third, prepare 30g honey; fourth, fry 1 to 2g salt on high heat. After the above ingredients are ready, boil the yellowish rice in 1 cup water until rice breaks to look like flowers. Add the ginger, salt and honey. Let the patient take 3 to 5 teaspoonfuls of this remedy at first and then continue to take more very slowly, about 10 minutes later; in general, vomiting should stop in half an hour.

Steam 2 teaspoonfuls fresh chive juice with 1 teaspoonful fresh ginger juice and 250ml fresh milk. Drink it warm before meals.

See the remedies under Hiccupping.

Chew a few preserved plums slowly, like chewing gum.

Grate 50g fresh ginger and make tea with 100g dried orange peel and water; drink it slowly. This is particularly recommended for people who develop the urge to vomit at the sight of foods.

In case of dry vomiting, mix a teaspoonful of honey with a small cup fresh ginger juice. Drink it slowly.

For chronic vomiting with cold sensations, prepare 7 black dates and a few whole cloves; crush the cloves and boil with the dates in water. Eat the dates and drink the soup on an empty stomach, once a day for 1 week, as a treatment program.

## NOSEBLEED

A Chinese physician writes, "In recent years, I have been treating cases of persisting nosebleed with a simple remedy and achieved instant results usually with a single treatment. Prepare a fresh tender onion leaf and cut it open, use a cotton ball to rub the inner surface of the onion leaf until the cotton ball becomes soaked with onion fluids; squeeze the cotton ball into the bleeding nose, which should stop the bleeding. This method is effective for nosebleed of various causes."

Wash fresh lotus roots with cold water; peel and crush them to squeeze out the juice. Drink 2 cups a day; this recipe is also a good remedy for coughing up blood resulting from pulmonary tuberculosis.

Crush a few garlic cloves and make a cake. Place it in the sole of the foot as an external treatment.

Squeeze the juice out of fresh chives. Drink a small cup of juice each time, twice a day.

## THE CHINESE THEORY OF OVERWEIGHT

Any useful or scientific theory should be based upon facts; otherwise, the theory is sheer speculation. But what are the facts?

It is a fact that Chinese emigrants do not become overweight as easily as their children born in the West. This phenomenon is obvious in Hawaii where there are as many overweight Orientals as Caucasians, which allows us to reason that obesity has no racial discrimination. In

# Chinese Diet for Weight Loss

other words, anyone—Oriental or Caucasian—born in the West has an equal opportunity to become overweight. But I have not met any Oriental immigrant who gained more than ten pounds after coming to the West. I have seen many immigrants gain eight pounds during the first year after their arrival. But their weight normally declined again within a year to maintain more or less the same as their weight in the Orient. A dramatic change in their diets caused the initial weight gain. Of course, a small number of Chinese immigrants remain overweight because they were overweight before they emigrated.

Since a person's native country should not influence his or her weight, I believe overweight in later life is already determined when a person has reached ten years of age. Similar to the theory in psychology that personality is already determined before ten years of age (or even earlier), I believe this concept is applicable also to obesity. Undoubtedly, some people have a greater tendency to become overweight due to hereditary factors; heredity plays a role in psychology and physiology. The crucial factors, however, are not the hereditary (predetermined) factors, but the environmental ones that may be altered and influenced. This does not mean that after age ten, a person will remain overweight or underweight, no matter what he or she eats or does; it only means that after age ten, an obese person will be heading in the direction of obesity and that a nonobese person will be moving away from obesity unless something is done to change the direction.

### HEADING TOWARDS OBESITY OR SLENDERNESS

What makes one person bound for obesity and another for slenderness? The growth of the human body may be compared to that of a tree. When the tree foundations are solidly built, the tree will be strong and more difficult to destroy at a later stage. In a similar way, when a person's internal organs are solidly built at an early age, the person will be strong and it will be more difficult to later weaken him or her. In other words, when the internal organs are nourished well in childhood, they tend to work hard afterwards and make you overweight; this is why the Chinese immigrants in the West do not become overweight easily; their internal organs were not overnourished when they were young.

There are always two factors at work when considering obesity: What you are and what you eat. Some people eat a lot but remain skinny; others eat a little but become overweight. I remember having a conversation with an excessively overweight gentleman in my Vancouver clinic who told me he was taking vitamins as food supplements every day. I saw no reason why it was necessary for him to take vitamins, particularly when he was so heavy. But this gentleman emphatically replied, "I do not believe vitamins will put on weight, do you?" The question is, do vitamins contribute to obesity?

If you think that only one factor (the foods you eat) contribute to obesity, it is obvious that vitamins have nothing to do with obesity; modern knowledge of vitamins indicates they will not contribute to obesity. But if you realize there are two factors contributing to obesity (what you are and what you eat), then you know that vitamins may contribute to obesity. If they are worth anything at all, vitamins must contribute to the body in a positive manner. For example, vitamin B-1 can increase appetite and absorption and vitamin D can promote normal growth of bone and teeth. This means that vitamins improve the conditions of the body and indirectly contribute to obesity, because when the body conditions are stronger they have a greater capacity to work hard during the digestion and absorption processes.

But it is not my intention to attack vitamins as culprits of obesity; my only purpose here is to point out the two factors that contribute to the problem of obesity and that both factors should be considered. When a person is overnourished at an early age, the internal organs in general and the digestive system in particular, will develop a far greater capacity for digestion and absorption, which make this person bound for obesity later in life. I deliberately use the word overnourished (as opposed to undernourished) because it indicates something undesirable. Under normal circumstances, we naturally think in terms of "the more, the better." For example, we believe that the stronger our body is, the better, that the more money we have, the better and that the longer we live, the better. And so, we have a natural tendency to think that the more our body is nourished, the better. This is a crucial error we make in nutrition and human health. It is not always true that the more our body is nourished, the better; we must add another condition to make it a true statement: The more our body is nourished, the better, provided the body is well balanced. A strong, imbalanced body is just as bad as a weak, balanced body.

## A WELL-BALANCED BODY

A well-balanced body means that the body is equally in shape in all respects. For example, a person with a strong stomach but a weak heart, or a strong heart but a weak liver, or who is strong and energetic but who suddenly dies of a heart attack is not wellbalanced; a person whose internal organs remain in good shape but suffers from hepatitis is not well-balanced.

It is interesting to see that our internal organs are not always cooperative with each other; when a given organ is excessively strong, it will weaken another organ or even cause harm to another organ. It would be nice if all of our internal organs could be equally nourished or even equally overnourished, because in that case, we would be very strong and live a long, happy life. Unfortunately, this has not happened before and is not happening now, even in this affluent society; on the contrary, far more cases of diabetes, hypertension, cancers and what not have developed, all of which point to the fact that as it is, our body is over-nourished but not balanced. This means that our internal organs are not overnourished equally. We have overnourished our digestive system at the expense of other internal organs, which is why we have more cases of heart, kidney and liver diseases, which are not directly related to the digestive system.

According to the Chinese theory of internal organs, when the stomach and spleen are over-nourished, it weakens the kidneys and bladder; when the kidneys and bladder are over-nourished, it weakens the lungs and large intestine; when the lungs and large intestine are overnourished, it weakens the liver and gall bladder; when the liver and the gall bladder are overnourished, it weakens the stomach and spleen. Under normal circumstances, we eat what we like most and the mouth is the final judge of our preferences and so, we eat according to our own taste dictated by the tongue or the mouth. But the mouth is only a representative of the stomach; it does not represent other organs, such as the liver or the heart or the lungs.

Ideally, all our internal organs should have equal representation in the mouth to guarantee fairness in the selection of foods, as in a democratic political system in which all regions of the nation should have representation in the central government. Since there is no equal representation of internal organs in the mouth, we eat just to please the mouth and the stomach it represents. Small wonder that we eat only for enjoyment and to put on weight. Sweet foods are pleasing to the mouth, so we eat them most frequently and in large quantities; bitter foods are good for the heart, but we seldom eat them, because they are not pleasing to the mouth; pungent foods are good for the lungs, but we don't eat them as often as sweet foods, because they are not particularly pleasing to the mouth; salty foods are good for the kidneys and gall bladder, but we do not particularly enjoy them, because they are not very pleasing to the mouth; sour foods are good for the liver and gall bladder, but we do not eat them often, because they are not particularly pleasing to the mouth. In short, we eat only to please the mouth and the stomach, which means to enjoy the taste and to gain weight as a result. This used to be good in the past when our stomaches were undernourished due to poverty, but now, in modern affluent society, it becomes bad.

## ENJOYING MEALS AND STAYING SLIM

It is not only possible but also realistic to enjoy your meals and stay slim at the same time. There are many possible ways of losing weight, but most are unrealistic and unworkable in real life: For example, losing weight by fasting is possible and effective, but unrealistic and dangerous in practice; losing weight by following those strict diet books is possible and may be effective, but it is not realistic because you eventually get sick of it and no doubt, you will quit; losing weight by going to weight control and diet clinics is possible and effective, but also unrealistic, because after a while, you will give up and gain back all the weight before you know it. As far as I can see, a realistic and long-term approach to weight loss is to be able to enjoy your meals and lose weight or stay slim at the same time. But can it be done? The answer is emphatically yes.

Expensive foods please our taste and overnourish our stomach, because the mouth (or taste) is a representative of the stomach. There are ways by which foods may be mixed to please the mouth without overnourishing the stomach, however and this is called the art of cooking. Let us assume that we have three ingredients: the first one is pleasing to the taste, the second is neutral and the third is repugnant to the taste. The three ingredients may be cooked together in such a way that they become pleasing to the taste and yet they do not overnourish the stomach. I will give a few examples to demonstrate how this is possible and also realistic.

CHINESE MEAT SAUCE: This standard recipe for meat sauce has ten ingredients listed below with their energies, flavors and organic actions:

*Dry orange peel*—warm; pungent and bitter; affects the spleen and lungs.

*Star anise*—warm; pungent and sweet; affects the spleen and kidneys.

*Cinnamon bark*—hot; pungent and sweet; affects the liver and kidneys.

*Cloves*—warm; pungent; affects the stomach, spleen and kidneys.

*Green onion white heads*—warm; pungent; affects the lungs and stomach.

*Fennel*—warm; pungent; affects the kidneys, bladder and stomach.

*Red chili*—hot; pungent; affects the heart and spleen.

*Black pepper*—hot; pungent; affects the stomach and large intestine.

*Nutmeg*—warm; pungent; affects the spleen and large intestine.

*Licorice*—neutral; sweet; affects the lungs, stomach and spleen.

Wrap the sauce ingredients in a clean cloth; boil in water with wine, soy sauce and some sugar. After the sauce is ready, the meat can be either soaked in the meat sauce for a few hours or simmered in the sauce for as long as two hours, which should thoroughly mix the meat with the sauce. But meat sauce is not meat soup and it cannot be drunk. The leftover sauce should be used in the next few days, but to preserve it, it is wise to boil the same sauce daily.

As you can see, many of the above ingredients by themselves are not pleasing to the taste at all. For example, few of us will like the taste of cloves or fennel or star anise. But when mixed with meat, they make a delicious dish. Moreover, virtually all internal organs and most flavors and energies are looked after. When this sauce is used to cook meat, the meat will not only be delicious, but will not put on weight because the warm, hot and pungent ingredients make it very yang. This is why I believe that it is not only possible, but also realistic to enjoy meals and stay slim at the same time.

SOUPS: Another example is the Chinese habit of making delicious soups — mushroom, chicken, beef, egg, pork, fish, clam soup and many others. Soups are delicious and will also help you lose weight. I have pointed out that it is the quality of foods not their quantity that really contributes to your gaining weight, but when the same foods are to be consumed, the quality does make a difference. For example, 1 pound of beef (450g) is certainly different from 100g, in terms of the effects on weight control. Everything else being equal, eating 1 pound of beef will put on more weight than eating 100g; and drinking soups will make you consume less foods without sacrificing your enjoyment of good meals. For example, 100g beef may seem like a very small quantity when it is used for a beefsteak, but when making soup, its quantity is significantly increased.

To make beef soup, cut up 100g beef into small pieces; place in a bowl, add a little wine and five small slices of fresh ginger and an adequate amount of water. Simmer the soup over low heat for an hour. This should make a delicious beef soup. Or, you can steam the ingredients for 2 hours. This beef soup will not put on weight. On the contrary, I believe it will make you lose weight and stay slim, because it will make you eat less as a result. Moreover, this beef soup contains wine and ginger, which act upon many other internal organs, in addition to the stomach, one of the best ways of eating beef without gaining weight. The same principle applies to making other soups to lose weight or stay slim.

How can soups promote good health?

Beef soup is good for weakness and anemia.

Chicken soup is good for fatigue and neurasthenia.

Mung bean soup is good for inflammation of the internal organs.

Mushroom soup is good for weak liver.

Clam soup is good for hypertension.

Longevity soup is made by using bones from chicken and pork legs. The bones should be crushed to extract the marrow, the essence of the bones, which is considered the most precious part of bone soup. In making the bone soup, soak the bones in the Chinese meat sauce (described above) and then simmer over low heat with other ingredients, such as peanuts, mushrooms, red beans, or radishes and then season with red chili powder or black pepper.

## ELIMINATING FAT IN MEATS

There are external and internal methods of eliminating meat fat. The external methods include cutting and discarding the fat before eating; and the use of meat sauce is partially intended to neutralize the effects of fat in meats. Also, in cooking pork (which contains a higher percentage of fat), boil pork for 20 to 30 minutes; remove the pork and wash it with cold water. This is one way of reducing fat in pork. Some fat will get into our body and something needs to be done about it and this is the internal method of removing or reducing fat in meats.

The Mongol people, who consume more meats than other people, rely on drinking large quantities of strong tea to counteract the effects of fat in meats. In Peking, for instance, customers served Mongolian roast meat are routinely offered a special wine believed to have the strong effect of dissolving the fat in the body; after the meal, a cup of strong tea is served as a way of reducing the effects of fat. As a test, next time you drink tea, don't throw away the tea leaves. Instead, use them to clean some fat from your hands to see how effective tea leaves are in removing grease. Then you can easily imagine the same effects taking place inside your body after you drink tea. Therefore, regular consumption of strong tea is another effective way of losing weight and staying slim. A doctor friend who recently returned from England said he was very surprised to find that the British people generally are much slimmer than their American and Canadian counterparts, which may be attributed to the British habit of tea-drinking.

For weight loss, green is better than black tea, because the effects of black tea are weakened by fermentation. In making tea, the water should be boiling; first, pour a little boiling water to warm up the teapot; then, measure the tea leaves in the teapot and quickly pour the boiling water into the teapot. Wait for a few minutes before drinking the tea. Expensive tea, like expensive foods, is not good for weight loss; the tea should be strong and bitter, which is less expensive. Expensive tea leaves can be used only once, but less expensive tea leaves may be used 2 or 3 times in a day, then discarded.

These broad principles may be generally useful to overweight people, but there are individual physical constitutions that should also be considered for a better solution to the problem of obesity. Two people may eat identical foods in identical quantity, but one may be overweight while the other may be underweight, due to the difference in their physical constitutions.

## PHYSICAL CONSTITUTIONS AND OBESITY

Two types of physical constitutions have a tendency to become obese: hot-damp and cold-damp types. People with hot-dry physical constitutions never become overweight no matter what or how much they eat; as a group, they are practically free of obesity. A rooster is the typical creature with a hot-dry physical constitution. Have you ever seen a fat rooster? I have not. When I was a little boy, I used to feed our chickens (and I always fed them equally without sexual discrimination, because I simply spread the rice on the ground and let them eat; whether roosters or hens was none of my business). I noticed that roosters always ate faster than hens, they were quicker and more aggressive. But to my great disappointment, hens easily became fat whereas roosters always remained skinny. I wished all of them would gain weight fast so that we could sell them and earn lots of money. Now you see, foods alone cannot be responsible for obesity; it is only when certain foods are consumed by certain people that obesity occurs.

The ultimate goal, therefore, is make the physical constitutions of overweight people hot and dry. Overweight people usually have a damp physical constitution; they retain an excessive amount of water in the body, making them overweight.

## DEALING WITH OBESITY

Chinese physicians developed four methods of drying the body, a prerequisite in dealing with obesity: The first is to promote urination, which may be compared to diuretics in Western medicine. Small red beans, corn and corn silk, Job's tears and the peel of wax gourd significantly promote urination.

Small red beans may be eaten often as a food. But it is frequently used in Chinese herbalism as an effective herb to promote urination, particularly in the treatment of edema in nephritis and beriberi. Small red beans look like ordinary red beans but are shaped longer and are more effective. They may be boiled with malt or red dates and a few garlic cloves.

Some people think that the more you eat, the more weight you will gain, which is not true. According to the traditional Chinese theory, it depends on what you are eating. The more small red beans you eat, for example, the more weight you will lose. Therefore, small red beans are absolutely not recommended for skinny people, particularly children, because a prolonged consumption of them will make them lose weight. If you look at a standard nutrition book, you read that 100g small red beans contain 319 calories, which is about the same as beefsteak. There is a basic difference between the two, however, in what the beans and steak can do, not what each of them has. It is true that both small red beans and beefsteak have about 300 calories per 100g but it is important to remember that small red beans can promote urination and dry up the body, which is lacking in beefsteak.

Job's tears is also used by the Chinese people both as a food and an herb to promote urination. In Chinese herbalism, Job's tears is considered an effective diuretic like small red beans. The Chinese people fry Job's tears, use it to make tea and drink it regularly, particularly when they have difficulty urinating or edema or feel unusually nervous. Job's tears can calm your nerves.

Corn and corn silk are also effective in promoting urination, particularly corn silk, which, according to one experiment, may be used when brewing coffee to promote urination with greater and longer effects.

Soybeans and garlic may also be used to promote urination. Boil 200g soybeans with 100g garlic until soft. Eat them at meals. If you don't like garlic, small red beans may be used as a substitute, but garlic is an energy tonic, which can make you feel more energetic and small red beans have no such effects.

The second method of getting rid of water in the body: Absorb tissue fluids in the body. Absorbing water inside the body is like using a cotton ball to soak up water in a glass; promoting urination removes water from the body through excretion. The majority of foods and herbs that can absorb the water inside the body are aromatic and the two used most frequently are broad beans and hyacinth beans. The aromatic foods not only can absorb water inside the body, but can stop diarrhea for the same reason. Diarrhea means discharge of extremely watery stools and when the water is absorbed, the stools dry and there will be no more diarrhea.

Broad beans may be ground into powder to be taken with warm water, but they can also be fried with oil and salt until they break and smell aromatic; use the beans without removing the shell, as the shell has a better effect of absorbing water inside the body and promoting urination.

As for hyacinth beans, use them the same as broad beans. In Chinese herbal therapy, hyacinth beans are very frequently used to relieve diarrhea and abdominal pain due to excessive water in the intestine. They may be used in soup or in powder form.

The third method of eliminating water is to cool the body to facilitate water passage. A dry-hot physical constitution is not prone to obesity as is a damp-hot physical constitution. This is how it works. What happens if you set fire to wet firewood? It won't burn quickly but can only produce smoke, which is bad. Similarly, when water and heat mix in the body, neither will go away. The result is difficulty when urinating or discharge of reddish urine in small quantities. The strategy, therefore, is to cool the body, allowing water to flow. Foods or herbs with a cold energy and a bitter flavor are used for this purpose, because cold energy can cool the body and bitter flavor can dry it.

Bitter gourd, which tastes extremely bitter, can significantly cool the body, reduce nervous tension due to its cold energy and also can soften the stools due to its bitter flavor. People with a hot-damp physical constitution often suffer from constipation, which may be effectively relieved by using bitter gourd in soup, as a vegetable, or as tea. Dry or canned bitter gourd may be used as substitutes.

Mung beans, mung bean sprouts or powder may also be used by people with a hot-damp physical constitution to rid the body of excessive water. Although mung bean has a cool energy and a sweet flavor, it is rather effective in removing water and reducing body heat. Mung bean also has an extremely strong detoxicating effect, useful in dealing with many hot symptoms, such as skin eruptions of a hot nature and inflammation of internal organs.

The fourth method of eliminating excessive body water is to warm the body. This method can be used by people with a cold-damp physical constitution, which may be compared to a mountain of ice. The strategy is to warm the body so that the water can flow out of the body, either through urination or perspiration. The foods producing best results should have a warm or hot energy and a pungent-sweet flavor. Hot or warm energy increases body heat, pungent flavor increases perspiration and a sweet or light flavor promotes urination. Cinnamon twig satisfies these three conditions. A time-honored Chinese herbal formula called five diuretics contains five ingredients: Two absorb water in the body, two promote urination and the last ingredient, cinnamon twig, is included to warm the body and facilitate water passage.

Regular consumption of fresh ginger can warm the body and induce perspiration simultaneously. Fresh ginger is used frequently to counteract cold particularly in winter and when it is used along with dry orange peel to make tea, its effects are significantly reinforced.

After the excessive water in the body has been removed and the body is dry, the person should be slim and stay in good shape. But how does a person remain slim and stay in good shape unless the body can stop retaining water?

## AVOIDING WATER RETENTION AND STAYING SLIM

An overweight person has two enemies in the body: fat and water. One important thing is to get rid of those enemies and the other is to keep them out of the body. Can and how can this be done? The Chinese believe one thing can do the job and it is called fire.

Many of my students in herbal therapy are at first puzzled by the concept of fire in Chinese medicine. They gradually become used to it and finally like and appreciate it as a very important and useful concept. Every science consists of concepts and theory; each concept is defined so that it can be used to present a theory. Fire is a concept in Chinese medicine and a very important one too. What is fire? It is a certain element in the body that functions like fire in cooking. How can fire get rid of fat? By burning it. How can fire get rid of water? By boiling it.

In cooking, fire can burn oil and bring water to a boil so that eventually the water will evaporate. This is a common phenomenon occurring in the human body as well. Is it really nonsensical for the Chinese people to believe that there is fire in the body that keeps burning excessive fat and steaming excessive water out of the body? Is there any fact to prove this is the case? Since I have lots of experiences raising chickens, I'll use them now to prove the point I am making about weight loss.

When you raise chickens for a livelihood as I did when I was a boy, you wish your chickens would quickly grow big and fat to produce a profitable business. But how can you achieve this goal? A hen will grow fat rather easily, but the Chinese people are not very fond of eating hens (their tough flesh is not easy to chew and their prices are much lower for that reason). On the other hand, a rooster will remain skinny and light as it grows. There is a way to make a rooster grow fat, however, by removing its testis. The rooster will then gain significant weight in a short time, making it even fatter than a hen. This was common knowledge and a common practice shared by all Chinese people when I raised chickens. I certainly did not realize that a few decades later I would use this knowledge about castrated roosters to prove an important point to my Western readers.

The crucial fact is that a castrated rooster is about twice as heavy as a rooster not castrated and the extra weight is put on soon after castration. Each rooster has one testis, but the presence of this testis in a rooster is crucial in weight control. We all know that in humans and in animals testes are responsible for sexual functions. Men cannot perform sex without testes. But how do the testes contribute to weight loss? In a man the testes heat the body as a heater heats a room. The Chinese physician calls this action the burning fire of the kidneys.

The testes, therefore, are the burning fire of the kidneys. Chinese physicians differentiate between internal (the two kidneys inside the body) and external kidneys (the two testes outside the body). Since women lack testes and their ovaries do not burn as violently as men's testes, small wonder there are more overweight women than men and that it is far easier for women to put on weight than men.

Everything may be classified into yin and yang, including the kidneys. There is kidney yin and kidney yang; kidney yin refers to water in the kidney while kidney yang refers to fire in the kidney. The concept of fire is a very important one in Chinese medicine as metioned earlier, but what is meant by "kidney fire"? It refers to the kidney's capacity to become energetic, active both in lifestyle and sexual performances. Therefore, in Chinese medicine, when a man becomes sexually impotent, it is attributed to "insufficient kidney fire"; when a man is sexually overactive, it is attributed to "excessive kidney fire".

When a man has a higher level of the burning fire of kidneys, he remains skinny and has a strong sexual capacity. To be slim is to be sexy. A fat fellow will not have a strong sexual capacity and a fellow with a strong sexual capacity will not be fat; nature does not mix sex with obesity. The burning fire of kidneys will keep burning fat and steaming water out of the body, keeping the body free of obesity. To remain slim and in good shape means you should increase the burning fire of the kidneys.

## INCREASING THE BURNING FIRE OF THE KIDNEYS

When I suggest to patients in my clinic that they try to increase the burning fire of their kidneys to lose weight, many jokingly ask me if they need an additional testis to lose weight more effectively. In fact, if this could be done, I imagine it would work in weight control; if someone wishes to lose weight, an extra testis is needed and to gain weight, one of the testes should be removed. I am amazed that our surgeons, so capable in cutting up the body, have not contemplated the possibility of testes transplantation, which should cure obesity and impotence at the same time and make the medical profession far more respectable. Some people think obesity and impotence are making a mockery of medical doctors as many obese and impotent patients are turned away every day as incurable by our doctors.

Foods called yang tonics can increase the burning fire of kidneys. In Chinese medicine, there are four basic tonics: energy tonics, blood tonics, yin tonics and yang tonics. A tonic is something that strengthens and energy tonic refers to something that strengthens the energy, blood tonic to something that strengthens the blood, yin tonic to something that strengthens the fluids, yang tonic to something that strengthens the burning fire of kidneys, also called yang energy in the body. In some cases, different kinds of tonics are used interchangeably, either because a certain food simultaneously performs two or more functions or because one food may be used as a substitute for another.

Animals' kidneys are highly recommended yang tonics, based on the traditional Chinese belief that when human internal organs are weakening, it is beneficial to eat the animal's corresponding organs. Thus, when your liver is weak, you should eat animal liver; when kidneys are weak, eat animal kidneys and so forth. At a lecture, I remember a lady half-jokingly asked me whether it is beneficial to eat animal's testes or penis when one suffers from impotence. My answer was emphatically yes, which was not a joke. As a matter of fact, when Chinese women with no physiological defects are unable to conceive, they eat animal testes cooked in rice wine (particularly pork testes, which are readily available). And when a Chinese woman consults a Chinese herbalist for infertility or a man for impotence, it is customary for the herbalist to present her or him with the following recipe: Prepare 2 lamb, pork, or beef testes, four kidneys and 50g black dates; stir them in rice wine until thoroughly soaked; then steam them. Place the steamed ingredients in a bottle of wine and store for three months before it is ready to drink. This is called yang tonic wine.

Eating kidneys (pork, beef, lamb, or chicken) has three advantages: kidneys have little fat, are easily digested and tone up the kidney functions. For people who don't like eating kidneys because of their taste, the flavor may be improved. First, cut the kidney in half, remove all unwanted parts and wash it; bring water to a boil and add a little wine; drop in the kidney and simmer until fully cooked; drain and slice into small pieces. Prepare a sauce with ginger, green onion, green pepper, soy sauce, sugar, sesame oil and vinegar. Pour the sauce over the kidney and it is ready to eat.

Another way to cook kidneys: Cut the kidney in large slices; put 1 tablespoonful oil in a wok or fry pan and as soon as the pan is hot, add sliced ginger, garlic and chive; stir-fry with the kidney for a few minutes. Garlic, ginger and chive are condiments and also yang tonics.

For treating impotence in men and frigidity in women, there is another Chinese recipe: cut 2 or 3 garlic cloves into small pieces; fry with 30g fresh ginger. In fact, if you wish to lose weight and stay slim, use ginger and garlic on a regular basis.

Liver (chicken, pork and beef) is the second food recommended as a yang tonic to increase the burning fire of the kidneys. Liver can also be cooked to make it pleasing to the taste. Fry the liver very quickly in vegetable oil with condiments, such as ginger, garlic, or celery; use black pepper and wine as seasonings.

Shrimps are the third food recommended as a yang tonic. A celebrated Chinese herbalist in the 16th century advised husbands not to eat shrimps on a journey, intended as a humorous remark to imply that shrimps can dramatically increase sexual desires and they may find themselves in desperation without a sexual partner when separated from their wives. Of course, this advice may not be valid today, because social environments have changed in the course of the past four centuries. Some Chinese herbalists believe that if one consumes too much shrimp without sexual intercourse, one may develop nosebleed due to excessive fire built up in the body.

Shrimps have the greatest capacity for reproduction, it is believed because one single sexual intercourse will produce thousands of eggs, far beyond the human capacity. There are different ways to eat shrimps. Try this traditional Chinese recipe called intoxicated shrimps. Wash the live shrimps and put them in a pan; pour in brandy or whisky, enough to cover the whole shrimps; then add some favorite seasonings, such as ginger, garlic and sesame oil. Immediately cover the pan because the shrimps will jump like crazy. When the shrimps calm down after a few minutes they are ready to eat. Shrimps may also be fried with garlic to make a strong yang tonic. The Chinese are particularly interested in shrimp's brain (which appears yellowish), shrimp's testes (located on the back), shrimp's liver (turns red immediately on cooking) and shrimp's eggs. The tiny black intestine on the back of the shrimp should be removed before cooking. If fresh shrimps are not available, dried shrimps may be used and cooked with other foods more as a condiment than as a main ingredient.

Mussel is also considered as an effective yang tonic. Mussel has a warm energy, unlike clam (sea or river clam), which has a cold energy. Mussel is a yang tonic; clam is a yin tonic. A Chinese diet classic says, "Cooked mussel can promote erection and heal lumbago." In fact, erection difficulty and lumbago are, in many cases, attributed to weakness of the kidneys and since mussel is a yang tonic, it should be beneficial to erection difficulty and lumbago. It is believed that mussel can raise body temperature, particularly in the genitals, which is why it is beneficial to sexual impotence in men and frigidity in women.

In China, many women cook mussel with rice wine, ginger and black soybeans to regulate menstrual flow, because irregular menstrual flow is often caused by coldness in the womb and mussel cooked with wine can significantly raise womb temperature. The same recipe may be used to warm the genital areas in men. In fact, dried mussel is an important food in Chinese medicine and is normally ground into powder for oral adminis-

tration. When using dried mussel, wash off the salt, fry and grind the mussel into powder, take 10g mussel powder with warm water or brandy each time, twice a day, to correct impotence and increase sexual capacity.

In addition to the above yang tonics from animals, the following fruits and vegetables may also be used as yang tonics, including raspberry (it must be dried green raspberry). In China, when summer begins, children pick green raspberries to be used as herbs. They clean the raspberries and soak them in boiling water for 1 to 2 minutes and then spread them on the ground to dry under the hot sun.

Raspberries can produce effects similar to those of a female hormone, according to an experiment on rabbits and rats. (A Chinese herbalist many centuries ago cautioned men that if they have excessively strong erections that last too long, they should stay away from raspberries.) Like mussel, raspberry can raise the body temperature, particularly in the genitals and for that reason, is beneficial to women who are unable to conceive due to coldness of the womb. Chinese people also believed that a prolonged consumption of raspberries can improve a woman's skin conditions and prevent hair from graying.

Other foods used as yang tonics include yam (which also acts on the kidneys and stops seminal emission in men and vaginal discharge in women and it stops frequent urination in both sexes); walnut (which tones up the kidneys and benefits the lungs), chive seed and bitter gourd seed (both good for a wide variety of purposes, particularly in relation to sexual weakness).

If my clinical experiences have taught me anything, it is that a large number of overweight people are not so much interested in a theory of obesity as in losing weight. Many of them ask me, "Can you simply tell me what foods to eat to lost weight?" For this reason I offer a simple and practical answer to the question in the form of a chart, Appendix A. To make use of this chart, determine your own type of physical constitution (as outlined in Chapter 3) and select foods that are good and avoid the foods that are bad for your type; as for foods listed as neutral, eat them whenever you please.

## IMMUNE DEFICIENCY AND CHINESE TONIC FOODS

The Chinese physicians of traditional medicine call the foods that can enhance the body's immune function food tonics. There are four categories of common food tonics that can strengthen the body's immune function: energy, blood, yin and yang tonics. In addition, there are organic tonics, namely, tonics that are considered effective in strengthening a specific internal organ;

# Deficiency and Excess Diseases and Chinese Foods

among the most common organic tonics are liver, lung, heart, stomach and spleen tonics. Kidneys are particularly important organs and yang and yin tonics are both for the kidneys.

The various categories of food tonics bear a resemblance to the five types of nutrients labelled by Western scientists. All of the tonics are designed to correct a particular deficiency. Just as a particular nutrient is beneficial to the body since it needs it, so a particular category of tonic is beneficial to the body that is suffering a specific deficiency. Vitamin A is beneficial to those with a vitamin-A deficiency; energy tonics are beneficial to those with an energy deficiency and so on. Specific tonic foods for deficiency diseases are discussed in Chapters 5 through 11.

### ENERGY TONICS

Energy deficiency refers to a low level of energy in the whole body, or an incomplete function of internal organs in general and the organs of the digestive system in particular. This deficiency may come about as a result of chronic illness, severe diseases, defective genetic factors and old age. A person with an energy deficiency may feel too lazy to talk, or speak in a feeble or low voice, feel fatigued and weak, have a poor appetite, perspire even at rest, or suffer abdominal swelling, chronic diarrhea or soft stools, prolapse of the uterus or the anus, or abnormal falling of the stomach or the kidney. A few common diseases are often indicative of an energy deficiency, including leukocytopenia (abnormal number of white blood cells), bronchial asthma, myasthenia gravis (muscular weakness and progressive fatigue) and frequent colds and skin infections.

The foods of energy tonics are beef, bird's nest, bitter gourd seed, broomcorn, cherries, chicken, coconut, crane meat, dates, eel, fermented glutinous rice, ginkgo, ginseng, goose, grapes, herring, honey, jackfruit, licorice, longan, lotus rhizome powder, mackerel, mandarin fish, octopus, pigeon egg and meat, sweet and white potatoes, rabbit,

red and black dates, glutinous and polished rice, rock sugar, shark's fin, shiitake mushrooms, squash, sturgeon, tofu and white string beans.

The foods for energy deficiency mostly affect the stomach, spleen and pancreas, all of which are regarded in Chinese medicine as the acquired sources of the immune function. When they are deficient, the body's immune function will be impaired, which is why energy tonics play an important role in enhancing the immune function. A Chinese physician in the third century named Zhang Zhong Jing said, "When the spleen and pancreas are full of energy, the body will be immune from disease."

### BLOOD TONICS

Blood deficiency refers to the symptoms that may result from an excessive loss of blood caused by severe bleeding or from a poor absorption of nutrients. When blood deficiency occurs, it may give rise to dizziness, palpitations, nervousness, pale complexion, white lips and nails, insomnia, forgetfulness, numbness in hands and feet and light menstrual flow in women. A few common diseases are often indicative of blood deficiency, including hemolytic anemia (anemia resulting from hemolysis of red blood cells), allergic and thrombocytopenic purpura and urticaria (a skin disease with severe itching and welts).

The foods of blood tonics are beef, beef liver, blood clams, chicken eggs, cuttlefish, donggui, grapes, ham, litchi nuts, longan, mandarin fish, human and mare's milk, octopus, oxtail, oysters, palm seed, pork liver and trotter, sea cucumber, sheep and goat's liver, black soybean skin and spinach.

Energy and blood deficiencies very often occur simultaneously, because deficiency in one may lead to deficiency in the other. The Chinese maintain that energy is the leader of the blood and that it is only when the body has sufficient energy that the blood can circulate properly. On the other hand, blood produces energy and it's only when the body has enough blood that it can produce sufficient energy. Those with both energy and blood deficiencies should consume both energy and blood tonics simultaneously.

### YIN TONICS (KIDNEY YIN TONICS)

Yin deficiency (also called kidney yin deficiency) refers to a shortage of body fluid, or a shortage of semen in men. It may result from chronic illness or excessive sex or frequent childbirths in women. A person with yin deficiency often displays a dry throat, thirst, dry skin, night sweats, cough with discharge of sputum or blood, constipation, urination in little amounts, red lips and cheeks, underweight body, blurred or poor vision, ringing in the ears, backache and premature ejaculation in men and menstrual disorders in women. A few common diseases are often indicative of yin deficiency, including allergic purpura, 1upus erythematosus (a chronic disease with a skin rash), rheumatism, rheumatoid arthritis, radiation damage, tuberculosis and chronic hepatitis.

The foods of yin tonics are abalone, air bladder of shark, apples, sweet apricot seed, asparagus, tofu, bird's nest, bitter gourd (balsam pear), brown sugar, cantaloupe (musk-melon), cheese, chicken eggs, saltwater clams, coconut milk, crab, cuttlefish, dates, duck and duck eggs, figs, freshwater clams, frog, white fungus, green turtle, honey, kidney beans, kumquats, lard, lemon, litchi nuts, loquat, maltose, mandarin oranges, mangoes, cow's milk, mussels, oysters, peas, pears, pineapples, pomegranates (sweet fruit), pork and pork marrow, rabbit, red bayberries, polished rice, royal jelly, sea cucumber, shrimp, star fruit (carambola), string beans, sugar cane, tomatoes, walnuts, watermelon, white sugar, whitebait and yams.

## YANG TONICS (KIDNEY YANG TONICS)

Yang deficiency, or kidney yang deficiency, refers to a lack of yang energy in the kidneys, which is essential in the maintenance of body warmth. Yang deficiency may result from old age, chronic illness and excessive sex. A person with yang deficiency often displays fatigue, cold limbs, backache, shortness of breath, frequent urination (especially at night), pale complexion, hair loss, edema, impotence in men and infertility and vaginal discharge in women, slow growth, soft bones, low spirits and diarrhea. A few common diseases are often indicative of yang deficiency, including bronchial asthma, asthmatic tracheitis, allergic rhinitis, chronic nephritis, vitiligo, psoriasis, tuberculosis of bones, osteoporosis and diabetes mellitus.

The foods of yang, tonics are air bladder of shark, beef kidney, Japanese cassia fruits, chestnuts, chive seeds, cinnamon, clove and clove oil, deer kidney, dill seeds, fennel seeds and roots, fenugreek seeds (Oriental fenugreek), green onion seeds, lobster, mandarin orange seeds, oxtail, pistachio nuts, pork testicles, prickly ash root, raspberries, sheep and goat kidney and testicles, shrimp, sparrow eggs, star anise, strawberries and sword beans (saber beans).

## LUNG TONICS

Lung tonics are good for lung deficiency, which may give rise to shortness of breath, coughing, fatigue, speaking in a weak voice, excessive perspiration, increased susceptibility to colds and flu, dry throat, night sweats and hot sensations in the palms or soles of the feet. A few common diseases are often indicative of lung deficiency, including chronic bronchitis, bronchial asthma, tuberculosis and emphysema.

The foods of lung tonics include air bladder of shark, cheese, garlic, ginkgo, ginseng, Job's tears, cow's milk, pork lungs and pancreas, glutinous rice, walnuts, whitebait and yams.

## LIVER TONICS

Liver tonics will help to prevent liver deficiency. Problems with the liver may cause headache, dizziness, pain in the ribs, ringing in the ears, insomnia, night sweats, hand and head tremors, dryness in the eyes and light menstrual flow or absence of it in women. A few common diseases often indicative of liver deficiency include neurosis, hypertension and nonjaundice hepatitis.

The foods of liver tonics include black sesame seeds, beef, chicken, pork, rabbit, sheep and goat liver, chive seeds, matrimony vine fruit, mulberries, mussels, perch, raspberries, royal jelly, sour dates, strawberries and turnip flowers.

## HEART TONICS

Heart tonics are good for deficiencies that may cause palpitations, shortness of breath, particularly when working, nervousness, forgetfulness, insomnia, nightmares, low-grade fever, tongue soreness and cold limbs. A few common diseases that often suggest heart deficiency include heart disease, heart failure, shock, neurosis and anemia.

Foods of heart tonics include air bladder of shark, ambergris, beer, chicory, coffee, ginkgo leaves, ginseng, longan with shell, lotus fruits and seeds, matrimony vine fruit, rock sugar, tea and wheat.

## STOMACH TONICS

Stomach tonics can prevent deficiencies that may lead to dry throat, stomachache, poor digestion and appetite, vomiting, underweight body and constipation. A few common diseases that indicate stomach deficiency include gastritis, morning sickness, diabetes mellitus and phrenospasm.

The foods of stomach tonics include areca nut male flowers, azalea root, beef, blood clams, cardamom seeds, grass carp, Japanese cassia bark and fruits, cherry leaves, chestnuts, cinnamon, clove oil, crown daisy, duck, fennel seeds, white fungus, hairtail, hyacinth bean flowers, Job's tears leaves, mangoes, cow's milk, perch, red and black dates, red bayberries, polished rice, shiitake mushrooms, trifoliate oranges, whitebait and whitefish.

## SPLEEN TONICS

Spleen tonics are good for spleen deficiencies that may give rise to poor appetite, bloated stomach after meals, fatigue, underweight or overweight conditions, diarrhea, stomachache, vomiting, edema, excessive menstrual flow and discharge of blood from the anus. A few common diseases that often indicate spleen deficiency are chronic gastritis, hepatitis and enteritis; prolapse of the uterus, stomach and anus; frequent urination; peptic ulcers; chronic nephritis; and viral hepatitis.

The foods of spleen tonics include apple cucumber, beef, bird's nest, broomcorn, caraway seeds, grass carp gall, carrots, Japanese cassia bark, cherry leaves, chestnuts, cinnamon, corn, crown daisy, dill seeds, dog's bone, frog, garlic, ham, horse beans, hyacinth beans and flowers, Job's tears root, longan, lotus fruits and seeds, mullet, pearl sago, perch, pheasant, pineapples, pistachio nuts, pork pancreas, red and black dates, glutinous and polished rice, rice sprouts, royal jelly, sheep or goat's blood, white and green string beans, whitefish and yams.

Foods classified as tonics may be consumed in large quantities to enhance the immune function in acute diseases in general and, also for acute consumptive diseases, such as cancer and hyperthyroidism, both of which use up a great deal of body energy and weaken the patient. Various types of cardiovascular malfunctions and incessant bleeding with profuse perspiration, cold limbs and shortness of breath may also be corrected by eating food tonics in large amounts. This is why when a patient suddenly collapses and loses consciousness, a Chinese physician often administers large amounts of ginseng to save the patient's life. Although ginseng is basically an herb, it's an energy tonic that can help restore the immune system of the body.

However, tonics are intended to enhance the immune function in order to correct immune deficiency and for that reason, there's no need for a person in good health to consume tonics in large amounts. The Chinese theory of tonics, like the Western theory of nutrition, is based upon the concept of balance, not excess. In the majority of cases, it is only when a person suffers from a severe disease or a chronic condition that tonics play a major role in restoring and enhancing the body's immune function.

There are three particular circumstances under which tonics may not be able to fulfill their functions. First of all, when people are suffering from illness due to external factors, such as microorganisms and viruses in infections and influenza, tonics will not help until the symptoms have improved substantially. The Chinese have coined the phrase "to lock in the thief" to describe the situation, because traditionally, microorganisms and viruses and all other factors that cause disease are referred to as "thieves" by the Chinese. When foreign agents enter the body and cause disease, they are like thieves who break into a house. Wise victims will not lock the doors before the thieves have left. Therefore, when a person is suffering from a disease that has nothing to do with immune deficiency, eating food tonics should be delayed until after the illness shows signs of improvement let the thieves leave the house before the door is locked.

In the second place, some people may not benefit from tonics if they have poor digestion, even though they have an immune deficiency. The Chinese describe this situation as "a deficiency disease that does not respond to tonics." The consumption of tonics may enhance the immune function provided they can be digested and absorbed. When people have poor digestion, eating tonics may prove counterproductive, since many tonics are difficult to digest. Thus, when people suffer from poor digestion, they should take tonics that are easily digestible.

And finally, tonics may not be effective for those who have taken them erroneously. For example, people with a vitamin-A deficiency should take vitamin A to benefit from it and those with a vitamin-C deficiency should take vitamin C. But when people with a vitamin-A deficiency take vitamin C, or vice versa, the deficiencies will not be corrected. By the same token, energy tonics are good only for people with an energy deficiency and so on. When people consume large amounts of yang tonics, they may develop a dry mouth, chapped lips and have trouble sleeping. This is because they do not have a yang deficiency, but instead have a yin deficiency. By consuming large amounts of yang tonics, they have boosted their yang energy excessively, which is unnecessary and contributes to a yin deficiency.

*I*mmune excess is the body's overreaction to the attack of foreign agents. In order to reduce immune excess, it is necessary to regulate the internal environments of the body so that the attack will be weakened and the body will not have to muster all its immune function to fight it. The Chinese call the foods that can control the internal environments to reduce immune excess "regulating foods." Specific regulating foods for excess diseases are discussed in Chapters 12 through 16.

internal organs. In patients with liver cancer, there may be hot sensations in the body, jaundice, vomiting of blood, or bleeding, from the anus; in patients with leukemia, we often see nosebleeds and skin eruptions.

A Chinese medical team in the city of Chongqing summed up the diseases associated with toxic heat in the internal environments: "Such diseases are mostly acute and contagious diseases, including Japanese B encephalitis, epidemic hemorrhagic fever, epidemic cerebrospinal meningitis, viral pneumonia, flu, acute viral hepatitis, lobar pneu-

# *Immune Excess and Regulating Foods*

## FOODS TO REDUCE TOXIC HEAT

There is little doubt that toxic heat in the internal environments contributes to disease caused by the attack of microorganisms. It's a well-known fact that smokers are much more susceptible to lung cancer than nonsmokers and from the traditional Chinese point of view, this is due to the lungs being under constant stimulation of the heat contained in the smoke. It has been discovered that heat from the external environment causes cancers in the body surface and in the regions that are most easily and constantly exposed to the heat. It's not difficult to imagine how toxic heat in the internal environments within the body can contribute to various types of diseases.

When people drink alcohol too frequently, or when they are in the habit of consuming very spicy foods, their internal environments will heat up to increase their susceptibility to the attack of diseases, both severe and minor. These conditions include carbuncles, constipation, hot sensations or pain on urination, vomiting of blood, nosebleeds, infections, boils, cellulitis, acute bacillary dysentery, acute lymphadenitis, sore throats, high fever, mumps, facial erysipelas, acute tonsillitis, mastitis, osteomyelitis, acute dacryocystitis, cystic hyperplasia of breasts and multilocular cysts.

The internal organs are much more delicate than the outer surface of the body, which is why they are much more vulnerable to the attack of toxic heat in the internal environments. There is reason to believe that internal toxic heat contributes to cancers of various organs in the same way that skin cancer is caused by excessive exposure to external heat. It is frequently observed that many cancer patients display the symptoms traditionally believed to be caused by toxic heat in the internal environments, such as burning pain, fever, thirst, constipation, or diarrhea. For example, patients with lung cancer, particularly in the late stages, often cough up blood and have fever, chest pain and tumors, all of which are considered symptoms associated with presence of toxic heat in the

monia, pulmonary abscess, acute bilary infections, acute urinary infections, acute leukemia, malignant tumors and chronic granulocytic leukemia."

The foods for reducing toxic heat in the internal environments are either cool or cold in nature. They include adzuki beans and flowers, aloe vera, asparagus, bamboo shoots, banana and rhizome, bear, cow, goose, pork and chicken gall bladder, bitter and Chinese endive, bitter gourd (balsam pear), brake, burdock, camphor mint, cattails, celery seeds, chicken egg whites, Chinese toon and leaf, chrysanthemums, clams, crabs, figs, frog, grapefruits, grape leaves, hair vegetable, honey, honeysuckle and stem-leaf, leaf beets, lemons, licorice, lily flowers, lotus rhizome and stem, mallow root, mung bean powder and sprouts, orchid leaves, pear peels, pearl, peppermint, potato, preserved duck eggs, pricking amaranth, purslane, rabbit, rambutan, romaine lettuce, Chinese rose, Russian olives (oleaster), safflower fruits, salt, soybean paste, squash, star fruit (carambola), strawberries, sweet basil, tangerine orange peels, tea melons, tea oil, tofu and wheat.

## FOODS FOR REDUCING DAMP HEAT

Dampness and heat may affect the internal environments of the body simultaneously. Hepatitis is one of the diseases associated with damp heat and treated by foods and herbs that can alleviate it. For example, 186 cases of hepatitis were treated by seven Chinese health units in China; the results showed 119 cured cases, which accounted for 63.9 percent and 67 deaths, which accounted for 36.1 percent. In order to compare the effects of different therapies, the Chinese Army Hospital treated 18 severe cases of hepatitis in 1970-1973 with Western medicine alone; the results showed eight cases cured, which accounted for 44.4 percent. The same hospital treated 21 severe cases of hepatitis in 1974-1975 with the combined therapy of Chinese and Western medicines, which resulted in 16 cured cases, or 76.2 percent. This is merely one of the many experiments that show a higher percentage of cures when Chinese and Western medicines are combined in the treatment.

Acute infection of the biliary tract is another disease caused by damp heat in the internal environments. This disease may include gallstones and cholecystitis (inflammation of the gallbladder), which used to be treated by surgery. However, Chinese doctors discovered that surgery was not always a good solution due to a higher recurrence rate. And so, the Nan-Kai Hospital in Tianjin, China, conducted an experiment in which 438 acute cases of biliary tract infections were treated with Chinese and Western medicines. The results showed 368 cured cases, which accounted for 84.5 percent; among them, 332 cases did not undergo surgical operations, which totaled 75.8 percent. The Chinese treatment of such symptoms always involves the use of foods and herbs to reduce damp heat in the body.

Damp heat in the internal organs is also associated with many skin diseases, including skin cancers. Chinese herbs and foods that can clear damp heat have been routinely used to treat these conditions. For example, the Health Hospital of Honan Province treated 200 cases of skin cancer with herbs and foods to reduce damp heat, including carcinoma of the mammary gland and penis. The results showed 122 cured cases, significant improvements in 33 cases, with an overall effective rate of 77.5 percent.

The foods for reducing damp heat in the internal environments include adzuki bean sprouts, alfalfa and brake roots, buckwheat, cantaloupe (muskmelon), carp, celery roots, Chinese cabbage, citron leaves, coconut shell, corn silk, cucumber vines and stems, day lilies, dried black soybean sprouts, eggplant (aubergine) and calyx, fig leaves, frog, glutinous rice stalk, green turtle, hawthorn fruits, Job's tears root, lard, olives, plantains, pricking amaranth, pumpkin root, snails, soybean oil, yellow soybeans, squash flowers and roots, star fruit (carambola), sunflowers, turnip seeds and wheat seedling.

## FOODS TO ELIMINATE SPUTUM (EXPECTORANT FOODS)

Another factor related to the conditions of the internal environments is presence of sputum in the body. Just as there is air and water pollution in the environment, so there is sputum in the human body. The presence of sputum is responsible for many diseases, including swellings in the body that are neither itchy nor painful, lumps in the breast, mucous discharge, vomiting of sputum, hard spots in the abdomen, gastric retention, intestinal obstruction with fluid retention, goiter, tuberculosis of the lymph nodes and breast, liver and stomach cancer.

According to modern research conducted in China, three types of diseases are most frequently associated with the presence of sputum in the internal environments: chronic tracheitis, hydrothorax (a noninflammatory collection of fluid in the pleural cavity) and Meniere's disease. The strategy to eliminate sputum in the body is eating the right foods, which may be compared to cleaning up environmental pollution.

The foods for eliminating the sputum include air bladder of shark, almonds, apple peels, apricot seeds, asafoetida, asparagus, azalea flowers, black sesame seeds, bamboo oil, bean drink, bottle gourds, brake, celery, chicken gall bladder, citron, clams, common button mushrooms, dates, eggplant root, epiphyllum, figs, fingered citron, garlic, ginkgo, grapefruit, hair vegetable, honey, jellyfish, kohlrabi leaves, kumquats, laver, leaf or brown mustard, lemon leaves and peels, licorice, limes, lobster, longevity fruit, loquat flower leaves and seeds, dried mandarin orange peels, wild marjoram, mustard seed, olives, onions, orange leaves and peels, oysters, oyster shells, peach blossoms, peanuts, pears, pearl, black and white pepper, peppermint, persimmon, plantains and seeds, plum blossoms, radish roots and seeds, rock sugar, salt, sea cucumber, seagrass, seaweed, shark's fin, shiitake mushrooms, sour and sweet green orange peels, squash calyx, tangerine seeds, tea, thyme, tofu, walnuts, water chestnuts, white or yellow mustard seed and white sugar.

## FOODS FOR PROMOTING ENERGY CIRCULATION

Poor energy circulation may occur in the human body, affecting various vital organs and causing pain. The symptoms arising from poor energy circulation are collectively called "energy congestion," which may give rise to chest pain and congestion, abdominal pain and swelling, hernias, cholecystitis, hepatitis, climacteric melancholia, furuncle, gastrointestinal disorders, peptic ulcers, retention of urine, ringing in the ears, stomachaches, urination difficulty and uterine bleeding.

Abdominal pain and swelling are two distinct symptoms due to poor energy circulation in the internal environments. The two symptoms are characterized by changes in their severity and the region affected often shifts around to different areas. Sometimes, abdominal pain and swelling may move upwards to cause pain and congestion in the chest or in the sides.

The foods for promoting energy circulation in the internal environments include ambergris, beef, camphor, caraway seeds, cardamom seeds, carrots, cherry roots, chicken eggs, chives, citrons, clams, common button mushrooms, dill seeds, fennel roots and seeds, fig roots, fingered citrons and roots, garlic, grapefruits including flowers and roots, green onion heads and fibrous roots, green turtle, hawthorn fruits, jasmine flowers, kumquats and roots, ladle gourd, leaf or brown mustard, lemon leaves, limes, litchi nuts, longan seeds, loquat seeds, lotus stems, malt, mango leaves, marjoram, muskmelon seeds, mussels, mustard seeds, orange leaves and peels, orchid leaves, radish leaves, rapeseed, red beans, roses, saffron, scallion bulbs, shiitake mushrooms, spearmint, star anise, string beans, sweet basil, sweet orange peels, sword bean roots, tangerine including peels and seeds, tea seeds, turmeric and vinegar.

## FOODS FOR PROMOTING BLOOD CIRCULATION

When poor blood circulation occurs in the internal environments, it may lead to blood coagulation, which results in persistent pricking pain in the local region and swelling, bleeding and blue spots in the skin. Blood coagulation may affect vital internal organs to cause heart pain, chest congestion, blue-purple lips, discharge of blood from the mouth, pain in the ribs, vomiting of blood or discharge of blood from the anus, pain in the lower abdomen, irregular menstruation in women with purple and dark menstrual blood clots and vaginal bleeding.

The foods for promoting blood circulation include ambergris, antler, arrowhead, bayberry roots, brown sugar, camellia, cantaloupe, castor bean roots, cattail pollen, celery including the roots, chestnuts, chicken blood, chili peppers including leaves and rhizome, chives including roots and bulbs, clams, coriander, corn roots, crabs including claws and shells, distillers' grains, dog's bone, eel blood, eggplant including leaves, fermented glutinous rice, fish air bladder, ginger leaves, green onion including white head and fibrous root and fresh juice, green turtle, hawthorn fruits, hemp, kiwifruit roots, leaf beets, leaf or brown mustard, lemon roots, lotus flowers including rhizome and sprouts, muskmelon seeds, peaches including blossoms and kernels and roots, peony flowers and root bark, plantains, plum kernels, pumpkin pedicel, purslane, radishes, rape, rapeseed, glutinous rice, Chinese rose including leaves and roses, safflower fruits, saffron, seagrass, shark, sheep or goat's blood, black and yellow soybeans, sturgeon, sweet basil, sword bean shells, tofu, turmeric, vinegar and white and yellow mustard seeds.

## AGING AS A FUNCTION OF IMMUNE DEFICIENCY

Why do people grow old? Research published in 1982 by the Chinese Academy of Medical Science pointed out that among 25 subjects over 60 years old and 20 subjects between 20 and 30 years old, the ratio of T cells (thymus-dependent cells) in the group of subjects over 60 years old had been found to be lower than in the group of subjects between 20 and 30 years old.

# Deficienct and Excess Diseases and Aging

This points to the connection between the aging process and immune deficiency. T cells comprise 70 percent of circulating lymphocytes in the blood with a life span up to 5 years. Each T cell is programmed to react to a number of antigens such as bacteria, bacterial toxins and foreign blood cells.

Longevity means to live long, but to do that, it is necessary to slow down the aging process of the body. Everyone would agree that aging is a natural process of life and that it is impossible for any human being to live forever. However, there is no question that the aging process can be slowed down, even though it cannot be avoided. Anyone who wishes to live a long life must fully understand how the aging process takes place before he or she can take effective steps to slow it down. Therefore, the first question to be raised is: How does the aging process take place?

The aging process is closely connected with the immune function of the body, so much so that all of us will stay alive and healthy as long as the immune function remains in good shape. As soon as the immune function is impaired, the survival of the body is in jeopardy. This is because the immune function guards against any harmful infections so that the body can function normally without disease.

According to a report presented by the Canton College of Chinese Medicine, those with various types of body deficiencies display a corresponding decrease in the number of leukocytes (white blood cells) that act as scavengers to combat infection. The same report also points out that when the body has a deficiency, the level of interferon (a protein formed when normal cells are exposed to viruses) is lowered so that the body becomes more susceptible to the attack of viruses.

Research conducted by the Hunan College of Chinese Medicine in 1977 indicates that among 37 subjects with chronic tracheitis and 20 people in good health, the average ratio of T cells among the cases of chronic tracheitis was 25.56 percent while that among the healthy people was 52.6 percent, which was statistically very significant ($p < 0.01$). After the patients recovered from chronic tracheitis, the ratio of T cells was returned to normal in the majority of cases.

Research conducted in 1982 by Dr. Liu Zheng-Cai in China involving 100 cases of chronic atrophic gastritis indicates that the vast majority of patients increased the ratio of T cells after they recovered from illness. A separate report prepared by the Army Hospital 302 in 1981 indicates that over 70 percent of 101 cases of chronic hepatitis showed a decrease in the ratio of T cells.

The body will muster its immune function to defend itself when it is under attack by foreign agents. For example, when the body is subjected to common cold and flu viruses or malignant cancer cells, the immune function will immediately try to resist such attacks or recover from them. Thus, when the body suffers immune deficiency, it will not have sufficient power to resist the attacks and so becomes more susceptible to various diseases.

Immunity consists of cellular and humoral immunity. Cellular immunity refers primarily to T cells and other nonspecific cells such as macrophage, which is a cell with the ability to ingest and destroy microorganisms (bacteria and protozoa) and neutrophil and reticuloendothelial cells, both of which can assist T cells in developing their immune capability. Humoral immunity consists primarily of various antibodies (such as IgA, IgG, IgE, IgM and IgD) produced by B cells (B lymphocytes) that comprise 30 percent of lymphocytes in the blood with a life span up to 15 days. Thus, by measuring such cells and antibodies in the body, scientists are able to determine the degree of the body's immune function.

There are many medical terms used to describe the various aspects of the body's immune function, such as "antibodies" that are developed in response to the presence of substances (antigens) harmful to the body and "immune surveillance" that refers to the body's ability to recognize the harmful elements and remove them accordingly. A well-known medical text contains a glossary of immunologic terminologies that lists over 100 terms and phrases related to the theory of immunity.

For the purpose of this book, immune deficiency simply means that people have become so weak that they get sick easily and frequently. To live long, it's necessary to make weak people stronger so that they don't become sick so often, which is the first and essential step to be taken in the pursuit of longevity.

Immune deficiency may be derived from genetic factors and it may also be developed from one's inability to look after one's body properly. Immune deficiency due to genetic factors may occur under different circumstances. For example, a baby may be born with a weak thymus gland. Since the thymus is responsible for the development of T cells, the baby may grow up with a shortage of T cells and become more susceptible to the attack of infectious diseases at a later time. Also, a baby may be born with only a small number of neutrophil cells in the blood and since these cells can assist T cells in developing the immune system, it may cause immune deficiency. This type of innate immune deficiency, like all other diseases associated with genetic factors, is more difficult to correct.

For example, some people do not gain any appreciable amount of weight, regardless of how much they eat, which is unquestionably associated with genetic factors. Other people do not eat much but still gain considerable weight, which is also apparently associated with genetic factors. It is more difficult for such people to lose or gain weight because of genetic factors.

Immune deficiencies due to genetic factors are, from the traditional Chinese point of view, associated with the condition of the kidneys: They are called kidney yin deficiency and kidney yang deficiency. Foods or herbs known as kidney yin tonics and yang tonics are normally used to correct the yin and yang deficiencies, respectively.

It is a historical fact that many Chinese scholars and physicians achieved longevity by eating kidney tonics. In his literary classic, entitled *My Teaching to Posterity*, a Chinese scholar by the name of Yan Zhi-Tui in the sixth century said, "I have been in the habit of eating kidney tonics throughout my life, which is why I could still read fine print when 70 years old with no gray hair on my head."

Two Chinese emperors were famous for their longevity due to their firm beliefs in Chinese medicine and to their regular practice of taking kidney tonics. The Emperor Jia-Jing (1507-1566), who had ruled the Chinese empire for 45 years (1521-1566), had lived 59 years and the Emperor Qian-Long (1711-1799), who had ruled for 61 years (1735-1796), had lived 88 years. Although their life spans may not seem very long today, the Chinese people during those periods of history had a much shorter average life span than now, particularly Chinese emperors, who lived between 45 and 50 years on the average.

As to immune deficiency, developed from one's inability to look after one's body properly, it should be enhanced by consumption of the right foods. A Chinese medical book published in the third century, entitled *Prescriptions for Acute Diseases*, said, "Good health is first and foremost to be found in foods; anyone who does not know how to eat the right foods cannot stay in good health." Today a prevailing belief among the Chinese people is that one should eat the right foods to maintain good health before trying to take natural herbs for the same purpose, that one should take natural herbs to maintain good health before resorting to chemical drugs and that one should take chemical drugs to maintain good health before undergoing surgical operations, which should be the last resort.

In short, when the immune function is defi-cient, the body will not be able to resist disease; if the body cannot resist disease, it cannot survive for long, since we live in environments full of potential enemies. Therefore, it is essential to enhance the immune function of the body if we wish to live a long life.

## IMMUNE DEFICIENCY AND NUTRIENTS

One important way of enhancing the immune function of the body is through the consumption of foods, because they are so essential to life that we cannot live without them. What do foods contribute to the body? In the twentieth century, we have come to know that there are five types of essential nutrients in foods: carbohydrates (sugars and starches), which are the body's principal source of energy; proteins, which are indispensable in building and repairing the tissues; fats, which are the body's secondary source of energy; vitamins, which are indispensable to the maintenance of the body's normal functions; and minerals, which also contribute to functions in a unique way. In about one century, scientists have discovered those five types of nutrients considered essential to the human body, which marks a significant advance in the field of health and nutrition.

Linus Pauling, who won a Nobel Prize, once maintained that vitamin C taken in large amounts prevents the onset of the common cold. Scientists subsequently pointed out that the effectiveness of vitamin C for this purpose has not been established. It all depends on whether the body suffers a vitamin-C deficiency; if it does, then it will definitely prevent the common cold, because, other things being equal, a person with a vitamin-C deficiency will certainly become more susceptible to a cold than another person without such a deficiency. In this sense, every nutrient can be used to prevent colds, depending on whether the body needs it. This is why vitamins and nutrients may be used to enhance the immune function when the body needs them.

On the other hand, if the body doesn't need them, such nutrients could be harmful to good health. At this writing, I read a report about vitamin A taken in excessive amounts being responsible for causing birth defects, according to American health officials. There seems little doubt that all nutrients may be used to enhance the immune function in order to correct immune deficiencies provided the body needs them. The question is not whether such nutrients can enhance the body's immune function, but under which circumstances they are effective in achieving this objective.

The five types ot nutrients represent only what scientists have discovered in foods. There are without doubt many more elements to be discovered in the future. For example, vitamins have existed in foods since the beginning of time and they have been consumed by people all over the world ever since, but they were not discovered by scientists until the twentieth century. But if the five types of nutrients are all that one needs in order to stay in good health, then why do we bother to eat foods at all? Why don't we simply eat those five nutrients?

In 1880, a Russian scientist had conducted an experiment in which he fed one group of rats fresh milk and other foods; another group was fed artificial extracts of carbohydrates, proteins, fats and minerals. He discovered that the rats in the first group grew satisfactorily, whereas those in the second group died very easily. This Russian scientist pointed out in his research report, "There are undoubtedly other things in foods that are equally essential to human health but that still remain unknown to us."

A similar experiment was conducted by Sir Frederick Hopkins in 1912 in which two groups of young rats were fed artificial foodstuffs consisting of only pure carbohydrates, protein and fats. It was found that the group of lab rats that were only fed the artificial food put on weight but became ill. Rats in the other group were fed the same diet but with a small amount of fresh milk and they all continued to grow.

These experiments were conducted in the late nineteenth and early twentieth centuries when vitamins had not yet been discovered. The death of the rats in the experimental group was subsequently attributed to a lack of vitamins in their diet. Now that vitamins have been discovered, can we safely, assume that the human body needs nothing else except the five types of nutrients so far discovered by scientists?

I haven't heard of or encountered any modern physician who advises his patients to eat the five types of nutrients alone, nor have I learned of anyone conducting experiments similar to those just mentioned. But virtually all of us can be absolutely certain that the body needs other things besides the five types of nutrients and that we would be better off and it would be safer to eat foods. What are the foundations of our belief that the body needs more than the five types of nutrients? The answer to this question may be expressed in two words: common experience. We are grateful to those scientists who have discovered various types of nutrients, but we know from our common experience that we need to eat foods to stay in good health.

## AGING AS A FUNCTION OF EXCESS DISEASES

When the body is suffering from immune deficiency, it will increase its susceptibility to disease, simply because the body is too weak to respond to the attack effectively. However, there is another type of disease that has nothing to do with the body's immune deficiency; a typical example is hypertension, or high blood pressure. When a person develops high blood pressure, there's no attacking foreign agent to take the blame for causing it.

Thus, we may classify diseases into two categories: deficiency diseases that occur as a result of immune deficiency and excess diseases that occur as a result of an excessive accumulation in the body such as water retention that causes eczema, dryness that causes itching, heat that causes skin eruptions and cholesterol that causes high blood pressure. Western nutrition is designed to combat deficiency diseases but remains mostly irrelevant to the treatment of excess diseases.

Chinese food cures are aimed at curing deficiency and excess diseases alike. The theory of Chinese medicine dealing with the internal environments of the body plays an important role in the treatment of excess diseases. Environments refer to the surrounding conditions that affect the body and according to this theory, a person lives in two different kinds of environments: external and internal. External environments are very familiar to all of us; they include climate, air, trees and water. When Chinese physicians talk about the internal environments, they mean the internal conditions of the body. When something has gone wrong in these environments, it will cause excess diseases and it will also create a favorable climate for the attack of disease-causing agents. Therefore, it's possible and desirable to create suitable environments within the body so that it will be free from excess diseases and foreign agents will find it difficult to survive or spread there. Foods that can achieve healthy internal environments are called regulating foods in Chinese theory. Thus, there are two categories of foods: tonic foods that are consumed to correct immune deficiency and regulating foods that balance the internal environments of the body.

Western doctors are preoccupied with destroying disease-causing agents and in the process of doing so, they sometimes also destroy the body and kill the patient. There is another way of dealing with diseases that can be illustrated with an analogy about migratory birds. It would be extremely difficult, if not impossible, for scientists to try to chase away a whole group of returning migratory birds and try to keep them away when they would prefer to stay because the climate is suitable to them. To do this would undoubtedly tap our human resources to an unthinkable extent even just to achieve a modest degree of success. But strangely enough, when the time comes and there is a change in climate, the migratory birds will leave voluntarily without the slightest effort on our part.

Another example is the common cold, which is caused by viruses according to Western medicine, but we do not have to kill viruses in treating a common cold. We either drive the viruses away or neutralize them by creating internal environments in which they cannot cause harm to the body. There are so many remedies for the common cold, Chinese or Western, but no manufacturers claim that their products are designed to kill the viruses that cause it. This clearly indicates that to kill the viruses is not the only method and not always the best way of treating diseases. There is a Chinese martial art that teaches you how to defend yourself without putting up a fight against your opponent, because you can simply let your opponent miss you and fall. The more force is involved the harder that selfdestruction will be. This is the secret weapon of Chinese medicine used to cure both deficiency and excess to diseases.

We are very aware of the negative impact of environmental factors on the body, including air and water pollution, toxins, cold air, humidity, among others. Doesn't it make sense to think in the same way when we talk about the internal environments? In point of fact, the conditions of external environments will not severely affect our health unless they become parts of our internal environments. Summer heat will irritate the skin for sure, but it's only after the heat penetrates into the body that it begins to have a real impact on our health. Therefore, it's important to pay close attention to the conditions of the internal environments of the body and regulate them accordingly if necessary.

The internal environments of the body may be regulated either before or after the diseases have occurred. For example, when we have the flu and a struggle between the body's immune function and the virus takes place, we can eat foods such as green onion and coriander to induce perspiration. When the fever is gone, the attack of the virus ceases and the body's immune function returns to normal. On the other hand, if we know that normally the internal environments of the body are both hot and damp, which tend to cause diseases of the gall bladder and liver, we can eat more cold and dry foods to cool and dry the internal environments to prevent the attack of such diseases. In short, both immune deficiency and excessive internal environmental factors are harmful to the longevity of the body. Immune deficiency should be corrected by eating tonic foods, while excessive factors in the internal environments can be remedied by eating regulating foods.

## MAKING AND STORING THE FOOD CURES

The preparation of Chinese food cures is not the same as general Chinese cooking. Unless it is specified, when making food cures and remedies in this book, no oil is used. In everyday cookery, "fry" usually means to fry in a large quantity of oil and sauté or stir-fry means to use a small quantity of oil or fat. In this book, the verb "fry" means to fry without oil. It is more like toasting a food in a pan, allowing the heat to penetrate the food to toast the surface.

Other cookery terms and methods are more familiar to both Chinese and Western readers: When a food is boiled, it is boiled in water, unless specified otherwise. Often the food or herb is strained and only the broth or liquid is consumed as soup or tea. For other remedies, after cooking the food in water, you may eat the food and drink the liquid as the recipe suggests.

The foods used for food cures are generally not kept for very long, except in powdered form. But even powder should be stored in the refrigerator. Make certain that the powder is really dry when you grind it.

As for the amounts, use common sense when following the suggestions in the subsequent chapters. It is important to emphasize that quantities given with each food are approximate only. You can make adjustments to meet your own needs. A person can eat one banana a day or three bananas a day for the hemorrhoid or constipation cures, which should not make a significant difference when recommending foods, not herbs or drugs.

When spoonfuls are suggested in this book, they always mean teaspoonfuls, unless otherwise specified. Other measurements and equivalents can be adjusted by referring to the Conversion Guides.

## SPECIAL PREPARATIONS

Rice wine, rice vinegar, fresh ginger juice, salt and honey are the five ingredients you can use to prepare foods to your specifications.

- Rice wine: In this book, always use rice wine when the recipe calls for wine. There are three ways you can use rice wine to prepare foods:
  1 While you are frying food, add wine in the process until it is dry; the quantity of wine may be individually adjusted.
  2 Soak foods in wine for a few hours before frying.
  3 When boiling foods, add some wine before removing from the heat. The purpose of using wine to prepare foods is to make them move upwards, which is good for symptoms in the upper body region, such as headache with a common cold.
- Rice vinegar: Use rice vinegar the same way as rice wine but for a different purpose. Rice vinegar is normally used to increase the constrictive effects of foods, which is particularly useful in curing diarrhea and stopping bleeding.
- Fresh ginger juice:
  1 Fresh ginger juice may be added to soup before it is removed from the heat.
  2 Foods may be cooked with a suitable amount of fresh ginger soup. The purpose of preparing foods with fresh ginger soup is to increase their yang nature so that the foods will move outward and become more effective for cold symptoms.
- Salt: Place an adequate amount of salt in a glass of water and stir it until completely dissolved; then pour the salt water into the pan while cooking the food; continue cooking until the water evaporates and the food becomes yellowish. The purpose of using salt to prepare foods is to make food move downwards— good for abdominal pain and constipation.
- Honey: Place a few tablespoonfuls of honey in the pan and heat it over low heat until honey becomes yellowish; add water and stir it. Then add the food and cook together until a little dry and very difficult to separate by hand. The purpose of preparing food with honey is to increase the degree of lubrication of the food, which is very desirable for curing a cough.

nergy tonics raise the level of energy in the body, especially in the internal organs of the digestive system. Energy deficiency may result from chronic illness, diseases, defective genetic factors and old age.

*Energy Tonic Foods*

## Beef

*Good for those who are underweight and for diabetes, edema.*

### DESCRIPTION

Neutral; sweet; used as a spleen, stomach, energy and blood tonic; affects the spleen and stomach.

### PREPARATION

- Eat regularly concentrated beef soup to relieve chronic diarrhea and prolapse of anus caused by chronic diarrhea.
- Mix together 1,000g beef, 10g ground black pepper, 5g dried orange peel powder; add 1 cup fresh ginger juice and an adequate amount of salt; marinate for 2 hours; cook the beef. Eat at meals to improve the conditions of stomach and stimulate the appetite. To make ginger juice, grate fresh ginger and boil it in water.

## Beef Liver

*Good for blurred vision, dizziness, night blindness, optic atrophy, dysentery, diarrhea.*

### PREPARATION

- Cut up beef liver to cook with matrimony vine fruits for dizziness and spots in front of the eyes. Boil beef liver in water until cooked; then cut it up and season it with vinegar to treat dysentery and diarrhea.

### CLASSICS

- A Chinese food classic written in 493 said, "When a person suffers night blindness, he cannot see at night like a bird. It should be treated by eating beef liver, because beef liver can sharpen the vision."

### NUTRITION

- One hundred grams of beef liver contains 18,300 I.U. of vitamin A, which accounts for its effectiveness in sharpening vision and treating night blindness.

## Bird's Nest

*Good for coughs, asthma, vomiting or coughing blood, chronic diarrhea, upset stomach or ulcers, frequent urination, incontinence, vaginal discharge, night sweats, chronic bronchitis, emphysema, lung or stomach disease, measles.*

### PREPARATION

- For a dry cough and night sweats, prepare 10g of bird's nest, 10g of white fungus and 2g of rock sugar. Soak the bird's nest and white fungus in water for 20 minutes; then wash and remove it and add the rock sugar. Steam it over water until cooked. Alternatively, prepare 5g of bird's nest and 5g of Western ginseng. Steam them over water until cooked; eat it at meals.
- For chronic bronchitis, emphysema and vomiting of blood, prepare a pear by coring it to remove seeds; then squeeze 4g of bird's nest inside the pear. Add 2g of rock sugar and steam it over boiling water. Eat once every morning without interruption.
- For an upset stomach and vomiting, soak 8g of bird's nest in water, then steam it over boiling water. Boil it in 2 cups of milk and drink the milk all at once.

- For stomach ulcers, cut up 20g of bird's nest and boil in a cup of water until cooked. Add 2g of rock sugar to the boiling water. Remove it from the heat, eat the bird's nest and drink the soup three times daily (20g of bird's nest is the average quantity for each meal per person).

## NUTRITION

- Bird's nest contains various proteins and mucin, which is a glycoprotein found in mucus and saliva. It also provides glucose (grape sugar), sulfur and nitrogen. Bird's nest is an important yin tonic due to the presence of mucin in it.

## Bitter Gourd Seeds (Balsam Pear Seeds)
*Good for fatigue and impotence.*

### PREPARATION

- Fry bitter gourd seeds and crush them into powder. Take 10g of powder each time with a little brandy three times daily for 10 days as a treatment for impotence. Don't drink more than half a glass of brandy in one day; the brandy is to reinforce the effects of bitter gourd seeds, not to induce intoxication.

### NUTRITION

- 8.6 percent water, 21.8 percent ash, 19.5 percent fibre, 16.4 percent carbohydrates, 31.0 percent fat and momordicine.

## Cherries
*Good for paralysis, numbness of arms and legs, rheumatism, lumbago, frostbite.*

### DESCRIPTION

- Warm; sweet.

### PREPARATION

- Chew 8 to 12 fresh cherries slowly like chewing gum, twice a day, to relieve pharyngolaryngitis at its early stage.
- Boil 1 K fresh cherries until very soft; remove and discard seeds. Add 500g sugar and boil to make jelly. Take a spoonful cherry jelly each time, twice a day, to relieve fatigue and improve your complexion.
- In a large jar, combine 500g fresh cherries and 4fi cups rice wine; cover and store for 10 days. Drink 30 to 60g cherry wine each time, twice a day, to alleviate numbness of joints and paralysis from rheumatism.

## Chicken
*Good for those who are underweight, have poor appetite, diarrhea, edema, frequent urination, vaginal bleeding and discharge, shortage of milk secretion after childbirth, weakness after childbirth.*

### DESCRIPTION

- Warm; sweet; used as an energy tonic; warms up the internal region; affects the spleen and stomach.

## PREPARATION

- Cut up a chicken and remove the skin; pat dry with a paper towel; heat and lightly oil a fry pan; drop chicken cubes into the pan, stirring constantly; add a little vegetable oil and 5 slices fresh ginger and continue to stir-fry for a while. Add 1 cup water and 1 cup rice wine; continue to cook for about 20 minutes; add more rice wine, if desired. Eat at meals to alleviate fatigue and increase milk secretion of lactating mothers.
- Cut up a chicken and remove the skin; wash chicken cubes with rice wine and place the cubes in a fry pan; stir-fry until dried. Steam the chicken cubes with 20g longans for 3 hours until reduced to half a cup of pure chicken and longan soup. Drink the strained soup (without eating the chicken or longans) to relieve neurasthenia and forgetfulness. This is an expensive recipe; dried longans are available in most Chinese foods shops.

## Coconut Meat
*Good for tapeworms and fasciolopsiasis, constipation, premature aging.*

### DESCRIPTION

- Warm (shell); neutral and obstructive (shell); sweet (coconut meat); the coconut meat produces fluids, promotes urination and destroys intestinal worms; the shell constricts and destroys intestinal worms and relieves itching.

### PREPARATION

- Consume coconut (meat and liquid) once a day, first thing in the morning on an empty stomach for 3 consecutive days, to relieve tapeworm and fasciolopsiasis.
- Eat meat of 1 coconut each time, in the morning and evening, to correct constipation.
- Cut the meat of a coconut into small cubes and mix with sugar. Put the coconut cubes in a jar; cover with sugar and store for 2 weeks. Eat 2 to 3 coconut sugar cubes each time, twice a day, to tone up weakness in the elderly and prevent premature aging.

## Cooked Ginkgo
*Good for pulmonary tuberculosis, tracheitis, coughs, frequent urination, asthma, seminal emission.*

### PREPARATION

- Boil 15g of ginkgo in 30g of wine. Eat the ginkgo and drink the wine to stop seminal emission.
- Boil 15g of ginkgo in a cup of water and eat it before bedtime to stop frequent urination and enuresis in children.
- Boil 9g of ginkgo and 9g of lotus seeds with 60g of chicken in 30g of wine. Eat once daily to stop vaginal discharge.
- Boil 10g of ginkgo in a cup of water until cooked. Add a teaspoon of honey or sugar. Drink it as a soup to stop cough with sputum and shortness of breath as in asthma.
- Fry 10g of ginkgo without oil; then boil it in a cup of water over low heat. Add a teaspoon of honey and drink as a soup to stop seminal emission, enuresis, vaginal discharge and frequent urination. Alternatively, grind the fried ginkgo into powder and take with warm water to produce similar effects.

## NUTRITION

- The food value of 100g of ginkgo: protein, 6.4g; fat, 2.4g; carbohydrates, 36g; calcium, 10mg; phosphorus, 218mg; iron, 1mg.

## Red and Black Dates

*Good for diarrhea, hepatitis, neurasthenia, insomnia, allergic purpura, anemia, chronic tracheitis.*

## PREPARATION

- Boil 10 dates in a half cup of water over low heat until the water is reduced by half. Drink the soup and eat the dates to stop chronic diarrhea.
- Boil 20 red dates with seven green onion wheat heads in 2 cups of water over low heat until the water is reduced to a half cup. Drink the soup without eating the dates or onions to cure insomnia.
- Use a knife to chop 30 very large black dates. Boil the dates in 3 cups of water until the water is reduced to one cup and drink it like tea. This is called black date tea and is considered beneficial for insomnia. When people continue to drink black date tea on a regular basis, many symptoms can be cured, including anemia, dry and coarse skin, cracked lips and chronic diarrhea.
- Boil 20g of black dates, 10g of longans and one teaspoonful of honey in 2 cups of water until the water is reduced to one cup. Drink it before bedtime to cure insomnia. This remedy may not be as strong as sleeping pills, but can induce sleep and produces no side effects. When you wake up in the morning, you won't feel thirsty or uncomfortable, which is often associated with taking sleeping pills.
- Red dates and walnuts are a good combination, because dates are an energy tonic while walnuts are a brain tonic. Boil the two ingredients, 30g each, in 2 cups of water until the water is reduced to one cup. Drink it as a soup to cure neurasthenia, which often involves low energy and poor brain functions.
- When children are underweight and have night sweats, they often have a poor appetite. If this occurs, boil an equal amount of hawthorn fruits and red dates to make soup and let them drink it like juice. Hawthorn fruits can improve digestion as a temporary measure; red dates can strengthen digestion as a long-term food cure.
- Red dates and dangguis are a good combination to cure anemia, because red dates are an energy tonic and dangguis are a blood tonic. When the two ingredients are combined, it can tone both energy and blood simultaneously. Boil 10 red dates with 3g of danggui in a cup of water over low heat until the water is reduced by half. Drink it once daily to improve the complexion, correct menstrual disorders and cure physical weakness, particularly after childbirth.

## CLASSICS

- A traditional Chinese song says, "Red dates in the north have a special flavor. It can tone energy and secure the body."
- *The Yellow Emperor's Classics*, written in the third century B.C., said, "Red dates are important spleen tonics. They benefit the spleen and the pancreas a great deal."
- Another Chinese classic in 1695 said, "Red dates are used as tonics in ancient China; but black dates may be used to tone the spleen and pancreas, because they are sweet and can produce fluids."
- *The Agriculture Emperor's Materia Medica*, published in the third century B.C., said, "Dates are good for all internal organs, particularly for the spleen."

in Nanking once conducted research about the effects of ginkgo and found that patients with pulmonary tuberculosis were cured by eating some each day for 30 to 100 days. It was reported that among the 400 patients, fever was reduced in 73 percent of cases, excessive perspiration was checked in 77 percent, coughing was stopped in 66 percent, discharge of blood from the mouth was halted in 85 percent and appetite was improved in 70 percent of cases.

Because of its color, ginkgo is called "silver-white fruit." It is sold in Chinese grocery stores and herb shops. Chinese chefs use it for seasoning in most restaurants.

### Notes

Dates have a mild nature among foods, comparable to a nice fellow in society. According to the theory of Chinese medicine, the liver is in charge of anger, which means that when a person gets mad very easily, something must be wrong with his liver. The reason that dates are good for liver disease is that as a mild food, it can calm the liver.

Chinese dates discussed here should be distinguished from Western dates, even though both are energy tonic foods. There are two kinds of Chinese dates: those produced in southern China are called south dates; those grown in northern China are called north dates. South dates are better than north dates. Dates have two different colors: red and black. When fresh dates are left to dry in the sun, they become red dates; when fresh dates are boiled or steamed and processed, they become black dates.

Red dates are better in quality than black dates, because only good fresh dates are dried in the sun. Dates that are not so good in shape and quality have to be boiled or steamed and processed. This is why red and black dates have different shapes, although both belong to the same fruit. As to their effects, red dates are also better for therapeutic purposes than black dates, which are much cheaper.

Strictly speaking, Chinese dates are foods, not herbs, but all Chinese herb shops carry dates and all Chinese herbalists use them in their clinical practice.

- A Chinese herbal classic in A.D. 992 presented a recipe for bronchial asthma: "Fry 20 red dates (with seeds removed) in 4 teaspoonfuls of butter over low heat. Let the dates gradually absorb the butter until all of it is gone. Put one date in the mouth at a time and chew it slowly. Chew five dates a day, which should relieve cough."

## NUTRITION

- Fresh dates contain 20 to 36 percent carbohydrates; dried dates contain 55 to 80 percent carbohydrates, which are higher than beets (19 to 20 percent) and sugar cane (12 percent).
- One hundred grams of dates contains 380 to 600mg of vitamin C, which is more than lemons have. This is why the Chinese call dates "living vitamin C tablets." Even 100g of fresh date leaves contain 1,200 to 1,500mg of vitamin C; 100g of dried date leaves contain 3,000mg of vitamin C. Research also indicates that when date leaves are soaked in hot water, the vast majority of vitamin C is soluble in water and is absorbed by the body in the same way as synthetic vitamin C.

## RESEARCH

- A team of Chinese researchers conducted an experiment on the effects of dates on rabbits whose livers had been damaged by carbon tetrachloride (a toxic substance that causes acute atrophy of the liver and kidneys). The result showed the quantity of serum albumins (the main proteins in the blood) in the experimental group of rabbits had increased much more than those in the control group. The rabbits in the experimental group also grew faster and became much stronger. Also, when laboratory rats were fed dates for three weeks, their body weight had increased substantially and they could also swim much longer.
- A Chinese researcher used a traditional herbal formula with dates to treat two groups of bronchitis patients. In the experiment, the researcher omitted the dates from the formula administered to the first group but included them with the second group. The results showed that coughing was significantly relieved among patients in the second group but not in the first group. Dates have been found to expand the bronchi to improve breathing.
- Research indicates that dates are effective for allergic and simple purpura and patients can either be cured or show significant improvements within a week. The research pointed out that the effects could be related to the fact that dates are an energy tonic.
- A traditional formula for red date and peanut soup can be used to treat patients with acute and chronic hepatitis and cirrhosis, since dates have the effect of improving the conditions of the liver. Red date and peanut soup contains three foods: red dates, peanuts and rock sugar. To prepare it, boil the three ingredients, 3g of each, in a cup of water over low heat until the water is reduced by half. Drink it all before bedtime.

*Eel*

*Good for fatigue, vaginal discharge, discharge of stools containing blood and pus, hemorrhoids.*

## DESCRIPTION

- Warm; sweet; used as an energy tonic, to counteract rheumatism and to strengthen the bones; affects the liver, spleen and kidneys.

## PREPARATION

- Bake an eel after discarding the internal organs; fry 10g brown sugar and grind with the eel to make a powder. Take the powder with warm water to relieve chronic diarrhea with discharge of stools containing blood and pus.
- Eat eel at meals to arrest bleeding of internal hemorrhoids.
- Boil an eel in an adequate amount of wine until the wine evaporates; bake the eel, including the skin and bones and grind into powder. Take 10g each time with a cup of wine in severe cases, or take 7g in light cases, to relieve difficulty when swallowing. Follow by drinking rice soup and avoiding meat or emotional disturbances and excessive sex.

## Ginseng

*Good for poor appetites, fatigue, upset stomachs, diarrhea, coughs, excessive perspiration, forgetfulness, impotence, frequent urination, diabetes, vaginal bleeding.*

### DESCRIPTION

- Warm; sweet and slightly bitter; tones up energy; produces fluids; calms the spirits; affects the spleen and lungs.

### PREPARATION

- Ginseng is one of the few Chinese herbs that is frequently applied alone. A traditional Chinese herbal formula — solitary ginseng soup — is made by steaming or boiling ginseng for consumption: Boil 5g ginseng in 1fi cups water over low heat until water is reduced to half. Drink it all within 1 day to cure prolapse and heart failure.
- Ginseng may be used with dry ginger to treat morning sickness and abdominal pain.

## Grape

*Good for blood and energy deficiency, cough, palpitations, night sweat, rheumatism, difficulty when urinating, edema.*

### DESCRIPTION

Neutral; sweet and sour; strengthens the tendons and bones; promotes urination; also used as blood tonic and energy tonic; affects the lungs, spleen and kidneys.

### PREPARATION

- Crush 500g fresh grapes; add 500g rice wine and mix thoroughly. Strain to make grape wine. Eat 30g of the soaked raisins or drink 30g grape wine in the morning and evening, to tone up energy after illness.
- Eat a large bunch of fresh grapes in the morning and evening, to relieve dry throat and thirst.
- Boil 30g raisins with 15g fresh ginger peel. Drink twice a day to cure nutritional edema.
- Squeeze juice from 250g fresh grapes and mix with an equal amount of warm water. Drink it all each time, once a day, to relieve pain on urination, difficult urination and discharge of short and reddish stream of urine.
- Crush 120g fresh grapes and 250g fresh lotus roots. Squeeze out the juice, drink it all each time, 3 times a day, to cure or prevent discharge of urine containing blood.
- Boil 30g raisins in water and drink it like soup. In addition, boil grapevine leaves and parsley and use the liquid to wash the body to promote the

### *Notes*

Ginseng is regarded as an important ingredient to perform the following groups of functions:

To excite the nervous system, improve working efficiency and reduce fatigue.

To stimulate blood forming organs and aid the blood production.

To increase the heart's contraction capacity and to tone up the heart (useful in the treatment of heart failure and shock).

To improve the sex gland functions in men and women in the treatment of hypogonadism.

To improve the functions of digestion, absorption and metabolism.

To act as an antidiuretic.

To lower blood sugar; this function is attributed to the presence of ginsenin in ginseng.

While ginseng has its important functions, there are also circumstances under which ginseng should not be used. Such circumstances may include the following:

Cough and coughing up blood. Vomiting of blood due to excessive indulgence in sexual intercourse.

Ginseng could cause encephalemia or cerebrovascular accidents in people suffering from hypertension.

Edema and incomplete functions of the kidneys with decreased urination, because ginseng is an antidiuretic that may cause edema to deteriorate.

Excessive type of insomnia, because ginseng can make an excessive condition even more excessive.

Common cold with fever, because ginseng can increase the production of extreme heat in the body, which can intensify the fever.

There are three basic kinds of ginseng with different functions: Chinese ginseng; Korean or red ginseng; and American ginseng. Chinese ginseng, more beneficial to the lungs and the digestive system, is more often used to benefit the lungs, produce fluids and hear other critical symptoms. Korean or red ginseng is warmer; it is most frequently used

to tone up energy and blood to improve the functions of the sex gland
and is less effective for other symptoms. American ginseng has a cool
energy. It tastes sweet and slightly
bitter, acting on the heart, the lungs
and the kidneys and is mostly used
for cough, thirst and alcoholism.

*Notes*

Eating excessive quantities of
grapes may decrease appetite.

outbreak of rash in measles.

- Boil 30g raisins with 15g red dates in water; drink like soup to relieve anxiety during quickening.

## *Honey*

*Good for dry coughs, constipation, stomachaches, sinusitis, mouth cankers, burns, neurasthenia, hypertension, pulmonary tuberculosis, heart disease, liver disease.*

### DESCRIPTION

- Neutral; sweet; detoxicates; lubricates dryness; relieves pain; affects the lungs, spleen and large intestine.

### PREPARATION

- Steam about half a cup honey. Eat it all at once on an empty stomach, 3 times a day, for 2 to 3 weeks on end, to relieve gastric and duodenal ulcers.
- Mix half a cup honey with warm water and drink once a day to treat hypertension, constipation, stomachache, neurasthenia, heart disease and coronary sclerosis.
- Drink a cup honey water at bedtime to cure insomnia due to neuras-thenia. Externally apply honey to the affected region to relieve burns.
- Mix 3 large spoonfuls honey in boiling water. Drink it in the morning and in the evening to relieve insomnia, headache and anemia; or eat honey at meals with other foods.
- Using a sterilized cotton ball, externally apply honey to the anus to heal cracked skin in hemorrhoids; or externally apply to the ear to relieve swelling of the ear.
- Mix 2 teaspoonfuls honey with warm water. Drink it first thing in the morning on an empty stomach to relieve chronic constipation.
- Mix 1 teaspoonful honey with warm water and drink it 3 hours after meals, 3 times a day, for 5 consecutive days, to relieve hoarseness caused by excessive fatigue but unrelated to common cold, with sufficient rest to produce best results.

### CLINICAL REPORT

- For treatment of gastric and duodenal ulcers; among 20 cases treated, the niche disappeared in 15 cases, showed progress in 3 cases (32 days on the average), pain completely disappeared in 18 and pain decreased in 2; pain was gone as quickly as 6 days and within 22 days on the aver-age. The method of treatment: each day, eat a third cup fresh honey before meals, 3 times a day; after the tenth day, increase the quantity of honey to half a cup each day.
- Clinical reports on treatment of other diseases showed good results: For treatment of acute bacillary dysentery, take 150g honey each day for adults (divide into 4 reduced dosages for children); for treatment of chronic and or temporary constipation in the elderly and in pregnant women, take honey first thing in the morning; for treatment of hypochromic anemia, take 80 to 100g honey each day, divided into 3 dosages; the results show an obvious increase in blood cells and hemoglobin.

## *Licorice*

*Good for abdominal pain, poor appetites, fatigue, fever, coughs, palpitations, convulsions, sore throats, digestive ulcers, drug poisoning, food poisoning.*

### DESCRIPTION

- Neutral; sweet; slows down acute diseases, lubricates lungs, counteracts toxic effects, coordinates the effects of other herbs; affects the spleen, stomach and lungs.

### PREPARATION

- Prepare 150g processed licorice and 80g dry ginger; boil in only enough water to cover the 2 ingredients; boil until the water is reduced by half; strain and drink 1 cup of the warm soup each time, twice a day, to cure abscessed lungs, suppurative pneumonia and bronchitis without cough.
- Boil 10g licorice with 20g whole wheat kernels and 5 Chinese red dates. Drink as soup to treat hysteria in women, anxiety and stress. This is a time-honored herbal formula in Chinese medicine.

## *Longan*

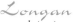

*Good for insomnia, forgetfulness, palpitations, nervousness.*

### DESCRIPTION

- Warm; sweet; used as a spleen tonic, heart tonic, blood tonic and energy tonic; affects the heart and spleen.

### PREPARATION

- Steam 15g longans with 30g lean pork, 2 fresh ginger slices and an adequate amount of rice wine. Eat once a day to relieve dizziness and underweight.
- Mix 500g longans with 500g sugar; steam them to make longan jelly.
- Take 1 spoonful longan jelly with warm water to relieve dizziness and edema after childbirth; or boil 15g longans with 5 red dates, 30g brown sugar and 6g fresh ginger. Drink it as soup once a day.

## *Pigeon Meat*

*Good for diabetes, menstrual disorders in women, discharge of blood from the anus.*

### CLASSICS

- A Chinese classic dating from 1695 said, "Pigeon meat is beneficial to those suffering from physical weakness, particularly in chronic cases."

### NUTRITION

- Pigeon meat contains 75.10 percent water, 22.14 percent protein, 1 percent fat and 1 percent ash.

## *Potatoes (Irish Potatoes)*

*Good for lack of energy, mumps, burns.*

### DESCRIPTION

- Neutral; sweet; heals inflammations; used as an energy tonic and a spleen tonic.

### PREPARATION

- Crush a potato and squeeze out the juice; mix it with vinegar.
- Apply the juice to the affected region to relieve mumps.

- Apply potato juice externally to burns.
- Prepare 5 potatoes (the size of eggs), 1 onion and an adequate amount of garlic and carrots. Wash and thoroughly clean the potatoes but do not peel them. Cut up the potatoes and onion; put all ingredients in about a few cups water; simmer over low heat until the water is reduced to half and add some salt. Drink 2 cups of the soup at each meal; or adjust the quantity and frequency according to individual needs. This soup is good for hypertension, malnutrition in infants, diarrhea, bronchial asthma, allergic skin, kidney disease and also for obesity.
- To relieve gastric and duodenal ulcers, eat a cupful of cooked potato liquid with a spoon once a day. To make the potato remedy, wash 30 fresh unpeeled potatoes and grate them to squeeze out the juice. Simmer the juice in an earthenware pot (not a metal one) over low heat without a cover until the water evaporates completely to form a thick layer at the bottom of the pot. This substance is called potato glue and is full of protein. By taking this sticky liquid you can relieve pain and heal a sensitive stomach. It is reported that gastric and duodenal ulcers may recover within 20 to 30 days by taking this glue.

## Sweet Potato

*Good for stomach weaknesses, kidney weaknesses, premature ejaculation.*

### DESCRIPTION

- Neutral; sweet; used as a spleen and an energy tonic and as a yin kidney tonic.

### PREPARATION

- Apply sweet potato soup to the affected region to heal frostbite; or apply the steam of the boiling sweet potato by holding to the frostbitten region over the steam.
- Bake sweet potato until the surface is charred; grind into powder. Take 10g of the powder dissolved in warm water to relieve common cold. Charred sweet potato can induce perspiration and reduce fever.

## Polished (White) Rice

*Good for diarrhea, morning sickness, difficult urination.*

### DESCRIPTION

Neutral; sweet; used as an energy tonic and a spleen tonic; affects the spleen and stomach.

### PREPARATION

- Fry 1 bowlful polished rice with fresh ginger juice until the rice becomes yellowish. Chew 20 to 30 grains before getting up in the morning to relieve morning sickness.
- Boil rice in water as you would normally, but cook it a little longer than usual to allow a thick crust of charred rice to form on the bottom of the pan; rice is neutral and bitter and sweet.
- Boil 150g browned crust of rice with an equal amount of lotus fruits and sugar in an adequate amount of water. Drink 2 teaspoonfuls each time, 3 times a day, to cure diarrhea, particularly in children.

*Notes*

When a child accidentally swallows a coin, feed the child large quantities of boiled sweet potatoes all at once; the coin will be coated by the sweet potatoes to discharge along with the stool.

## Sweet (Glutinous) Rice

*Good for excessive urination, excessive perspiration, diarrhea.*

### DESCRIPTION

- Warm; sweet; used as an energy tonic; affects the spleen, stomach and lungs.

### PREPARATION

- Fry sweet rice with wheat bran and grind into powder. Take 10g powder in warm water each time, 3 times a day, to stop excessive perspiration.
- Cook 50g sweet rice with 60g Job's tears and 8 red dates. Eat at meals to relieve pulmonary tuberculosis, neurasthenia, anemia and various kinds of chronic diseases.
- Boil sweet rice sprouts in water with malt. Drink the soup to relieve indigestion and to promote appetite.

## Shiitake Mushrooms

*Good for prevention of rickets, anemia, measles.*

### DESCRIPTION

- Neutral; sweet; affects the stomach.

### PREPARATION

- Boil some shiitake mushrooms in water until the soup becomes yellowish. Drink only the liquid (without eating the mushrooms) to relieve vomiting caused by careless eating; another alternative is to place shiitake mushrooms in boiling water and steep until the soup becomes yellowish. Drink it as tea.
- Dissolve some sugar or honey in the shiitake mushroom soup to treat coughing.
- Drink shiitake mushroom soup, or dissolve shiitake mushroom powder in hot water and drink it as tea to relieve fish poisoning. A prolonged consumption by this method is believed to prevent arteriosclerosis.
- In case of difficult urination or discharge of urine containing blood, bake some shiitake mushroom until it appears burned on the surface. Eat 10g each time, twice a day, or eat fresh shiitake mushrooms.

### EXPERIMENT

Studies with rats show shiitake mushroom lowers blood fat levels.

### CLINICAL REPORT

Shiitake mushroom counteracts cholesterol, a recent report indicates.

## Squash

*Good for pulmonary abscessed, bronchiectasis, roundworms, opium addiction.*

### DESCRIPTION

- Warm; sweet; heals inflammation; relieves pain; affects the spleen and stomach.

### PREPARATION

- Drink fresh squash juice frequently to relieve opium addiction.
- Cook 400g squash with 200g beef without salt or oil. Eat it to cure pulmonary abscess and bronchiectasis.

### Notes

Shiitake mushroom is believed to counteract stomach and cervical cancers. (When I visited Japan in October 1985, I learned that a new product containing the extract from shiitake mushroom had been approved by the Japanese government as an anti-cancerous agent.) The Chinese people are very fond of mushrooms, including shiitake mushrooms, which are produced primarily in Japan. Shiitake mushroom may be cooked by itself and it may also be cooked with other vegetables. In either case, avoid excessive amounts of soy sauce and salt because they are quickly absorbed by the mushroom and spoil its good taste.

### Notes

Squash is not recommended for people suffering from chest congestion or water retention.

- Apply fresh squash juice to burns.

## CLINICAL REPORT

- Consumption of 400g fresh squash (reduced by half in children) followed by taking a purgative 2 hours later, once a day for 2 consecutive days, was found to expel roundworms (from 2 to over 100) in 6 out of 10 cases.
- Squash seeds have been found to expel tape worms, roundworms and blood flukes.
- Prepare 20g squash seeds and remove the shells; wrap the seeds in a cloth and crush them. Mix it with water or with a little soy sauce or sugar. Drink it in the morning and evening for 3 to 5 days. This has been found to promote milk secretion after childbirth; but fully cooked seeds have not been found effective.
- Squash leaves are effective for dysentery. Boil 10 leaves with a little salt. Drink it as tea twice a day to relieve dysentery.
- Squash flowers may be boiled to drink as tea to cure jaundice and cough.

## *Vinegar*

*Good for jaundice, vomiting of blood, nosebleeds, discharge of blood from anus, itching in the genital region, fish, meat and vegetable poisoning.*

## DESCRIPTION

Warm; sour and bitter; disperses coagulations; detoxicates; arrests bleeding; affects the liver and stomach.

## PREPARATION

- Crush a small piece fresh ginger and mix it with 1 or 2 cups rice vinegar; drink it to correct indigestion caused by an excessive consumption of fish, salads and fruits.
- Add some vinegar to meats when cooking to promote digestion and stimulate the appetite.
- Cook celery with vinegar as a seasoning to treat hypertension with headache.
- In Chinese folk medicine, when a child suffers from convulsions and faints, with body temperature decreasing rapidly, vinegar is boiled at high heat with the doors closed so that the patient will inhale the vinegar vapor to regain consciousness. The same method may be used to arouse women who faint following childbirth.
- Drink a cup of hot vinegar to relieve pain caused by binary ascariasis and intestinal ascariasis.
- Combine half a bowl of vinegar, 70g brown sugar and 35g sliced fresh ginger; bring to a boil twice and strain it. Drink 1 small cup of the liquid each time with warm water, 3 times a day, to relieve itchiness and skin eruptions from allergic reactions after eating fish and crab.
- Soak overnight 10 peanuts in a small cup of vinegar. Drink the vinegar and eat the peanuts the next morning to treat hypertension; repeat for 10 to 15 days as a treatment program.

## CLINICAL REPORT

- A child was suffering from epidemic encephalitis and the Chinese doctor told the patient's father that it was necessary to use lactic acid sterilization; but lactic acid was not readily available. So the father used vinegar as a substitute and obtained good results.

*Notes*

Vinegar is called bitter wine in the Chinese language and vinegar and wine are considered the 2 friends of Chinese herbs. Why? Vinegar and wine are very frequently used to process Chinese herbs, not only to inhibit the side effects of herbs but also to increase their effects.

Drink between 30 to 50ml vinegar or more, according to your age, to alleviate the pain caused by biliary ascariasis. This treatment may be repeated until pain is gone. After pain is significantly reduced, apply anthelmintic as usual. Among the 15 cases of biliary ascariasis observed, with a total of 300 to 500ml vinegar administered in each case, pain stopped completely in 12 cases within 2 days and pain stopped within 3 to 4 days in 3 cases.

- Once a Chinese food factory reported an epidemic of influenza. All workers in the factory were stricken except the workers in the vinegar division; none of them became ill.
- According to a report from a Chinese food-processing plant, an average 8 percent of the factory workers are sick with respiratory infections yearly; but only 1 percent of the workers in the vinegar division have suffered from respiratory infections each year. Moreover, when the workers in the vinegar division do suffer from respiratory infections, the attack is lighter, too.
- Boil 500g pork bones and 100g white sugar in 4 cups vinegar for 30 minutes; strain it. Adults take 30 to 40 ml and children take 10 to 15 ml each time after meals, 3 times a day for 1 month as a treatment program. Chronic patients undergo 2 to 3 treatment programs (except patients with high fever who should not be treated by this method). Among the 3 cases of acute and chronic contagious hepatitis treated, all recovered within 40 to 60 days.
- In Hu Bei Yeecang People's Hospital in China, 51 cases of acute contagious jaundice-type hepatitis were treated with 10 ml rice vinegar and 2 vitamin B-1 tablets. All patients recovered from the illness within an average of 4 days and their poor appetites were significantly improved.

## EXPERIMENT

- In an experiment conducted by the Research Institute of Epidemic Diseases at the Chinese Academy of Medical Science, 200 bacteria colonies were cultured, consisting of 5 bacteria most frequently causing respiratory infections, such as pneumonia, catarrh and influenza. It was found that all but a few isolated bacteria colonies were exterminated within 30 minutes by vinegar vaporized at 100 degrees C; the same experiment also indicated that vinegar has no obvious bacteria-exterminating power when vaporized below 100 degrees C.

## Tofu (Bean Curd)

*Good for dysentery, diarrhea, intoxication, stomach bleeding, shortage of milk secretion after childbirth, anemia, irregular menstruation, diabetes, abdominal obstruction, tinea, whooping cough.*

## PREPARATION

- Boil a piece of tofu and slice it. Apply the slices to the skin eruptions of alcoholics as if using a bandage to cover them.
- Boil tofu with vinegar in water over low heat. Eat the tofu and drink the soup to cure chronic diarrhea and dysentery.
- Boil 500g of tofu and 120g of brown sugar in 2 cups of water. Continue to cook for another 10 minutes. Drink it all slowly within 2 hours to stop stomach bleeding.
- Prepare five cubes of tofu, 20g of dried shiitake mushrooms and one pork trotter. Boil the pork trotter and shiitake mushrooms first, season with salt and ginger, then add tofu and bring to a boil until cooked. Eat it at meals in one day. Alternatively, boil four cubes of tofu with 30g of brown sugar in a cup of water. Add a half cup of wine and remove it from the heat. Drink in one day. Both preparations are good for promoting milk secretion in nursing mothers.
- Slowly boil two cubes of tofu, 40g of mutton and 10 fresh ginger slices, in 2 cups of water over low heat. Season it with a little salt; eat at meals within one day to cure irregular menstruation and cold sensations in the stomach.

- Tofu may be eaten by patients with gastrointestinal diseases without causing digestive disorders. Since tofu contains unsaturated fat, it is safe for those with arteriosclerosis and heart disease.
- There is a disease known in Chinese medicine as "running fire," which refers to swollen eruptions in the legs and feet. In fact, this symptom is due to a stream of toxic heat running downwards to cause the eruption. One way to treat this symptom is to eliminate toxic heat in the body; another way is to crush a few cubes of tofu and apply it to the affected region like an ointment. Traditionally, the Chinese use jellyfish skin as a bandage to wrap the crushed tofu, because jellyfish skin itself can also heal swelling and relieve pain, but a cloth may also be used.

## CLASSICS

- An herbal classic dating from 1590 said, "Tofu can eliminate toxic heat from the body and promote blood circulation."
- A food classic published in 1861 listed seven functions of tofu: "To eliminate toxic heat, lubricate dryness, produce fluids, detoxify, tone the body, strengthen the intestines and eliminate water."
- A book written in 1641 said, "Whenever you go to a new place and cannot get used to the foods the local people eat, you should eat tofu, which will give you time to adjust yourself to the new foods."
- A celebrated Chinese poet named Dong-Po Su (1037-1101) wrote, "Tofu may be compared to milk, its skin to butter." The skin refers to the boiled soybean top layer, because when bean drink is boiled, a layer is formed on the top like skin. Modern Chinese physicians agree that the Chinese poet had a good point, because tofu is comparable to milk and its skin to butter, as shown in the following chart.

## NUTRITION

The chart compares the nutritional values of 100g of tofu and its skin with those of milk and butter:

|  | TOFU | MILK | SKIN | BUTTER |
|---|---|---|---|---|
| *Protein (g)* | 10.7 | 2.9 | 47.7 | 1.1 |
| *Fat (g)* | 2.1 | 1.8 | 28.0 | 90.2 |
| *Carbohydrates (g)* | 2.0 | 2.7 | 13.5 | 0.3 |
| *Calories* | 70 | 39 | 504 | 817 |
| *Ash (g)* | 0.9 | 0.6 | 2.1 | 0.2 |
| *Calcium (mg)* | 200 | 102 | 319 | 38 |
| *Phosphorus (mg)* | 89 | 17 | 43.6 | — |
| *Iron (mg)* | 3.1 | trace | 9.6 | — |

In addition, tofu is rich in calcium and magnesium because it is made of soybeans with gypsum (calcium sulfate) or bittern (magnesium chloride). Soybeans are also very rich in both calcium and magnesium.

Tofu contains a high concentration of purines (over 150mg per 100g), which may not be good for patients with gout, gouty arthritis and hyperurincernia (high levels of uric acid in the blood).

Tofu was invented in China over twenty centuries ago, but it was not until less than a decade ago that people in North America began to realize how good it is. There can be no doubt that there are a vast number of other Chinese foods still to be discovered by Western people in pursuit of longevity. The following chart lists some of these foods and the symptoms that can be treated with them.

*Notes*

To make tofu, soak soybeans in water for one day until they swell. Crush them with water; then drain it and discard the roughage. Boil the liquids to become bean drink. Add gypsum or bittern to coagulate it into tofu flowers, which are then shaped into cubes of tofu.

Tofu is a chief ingredient in many dishes. Being vegetarians, Chinese Buddhists have invented many refined methods of cooking tofu to make it look like meat and it has been called "vegetable meat" ever since.

When a group of Chinese students went to study in France at the start of the twentieth century, they brought a few expert tofu makers with them to manufacture tofu in France, which became the first European country to be introduced to it. The Chinese have a saying that tofu is everyone's favorite food, whether young or old, rich or poor, good or bad.

| FOODS | SYMPTOMS |
|---|---|
| *Coconut meat* | Fasciolopsiasis, used as a taeniafuge (to expel tapeworms) |
| *Crane meat* | Diabetes, fatigue |
| *Dates* | Weakness, coughing, indigestion |
| *Fermented glutinous rice* | External application for mastitis, helps eruptions in measles and chicken pox |
| *Goose meat* | Thirst, upset stomach, low energy |
| *Herring* | Fatigue, lung and spleen disease |
| *Jackfruits* | Jaundice, pneumonia, intoxication, indigestion, hypoglycemia |
| *Lotus rhizome powder* | Indigestion, diarrhea, intestinal roundworms |
| *Mackerel* | Beriberi, rheumatism, blurred vision, swelling, urination difficulty, diarrhea, dysentery |
| *Mandarin fish* | Fatigue, underweight body, discharge of blood from the anus |
| *Octopus* | Underweight body, carbuncle, healing of wounds |
| *Pigeon eggs* | Prevention of measles |
| *Polished rice* | Diarrhea, underweight body, blurred vision, thirst, urination difficulty, gastritis, hiccups, vomiting |
| *Rabbit* | Diabetes, underweight body, vomiting, discharge of blood from the anus, incontinence, pulmonary tuberculosis |
| *Rock sugar* | Night sweats in children, coughing, sputum, diarrhea |
| *Shark's fin* | Urination difficulty, sputum, poor appetite |
| *Sturgeon* | Stomach weakness, urination difficulty, blood in the urine |

Blood tonics treat symptoms that may result from an excessive loss of blood or poor absorption of nutrients.

# Blood Tonic Foods

## Beef

*Good for those who are underweight and for diabetes, edema.*

### DESCRIPTION

- Neutral; sweet; used as a spleen, stomach, energy and blood tonic; affects the spleen and stomach.

### PREPARATION

- Eat regularly concentrated beef soup to relieve chronic diarrhea and prolapse of anus caused by chronic diarrhea.
- Mix together 1,000g beef, 10g ground black pepper, 5g dried orange peel powder; add 1 cup fresh ginger juice and an adequate amount of salt; marinate for 2 hours; cook the beef. Eat at meals to improve the conditions of stomach and stimulate the appetite. To make ginger juice, grate fresh ginger and boil it in water.

## Black Soybean Skin

*Nourishes the blood, relieves gas; good for night sweats, headache, dizziness.*

## Blood Clams

*Tone the blood, warm the internal region and strengthen the stomach; shells can balance the stomach, control acid production, remove phlegm, soften hard spots, disperse coagulation and eliminate accumulation.*

### PREPARATION

- To cure peptic ulcers, bake blood clam shells thoroughly and grind into powder. Mix it with licorice powder in equal amount. Take 2g of powder three times daily, or take it 20 minutes before pain occurs.

## Broomcorn

*Tones the internal region, increases body energy; good for diarrhea, thirst, vomiting, coughing, stomachache.*

## Chicken Eggs

*Good for dry cough, hoarseness, pink eyes, sore throat, quickening, diarrhea, burns.*

### DESCRIPTION

- Neutral; sweet; used as a blood tonic; lubricates dryness.

### PREPARATION

- Egg may be eaten fresh or mixed with hot water; or use a mixture of egg white and yolk for external applications.
- Break an egg into a cup and mix with a few teaspoonfuls rice wine. Drink it to relieve heart pain in pregnant women.
- Boil 20 chicken eggs in their shells until fully cooked. Crush the eggs, including the shell; boil the eggs again in water with 500g black soybeans for 2 or 3 hours until the eggs and beans are thoroughly mixed and become black; remove and discard the black soybeans. Store the eggs in a container until needed. Peel the eggs and eat 2 to 3 warm eggs each time, once a day, for as long as necessary, to sharpen vision and correct blurred vision.

*Notes*

Beef kidney is used as kidney tonic to improve sexual capacity and to cure temporary and permanent impotence in men; cut a kidney into small pieces to boil with one bowl of rice and when the kidney is cooked, add five green onion white heads.

Beef liver is neutral and sweet, is used as a liver tonic and to sharpen the vision and relieve glaucoma and night blindness.

*Notes*

Salted foods travel to the blood and can soften hard spots, which is why blood clam shells can dissolve blood coagulation and eliminate accumulation of phlegm.

### CLINICAL REPORT

- For treatment of neurodermatitis and psoriasis, sterilize 2 chicken eggs with alcohol and place in a jar slightly larger than the eggs; add vinegar to cover the eggs and seal; set aside for 7 days. Break the eggs and pour the egg white and egg yolk into another sterilized jar and seal the jar. Use a cotton ball to rub the egg on the affected region for 1 to 2 minutes each time, several times a day; the treatment should continue without interruption. In general, scales begin to fall off after a number of treatments; severe itching either improves or stops completely. If treatment continues, then the focus of the skin ailment will gradually be reduced in size; but if treatment is interrupted at this point, symptoms will recur. The longer the history of symptoms, the longer the treatment needed. Among the 12 cases of neurodermatitis treated, 9 cases recovered completely and 3 cases improved; among the 5 cases of psoriasis treated, 2 cases recovered completely and 3 cases improved.

## Cuttlefish

*Cuttlefish are good for anemia, vaginal bleeding and discharge and suppression of menstruation; cuttlebone for stomachache, excessive gastric acid, vomiting of blood, discharge of blood from anus, vaginal bleeding and discharge, abdominal pain, suppression of menstrual flow, diarrhea, ulcers and blisters.*

### DESCRIPTION

- Cuttlefish—neutral, salty, used as a blood tonic, sharpens vision, acts on liver and kidneys; cuttlebone—slightly warm, salty, used to facilitate water passage, check acid and skin blisters, arrests bleeding, acts on liver and kidneys.

### CLINICAL REPORT

- For treatment of gastric and duodenal ulcers with cuttlebone, use cuttlebone as the key ingredient; cuttlebone is effective for bleeding and perforation due to ulcers, for checking acid and to arrest bleeding and minimize pain due to ulcers.
- For treatment of asthma, mix 500g cuttlebone powder and 1,000g sugar for oral administration. Take 20g each time for adults or a reduced quantity for children, 3 times a day; in general, the treatment takes effect in 2 weeks. Among the 8 cases treated with a history of 3 to 27 years (all treated many times by Western medicine without results), 7 cases were brought under control and the asthma attacks have not recurred despite many changes in weather and 1 case showed improvements.

## Donggui (Lovage)

*Tones the blood, regulates menstruation and menses, relieves abdominal and intestinal pain, lubricates dryness, suppresses vaginal bleeding, headache and constipation.*

## Grape

*Good for blood and energy deficiency, cough, palpitations, night sweat, rheumatism, difficulty when urinating, edema.*

### DESCRIPTION

- Neutral; sweet and sour; strengthens the tendons and bones; promotes

*Notes*

Eating excessive quantities of grapes may decrease appetite.

urination; also used as blood tonic and energy tonic; affects the lungs, spleen and kidneys.

## PREPARATION

- Crush 500g fresh grapes; add 500g rice wine and mix thoroughly. Strain to make grape wine. Eat 30g of the soaked raisins or drink 30g grape wine in the morning and evening, to tone up energy after illness.
- Eat a large bunch of fresh grapes in the morning and evening, to relieve dry throat and thirst.
- Boil 30g raisins with 15g fresh ginger peel. Drink twice a day to cure nutritional edema.
- Squeeze juice from 250g fresh grapes and mix with an equal amount of warm water. Drink it all each time, once a day, to relieve pain on urination, difficult urination and discharge of short and reddish stream of urine.
- Crush 120g fresh grapes and 250g fresh lotus roots. Squeeze out the juice, drink it all each time, 3 times a day, to cure or prevent discharge of urine containing blood.
- Boil 30g raisins in water and drink it like soup. In addition, boil grapevine leaves and parsley and use the liquid to wash the body to promote the outbreak of rash in measles.
- Boil 30g raisins with 15g red dates in water; drink like soup to relieve anxiety during quickening.

## *Ham*

*Strengthens the spleen, improves appetite, produces fluids, improves the condition of blood; good for deficiency, fatigue, nervousness, chronic diarrhea.*

## *Human Milk*

*Tones the blood, lubricates dryness; good for deficiency, paralysis, diabetes, constipation and blurred vision.*

## *Litchi (Lychee)*

*Good for hiccupping, stomachache, diarrhea, asthma, hernial pain.*

## DESCRIPTION

- Warm; sweet and sour; produces fluids; stimulates energy; relieves pain; affects the spleen and liver.

## PREPARATION

- Eat 60 to 150g fresh litchis to improve physical conditions after prolonged illness.
- Fresh litchis may be left in the sun to dry. Dried litchis are widely used in the Chinese diet.
- Boil 30 to 60g dried litchis and 5 dried red dates with adequate water. Drink the soup twice a day to cure chronic diarrhea.
- Steam 120g dried litchis and eat once a day to cure asthma.
- Collect litchi seeds and leave them in the sun to dry to use in remedies.
- Crush 30g dried litchi seeds; boil in water with 6g fresh ginger or dried orange peels. Drink it once a day to relieve stomachache and abdominal pain.
- Crush 60g dried litchi seeds and 15g caraway seeds; boil them in an adequate amount of water. Drink the soup once a day to relieve hernial pain, elephantiasis, hydrocele of tunica vaginalis and swelling and pain in the testes.

*Notes*

Ham can produce fluids, improve the condition of blood vessels, solidify bones and marrow, increase sex drive, stop diarrhea caused by weakness, relieve nervousness, improve appetite and calm the spirits.

When one has a common cold, one should refrain from eating ham.

## *Litchi Nuts*

*Produce body fluids, improve the spirits and intelligence, beautify the complexion; used to treat scrofula, tumors, swelling and measles in children.*

### PREPARATION

- Although litchi nuts are beneficial in many ways, one should not eat too many, because they may cause hypoglycemia with such symptoms as acute fatigue, malaise and coma.
- To facilitate eruptions of measles, boil 9g of litchi nuts in water and drink. To correct enuresis in children, let them eat 10 dried litchi nuts every day. To reduce anemia in women, boil seven litchi nuts and red dates in water for one-day consumption.
- To stop diarrhea due to spleen deficiency, boil 15g of dried litchi nuts with three to five red dates in water for regular consumption. To warm the stomach and increase stomach energy, boil five litchi nuts in a glass of wine over low heat; drink the wine and eat the nuts on a regular basis. For older persons who have diarrhea early in the morning, boil five dried litchi nuts with half a glass of rice for regular consumption.

## *Longan*

*Good for insomnia, forgetfulness, palpitations, nervousness.*

### DESCRIPTION

- Warm; sweet; used as a spleen tonic, heart tonic, blood tonic and energy tonic; affects the heart and spleen.

### PREPARATION

- Steam 15g longans with 30g lean pork, 2 fresh ginger slices and an adequate amount of rice wine. Eat once a day to relieve dizziness and underweight.
- Mix 500g longans with 500g sugar; steam them to make longan jelly.
- Take 1 spoonful longan jelly with warm water to relieve dizziness and edema after childbirth; or boil 15g longans with 5 red dates, 30g brown sugar and 6g fresh ginger. Drink it as soup once a day.

## *Mare's Milk*

*Tones the blood, lubricates dryness, reduces internal heat and quenches thirst; good for burning sensations coming from the bones and for diabetes.*

## *Oxtail*

*Good for edema and diminished urination.*

## *Oyster and Shell*

*Oyster is good for insomnia, stress and nervousness; oyster shell good for excessive perspiration, night sweat, premature ejaculation, vaginal bleeding and discharge, tuberculosis of lymph node, goitre.*

### DESCRIPTION

- Oyster—neutral, sweet and salty, used as a blood tonic; oyster shell—cool, salty, obstructive, checks excessive perspiration and premature ejaculation, softens hardness, acts on the liver and kidneys.

*Notes*

Litchi nuts are sweet and warm. They can lubricate the body and are ideal for improving the conditions of the spleen and liver and for increasing semen and blood. When yang energy in the body is in decline with cold blood, litchi nuts are recommended. In case of hot blood, longans are preferred. Dried litchi nuts are not as sweet as fresh ones, but the former are relatively mild and do not produce excessive heat in the body.

## PREPARATION

- Eat 15 to 25 oysters at meals to cure tuberculosis of the lymph node and goitre; or use oyster sauce as seasoning if fresh oyster is not readily available.
- Crush oyster shell into powder and wrap 15g of the powder in a cloth. Boil in 3 cups water over low heat until the water is reduced to 1 cup. Drink as tea before a meal, once a day, to relieve excessive gastric acid; or grind the shell into very fine powder and take 3g of the powder, each time with warm water, 3 times a day.

## CLINICAL REPORT

- For treatment of night sweat in pulmonary tuberculosis, boil 20g oyster shell in 500 ml water until the water is reduced to 200ml. (Sugar may be added, if desired.) Divide into 2 dosages and drink in the morning and in the evening for a few consecutive days. After the night sweat stops, the treatment continues for another 2 to 3 days to stabilize the effects. Herbal therapy may be used in combination, if no satisfactory results are obtained. In the 10 cases treated, after taking 2 to 3 dosages night sweat disappeared in 7 cases, 3 showed no obvious results, but 2 recovered after being treated in combination with other herbs. No side effects were observed.

## Palm Seed

*Restricts intestinal movements and checks diarrhea.*

## Pork Liver

*Strengthens the liver, nourishes the blood and sharpens vision.*

## PREPARATION

- To cure edema with congested chest and poor appetite, cut up a pork liver and boil in water; add green onion, ginger and prickly ash to season it before eating.
- To cure edema with urination difficulty, boil three pork liver tips, 200g of mung beans and 150g of rice in water and eat at meals.
- To cure night blindness and pellagra, boil pork liver and eat on a regular basis.
- To cure anemia, boil 70g of pork liver with 300g of spinach and eat at meals.

## Pork Trotter

*Promotes milk secretion in breastfeeding mothers, smooths muscles, counteracts cold and reduces heat in the body, heals carbuncles and detoxicates.*

## PREPARATION

- Pork trotter and pork skin have similar effects; both are full of protein and fat and also contain animal colloid.
- To cure hemophilia, nosebleed, bleeding from gums and purpura, boil a piece of pork skin or one pork trotter with 10 to 15 red dates until the dates are extremely soft. Eat at meals once a day.
- To cure anemia due to loss of blood, bleeding in hemorrhoids, discharge of blood from the anus and vaginal bleeding in women, boil 60 to 90g of pork skin in water with a little rice wine over low heat until it becomes very soft. Add a teaspoon of brown sugar and drink.

To promote milk secretion, boil a pork trotter in water until the water is reduced by half. Drink it at meals. Or, boil one to two trotters and season with salt, or add 100g of peanuts and boil together.

## Sea Cucumber

*Tones the kidneys, increases sexual potency in men, strengthens body and yin energy, lubricates the intestine to promote bowel movements, stops bleeding, heals inflammation.*

### PREPARATION

Sea cucumber is called "sea ginseng," because its effects are similar to those of Chinese ginseng. After a sea cucumber is caught, its organs are removed and internal region washed; then boil it in salt water for about an hour. Remove from the water to cool, dry in the sun or bake to about 80 to 90 percent dry and then boil again for a short while and dry in the sun.

## Sheep or Goat's Liver

*Tones the liver, sharpens vision and improves the conditions of blood.*

### PREPARATION

- To cure hot sensations in the eyes with pain and blurred vision, cook a sheep or goat's liver with other foods and eat. To cure nearsightedness, cut up a sheep or goat's liver and fry with green onion seeds until dry. Boil and strain it to cook with rice to eat at meals.
- To cure anemia, boil sheep or goat's liver until cooked; then add spinach and boil again. Mix a chicken egg into the soup and eat.

## Spinach

*Good for anemia, bleeding, thirst, constipation and can also stimulate the pancreas to assist in digestion. As spinach is a cool food, it can relieve hypertension, headaches, dizziness, pink eye, diabetes and constipation.*

### PREPARATION

- To treat hypertension, headaches, dizziness and constipation, soak spinach in hot water for 3 minutes. Season it with sesame oil and eat at meals.
- To cure night blindness, crush 450g of spinach to make juice; divide it into two dosages for one-day consumption.

*Notes*

Sea cucumber may also be used to treat impotence. Sea cucumber can increase yin and yang energy, regulate menstruation, nourish the fetus and facilitate labor. It is wise to cook sea cucumber with ham, pork, or mutton to ease general fatigue after a prolonged illness or after childbirth.

*Notes*

Since sheep or goat's liver resembles the human liver, it may be used to treat liver diseases.

*Notes*

Spinach was originally imported into China from southern Asia in the Tang dynasty (a.d. 618-907). Spinach contains lutein, chlorophyll, folic acid and oxalic acid. Many proteins contained in spinach are essential amino acids that can only be obtained from foods.

Spinach is beneficial to the internal organs, promotes intestinal movements, reduces heat in the stomach, relieves alcoholism and cools the intestines. Spinach promotes blood circulation, expands the chest, regulates internal energy, quenches thirst and lubricates dryness.

*Y*in tonic foods, also called

kidney yin tonics, restore

yin deficiencies, such as a shortage of

body fluids in both men and women.

*Yin Tonic Foods*

## Abalone

*Good for relieving hot sensations, coughs, vaginal bleeding, vaginal discharge, urinary strains, glaucosis, cataract.*

### DESCRIPTION

Neutral; sweet and salty; detoxicates; sharpens vision.

*Notes*

Abalone is difficult to digest.

## Apple

*Good for indigestion, low blood sugar, morning sickness, chronic enteritis.*

### DESCRIPTION

- Cool; sweet and sour; produces fluids; lubricates the lungs; promotes digestion; relieves intoxication.

### PREPARATION

- Peel and core a few half-ripe apples and press or crush them to squeeze out the juice. Drink half a cup of juice each time, 3 times a day for 3 consecutive days, to remedy indigestion.
- Eat 2 peeled apples each time, twice a day for 3 consecutive days as a treatment program to treat low blood sugar.
- Prepare 6 fresh apples: Peel, core and remove seeds; crush apples and steam them with 500g honey until as soft as jelly. Take 2 teaspoonfuls each time 3 times a day, to treat cough due to hot lungs and dry sensations in the mouth and tongue. This remedy is also good for neutralizing the effects of smoking.
- Prepare 30 to 60g fresh apple peel. Fry 30g rice until yellowish; mix the rice with apple peel to make tea to alleviate morning sickness.
- Cut a few unripe apples into 4 slices; dry the slices in the sun; grind into powder. Take 15g apple powder with 1 cup warm water, twice a day, to cure chronic enteritis, abdominal pain and diarrhea.

## Bean Curd (Tofu)

*Good for pink eye, diabetes, periodic diarrhea, sulfur poisoning.*

### DESCRIPTION

- Cool; sweet; used as an energy tonic; produces fluids; lubricates dryness; detoxicates; affects the spleen, stomach and large intestine.

### PREPARATION

- Prepare 1 bowl bean curd, 70g maltose and half a cup of fresh radish juice; combine the 3 ingredients in a pan, add half a cup of water and bring to a boil once. Divide the soup into 2 dosages and drink twice a day to treat asthma with mucous discharge, including acute bronchial asthma.
- Crush a number of bean curds and apply the mash to the legs to heal erysipelas on the legs; change the dressing as soon as the mash dries.

## Bitter Gourd (Wild Cucumber)

*Good for sunstroke, dysentery, pink eyes and pain in eyes.*

## DESCRIPTION

- Cold; bitter; detoxicates; sharpens the vision; affects the heart, spleen and stomach.

## PREPARATION

- Fry bitter gourd seeds and grind into powder. Take 10g of the powder dissolved in wine each time, twice a day, to cure impotence.
- Regular consumption of bitter gourd improves eyesight.

## Brown Sugar

*Good for abdominal pain, dysentery, lochiastasis.*

## DESCRIPTION

- Warm; sweet; used as an energy tonic; promotes blood circulation; counteracts or eliminates blood coagulations; affects the liver, spleen and stomach.

## PREPARATION

- Mix brown sugar with rice wine. Drink it to relieve lochiostasis and faintness after childbirth due to excessive loss of blood.
- Boil brown sugar with 2 plums and drink as tea to relieve dysentery.

## Cantaloupe (Muskmelon)

*Quenches thirst, reduces internal heat, promotes urination; an ideal food for people with a hot constitution that may cause constipation and urination difficulty; but those with a cold constitution may develop edema and diarrhea.*

## Chicken Eggs

*Good for dry cough, hoarseness, pink eyes, sore throat, quickening, diarrhea, burns.*

## DESCRIPTION

- Neutral; sweet; used as a blood tonic; lubricates dryness.

## PREPARATION

- Egg may be eaten fresh or mixed with hot water; or use a mixture of egg white and yolk for external applications.
- Break an egg into a cup and mix with a few teaspoonfuls rice wine. Drink it to relieve heart pain in pregnant women.
- Boil 20 chicken eggs in their shells until fully cooked. Crush the eggs, including the shell; boil the eggs again in water with 500g black soybeans for 2 or 3 hours until the eggs and beans are thoroughly mixed and become black; remove and discard the black soybeans. Store the eggs in a container until needed. Peel the eggs and eat 2 to 3 warm eggs each time, once a day, for as long as necessary, to sharpen vision and correct blurred vision.

## CLINICAL REPORT

- For treatment of neurodermatitis and psoriasis, sterilize 2 chicken eggs with alcohol and place in a jar slightly larger than the eggs; add vinegar to cover the eggs and seal; set aside for 7 days. Break the eggs and pour the egg white and egg yolk into another sterilized jar and seal the jar.

*Notes*

Bitter gourd is regarded as the king of bitter foods. It is bad for people with a weak stomach because it could cause vomiting. But it is good for those with a hot physical constitution as it can cool down the internal region and relieve hot constipation.

According to Chinese medical theory, bitter foods can improve the conditions of the liver (which is why bitter gourd is good for liver disease).

*Notes*

Both white (granulated) and brown sugar are obtained from the juice of the sugar cane.

*Notes*

There are many varieties of cantaloupe in China; the Chinese call it "aromatic melon" or "melon of fruits." Cantaloupes cultivated in the Yellow River valley where the climate is relatively dry are among the best. A place in China named Tun-Huang is often referred to as "cantaloupe city" because it produces the best quality in the country.

Cantaloupe contains peptones that are not coagulated by boiling and make proteins soluble as well; it also contains large amounts of carbohydrates, ranging from 4.2 to 18 percent.

It is good to eat cantaloupes in small quantity, since excessive amounts can cause low energy, forgetfulness and weak limbs.

Use a cotton ball to rub the egg on the affected region for 1 to 2 minutes each time, several times a day; the treatment should continue without interruption. In general, scales begin to fall off after a number of treatments; severe itching either improves or stops completely. If treatment continues, then the focus of the skin ailment will gradually be reduced in size; but if treatment is interrupted at this point, symptoms will recur. The longer the history of symptoms, the longer the treatment needed. Among the 12 cases of neurodermatitis treated, 9 cases recovered completely and 3 cases improved; among the 5 cases of psoriasis treated, 2 cases recovered completely and 3 cases improved.

## Coconut Milk
*Good for diabetes, edema and vomiting of blood.*

### DESCRIPTION

- Warm; slightly sweet and aromatic; the liquid produces fluids, promotes urination and destroys intestinal worms

### PREPARATION

- Drink coconut liquid to relieve thirst, sunstroke, fever, diabetes, edema.
- Drink a glass of coconut liquid with 30g sugar and a little salt, 3 times a day for 3 consecutive days and then once a day afterwards, to relieve vomiting and weakness after severe bleeding and dehydration after severe diarrhea.
- Consume coconut (meat and liquid) once a day, first thing in the morning on an empty stomach for 3 consecutive days, to relieve tapeworm and fasciolopsiasis.

## Crabs
*Good for fractures and dislocations, tinea, skin eruption caused by lacquer.*

### DESCRIPTION

- Cold; salty; relieves blood coagulations; cools hot sensations; facilitates recovery of dislocations; affects the liver and stomach.

### PREPARATION

- Crush a fresh crab to mix with hot broth. Drink it frequently and apply remaining crab to the affected region to restore dislocations; or mix ash of burned crab with liquor for oral consumption to restore dislocations and heal fractures.
- Crush a fresh crab and apply it to the affected region to relieve lacquer-induced skin eruptions and tinea.
- Bake a crab until charred and grind into powder and mix with rice wine. Take 10g of the powder and wine each time, twice a day, to relieve jaundice.
- Roast a few crabs until charred and grind into powder. Take 10g powder with rice wine each time, twice a day, to relieve hypogastric pain after childbirth.
- Bake 1 male crab and 1 female crab and grind into powder; take the powder with wine all at once to facilitate the healing of breast cancer.
- Wrap a fresh crab in a clean cloth, crush it to squeeze out the juice; apply the juice to the affected region for relief of lacquer-induced skin eruptions, or drink the juice all at once to stop or suppress coughing.

## Cuttlefish

*Cuttlefish are good for anemia, vaginal bleeding and discharge and suppression of menstruation; cuttlebone for stomachache, excessive gastric acid, vomiting of blood, discharge of blood from anus, vaginal bleeding and discharge, abdominal pain, suppression of menstrual flow, diarrhea, ulcers and blisters.*

### DESCRIPTION

- Cuttlefish—neutral, salty, used as a blood tonic, sharpens vision, acts on liver and kidneys; cuttlebone—slightly warm, salty, used to facilitate water passage, check acid and skin blisters, arrests bleeding, acts on liver and kidneys.

### CLINICAL REPORT

- For treatment of gastric and duodenal ulcers with cuttlebone, use cuttlebone as the key ingredient; cuttlebone is effective for bleeding and perforation due to ulcers, for checking acid and to arrest bleeding and minimize pain due to ulcers.
- For treatment of asthma, mix 500g cuttlebone powder and 1,000g sugar for oral administration. Take 20g each time for adults or a reduced quantity for children, 3 times a day; in general, the treatment takes effect in 2 weeks. Among the 8 cases treated with a history of 3 to 27 years (all treated many times by Western medicine without results), 7 cases were brought under control and the asthma attacks have not recurred despite many changes in weather and 1 case showed improvements.

## Date

*Good for weak stomachs, palpitations, nervousness, hysteria in women, allergic purpura.*

### DESCRIPTION

- Warm; sweet; used as a spleen tonic, energy tonic and blood tonic; produces fluids; detoxicates; affects the spleen and stomach.

### PREPARATION

- Boil 30g red dates with 1 whole chicken egg, 4 fresh ginger slices and 30g brown sugar in water. Eat at meals to relieve weakness after childbirth.
- Prolonged consumption of 30g red dates in the evening every day improves physical conditions, such as skinniness and weakness.
- Boil 30g red dates with 5 green onion white heads. Eat it at bedtime to relieve insomnia.
- Eat 30 to 60g red dates each time, 3 times a day for 15 consecutive days, to cure allergic purpura.
- Boil 30g red dates and 30g yam with 2 fresh ginger slices until soft. Eat it once a day for 10 consecutive days to treat cold stomachache, abdominal pain and diarrhea due to digestive weakness.
- Boil 30g dried red dates with 15g yam, 15g whole wheat and 15g processed licorice. Drink the juice in the morning and evening to treat hysteria in women and jumpiness in women during menopause.
- Boil 15g black dates with 9g longans and 30g brown sugar. Eat the stewed fruit at meals on a long-term basis to treat anemia.
- To prepare date jelly, boil 1,500g fresh dates, seeded, or 500g red dates, seeded, until they look like jelly; add 500g sugar and stir until dissolved.
- Take a teaspoonful of date jelly with warm water on a long-term basis to relieve hepatitis, pulmonary tuberculosis and weakness after illness.

*Notes*

Fresh dates may be left in the sun to dry until red to make dried red dates.

Fresh red dates may be boiled and left in the sun to dry, then steamed and baked a few times until the surface becomes quite black; these are called black dates.

### Duck
*Good for relieving hot sensations, cough, edema.*

## DESCRIPTION

- Neutral; sweet and salty; facilitates water passage and heals swelling; affects the lungs and kidneys.

## PREPARATION

- Cook a duck with suitable quantities of ham. Eat at meals to relieve diarrhea, particularly chronic diarrhea after childbirth.
- Place 4 to 5 garlic cloves inside a prepared duck; simmer duck in water until very soft. Eat the duck and garlic and drink the soup without salt to relieve chronic nephritis and edema.

### Duck Eggs
*Increase yin energy in the body, clear heat in the lungs, tone the heart, stop hot cough, cure sore throat and toothache.*

## PREPARATION

- To cure diarrhea in women before and after childbirth, mix a duck egg in a container with fresh ginger juice. Boil the mixture until it is reduced by 20 percent. Drink it on an empty stomach.

### Figs
*Good for enteritis, dysentery, constipation, hemorrhoids, sore throat, diarrhea.*

## DESCRIPTION

- Neutral; sweet; detoxicates; used as stomachic tonic; affects the spleen and large intestine.

## PREPARATION

- Eat 1 to 2 fresh figs each time, in the morning and evening, to wake up appetite and correct indigestion.
- Eat 1 to 2 fresh figs at bedtime to relieve constipation, particularly in the elderly.
- Steam until very soft 1 to 2 fresh figs and 2 honey dates (processed in honey). Eat 1 to 2 figs each day to relieve dry cough and sore throat.
- Boil 1kg dry figs in water at low heat until they are soft as jelly. Add 750g sugar and heat until sugar dissolves. Then mix all the ingredients; take 1 teaspoonful fig jelly each time, in the morning and evening, to correct weakness after illness. Fig jelly is also used as adjuvant therapy for pulmonary tuberculosis and hepatitis.
- Boil until very soft 1 to 3 fresh figs or 30g dry figs with 60g lean pork and 2 red dates; eat once a day to increase milk secretion in women after childbirth.
- Boil 60g fresh figs with 60g pork or with 1 chicken egg and 15g rice wine. Eat once a day to relieve pain in muscles and bones and numbness from rheumatism.
- Fry 30g dry figs until aromatic; separately, fry 9g dry ginger until it looks like charcoal. Boil together the figs and ginger. Eat 3 times a day, to cure chronic diarrhea.
- Eat 2 unripe fresh figs in the morning and evening to alleviate pain and bleeding in hemorrhoids.

*Notes*

Duck is good for hot symptoms, such as the presence of internal heat. But it may not be easily digested and is considered bad for hemorrhoids.

Duck egg is cool and sweet, is used to reduce heat in the lungs and also to relieve cough, sore throat, toothache and diarrhea.

Lime, salt and other ingredients may be used to preserve duck egg to make preserved duck egg, which has a cold energy and pungent and sweet and salty flavors; eat 2 to 3 preserved duck eggs every day (with sugar and vinegar, if desired) to relieve hypertension; or eat 2 preserved duck eggs to check diarrhea and to relieve a hangover. Preserved duck eggs are available in most Chinese food shops.

*Notes*

Other diseases that can be treated with duck eggs are neurosis, bronchial asthma, hypertension, malnutrition in children and chronic gastritis.

*Notes*

Fig leaf is neutral in energy and tastes sweet and slightly pungent; it can heal hemorrhoids and heart pain and swelling.

## Freshwater Clams

*Reduce internal heat, increase yin energy in the body, sharpen vision and detoxicate; good for diabetes, vaginal bleeding and discharge, hemorrhoids, pink eye and eczema.*

## Honey

*Good for dry coughs, constipation, stomachaches, sinusitis, mouth cankers, burns, neurasthenia, hypertension, pulmonary tuberculosis, heart disease, liver disease.*

### DESCRIPTION

- Neutral; sweet; detoxicates; lubricates dryness; relieves pain; affects the lungs, spleen and large intestine.

### PREPARATION

- Steam about half a cup honey. Eat it all at once on an empty stomach, 3 times a day, for 2 to 3 weeks on end, to relieve gastric and duodenal ulcers.
- Mix half a cup honey with warm water and drink once a day to treat hypertension, constipation, stomachache, neurasthenia, heart disease and coronary sclerosis.
- Drink a cup honey water at bedtime to cure insomnia due to neurasthenia. Externally apply honey to the affected region to relieve burns.
- Mix 3 large spoonfuls honey in boiling water. Drink it in the morning and in the evening to relieve insomnia, headache and anemia; or eat honey at meals with other foods.
- Using a sterilized cotton ball, externally apply honey to the anus to heal cracked skin in hemorrhoids; or externally apply to the ear to relieve swelling of the ear.
- Mix 2 teaspoonfuls honey with warm water. Drink it first thing in the morning on an empty stomach to relieve chronic constipation.
- Mix 1 teaspoonful honey with warm water and drink it 3 hours after meals, 3 times a day, for 5 consecutive days, to relieve hoarseness caused by excessive fatigue but unrelated to common cold, with sufficient rest to produce best results.

### CLINICAL REPORT

- For treatment of gastric and duodenal ulcers; among 20 cases treated, the niche disappeared in 15 cases, showed progress in 3 cases (32 days on the average), pain completely disappeared in 18 and pain decreased in 2; pain was gone as quickly as 6 days and within 22 days on the average. The method of treatment: each day, eat a third cup fresh honey before meals, 3 times a day; after the tenth day, increase the quantity of honey to half a cup each day.
- Clinical reports on treatment of other diseases showed good results: For treatment of acute bacillary dysentery, take 150g honey each day for adults (divide into 4 reduced dosages for children); for treatment of chronic and or temporary constipation in the elderly and in pregnant women, take honey first thing in the morning; for treatment of hypochromic anemia, take 80 to 100g honey each day, divided into 3 dosages; the results show an obvious increase in blood cells and hemoglobin.

## Milk

*Cow's milk is good for an upset stomach, difficulty swallowing, diabetes, constipation; human milk is good for fatigue, skinniness, diabetes, difficulty swallowing, dry stools.*

## DESCRIPTION

- Cow's milk—neutral; sweet; pushes downwards; is used as a lung and stomach tonic; and is used to produce fluids and lubricate the intestines; affects the heart, lungs and stomach. Human milk — neutral; sweet and salty; is used as a blood tonic and to lubricate dryness; affects the heart, lungs and stomach.

## PREPARATION

- Boil 1 glass cow's milk in 4 glasses water over low heat until water is reduced to 1 cup. Drink it slowly on an empty stomach to improve physical conditions after a prolonged illness.
- Mix 1 glass cow's milk with half a glass fresh chive juice and 3 teaspoonfuls fresh ginger juice; heat in a small pan. Drink to relieve an upset stomach.
- Mix equal amounts of cow's and sheep's milks. Drink the milk as a substitute for tea or juice to improve the physical condition of diabetes patients and frequent urination.

## CLINICAL REPORT

- For treatment of electric ophthalmia by human milk, squeeze fresh human milk directly into a sterilized bottle or sterile eyedrop bottle; apply 2 to 3 drops on the bulbar conjunctiva of the lateral angle of each eye at 5- to 15-minute intervals; close the eyes and rest for a while. In general, discomfort or pain will disappear or decrease within 8 to 16 hours with neither side effects nor discomfort.

## White Fungus

*Good for coughs, discharge of mucus with blood, chronic constipation.*

## DESCRIPTION

- Neutral; sweet with a light taste; glossy; produces fluids and lubricates the lungs.

## Green Turtle

*Increases yin energy, cools the blood and tones deficiency.*

## PREPARATION

- To cure dizziness with spots before the eyes, lumbago and seminal emission, boil green turtle and eat at meals on a regular basis.
- To cure chronic nephritis, cook 450g of green turtle with 60g of garlic; then add some white sugar and wine.
- To suppress menses, cook green turtle with pork and eat at meals.

## Kidney Beans

*Good for edema, beriberi.*

## DESCRIPTION

- Neutral; sweet and light taste; promotes urination; heals swelling.

## PREPARATION

- Boil 150g kidney beans with 15g garlic and 40g sugar in water. Drink as soup at meals to relieve edema.

*Notes*

Cow's milk is not recommended for people with diarrhea or mucous discharge.

*Notes*

White fungus is also called snow fungus. It is considered an important yin tonic, good for insomnia, lung disease, liver disease and poor appetite. As white fungus is glossy, it is not recommended for those suffering from diarrhea or seminal emission.

It is customary to cook white fungus with lean pork over low heat for as long as 3 hours; or boil white fungus in water with rock sugar. Some people prefer to boil white fungus in chicken soup, which makes it more delicious.

White fungus should not be used to relieve cough due to common cold.

*Notes*

Green turtle can increase yin energy in the liver and kidneys and reduce internal heat. It's also good for prolapse of the anus, vaginal discharge, scrofula and abdominal swelling.

Green turtle is an excellent remedy for fatigue and sexual dysfunction in men.

## Kumquats

*Treat acute hepatitis, cholecystitis, gallstones, stomachache, hernia, chronic tracheitis, prolapse of the anus and uterus.*

### PREPARATION

- To cure cough and asthma, wash two to three kumquats and cut them open with a knife. Squeeze out all seeds and place the kumquats in water. Add some rock sugar and boil over low heat. Eat the contents and drink the soup in three dosages in one day.

## Lard

*Tones deficiency, lubricates dryness and detoxifies; good for dry skin, dry cough and constipation.*

## Lemons

*Good for coughs with mucous discharge, indigestion, diabetes, pharyngolaryngitis.*

### DESCRIPTION

- Extremely sour; produces fluids; secures fetus in quickening, considered good for pregnant women.

### PREPARATION

- To make preserved lemons, place 500g fresh lemons in a large earthenware container; add 250g salt and leave the container in the sun to dry until the peels become wrinkled and soft with the juices flowing out. The older preserved lemons are the best. Eat preserved lemons with meals to relieve indigestion.
- Peel a lemon and squeeze it to make lemonade for relief of summer heat, diabetes and pharyngolaryngitis.
- Steam a fresh lemon with an adequate amount of rock sugar. Eat it in the morning and evening to relieve cough with plenty of mucous discharge and whooping cough in children.

## Litchi (Lychee)

*Good for hiccupping, stomachache, diarrhea, asthma, hernial pain.*

### DESCRIPTION

- Warm; sweet and sour; produces fluids; stimulates energy; relieves pain; affects the spleen and liver.

### PREPARATION

- Eat 60 to 150g fresh litchis to improve physical conditions after prolonged illness.
- Fresh litchis may be left in the sun to dry. Dried litchis are widely used in the Chinese diet.
- Boil 30 to 60g dried litchis and 5 dried red dates with adequate water. Drink the soup twice a day to cure chronic diarrhea.
- Steam 120g dried litchis and eat once a day to cure asthma.
- Collect litchi seeds and leave them in the sun to dry to use in remedies.
- Crush 30g dried litchi seeds; boil in water with 6g fresh ginger or dried orange peels. Drink it once a day to relieve stomachache and abdominal pain.
- Crush 60g dried litchi seeds and 15g caraway seeds; boil them in an

### Notes

Kumquats may be eaten with the peel, which smells more aromatic than the kumquat itself.

Kumquats can regulate energy flow in the body, relieve congestion, remove phlegm and relieve intoxication.

Kumquats can quench thirst and neutralize foul odors, particularly using the peel.

One hundred grams of kumquats contain 49 milligrams of vitamin C, 80 percent of which is found in the peel, which can promote vascular functions, also good for hypertension, arteriosclerosis and coronary heart disease.

### Notes

Lemon is not recommended for people with gastric or duodenal ulcers and excessive gastric acid.

Lemon seed is neutral and bitter and good to use to stimulate energy and relieve pain.

Crush 15g lemon seeds and grind into powder. Dissolve 3g lemon seed powder in water each time, once a day, for 5 consecutive days, to relieve blurred vision.

Grind lemon seeds into powder. Dissolve 3g lemon seed powder in a little rice wine. Drink at bedtime to relieve body pain from excessive fatigue.

adequate amount of water. Drink the soup once a day to relieve hernial pain, elephantiasis, hydrocele of tunica vaginalis and swelling and pain in the testes.

## *Loquat*

*Good for pharyngolaryngitis, cough, thirst, constipation.*

### DESCRIPTION

- Cool; sweet and sour; lubricates the lungs; quenches thirst; pushes downwards; affects the spleen, lungs and liver.

### PREPARATION

- Steam 90g fresh seeded loquats along with 15g rock sugar for half an hour. Eat the loquats and drink soup to cure acute and chronic pharyngolaryngitis.
- Eat 250g fully ripe loquats each time, in the morning and evening, to relieve dry throat and thirst and difficult urination.
- Crush 15g loquat seeds; boil in water with 3 fresh ginger slices. Drink 1 cup of the juice each time, twice a day, to relieve coughing. Crush 9 to 15g loquat seeds; boil seeds in water; strain and add 30g honey and mix thoroughly. Drink once a day to cure senile constipation, cough and asthma.

## *Lucid Asparagus*

*Increases yin energy in the body, lubricates dryness, reduces heat in the lungs, good for fever, coughing, vomiting of blood, pulmonary tuberculosis, diabetes, sore throat and constipation.*

## *Maltose*

*Good for fatigue, abdominal pain, dry cough, thirst, vomiting of blood, sore throat, constipation.*

### DESCRIPTION

- Warm; sweet; slows down the attack of acute symptoms; produces fluids; lubricates dryness; also used as an energy tonic; affects the spleen, stomach and lungs.

### PREPARATION

- Take a few teaspoonfuls of maltose with warm water several times a day to neutralize the effects of drug overdose and to relieve pain from chronic gastric and duodenal ulcers and stomachache.
- Shape maltose into a ball as large as an egg yolk and swallow it to dislodge a fishbone stuck in the throat; a few balls may be necessary and the ball of maltose gradually may be increased in size each time.
- Bake maltose until partially browned. Take 1 teaspoonful dissolved in warm water each time, twice a day, to relieve a sore throat; or, mix maltose with crushed carrot; marinate overnight; next day, mix with water and drink 1 glass each time, 3 times a day.

## *Mango*

*Good for coughs, indigestion, bleeding from gums.*

### DESCRIPTION

- Cool; sweet and sour; quenches thirst; strengthens the stomach; relieves

### Notes

Loquat is not recommended for people with weak digestions.

Dried loquat leaf is an important Chinese herb with a cool energy and bitter flavor. It is used to relieve cough and nosebleed and coughing up blood.

vomiting; promotes urination.

### PREPARATION

- Eat a fresh mango with peel each time, 3 times a day, to relieve cough with mucous discharge and asthma.
- Eat a fresh mango with peel in the morning and evening to relieve indigestion, chest congestion and abdominal swelling.
- Eat 2 mangoes every day to relieve bleeding from gums.

## Mandarin Orange

*Good for thirst, intoxication, urination difficulty, emphysema.*

### DESCRIPTION

- Cool; sweet and sour; promotes urination; lubricates the lungs; relieves cough; eliminates mucus.

### PREPARATION

- Eat a few fresh mandarin oranges to relieve thirst from a fever or painful urination. Repeat 4 hours later.
- Steam a fresh unpeeled mandarin orange with 15g rock sugar and 2 fresh ginger slices for 1 hour. Eat the orange with peel to treat senile and chronic cough.
- Drink fresh mandarin orange juice to relieve a hangover.
- Steam a fresh unpeeled mandarin orange with 5 red dates for half an hour. Eat the orange and dates to relieve symptoms of emphysema.
- Slowly chew the peel of a fresh mandarin orange to relieve chest congestion and abdominal swelling due to indigestion.
- Mandarin orange seeds may be left in the sun to dry for use in remedies.
- Fry 30g mandarin orange seeds; boil the seeds in 3 cups water with 9g caraway seeds until the water is reduced to 2 cups. Drink 1 cup of the juice each time, in the morning and evening, to cure hernia and painful swelling in the testes.
- Crush 15g mandarin orange seeds and boil them in 30g rice wine. Drink the juice twice a day to promote milk secretion and to soften a lump in breast.
- Collect mandarin orange peels and dry them in the sun to make dried mandarin orange peels.

## Mussel

*Good for night sweats, lumbago, impotence, vomiting of blood, vaginal discharge, goiter.*

### DESCRIPTION

Warm; salty; increases the energy of kidneys and liver; cures simple goiter; affects the liver and kidneys.

### PREPARATION

- Bake 100g mussels and grind into powder. Grind into powder 10g dried orange peel. Mix the two powders with honey. Dissolve 3 teaspoonfuls in water each time, 3 times daily, to cure insomnia and dizziness.
- Use rice wine to wash mussels and cook with chive. Eat to cure lumbago and to counteract cold sensations in the lower abdomen in women.
- Boil 10g mussels with 30g celery. Eat at meals to lower blood pressure.

### Notes

An excessive consumption of mango is reported to have caused nephritis.

Eating mango after a full meal will cause swelling of the stomach.

Mango should not be eaten with foods that have a pungent flavor, such as garlic or green onion, as it will cause skin itching and jaundice. One day I intentionally ate 5 large mangoes with a small quantity of green onion, partly to determine the validity of this centuries-old belief and partly to enjoy the taste of mango. I developed severe skin itching within 5 hours, but no sign of jaundice, because it takes longer for a person to develop jaundice.

Mango kernel is neutral, tastes sweet and bitter and stimulates energy and relieves pain. To use the mango kernel, dry the large, flat seed first and break it up.

Crush 15g mango kernels and 15g longan seeds; add 5 red dates and boil together in 3 cups water until the water is reduced to 1 cup. Drink 1 cup of juice each time, in the morning and evening, to relieve hernial pain and orchitis.

Boil 15g mango peel with 30g of mango kernel in the amount of water sufficient to cover the two ingredients; drink two cups of juice each time, once a day, to relieve skin edema.

## Oyster and Shell

*Oyster is good for insomnia, stress and nervousness; oyster shell good for excessive perspiration, night sweat, premature ejaculation, vaginal bleeding and discharge, tuberculosis of lymph node, goiter.*

### DESCRIPTION

- Oyster—neutral, sweet and salty, used as a blood tonic; oyster shell—cool, salty, obstructive, checks excessive perspiration and premature ejaculation, softens hardness, acts on the liver and kidneys.

### PREPARATION

- Eat 15 to 25 oysters at meals to cure tuberculosis of the lymph node and goitre; or use oyster sauce as seasoning if fresh oyster is not readily available. Crush oyster shell into powder and wrap 15g of the powder in a cloth. Boil in 3 cups water over low heat until the water is reduced to 1 cup. Drink as tea before a meal, once a day, to relieve excessive gastric acid; or grind the shell into very fine powder and take 3g of the powder, each time with warm water, 3 times a day.

### CLINICAL REPORT

For treatment of night sweat in pulmonary tuberculosis, boil 20g oyster shell in 500ml water until the water is reduced to 200ml. (Sugar may be added, if desired.) Divide into 2 dosages and drink in the morning and in the evening for a few consecutive days. After the night sweat stops, the treatment continues for another 2 to 3 days to stabilize the effects. Herbal therapy may be used in combination, if no satisfactory results are obtained. In the 10 cases treated, after taking 2 to 3 dosages night sweat disappeared in 7 cases, 3 showed no obvious results, but 2 recovered after being treated in combination with other herbs. No side effects were observed.

## Pear

*Good for cough with mucus, constipation, difficulty when swallowing, alcoholism, difficult urination, indigestion.*

### DESCRIPTION

- Cool; sweet and slightly sour; produces fluids; lubricates dryness; eliminates mucus; affects the lungs and stomach.

### PREPARATION

- Drink a glass of fresh pear juice in the morning and evening to relieve cough and thirst from fever. Soak fresh unpeeled pears in vinegar to make vinegar pears. Peel 2 vinegar pears and eat them to relieve indigestion and alcoholism.
- Crush 2 vinegar pears to squeeze out the juice. Drink the juice slowly in the morning and evening to cure sore throat and difficulty when swallowing.
- Boil 60g dried pear peels in water. Drink the juice to relieve difficult urination and pain when urinating.

## Peas

*Balance the internal organs, produce body fluids, quench thirst, relieve coughs and hiccups, promote milk secretion in breastfeeding mothers and reduce swelling.*

*Notes*

Peas may be boiled, fried, or ground into powder for consumption. They are about the best foods on earth.

Peas may be cooked with mutton to boost body energy. Diabetes is also among the symptoms most frequently treated with peas.

## Pineapples

*Good for edema, indigestion, diarrhea, vomiting, abdominal swelling.*

### DESCRIPTION

- Neutral; sweet and sour; promotes urination and digestion; quenches thirst; heals swelling.

### PREPARATION

- Fry 250g fresh pineapple, sliced, with 60g chicken in oil, seasoned with pepper and salt. Eat every day, or every other day, to relieve dizziness due to low blood pressure.
- Eat 4 slices fresh pineapple or drink a glass of fresh pineapple juice each time, twice a day, to relieve indigestion, abdominal swelling, vomiting, or diarrhea.
- Drink a glass of fresh pineapple juice seasoned with a little salt each time, twice a day, to relieve thirst from fever.

## Polished (White) Rice

*Good for diarrhea, morning sickness, difficult urination.*

### DESCRIPTION

- Neutral; sweet; used as an energy tonic and a spleen tonic; affects the spleen and stomach.

### PREPARATION

- Fry 1 bowlful polished rice with fresh ginger juice until the rice becomes yellowish. Chew 20 to 30 grains before getting up in the morning to relieve morning sickness.
- Boil rice in water as you would normally, but cook it a little longer than usual to allow a thick crust of charred rice to form on the bottom of the pan; rice is neutral and bitter and sweet.
- Boil 150g browned crust of rice with an equal amount of lotus fruits and sugar in an adequate amount of water. Drink 2 teaspoonfuls each time, 3 times a day, to cure diarrhea, particularly in children.

## Pomegranates (Sweet Fruit)

*Produce fluids and quench thirst; good for dry throat and chronic diarrhea.*

## Pork

*Good for diabetes, underweight, dry cough, constipation.*

### DESCRIPTION

- Neutral, sweet and salty; used to lubricate dryness; affects the spleen, stomach and kidneys.

### PREPARATION

- Boil 500 to 1,000g pork; skim off and discard the floating fat. Drink the soup to relieve dry cough and constipation.
- Cut up 100g lean pork (red meats) to boil in water with 100g Job's tears over low heat for 2 hours. Eat it at meals to moisten the skin; this is considered a good remedy for dry skin.

## Pork Marrow

*Increases yin energy and marrow in the body, reduces burning sensations, cures vaginal discharge in women and seminal emission in men. Pork marrow is an ideal food for the elderly.*

### PREPARATION

- The Chinese are very fond of using pork bones to make various kinds of soup, because the marrow is good for facilitating the growth of bones in children, particularly when mixed with vegetables with a high level of calcium, such as peas, seaweed, spinach and tofu. It's an ideal recipe for rickets in children.
- When preparing bone soup, it's wise to add vinegar, fresh ginger and black pepper, since they can make the marrow separate from the bones more easily.

## Red Bayberries

*Quench thirst, promote digestion, cleanse the stomach and intestines, balance the internal organs, stop vomiting and diarrhea.*

### PREPARATION

- To cure chronic diarrhea, bake red bayberries until burned on the surface; then grind into powder. Take 6g of powder with rice soup two times daily. Or, soak red bayberries in wine; eat one to two berries two times daily.
- To cure chronic headaches, bake red bayberries and grind into powder. Take 6g of powder with peppermint tea two times daily.

## Royal Jelly

*Good for those suffering from underdevelopment, loss of weight, poor appetite, hepatitis, neurasthenia, nodular phlebitis, malnutrition, rheumatoid arthritis, anemia, gastric ulcers.*

### DESCRIPTION

- Royal jelly, a modern product not recorded in traditional Chinese diet classics, is now widely used to promote growth, slow down the aging process and prevent loss of hair; it is produced from a secretion of the worker bees' salivary glands and fermented with honey pollen and other ingredients and specially used as food for the queen bees. This explains why virtually all queen bees are able to live up to 5 years whereas worker bees can live only 2 to 4 months. On top of that, at the height of the laying season, a single queen bee can lay 2,500 to 3,000 ovules that weigh more than the queen bee's own body.

## Saltwater Clams

*Increase yin energy, promote urination, remove sputum, soften hard spots in the body; their shell can reduce internal heat and remove dampness from the body.*

## Shrimp

*Fresh shrimp are good for impotence and dry shrimp for shortage of milk secretion.*

### DESCRIPTION

- Warm; sweet; used to increase yang energy.

*Notes*

Royal jelly is available in tablet form.

*Notes*

Saltwater clams are watery and lubricating, which can generate fluids, lubricate the internal organs, relieve diabetes and increase appetites. The salt in clams is most beneficial to blood clots in women with cold and hot sensations.

Cold foods can control fire; salted foods can lubricate and travel downwards. When the body develops hard spots, it is necessary to soften them by eating salted foods.

Saltwater clams are often used to treat jaundice, edema, pulmonary tuberculosis, diabetes, chronic tracheitis and vaginal bleeding. Clams can be baked and ground into powder for applications.

*Notes*

Shrimp is bad for men with seminal emission or premature ejaculation.

### PREPARATION

- Crush 500g shrimps and mix with hot rice wine. Drink it to increase milk secretion; or drink this with soup made from pork leg to reinforce the effects.

## Spinach
*Good for nosebleeds, discharge of blood from anus, thirst in diabetes, constipation, alcoholism, scurvy, hemorrhoids.*

### DESCRIPTION

- Cool; sweet; glossy; lubricates dryness, arrests bleeding, used as a blood tonic; affects the large and small intestines.

### PREPARATION

- Immerse spinach in boiling water for 3 minutes and eat it with a little sesame oil to treat hypertension, constipation, headache and dizziness.
- Simmer large quantities of spinach, including roots and heads, over low heat for 2 or 3 hours. Drink it as tea to relieve a hangover and alcoholism.

### REMARKS

- Spinach is not recommended for persons with premature ejaculation and diarrhea because it is glossy (sliding). But it is good for skin eruptions caused by a hot physical constitution.
- Spinach can cleanse the blood and is good for many hot skin eruptions and itchy skin, which are caused by hot blood in many instances. Spinach also has a cool energy. To treat hot skin diseases, spinach may be cooked with seaweed or kelp, which also can cleanse the blood.
- In summer when the weather is really hot, if some people develop sore throat or chest congestion after eating fried foods, it is beneficial to drink some spinach soup.

## Star Fruit (Carambola)
*Good for coughs and fevers from a common cold, toothache, kidney and bladder stones, hemorrhoids, mouth canker, indigestion, hangover.*

### DESCRIPTION

- Cold; sweet and sour; reduces fever; produces fluids; promotes urination; detoxicates.

### PREPARATION

- Eat a fresh star fruit each time, twice a day, to relieve fever and cough in common cold.
- Boil 3 fresh star fruits with 2 teaspoonfuls honey. Eat the fruits and drink the juice once a day to relieve kidney and bladder stones and difficult urination.
- Crush 3 fresh star fruits to make juice. Drink it twice a day to relieve pharyngolaryngitis, mouth canker and toothache.
- Crush 3 fresh star fruits and mix the juice with cold water. Drink it 3 times a day to relieve painful urination and discharge of red urine.
- Eat 2 fresh star fruits each time, twice a day, first thing in the morning on an empty stomach and in the evening, to relieve hemorrhoids.

## String Bean (Green Bean)

*Good for diarrhea, vomiting, diabetes, seminal emission, whitish vaginal discharge, frequent urination.*

### DESCRIPTION

- Neutral; sweet; used as a kidney tonic and a spleen tonic; affects the spleen and kidneys.

### PREPARATION

- Boil 50g dried string beans (with the shells) in water. Drink as soup once a day to relieve diabetes, thirst and frequent urination.

## Sugar Cane

*Good for vomiting, dry cough, constipation, alcoholism.*

### DESCRIPTION

- Cold; sweet; lubricates dryness; promotes urination; produces fluids, pushes downwards; affects the lungs and stomach.

### PREPARATION

- Drink sugar cane juice to relieve fever, difficult urination and thirst.
- Mix half a glass sugar cane juice with 3 teaspoonfuls fresh ginger juice. Drink it to relieve vomiting.
- Drink 1 glass fresh sugar cane juice, 3 times a day, to cure light edema during pregnancy.

## Sweet Apricot Seed

*Lubricates the lungs and stops asthma; good for coughs and for constipation due to intestinal dryness.*

## Tomatoes

*Good for thirst, poor appetite, hypertension, constipation.*

### DESCRIPTION

- Slightly cold; sweet and sour; produces fluids; promotes digestion.

### PREPARATION

- Eat 1 or 2 fresh tomatoes first thing in the morning on an empty stomach to relieve hypertension and bloodshot eyes.
- Boil tomato juice with ginger juice and drink it as soup to prevent blood coagulations after injuries.
- Cook 2 tomatoes with 60g pork liver to relieve night blindness.
- Eat 1 fresh tomato sweetened with sugar twice a day to relieve bleeding gums.
- Eat 1 or 2 fresh tomatoes twice a day; or cook tomatoes with pork and eat it to quench thirst and improve appetite.

## Walnut

*Good for coughs, lumbago, impotence, seminal emission, frequent urination, kidney and bladder stones, constipation.*

### Notes

Sugar may be boiled and made into the shape of a rock; this is called rock sugar (rock candy) with a neutral energy and sweet flavor. Rock sugar is regarded as the best quality of sugar and is frequently used in combination with other foods in Chinese remedies.

## DESCRIPTION

- Warm; sweet; used as kidney tonic and to lubricate intestines and check seminal emission; affects the kidneys and lungs.

## PREPARATION

- Steam 30g walnuts with 15g rock sugar and 6g radish seeds for half an hour. Eat the mixture twice a day to cure chronic asthma and cough.
- Chew 90g of walnuts slowly each day to relieve sore throat, hoarseness, constipation and gastric and duodenal ulcers.
- Boil 15g walnut with 15g crushed fresh ginger. Drink it twice a day to relieve headache and fever and fear of cold due to common cold and also to induce perspiration in common cold.
- Steam 250g walnuts and persimmon cakes each for 1 hour. Divide into 3 portions and eat 1 portion each time, 3 times a day, for 1 month to relieve cough and underweight due to pulmonary tuberculosis.
- Prepare 30g walnuts, 2 pork kidneys, sliced and a little lard; fry them together. Eat it hot every day at bedtime for 3 days to cure seminal emission with sudden urination.
- Fry 120g walnuts in vegetable oil until crunchy. Mix walnuts with some sugar and water to make syrup. Eat it within 2 days to relieve stones in urinary tract.

## CLINICAL REPORT

- For the treatment of kidney and bladder stones: Fry 120g walnuts in vegetable oil until crunchy. Add sugar and grind into an emulsion or cream. Eat the walnuts within 1 to 2 days. (Reduce the dosage for children.) Treatment continues until stones are passed or the symptoms disappear. In general, stones are passed once or several times within a few days. They also appear smaller and softer than earlier stones or they are dissolved in urine to look like cream. Thus, walnut is considered effective for dissolving the stones.

## Watermelon

*Good for diminished urination, sore throat, mouth canker.*

## DESCRIPTION

- Cold; sweet; promotes urination and lubricates intestines; affects the heart, stomach and bladder.

## PREPARATION

- Drink a glass of fresh watermelon juice to relieve dizziness in sunstroke and vomiting. Eat 500 to 1,000g fresh watermelon each time, twice a day, to relieve thirst, bitter taste in mouth, bad breath, discharge of yellowish urine, pain in urethra and a hangover.
- Cut off watermelon peels about 0.5 cm thick and put them in the sun to dry, which become dry watermelon peels widely used as herb in Chinese herbalism.
- Boil 50g of dry watermelon peels in water and drink as tea to treat hypertension, diabetes, nephritis and a hangover.

## Whitebait

*Tones deficiency, strengthens the stomach, benefits the lungs, promotes urination.*

## White Sugar

*Good for dry coughs, thirst, stomachaches.*

### DESCRIPTION

- Neutral; sweet; lubricates the lungs; produces fluids; affects the spleen.

### PREPARATION

- Boil 3 spoonfuls sugar in 1 glass rice wine over low heat. Drink it to relieve a tight sensation in the abdomen.
- Mix sugar with red dates and chew 2 dates after meals like chewing gum to relieve a dry cough.
- Boil sugar in water to make concentrated syrups to treat stomachache, abdominal discomfort caused by eating fish and crabs and bad breath caused by eating garlic and onion.

## Yam

*Good for chronic diarrhea, coughs, diabetes, seminal emission, vaginal discharge, frequent urination.*

### DESCRIPTION

- Neutral; sweet, spleen tonic, lung tonic and kidney tonic; affects the lungs, spleen and kidneys.

### PREPARATION

- Prepare 80g raw yam and grind into powder. Wash an equal amount of glutinous (sweet) rice and drain it; put rice in the sun to dry. Toast the rice in a pan, shaking or stirring, until yellowish and grind into powder. Mix the yam and rice. Take 4 spoonfuls of the powder, some sugar and black pepper dissolved in warm water each morning to treat chronic diarrhea and poor appetite.
- Boil yam with ginseng for 30 minutes and drink it as tea. Or make a soup with yam and beef or pork.

Yang tonic foods, or kidney yang tonics, restore yang energy in the kidneys, which is essential in the maintenance of body warmth.

# Yang Tonic Foods

## Beef Kidneys

*Tone the kidneys and increase the level of semen; good for impotence and rheumatism.*

## Chestnuts

*Increase energy in the body and strengthen the stomach, intestines and kidneys.*

## Chive Seeds

*Tone the liver and kidneys, warm the loins and knees, boost yang energy in the body and solidify semen; good for impotence, frequent urination, enuresis, vaginal discharge and diarrhea.*

## Cinnamon Bark

*Good for cold limbs, abdominal pain, diarrhea, hot sensations in the upper region with cold sensations in the lower region.*

### DESCRIPTION

- Hot; pungent and sweet; affects the kidneys, spleen and bladder.

### PREPARATION

- Grind dry cinnamon bark into powder; dissolve 5g of the powder in warm water and drink each time, 3 times a day, to cure various types of cold symptoms (including cold abdominal pain, cold abdominal swelling and cold stomachache).
- Dissolve 5g of the powder in rice wine and drink each time, 3 times a day, to alleviate abdominal pain in women after childbirth.
- Dissolve 3g cinnamon-bark powder in warm water to correct excessive gastric acid and vomiting of acid.
- Use cinnamon bark as a seasoning in cooking to warm up the body.

### EXPERIMENT

- Effects of cinnamon bark on animals indicate it calms the central nervous system in rats and also reduces their blood pressure.

## Clove Oil

*Warms the stomach and kidneys; good for cold stomachaches, hiccups, vomiting, diarrhea, rheumatic pain, hernia pain, toothaches and bad breath.*

## Clove

*Good for vomiting, hiccupping, upset stomach, diarrhea, abdominal pain, hernia.*

### DESCRIPTION

- Warm; pungent; pushes downward, warms internal region in general and kidneys in particular; affects the stomach, spleen and kidneys.

### PREPARATION

- Chew 1 or 2 cloves to get rid of bad breath.
- Apply ground cloves to nipples to heal cracked nipples.
- Grind cloves and persimmon calynx into powder; take 2g each time in water, twice a day, to relieve hiccupping.

- Boil 4g cloves with 6g persimmon calyx and 4g fresh ginger in 2 cups water over low heat until water is reduced to 1 cup; drink half a cupful each time, twice a day, to stop vomiting.
- A traditional Chinese formula to relieve hiccupping: Combine 2g cloves, 3g persimmon calyx (available in most Chinese herb shops), 3g ginseng and 2g dried ginger and boil; divide into 2 dosages and drink in 1 day. In my experience, this has never failed to produce instant results.
- Boil 20 cloves with red tea leaves and enough water to cover; drink it as tea to correct poor appetite and discomfort in the stomach from indigestion and also to correct excessive gastric acid.

## Deer's Kidneys

*Tone the kidneys, improve sexual capacity, produce semen; good for fatigue, lumbago, ringing in the ears, deafness, impotence and infertility in women due to cold womb.*

## Dillseed

*Good for abdominal pain, poor appetite, shortage of milk secretion after childbirth.*

### DESCRIPTION

- Warm; pungent; warms the body, promotes energy circulation and counteracts fish and meat poisoning; affects the spleen and kidneys.

### PREPARATION

- Fry dillseeds until aromatic and grind into powder; dissolve 5g of the powder in warm rice wine and drink each time to cure lumbago due to twisted muscles.

## Fennel Roots

*Warm the kidneys, balance the internal region, promote energy circulation and relieve pain; good for arthritis, rheumatism, abdominal pain, stomachaches.*

## Fennel Seed

*Good for hernias, cold pain in lower abdomen, lumbago, stomachache, vomiting, dry and wet beriberi.*

### DESCRIPTION

- Warm; pungent; warms the internal region and promotes energy circulation; affects the kidneys, the bladder and stomach.

### PREPARATION

- Prepare 40g apricot seeds; crush 20g fresh green onion white heads with roots and bake until dry; prepare 40g fennel seed; grind all the ingredients into a powder. Drink 10g of the powder dissolved in rice wine each time, twice a day, to relieve pain in hernia of small intestine.
- Fry equal amounts of fennel and litchi seeds and grind into powder; dissolve 10g of the powder in rice wine and drink each time, twice a day, to relieve pain in hernia of the small intestine.
- Measure equal amounts fennel and black pepper and grind them into

Cinnamon bark is such a powerful herb, the Chinese herbalists have listed more than 30 conditions as contraindications of cinnamon bark. Persons with any of these conditions should avoid this herb. The conditions listed as contraindications of cinnamon bark include: hot conditions (including excessive menstrual flow), discharge of urine containing blood, nosebleed, urination difficulty, discharge of dry stools, cough due to hot lungs, fever, loss of voice, hemorrhoids and other ailments. And anyone suffering from common cold should avoid cinnamon bark. This spice should also be avoided by pregnant women.

Cinnamon Forests, a city in China named for its ubiquitous cinnamon trees, also has the most beautiful scenic views in the country. When I recently visited Cinnamon Forests I could smell cinnamon everywhere, including the downtown area and I was pleased as much by the plentiful cinnamon trees in the city as by its beautiful scenery.

### Notes

Clove is a very warm spice and as such can warm the stomach and relieve vomiting, hiccupping and hernia pain. But sometimes vomiting and hiccupping are due to hot energy and clove should not be used. If you develop hiccupping and take clove for relief, normally it will take effect in a few minutes, or at most, a few hours. But if clove does not relieve the symptoms, then most probably, they are hot symptoms. Most symptoms of vomiting and hiccupping are cold symptoms, however and clove may be used for relief.

### Notes

Dill leaf is warm, pungent and oppressive. According to 1 experiment, dill leaf is found to have the effect of lowering blood pressure and expanding blood vessels in animals.

powder; dissolve 10g of the powder in rice wine each time, twice a day, to relieve pain in small intestine.

- For lumbago, when unable to turn sideways and extreme fatigue, cook slices of pork kidneys with fried fennel and eat at meals.
- To heal cold stomachache and abdominal pain, use fennel and ginger as seasonings when preparing meals.

## CLINICAL REPORT

- For treatment of incarcerated hernia of small intestine, use 10 to 20g fennel (less for children) to make tea; drink it hot; if no effects are shown within 15 to 30 minutes, repeat once more. Or, use hot water to make fennel soup (4 to 8g fennel seed for adults and 2g for children) and drink the soup; 10 minutes later, repeat and drink once more, then lie down on your back with your legs together and knees half bent for 40 minutes. In general, the incarcerated hernia should restore itself within half an hour and the pain should disappear or improve, otherwise, surgery is indicated, according to this clinical report. Among the 26 cases treated from 2 hours to 3 days, 22 cases have recovered and 4 cases have shown no effects (3 cases of incarcerated omenturn majus and 1 case of parietal necrosis). The report also indicates that the treatment results are better in cases with a shorter history of the disease; if the symptoms have a long history, necrosis and perforation may have already occurred and they should not be treated by this method. In case of incarcerated momentum majus, surgery should be considered, according to this report.
- For treatment of hydrocele of tunica vaginalis and elephantiasis scroti: Fry 16g fennel and 5g salt until black; grind them into powder to make cakes with 2 raw duck eggs; eat the cakes while drinking warm rice wine at bedtime. Each treatment program continues for 4 days; the second treatment program begins 2 to 5 days after completing the first program. Treatment may continue, if necessary. Among the 64 cases of hydrocele of tunica vaginalis treated for
1 to 6 programs, 59 cases recovered, 1 case has shown progress, 4 cases have shown no results. The majority of patients suffering from elephantiasis scroti have shown results only after 4 treatment programs; the results are rather satisfactory with no side effects (except the cases in which the scrotum was as hard as stone).

### Fenugreek Seeds (Oriental Fenugreek)
*Tone the kidney yang, remove cold and dampness; good for abdominal pain and swelling, wet beriberi, lumbago and impotence.*

### Green Onion Seeds
*Warm the kidneys, sharpen vision; good for impotence dizziness, blurred vision.*

### Japanese Cassia Fruits
*Warm the internal region, particularly the stomach, calm the liver, strengthen the kidneys, disperse cold.*

### Pistachio Nuts
*Warm the kidneys and spleen; good for impotence and cold diarrhea.*

## Pork Testes
*Good for tracheitis, asthma, hernia and blocked urination.*

## Prickly Asg Root
*Good for cold bladder and for blood in urine.*

## Raspberry
*Good for frequent urination, dizziness.*

### DESCRIPTION

- Warm; sweet and sour; used as a liver tonic and kidney tonic to control urination.

### PREPARATION

- Drink fresh raspberry juice to stop frequent urination and dizziness due to motion sickness.
- Mix fresh raspberry juice with honey as a remedy to cure dry cough due to cold.

**Notes**

Dry green (unripe) raspberry is an important Chinese herb with a neutral energy and sweet-sour flavor. It acts on the liver and kidneys, is used to correct impotence, seminal emission, frequent urination, blurred vision and is reported to produce similar effects as those of a female sex hormone.

## Shark Air Bladder
*Strengthens the lungs, tones the heart, removes phlegm, nourishes semen, increases yin and yang energies in the body.*

## Star Anise
*Good for hernias, abdominal pain, lumbago, beriberi, vomiting.*

### DESCRIPTION

- Warm; pungent and sweet; warms up yang energy (energy that travels in the skin and muscles as opposed to yin energy that travels through internal organs) and promotes energy circulation; affects the spleen, kidneys and liver.

### PREPARATION

- Crush 7 star anises and 7 fresh onion white heads and boil them in 3 cups water over low heat until liquid is reduced to 1 cup. Drink it like tea, twice a day, to cure constipation, urination difficulty and abdominal swelling.
- Bake 40g star anise and grind into powder; drink 5g of the powder dissolved in warm rice wine each time, twice a day, to relieve hernia of the small intestine.
- Fry star anise and grind into powder; dissolve 7g of the powder with a little salt in warm water before meals, twice a day, to cure lumbago.

**Notes**

According to traditional Chinese theory, star anise heals all sorts of cold symptoms, as well as hernia, swollen scrotum, lumbago and beriberi. It is wise to take star anise with a little salt, rice wine and cinnamon for better results. If you have an eye or skin disease, you should avoid star anise.

## Sword Beans
*Good for hiccupping, vomiting, abdominal swelling, lumbago due to kidney deficiency, mucous discharge.*

### DESCRIPTION

- Warm; sweet; pushes downwards; warms the internal region; used as a kidney tonic; affects the stomach and large intestine.

## PREPARATION

- Boil 30g old dried sword beans with shell, along with 3 slices fresh ginger; strain it to obtain juice and add some brown sugar. Drink 1 cup each time, 3 times a day, to relieve hiccupping and coughing.
- Cook 50g sword beans with a pork kidney. Eat them at meals once every other day to relieve lumbago due to weak kidneys and during pregnancy.
- Fry sword beans until browned; grind into powder. Take 4g powder each time with rice wine, 3 times a day, to cure headache, intercostal neuralgia and pain caused by injuries.
- Boil 20g sword beans in water; strain and add rock sugar or honey. Drink it as tea once a day to relieve whooping cough in children and asthma and cough in the elderly.

These foods restore deficiencies that may result in dysfunctions or diseases of the lungs and liver.

# Lung & Liver Tonic Foods

## Black Sesame Seed

*Good for constipation, dry skin, grey hair, shortage of milk secretion.*

### DESCRIPTION

- Neutral; sweet; used as a liver tonic and a kidney tonic; affects the liver and kidneys.

### PREPARATION

- Fry 15g black sesame seeds; add some salt. Eat it to increase milk secretion.
- Soak 1 cup rice for a few hours; drain and crush the rice; boil it with 1 cup black sesame seeds in water to make soup. Drink the soup at meals to correct constipation.

## Cheese

*Tones the lungs, lubricates the intestines, nourishes yin energy in the body, quenches thirst; good for constipation and dry and itchy skin.*

## Chicken Liver

*Vitalizes yang energy, tones the kidneys, sharpens vision.*

### PREPARATION

- To cure enuresis at night, mix the liver of a rooster with cinnamon in equal amounts, forming into small tablets. Take one tablet with rice soup three times daily.
- To cure blurred vision in the elderly, cut up a chicken liver and mix with processed black soybean seeds and rice. Make the mixture into cake and eat at meals.

## Garlic

*Good for cold abdominal pain, edema, diarrhea, dysentery, whooping cough.*

### DESCRIPTION

- Warm; pungent; promotes energy circulation, warms the stomach and spleen, destroys worms; affects the spleen, stomach and lungs.

### PREPARATION

- Boil 3 garlic cloves in water and eat with soy sauce at meals to relieve cough and abdominal pain and also to promote blood circulation and urination.
- For women, to relieve itch in the genital region, boil a few garlic cloves and use the liquid to wash the genital region.
- Crush a few garlic cloves to mix with mustard (powder or paste) and eat it with rice wine. Or, boil a few garlic cloves in water and drink it as tea to correct chronic cold sensations, particularly in women. If wine is desired, make garlic wine: Simply cut up a garlic clove in large pieces, drop into a small bottle of wine; put away for 1 month and it is ready to drink as a wine tonic.
- Eat 1 to 3 fresh garlic cloves daily by dividing them into 3 dosages; continue treatment for 5 to 10 consecutive days to heal amebic dysentery.
- Take 2 teaspoonfuls 10 to 20 percent garlic solution every 2 hours (mixed with some syrup or orange tincture to make it more appetizing) to relieve whooping cough in children.

- Eat garlic cloves regularly to prevent bacillary dysentery when it is widespread.
- Cut up a garlic clove and use the juicy slice to rub the skin to relieve pain caused by insect bite (such as bee sting) as an emergency measure.
- Garlic may be cooked with soybeans: Soak the soybeans overnight; cook soybeans with 5 to 10 garlic cloves. Eat as a tonic and also to promote urination, relieve edema and chronic nephritis.
- Another way to use garlic: Fry garlic cloves in vegetable oil with black pepper, sliced fresh ginger and salt; add dry shrimps, then sprinkle with sugar, vinegar and green onion. Add some tomato ketchup and flour to thicken, if desired. This recipe contains almost all the needed flavors—sweet, sour, pungent and salty.

### CLINICAL REPORT

- For treatment of lobar pneumonia; 1 tablespoon garlic syrup every 4 hours (in general 10 percent, but sometimes 100 percent). Among the 9 people treated, 6 cases show complete recovery, 3 show no satisfactory results.

## Job's Tears

*Good for diarrhea, rheumatism, muscular twitching, difficulty in movements of joints, edema, beriberi, lung diseases, whitish vaginal discharge.*

### DESCRIPTION

- Cool; sweet and light flavor; detoxicates; used as a spleen tonic and a lung tonic; diuretic, affects the spleen, lungs and kidneys.

### PREPARATION

- Boil an equal amount of Job's tears, peanuts and brown sugar. Drink as tea to relieve edema, promote urination and tone up the stomach.
- Boil 40g Job's tears to be divided into 2 dosages for consumption twice a day, for 10 days, as a treatment program to relieve flat wart and common wart.

### CLINICAL REPORT

- For the treatment of a flat wart: Cook 60g fresh Job's tears with husked rice in water. Eat it once a day until recovered. Among the 23 cases treated for 7 to 16 days, 11 cases recovered completely, 6 cases showed no clear results and 6 cases had no results; the majority of patients showed some reactions during the periods between the beginning of treatment and disappearance of the skin rash, including enlargement of the wart focus, which turned red with increased inflammation; but as treatment continued for several days, the damaged focus became dry and desquamative until completely gone.

## Matrimony Vine Fruits

*Lower the level of blood sugar, inhibit the growth of many bacteria.*

## Milk

*Cow's milk is good for an upset stomach, difficulty swallowing, diabetes, constipation; human milk is good for fatigue, skinniness, diabetes, difficulty swallowing, dry stools.*

strong smell of meats or fish. It is believed that a small quantity of garlic can counteract cancer, but an excessive quantity of garlic can cause cancer (based on the Chinese theory that excessive garlic is bad for the stomach and liver).

Chinese people eat large quantities of garlic only under special circumstances, such as severe malnutrition or edema.

In recent years, garlic has emerged as an important ingredient in Chinese medicine, mostly due to its powerful effects in treating dysentery and destroying germs. In fact, many modern medicines contain garlic as an important ingredient. For dysentery at its early stage, chew a garlic clove five or six times a day every four hours.

Contraindications of garlic include eye diseases and sore throat.

### Notes

Job's tears is reported to inhibit the growth of and destroy cancer cells. For example, according to a report in the first issue of Jiangsu Chinese Medical Journal (1962), a patient suffering from throat cancer was treated with Job's tears in the hospital, because the cancer was located in the deep region of the throat, which was rather difficult to be treated by surgery. The patient was treated with Job's tears every day and the treatment produced significant effects within 2 months; the patient recovered completely within 6 months.

### Notes

Matrimony vine fruits may be eaten as fruits or cooked as vegetables. It is commonly used as an herb for hypertension and diabetes. It is also a famous remedy for eye disease, because it acts on the liver, which is considered the organ responsible for the eyes.

## DESCRIPTION

- Cow's milk—neutral; sweet; pushes downwards; is used as a lung and stomach tonic; and is used to produce fluids and lubricate the intestines; affects the heart, lungs and stomach. Human milk—neutral; sweet and salty; is used as a blood tonic and to lubricate dryness; affects the heart, lungs and stomach.

## PREPARATION

- Boil 1 glass cow's milk in 4 glasses water over low heat until water is reduced to 1 cup. Drink it slowly on an empty stomach to improve physical conditions after a prolonged illness.
- Mix 1 glass cow's milk with half a glass fresh chive juice and 3 teaspoonfuls fresh ginger juice; heat in a small pan. Drink to relieve an upset stomach.
- Mix equal amounts of cow's and sheep's milks. Drink the milk as a substitute for tea or juice to improve the physical condition of diabetes patients and frequent urination.

## CLINICAL REPORT

- For treatment of electric ophthalmia by human milk, squeeze fresh human milk directly into a sterilized bottle or sterile eyedrop bottle; apply 2 to 3 drops on the bulbar conjunctiva of the lateral angle of each eye at 5- to 15-minute intervals; close the eyes and rest for a while. In general, discomfort or pain will disappear or decrease within 8 to 16 hours with neither side effects nor discomfort.

*Notes*

Cow's milk is not recommended for people with diarrhea or mucous discharge.

## Mulberries

*Mulberries are often made into ointment for internal consumption to reduce fever, quench thirst, improve spirits and reduce heat in the small intestines; beneficial to the internal organs, good for the joints, effective in promoting blood circulation, increase yin energy in the body; frequently used to treat diabetes, dizziness, insomnia and constipation.*

## PREPARATION

- To cure rheumatoid arthritis, paralysis of limbs and various kinds of neuralgia, boil 50g of fresh mulberries in water and drink like soup.

*Notes*

Mulberries can improve the condition of the liver and kidneys, increase the quantity of blood, counteract alcoholism, relieve rheumatism, sharpen vision and improve hearing

## Mussel

*Good for night sweats, lumbago, impotence, vomiting of blood, vaginal discharge, goitre.*

## DESCRIPTION

- Warm; salty; increases the energy of kidneys and liver; cures simple goitre; affects the liver and kidneys.

## PREPARATION

- Bake 100g mussels and grind into powder. Grind into powder 10g dried orange peel. Mix the two powders with honey. Dissolve 3 teaspoonfuls in water each time, 3 times daily, to cure insomnia and dizziness.
- Use rice wine to wash mussels and cook with chive. Eat to cure lumbago and to counteract cold sensations in the lower abdomen in women.
- Boil 10g mussels with 30g celery. Eat at meals to lower blood pressure.

## Pork Lung

*Good for coughs and for discharge of blood from the mouth.*

## Pork Pancreas

*Heals pulmonary tuberculosis with cough; when it is cooked with red dates and wine, it cures weakness and skinniness.*

### PREPARATION

- To cure coughs, cut up a pork pancreas in thin slices; boil it with vinegar and eat at meals.
- To cure vitiligo, soak a pork pancreas in wine for an hour; then steam it. Eat at meals, once a day, for a maximum of 10 days.
- To treat diabetes, soak a fresh pork pancreas in boiling water until it is half cooked, then season it with soy sauce. Or, boil a pork pancreas with 40g of corn silk. Drink the soup and eat the pancreas once a day for 7 days.

## Rabbit Liver

*Tones the liver, sharpens vision; good for dizziness, film or pain in the eyes.*

## Raspberry

*Good for frequent urination, dizziness.*

### DESCRIPTION

- Warm; sweet and sour; used as a liver tonic and kidney tonic to control urination.

### PREPARATION

- Drink fresh raspberry juice to stop frequent urination and dizziness due to motion sickness.
- Mix fresh raspberry juice with honey as a remedy to cure dry cough due to cold.

## Royal Jelly

*Good for those suffering from underdevelopment, loss of weight, poor appetite, hepatitis, neurasthenia, nodular phlebitis, malnutrition, rheumatoid arthritis, anemia, gastric ulcers.*

### DESCRIPTION

- Royal jelly, a modern product not recorded in traditional Chinese diet classics, is now widely used to promote growth, slow down the aging process and prevent loss of hair; it is produced from a secretion of the worker bees' salivary glands and fermented with honey pollen and other ingredients and specially used as food for the queen bees. This explains why virtually all queen bees are able to live up to 5 years whereas worker bees can live only 2 to 4 months. On top of that, at the height of the laying season, a single queen bee can lay 2,500 to 3,000 ovules that weigh more than the queen bee's own body.

*Notes*

Dry green (unripe) raspberry is an important Chinese herb with a neutral energy and sweet-sour flavor. It acts on the liver and kidneys, is used to correct impotence, seminal emission, frequent urination, blurred vision and is reported to produce similar effects as those of a female sex hormone.

*Notes*

Royal jelly is available in tablet form.

## Sour Dates (Chinese or Wild Jujubes)

*Nourish the liver, secure the heart, calm spirits, check perspiration; good for insomnia, palpitations, nervousness, thirst and excessive perspiration.*

## Strawberries

*Good for dry coughs, thirst, sore throats, hoarseness, indigestion, difficulty when urinating, hangover.*

### DESCRIPTION

- Cool; sweet and sour; lubricates the lungs, produces fluids, strengthens spleen, relieves intoxication.

### PREPARATION

- Steam 60g fresh strawberries with 30g rock sugar. Eat 3 times a day to treat dry cough which drags on and on.
- Drink a glass of fresh strawberry juice in the morning and evening, to relieve thirst in fever, sore throat and hoarseness.
- Eat 60g fresh strawberries before meals, 3 times a day, to relieve indigestion and abdominal pain and swelling and to improve appetite.
- Crush 60g fresh strawberries and mix with cold water. Drink a glass of the juice each time, 3 times a day, to relieve difficult and painful urination and discharge of red urine.
- Eat 8 to 10 fresh strawberries all at once to relieve hangover.
- Mix fresh strawberry juice with an equal amount of rice wine. Drink it to correct malnutrition and for weakness after illness.

## Sweet (Glutinous) Rice

*Good for excessive urination, excessive perspiration, diarrhea.*

### DESCRIPTION

- Warm; sweet; used as an energy tonic; affects the spleen, stomach and lungs.

### PREPARATION

- Fry sweet rice with wheat bran and grind into powder. Take 10g powder in warm water each time, 3 times a day, to stop excessive perspiration.
- Cook 50g sweet rice with 60g Job's tears and 8 red dates. Eat at meals to relieve pulmonary tuberculosis, neurasthenia, anemia and various kinds of chronic diseases.
- Boil sweet rice sprouts in water with malt. Drink the soup to relieve indigestion and to promote appetite.

## Turnip Flowers

*Tone the liver, sharpen vision.*

## Walnut

*Good for coughs, lumbago, impotence, seminal emission, frequent urination, kidney and bladder stones, constipation.*

### DESCRIPTION

- Warm; sweet; used as kidney tonic and to lubricate intestines and check seminal emission; affects the kidneys and lungs.

## PREPARATION

- Steam 30g walnuts with 15g rock sugar and 6g radish seeds for half an hour. Eat the mixture twice a day to cure chronic asthma and cough.
- Chew 90g of walnuts slowly each day to relieve sore throat, hoarseness, constipation and gastric and duodenal ulcers.
- Boil 15g walnut with 15g crushed fresh ginger. Drink it twice a day to relieve headache and fever and fear of cold due to common cold and also to induce perspiration in common cold.
- Steam 250g walnuts and persimmon cakes each for 1 hour. Divide into 3 portions and eat 1 portion each time, 3 times a day, for 1 month to relieve cough and underweight due to pulmonary tuberculosis.
- Prepare 30g walnuts, 2 pork kidneys, sliced and a little lard; fry them together. Eat it hot every day at bedtime for 3 days to cure seminal emission with sudden urination.
- Fry 120g walnuts in vegetable oil until crunchy. Mix walnuts with some sugar and water to make syrup. Eat it within 2 days to relieve stones in urinary tract.

## CLINICAL REPORT

- For the treatment of kidney and bladder stones: Fry 120g walnuts in vegetable oil until crunchy. Add sugar and grind into an emulsion or cream. Eat the walnuts within 1 to 2 days. (Reduce the dosage for children.) Treatment continues until stones are passed or the symptoms disappear. In general, stones are passed once or several times within a few days. They also appear smaller and softer than earlier stones or they are dissolved in urine to look like cream. Thus, walnut is considered effective for dissolving the stones.

## Western Ginseng

*Increases yin energy in the lungs, reduces internal heat, produces fluids, quenches thirst; good for coughs, loss of blood, dry throat and fatigue.*

## Yam

*Good for chronic diarrhea, coughs, diabetes, seminal emission, vaginal discharge, frequent urination.*

## DESCRIPTION

- Neutral; sweet, spleen tonic, lung tonic and kidney tonic; affects the lungs, spleen and kidneys.

## PREPARATION

- Prepare 80g raw yam and grind into powder. Wash an equal amount of glutinous (sweet) rice and drain it; put rice in the sun to dry. Toast the rice in a pan, shaking or stirring, until yellowish and grind into powder. Mix the yam and rice. Take 4 spoonfuls of the powder, some sugar and black pepper dissolved in warm water each morning to treat chronic diarrhea and poor appetite.
- Boil yam with ginseng for 30 minutes and drink it as tea. Or make a soup with yam and beef or pork.

*T*hese foods are used to treat disorders and strengthen the condition of the heart and stomach.

# Heart & Stomach Tonic Foods

## Ambergris

*Promotes energy and blood circulation, relieves pain, promotes urination; good for coughs, asthma and abdominal pain.*

## Areca Nut Male Flowers

*Cool the blood and quench thirst; good for coughs.*

## Azalea Roots

*Arrest bleeding and relieve pain; good for nosebleeds, vomiting blood, irregular menstruation and rheumatic pain.*

## Beef

*Good for those who are underweight and for diabetes, edema.*

### DESCRIPTION

- Neutral; sweet; used as a spleen, stomach, energy and blood tonic; affects the spleen and stomach.

### PREPARATION

- Eat regularly concentrated beef soup to relieve chronic diarrhea and prolapse of anus caused by chronic diarrhea.
- Mix together 1,000g beef, 10g ground black pepper, 5g dried orange peel powder; add 1 cup fresh ginger juice and an adequate amount of salt; marinate for 2 hours; cook the beef. Eat at meals to improve the conditions of stomach and stimulate the appetite. To make ginger juice, grate fresh ginger and boil it in water.

## Beer

*Promotes urination and calms the spirits.*

## Cardamon Seeds

*Promote energy circulation in the body, warm the stomach, aid digestion, expand the chest; good for poor circulation, congested chest, abdominal swelling and hiccups.*

## Chicory

*Reduces heat in the liver and benefits the gallbladder; good for jaundice-type hepatitis.*

## Chinese Magnolia Fruits

*Produce fluids and constrict semen; good for excessive perspiration and seminal emission.*

### Notes

Beef kidney is used as kidney tonic to improve sexual capacity and to cure temporary and permanent impotence in men; cut a kidney into small pieces to boil with one bowl of rice and when the kidney is cooked, add five green onion white heads.

Beef liver is neutral and sweet, is used as a liver tonic and to sharpen the vision and relieve glaucoma and night blindness.

## *Clam*

*Saltwater clams good for edema, mucous discharge, goiter, vaginal discharge, hemorrhoids; freshwater clams good for vaginal bleeding and discharge, pink eyes, eczema and hemorrhoids; saltwater clamshell powder good for diabetes, edema, goiter and hemorrhoids; freshwater clam saliva good for diabetes, pink eyes and burns; freshwater clamshell powder good for cough with mucous discharge, stomachache, hiccupping, vomiting, whitish vaginal discharge, eczema, swelling.*

### DESCRIPTION

- Sea (saltwater) clam—cold, salty, acts on the stomach, promotes water passage, eliminates mucus and softens hardness; freshwater clam—cold, sweet and salty, detoxicates, sharpens the vision, acts on the liver and kidneys. Sea clamshell powder-cold, salty, promotes water passage, softens hardness, eliminates mucus, acts on the lungs and kidneys; river clam saliva—sharpens vision; freshwater clam-shell powder—cold, salty, eliminates mucus and dries dampness, acts on the lungs, liver and stomach.

### PREPARATION

- Sea clamshell may be baked and ground into very fine powder to make sea clamshell powder. Freshwater clamshell may be washed clean (with the black skin removed) and ground into powder or baked and ground into powder to make freshwater clamshell powder. Apply saltwater clam's saliva externally to the affected region to relieve itching and pain and swelling of the vaginal orifice.
- Crush a few garlics to mix with clamshell powder and make into tablets of a normal size. Take 10 tablets with warm water each time, once a day, to relieve edema in weak persons.
- Mix clamshell powder with lard for external application to the affected region to relieve burns.
- Mix fine clamshell powder with an equal amount of raw licorice powder, take 7g each time with warm water, twice a day, to cure gastric ulcer and excessive gastric acid.
- Regular consumption of clam meat at meals relieves lymphadenitis scrofula in the neck and goiter.
- Cook clam with chive. Eat at meals to relieve pulmonary tuberculosis and night sweat.
- Boil 30g fine clamshell powder with 4g outer layer of peanuts and 6 red dates to make concentrated soup. Drink the soup once a day to relieve nosebleed, bleeding from gums and purpura hemorrhagica.
- Roast a whole freshwater clam until its outer part is charred and the inner part becomes yellow-brown with its original shape remaining intact; grind into fine powder and mix with sesame oil for external application to relieve eczema in infants.

### CLINICAL REPORT

- For treatment of gastric and duodenal ulcers, fry freshwater clamshell powder in a bronze fry pan (or any earthenware fry pan) until it becomes yellow-brown with the fishy smell gone; strain it before using. Take 1 to 2g each time mixed with warm water, once every hour during the daytime, 12 to 14 times a day, for 4 to 8 weeks. Among the 41 cases treated from 14 to 79 days, 28 cases showed disappearance of pain in the upper abdomen and 7 cases a decrease, 23 cases showed disappearance of pressure pain in the upper abdomen (pain that occurs on pressure by hand) and 6 cases a decrease; 21 cases had a follow-up X-ray examination, which indicated disappearance of the niche in 9 cases, disappearance of deformity in 1 case and a reduction in the size of the niche in 6 cases.

## Coffee

*Good for bronchitis, emphysema, cor pulmonale, intoxication.*

### DESCRIPTION

- Warm; sweet and bitter; used as a stimulant, heart tonic and diuretic.

### PREPARATION

- Drink strong black coffee to relieve intoxication.
- Boil 10g roasted coffee beans in water. Drink each day to relieve chronic bronchitis, emphysema and cor pulmonale.

## Corn (Maize)

*Good for difficult urination, weak heart.*

### DESCRIPTION

- Neutral; sweet; used as a stomach tonic; promotes urination; affects the stomach and large intestine.

## Duck

*Good for relieving hot sensations, cough, edema.*

### DESCRIPTION

- Neutral; sweet and salty; facilitates water passage and heals swelling; affects the lungs and kidneys.

### PREPARATION

- Cook a duck with suitable quantities of ham. Eat at meals to relieve diarrhea, particularly chronic diarrhea after childbirth.
- Place 4 to 5 garlic cloves inside a prepared duck; simmer duck in water until very soft. Eat the duck and garlic and drink the soup without salt to relieve chronic nephritis and edema.

## Fennel Seed

*Good for hernias, cold pain in lower abdomen, lumbago, stomachache, vomiting, dry and wet beriberi.*

### DESCRIPTION

- Warm; pungent; warms the internal region and promotes energy circulation; affects the kidneys, the bladder and stomach.

### PREPARATION

- Prepare 40g apricot seeds; crush 20g fresh green onion white heads with roots and bake until dry; prepare 40g fennel seed; grind all the ingredients into a powder. Drink 10g of the powder dissolved in rice wine each time, twice a day, to relieve pain in hernia of small intestine.
- Fry equal amounts of fennel and litchi seeds and grind into powder; dissolve 10g of the powder in rice wine and drink each time, twice a day, to relieve pain in hernia of the small intestine.
- Measure equal amounts fennel and black pepper and grind them into powder; dissolve 10g of the powder in rice wine each time, twice a day, to relieve pain in small intestine.
- For lumbago, when unable to turn sideways and extreme fatigue, cook slices of pork kidneys with fried fennel and eat at meals.

### Notes

One source indicates that a regular consumption of corn makes the heart stronger and increases sexual capacities, according to an experiment on swallows.

Boil 15g corn kernels in 3 glasses water over low heat until water is reduced to 1 glass, or until water becomes reddish brown. Drink half a glass of the soup each time, twice a day, to relieve kidney disease.

Boil 30g fresh corn leaves over low heat for 20 minutes. Drink the soup to relieve difficulty when urinating.

### Notes

Duck is good for hot symptoms, such as the presence of internal heat. But it may not be easily digested and is considered bad for hemorrhoids.

Duck egg is cool and sweet, is used to reduce heat in the lungs and also to relieve cough, sore throat, toothache and diarrhea.

Lime, salt and other ingredients may be used to preserve duck egg to make preserved duck egg, which has a cold energy and pungent and sweet and salty flavors; eat 2 to 3 preserved duck eggs every day (with sugar and vinegar, if desired) to relieve hypertension; or eat 2 preserved duck eggs to check diarrhea and to relieve a hangover. Preserved duck eggs are available in most Chinese food shops.

### Notes

Chinese herbalists believe that fennel travels very fast in the body and it can quickly warm up the internal re-gion. Therefore, fennel can treat cold pain in the body; but since it is warm in nature, fennel should not be used to treat any hot disease, such as hot diarrhea

- To heal cold stomachache and abdominal pain, use fennel and ginger as seasonings when preparing meals.

## CLINICAL REPORT

- For treatment of incarcerated hernia of small intestine, use 10 to 20g fennel (less for children) to make tea; drink it hot; if no effects are shown within 15 to 30 minutes, repeat once more. Or, use hot water to make fennel soup (4 to 8g fennel seed for adults and 2g for children) and drink the soup; 10 minutes later, repeat and drink once more, then lie down on your back with your legs together and knees half bent for 40 minutes. In general, the incarcerated hernia should restore itself within half an hour and the pain should disappear or improve, otherwise, surgery is indicated, according to this clinical report. Among the 26 cases treated from 2 hours to 3 days, 22 cases have recovered and 4 cases have shown no effects (3 cases of incarcerated omenturn majus and 1 case of parietal necrosis). The report also indicates that the treatment results are better in cases with a shorter history of the disease; if the symptoms have a long history, necrosis and perforation may have already occurred and they should not be treated by this method. In case of incarcerated momentum majus, surgery should be considered, according to this report.
- For treatment of hydrocele of tunica vaginalis and elephantiasis scroti: Fry 16g fennel and 5g salt until black; grind them into powder to make cakes with 2 raw duck eggs; eat the cakes while drinking warm rice wine at bedtime. Each treatment program continues for 4 days; the second treatment program begins 2 to 5 days after completing the first program. Treatment may continue, if necessary. Among the 64 cases of hydrocele of tunica vaginalis treated for 1 to 6 programs, 59 cases recovered, 1 case has shown progress, 4 cases have shown no results. The majority of patients suffering from elephantiasis scroti have shown results only after 4 treatment programs; the results are rather satisfactory with no side effects (except the cases in which the scrotum was as hard as stone).

## White Fungus

*Good for coughs, discharge of mucus with blood, chronic constipation.*

## DESCRIPTION

- Neutral; sweet with a light taste; glossy; produces fluids and lubricates the lungs.

## Ginkgo Leaves

*Tone the heart, control the lungs, remove dampness, check diarrhea; good for heart pain, palpitations, coughs, vaginal discharge and coronary heart disease.*

## Ginseng

*Good for poor appetites, fatigue, upset stomachs, diarrhea, coughs, excessive perspiration, forgetfulness, impotence, frequent urination, diabetes, vaginal bleeding.*

## DESCRIPTION

- Warm; sweet and slightly bitter; tones up energy; produces fluids; calms the spirits; affects the spleen and lungs.

or pain that occurs on exposure to hot surroundings (sunburn, burn, or warm temperatures). Fennel is not recommended for men with excessively strong erection and premature ejaculation. Fennel should be of the best quality, fresh and aromatic; it is considered an aromatic digestive and carminative, good for regulation of intestines, expelling intestinal gas, warming up internal region and exciting the nervous system. Fennel root is warm and tastes pungent and sweet, it can warm the kidneys and promote energy circulation to relieve pain; good for cold pain in hernia, cold vomiting, abdominal pain and arthritis.

*Notes*

White fungus is also called snow fungus. It is considered an important yin tonic, good for insomnia, lung disease, liver disease and poor appetite. As white fungus is glossy, it is not recommended for those suffering from diarrhea or seminal emission.

It is customary to cook white fungus with lean pork over low heat for as long as 3 hours; or boil white fungus in water with rock sugar. Some people prefer to boil white fungus in chicken soup, which makes it more delicious.

White fungus should not be used to relieve cough due to common cold.

*Notes*

To improve the sex gland functions in men and women in the treatment of hypogonadism.

To improve the functions of digestion, absorption and metabolism.

To act as an antidiuretic.

To lower blood sugar; this function is attributed to the presence of ginsenin in ginseng.

While ginseng has its important functions, there are also circumstances under which ginseng should not be used. Such circumstances may include the following:

## PREPARATION

- Ginseng is one of the few Chinese herbs that is frequently applied alone. A traditional Chinese herbal formula—solitary ginseng soup—is made by steaming or boiling ginseng for consumption: Boil 5g ginseng in 1.5 cups water over low heat until water is reduced to half. Drink it all within 1 day to cure prolapse and heart failure.
- Ginseng may be used with dry ginger to treat morning sickness and abdominal pain.

### Grass Carp

*Warms the stomach and balances the internal region; good for rheumatism, headaches and liver disease.*

### Hairtail

*Warms the stomach, tones deficiency and lubricates the skin.*

### Job's Tears Leaves

*Warm the stomach, beneficial to the blood, increase energy.*

### Longan

*Good for insomnia, forgetfulness, palpitations, nervousness.*

## DESCRIPTION

- Warm; sweet; used as a spleen tonic, heart tonic, blood tonic and energy tonic; affects the heart and spleen.

## PREPARATION

- Steam 15g longans with 30g lean pork, 2 fresh ginger slices and an adequate amount of rice wine. Eat once a day to relieve dizziness and underweight.
- Mix 500g longans with 500g sugar; steam them to make longan jelly.
- Take 1 spoonful longan jelly with warm water to relieve dizziness and edema after childbirth; or boil 15g longans with 5 red dates, 30g brown sugar and 6g fresh ginger. Drink it as soup once a day.

### Longan Shells

*Arrest bleeding, relieve pain, regulate energy, remove dampness; good for bleeding due to injuries, hernias, scrofula and eczema.*

### Lotus Fruit, Lotus Seed and Lotus Root

*Good for dreaminess, seminal emission, chronic diarrhea, vaginal bleeding and discharge.*

## DESCRIPTION

- Neutral; sweet; obstructive; used as a spleen tonic, heart tonic and kidney tonic; lotus root is also used as calmative; affects the heart, spleen and kidneys.

Cough and coughing up blood. Vomiting of blood due to excessive indulgence in sexual intercourse.

Ginseng could cause encephalemia or cerebrovascular accidents in people suffering from hypertension.

Edema and incomplete functions of the kidneys with decreased urination, because ginseng is an antidiuretic that may cause edema to deteriorate.

Excessive type of insomnia, because ginseng can make an excessive condition even more excessive.

Common cold with fever, because ginseng can increase the production of extreme heat in the body, which can intensify the fever.

There are three basic kinds of ginseng with different functions: Chinese ginseng; Korean or red ginseng; and American ginseng. Chinese ginseng, more beneficial to the lungs and the digestive system, is more often used to benefit the lungs, produce fluids and heal other critical symptoms. Korean or red ginseng is warmer; it is most frequently used to tone up energy and blood to improve the functions of the sex gland and is less effective for other symptoms. American ginseng has a cool energy. It tastes sweet and slightly bitter, acting on the heart, the lungs and the kidneys and is mostly used for cough, thirst and alcoholism.

### Notes

The scales of a hairtail contain various unsaturated acids; in an experiment, the oil from hairtail scales was found to reduce cholesterol levels in rats.

Another report indicated when rats were fed the oil from hairtail scales, their hair grew faster and thicker. When some people applied the oil on the withered hair on children's heads, the hair began to grow in its original color within one month.

In a factory in Shanghai, extracts from hairtail scales are used to treat acute leukemia and other cancers with good results, but the patients show some side effects, such as nausea, loss of appetite and a rise in transaminase. Therefore, patients with liver or kidney disorders shouldn't use hairtail extracts. When the extracts are used in combination with other anticancerous drugs, they may be effective in the treatment of stomach cancer, lymphatic tumors and villoma.

## PREPARATION

- Boil 30g dried lotus fruits and 30g brown sugar in 30g rice wine; add 1 chicken egg as in egg-drop soup. Drink the soup every evening for 1 month to improve physical conditions after childbirth or excessive fatigue due to old age.
- Steam lotus fruits until cooked. Leave them in the sun to dry; grind into powder. Take 15g of the powder each time, 3 times a day, to cure chronic diarrhea.
- Steam 250g dried lotus fruits with 6g rice wine and 6g lard. Take the entire dosage 3 times a day for 1 month to cure ulcers or during the recovery stage after stomach bleeding.
- Mix 180g lotus seeds and 30g licorice and grind into powder. Take 3 to 6g powder each time with warm water, 3 times a day, to relieve discharge of a short stream of red urine.
- Crush a few fresh lotus roots; squeeze out the juice. Drink a glass of the juice each time to stop bleeding of various kinds, including nosebleed, vaginal bleeding, discharge of blood from anus and vomiting of blood.

## *Lotus Plumule*

*Good for seminal emission, hypertension, blurred vision, swelling and pain in eyes.*

### DESCRIPTION

- Cold; bitter; obstructive; arrests bleeding; stops seminal emission; also used as a heart tonic; affects the heart, lungs and kidneys.

### PREPARATION

- Boil 3g lotus plumule and drink it all at once to relieve seminal emission with or without dreams.
- Chew 1.5g lotus plumule slowly and wash down with water to relieve hypertension.
- Boil 3g lotus plumule and 3g licorice with water. Drink it as tea, twice a day, to relieve anxiety and mouth canker.

### EXPERIMENT

- An experiment on animals shows that lotus plumule can lower blood pressure.

### REMARKS

- Lotus plumule refers to the green bud of a ripe dry lotus seed.

## *Mango*

*Good for coughs, indigestion, bleeding from gums.*

### DESCRIPTION

- Cool; sweet and sour; quenches thirst; strengthens the stomach; relieves vomiting; promotes urination.

### PREPARATION

- Eat a fresh mango with peel each time, 3 times a day, to relieve cough with mucous discharge and asthma.
- Eat a fresh mango with peel in the morning and evening to relieve indigestion, chest congestion and abdominal swelling.

*Notes*

It is interesting to note that lotus was referred to in Greek legend as yielding a fruit which induced a state of dreamy and contented forgetfulness in those who ate it. But in Chinese herbal remedies, it is believed that lotus fruit may be eaten to relieve dreaminess.

*Notes*

An excessive consumption of mango is reported to have caused nephritis.

Eating mango after a full meal will cause swelling of the stomach.

Mango should not be eaten with foods that have a pungent flavor, such as garlic or green onion, as it will cause skin itching and jaundice. One day I intentionally ate 5 large mangoes with a small quantity of green onion, partly to determine the validity of this centuries-old belief and partly to enjoy the taste of mango. I developed severe skin itching within 5 hours, but no sign of jaundice, because it takes longer for a person to develop jaundice.

Mango kernel is neutral, tastes sweet and bitter and stimulates energy and relieves pain. To use the mango kernel, dry the large, flat seed first and break it up.

Crush 15g mango kernels and 15g longan seeds; add 5 red dates and boil together in 3 cups water until the water is reduced to 1 cup. Drink 1 cup of juice each time, in the morning and evening, to relieve hernial pain and orchitis.

Boil 15g of mango peel with 30g of mango kernel in the amount of water sufficient to cover the two ingredients; drink two cups of juice each time, once a day, to relieve skin edema.

○ Eat 2 mangoes every day to relieve bleeding from gums.

## Milk

*Cow's milk is good for an upset stomach, difficulty swallowing, diabetes, constipation; human milk is good for fatigue, skinniness, diabetes, difficulty swallowing, dry stools.*

### DESCRIPTION

○ Cow's milk—neutral; sweet; pushes downwards; is used as a lung and stomach tonic; and is used to produce fluids and lubricate the intestines; affects the heart, lungs and stomach. Human milk—neutral; sweet and salty; is used as a blood tonic and to lubricate dryness; affects the heart, lungs and stomach.

### PREPARATION

○ Boil 1 glass cow's milk in 4 glasses water over low heat until water is reduced to 1 cup. Drink it slowly on an empty stomach to improve physical conditions after a prolonged illness.

○ Mix 1 glass cow's milk with half a glass fresh chive juice and 3 teaspoonfuls fresh ginger juice; heat in a small pan. Drink to relieve an upset stomach.

○ Mix equal amounts of cow's and sheep's milks. Drink the milk as a substitute for tea or juice to improve the physical condition of diabetes patients and frequent urination.

### CLINICAL REPORT

○ For treatment of electric ophthalmia by human milk, squeeze fresh human milk directly into a sterilized bottle or sterile eyedrop bottle; apply 2 to 3 drops on the bulbar conjunctiva of the lateral angle of each eye at 5- to 15-minute intervals; close the eyes and rest for a while. In general, discomfort or pain will disappear or decrease within 8 to 16 hours with neither side effects nor discomfort.

*Notes*
_____

Cow's milk is not recommended for people with diarrhea or mucous discharge.

## Polished (White) Rice

*Good for diarrhea, morning sickness, difficult urination.*

### DESCRIPTION

○ Neutral; sweet; used as an energy tonic and a spleen tonic; affects the spleen and stomach.

### PREPARATION

○ Fry 1 bowlful polished rice with fresh ginger juice until the rice becomes yellowish. Chew 20 to 30 grains before getting up in the morning to relieve morning sickness.

○ Boil rice in water as you would normally, but cook it a little longer than usual to allow a thick crust of charred rice to form on the bottom of the pan; rice is neutral and bitter and sweet.

○ Boil 150g browned crust of rice with an equal amount of lotus fruits and sugar in an adequate amount of water. Drink 2 teaspoonfuls each time, 3 times a day, to cure diarrhea, particularly in children.

## Shiitake Mushrooms
*Good for prevention of rickets, anemia, measles.*

### DESCRIPTION

- Neutral; sweet; affects the stomach.

### PREPARATION

- Boil some shiitake mushrooms in water until the soup becomes yellow-ish. Drink only the liquid (without eating the mushrooms) to relieve vomiting caused by careless eating; another alternative is to place shi-itake mushrooms in boiling water and steep until the soup becomes yellowish. Drink it as tea.
- Dissolve some sugar or honey in the shiitake mushroom soup to treat coughing.
- Drink shiitake mushroom soup, or dissolve shiitake mushroom powder in hot water and drink it as tea to relieve fish poisoning. A prolonged consumption by this method is believed to prevent arteriosclerosis.
- In case of difficult urination or discharge of urine containing blood, bake some shiitake mushroom until it appears burned on the surface. Eat 10g each time, twice a day, or eat fresh shiitake mushrooms.

### EXPERIMENT

- Studies with rats show shiitake mushroom lowers blood fat levels.

### CLINICAL REPORT

- Shiitake mushroom counteracts cholesterol, a recent report indicates.

## Tea
*Good for headaches, blurred vision, sleepiness, thirst, indigestion, enteritis, bacillary dysentery, edema in heart disease, herpes zoster.*

### DESCRIPTION

- Bitter; sweet; slightly cold; quenches thirst; wakes up the spirits; pro-motes digestion and urination; affects the heart, lungs and stomach.

### PREPARATION

- Grind into powder 10g tea leaves and 10g dried ginger. Take one tea-spoonful powder with warm water each time, 2 to 3 times daily, to cure acute gastroenteritis.
- Grind tea leaves into powder; dissolve the powder in strong tea and apply externally to the affected region 2 to 3 times daily to cure herpes zoster.

### CLINICAL REPORT

- It is reported that among 168 cases of bacillary dysentery treated by drinking 2 ml strong tea 3 to 4 times daily, 40.6 percent recovered within a few days to a few weeks.
- Strong tea was also used to treat 87 cases of acute enteritis and more than 90 percent of patients recovered within 2 days; the same method was used to treat 12 cases of chronic enteritis. Ten cases completely recovered within 4 to 21 days with stools returning to normal; 2 cases improved to a very significant degree. The method of treatment: Drink 2 to 5 ml of very strong tea 3 to 4 times a day. (Tea leaves are boiled over low heat to make very strong tea, which is different from the nor-mal way of making tea by pouring hot water over tea leaves.)

*Notes*

Shiitake mushroom is believed to counteract stomach and cervical cancers. (When I visited Japan in October 1985, I learned that a new product containing the extract from shiitake mushroom had been approved by the Japanese government as an anti-cancerous agent.) The Chinese people are very fond of mushrooms, including shiitake mushrooms, which are produced primarily in Japan. Shiitake mushroom may be cooked by itself and it may also be cooked with other vegetables. In either case, avoid excessive amounts of soy sauce and salt because they are quickly absorbed by the mushroom and spoil its good taste.

## Trifoliate Orange

*Disperses liver energy, balances the stomach, regulates energy, relieves pain; good for abdominal swelling, stomachaches, hernia, pain, swollen testes and breast and prolapse of the uterus.*

## Wheat

*Nourishes heart energy, good for people with heart disease, insomnia, palpitations and hysteria.*

### PREPARATION

- Wheat may also be used for stomach weakness and diarrhea by preparing this simple recipe: Remove seeds from red dates and bake dry. Fry wheat flour and glutinous rice powder together without oil until they are yellowish. Grind dry red dates into powder. Mix the three ingredients together and take 30g of the mixture each time with warm water.

## White Fungus

*Increases yin energy in the body, lubricates the lungs, nourishes the stomach and produces fluids; good for coughs due to fatigue and body deficiency, blood in phlegm, thirst and hot sensations. However, coughs from the common cold should not be treated with white fungus.*

### PREPARATION

- To stop bleeding in hemorrhoids, boil 6g of white fungus with a persimmon cake in water until the fungus is extremely soft. Eat as a snack.

### Notes

Wheat that floats in water is dried and used as an important Chinese herb, which is called "floating wheat." It is stronger than wheat as a remedy. Floating wheat can increase energy, relieve mental depression, stop excessive perspiration and night sweats and cool burning sensations in the bones and in women with fatigue.

### Notes

White fungus can reduce heat and lubricate dryness in the lungs. It is often used to treat dry coughs, coughs with a little phlegm, nosebleeds and discharge of blood from the mouth.

White fungus is considerably more expensive than black fungus, but their functions are basically the same.

*F*ood cures for the spleen will treat and prevent deficiencies in this vital internal organ.

# Spleen Tonic Foods

## Apple Cucumbers

*Quench thirst, produce fluids, strengthen the spleen; good for edema and sunstroke.*

## Beef

*Good for those who are underweight and for diabetes, edema.*

### DESCRIPTION

- Neutral; sweet; used as a spleen, stomach, energy and blood tonic; affects the spleen and stomach.

### PREPARATION

- Eat regularly concentrated beef soup to relieve chronic diarrhea and prolapse of anus caused by chronic diarrhea.
- Mix together 1,000g beef, 10g ground black pepper, 5g dried orange peel powder; add 1 cup fresh ginger juice and an adequate amount of salt; marinate for 2 hours; cook the beef. Eat at meals to improve the conditions of stomach and stimulate the appetite. To make ginger juice, grate fresh ginger and boil it in water.

## Caraway Seeds

*Good for stomachaches, abdominal pain, hernias, lumbago.*

### DESCRIPTION

- Warm; slightly pungent; promotes energy circulation; good for the stomach; affects the kidneys and stomach.

### PREPARATION

- Boil 10g caraway seed with 5g cinnamon and 5g dried ginger; drink it as soup to treat vomiting and hiccupping.
- Boil 10g fennel seed in 3 cups water over low heat until water is reduced to 1 cup. Drink a cupful each time, twice a day, to relieve cough.

### EXPERIMENT

- Caraway has been found to relieve asthma in rats.

## Carrot

*Good for chronic diarrhea; coughs; indigestion; difficulty when urinating.*

### DESCRIPTION

- Neutral; sweet; pushes downwards; used as a diuretic and digestive; affects the lungs and spleen.

### PREPARATION

- Regular consumption of fresh or cooked carrot prevents night blindness.
- Boil carrot and red dates in water to make soup to treat whooping cough in children.
- Carrot may be cooked with parsley and water chestnut for facilitating eruption in measles.
- Fresh carrot juice may be used for external application to heal burns.
- Boil 5g carrot seeds in 2 glasses water over low heat until water is reduced to 1 glass. Drink the soup to promote urination for treatment of edema.

- Bake the peels of carrots until they appear burned. Eat the peels while hot to relieve frequent urination at night. Divide 1 carrot into 3 dosages and eat them 3 times a day.
- To use carrot as a blood tonic, cook it with spinach and lotus roots in soup; or, cook carrot with tomatoes, onion and beef; or, cook carrot with pork liver.
- For sharpening the vision, cook carrot with chicken liver or duck liver.

### EXPERIMENT

- Shows the effect of lowering blood sugar in animals.

## Cherry Leaves

*Warm the stomach, strengthen the spleen, stop bleeding; good for indigestion, diarrhea, vomiting of blood and hemorrhoids.*

## Cinnamon Bark

*Good for cold limbs, abdominal pain, diarrhea, hot sensations in the upper region with cold sensations in the lower region.*

### DESCRIPTION

- Hot; pungent and sweet; affects the kidneys, spleen and bladder.

### PREPARATION

- Grind dry cinnamon bark into powder; dissolve 5g of the powder in warm water and drink each time, 3 times a day, to cure various types of cold symptoms (including cold abdominal pain, cold abdominal swelling and cold stomachache).
- Dissolve 5g of the powder in rice wine and drink each time, 3 times a day, to alleviate abdominal pain in women after childbirth.
- Dissolve 3g cinnamon-bark powder in warm water to correct excessive gastric acid and vomiting of acid.
- Use cinnamon bark as a seasoning in cooking to warm up the body.

### EXPERIMENT

- Effects of cinnamon bark on animals indicate it calms the central nervous system in rats and also reduces their blood pressure.

## Corncobs

*Strengthen the spleen and remove dampness; good for diminished urination, edema, beriberi and diarrhea.*

## Crown Daisies

*Strengthen the spleen and stomach, increase memory, promote bowel movements and lubricate and remove phlegm from the lungs.*

### PREPARATION

- To suppress cough and remove phlegm, boil 90g of fresh crown daisies in water. Add some rock sugar and divide it into two dosages for one-day consumption.

To treat hypertension with headache, squeeze the juice from fresh crown daisies and drink a glass of juice two times daily.

## *Dillseed*

*Good for abdominal pain, poor appetite, shortage of milk secretion after childbirth.*

### DESCRIPTION

Warm; pungent; warms the body, promotes energy circulation and counteracts fish and meat poisoning; affects the spleen and kidneys.

### PREPARATION

Fry dillseeds until aromatic and grind into powder; dissolve 5g of the powder in warm rice wine and drink each time to cure lumbago due to twisted muscles.

## *Dog's Bone*

*Strengthens the spleen, activates the blood, builds muscles; used to treat rheumatic pain, weak loins and legs, numbness of limbs, chronic diarrhea and frostbite.*

## *Frog*

*Reduces internal heat, detoxifies and eliminates water in the body. When a frog is baked and reduced to ash, it can heal carbuncle with external applications. When it is cooked and eaten, it can correct weakness and tone deficiency; particularly good for women after childbirth. The juice relieves a red face and swollen neck.*

### PREPARATION

To cure a red face and swollen neck, crush a frog and squeeze the juice from it. Mix the juice with water and drink on an empty stomach.

To suppress menses, bake a frog and grind it into powder. Add a little wine and take 9g each time. Or, steam a frog with 90g of yellow soybeans. Eat at meals for three days in a row.

## *Garlic*

*Good for cold abdominal pain, edema, diarrhea, dysentery, whooping cough.*

### DESCRIPTION

Warm; pungent; promotes energy circulation, warms the stomach and spleen, destroys worms; affects the spleen, stomach and lungs.

### PREPARATION

Boil 3 garlic cloves in water and eat with soy sauce at meals to relieve cough and abdominal pain and also to promote blood circulation and urination.

For women, to relieve itch in the genital region, boil a few garlic cloves and use the liquid to wash the genital region.

Crush a few garlic cloves to mix with mustard (powder or paste) and eat it with rice wine. Or, boil a few garlic cloves in water and drink it as tea to correct chronic cold sensations, particularly in women. If wine is

Cinnamon Forests, a city in China named for its ubiquitous cinnamon trees, also has the most beautiful scenic views in the country. When I recently visited Cinnamon Forests I could smell cinnamon everywhere, including the downtown area and I was pleased as much by the plentiful cinnamon trees in the city as by its beautiful scenery.

*Notes*

Crown daisies contain plenty of carotene, in addition to essential oil and choline.

*Notes*

Dill leaf is warm, pungent and oppressive. According to 1 experiment, dill leaf is found to have the effect of lowering blood pressure and expanding blood vessels in animals.

*Notes*

People in southern China eat frog and call it a farm chicken, because its meat tastes like chicken meat.

desired, make garlic wine: Simply cut up a garlic clove in large pieces, drop into a small bottle of wine; put away for 1 month and it is ready to drink as a wine tonic.

- Eat 1 to 3 fresh garlic cloves daily by dividing them into 3 dosages; continue treatment for 5 to 10 consecutive days to heal amebic dysentery.
- Take 2 teaspoonfuls 10 to 20 percent garlic solution every 2 hours (mixed with some syrup or orange tincture to make it more appetizing) to relieve whooping cough in children.
- Eat garlic cloves regularly to prevent bacillary dysentery when it is widespread.
- Cut up a garlic clove and use the juicy slice to rub the skin to relieve pain caused by insect bite (such as bee sting) as an emergency measure.
- Garlic may be cooked with soybeans: Soak the soybeans overnight; cook soybeans with 5 to 10 garlic cloves. Eat as a tonic and also to promote urination, relieve edema and chronic nephritis.
- Another way to use garlic: Fry garlic cloves in vegetable oil with black pepper, sliced fresh ginger and salt; add dry shrimps, then sprinkle with sugar, vinegar and green onion. Add some tomato ketchup and flour to thicken, if desired. This recipe contains almost all the needed flavors—sweet, sour, pungent and salty.

### CLINICAL REPORT

- For treatment of lobar pneumonia; 1 tablespoon garlic syrup every 4 hours (in general 10 percent, but sometimes 100 percent). Among the 9 people treated, 6 cases show complete recovery, 3 show no satisfactory results.

## Grass Carp Gall

*Good for sore throats.*

## Fresh Ham

*Good for diarrhea, nervousness, poor appetite.*

### DESCRIPTION

- Warm; salty; used as a spleen tonic; stimulates the appetite; produces fluids; pushes downwards.

### PREPARATION

- Boil ham in water with red pepper to make soup; skim off and discard the floating fat. Drink the hot soup to relieve hiccupping and abdominal pain that has lasted for 3 to 4 days.
- Boil 200g ham in water over low heat for a full day until extremely tender; discard the fat from the surface. Drink as soup to relieve chronic diarrhea.

## Horse Bean

*Good for edema, tinea capitis.*

### DESCRIPTION

- Neutral; sweet; used as a spleen tonic; eliminates water retention; affects the spleen and stomach.

*Notes*

There have been fewer cases of pulmonary tuberculosis in Sandong, a province of China where people consume more garlic than in any other province. As a result of these findings, garlic has been made into tablets and used with good results.

In the northern provinces of China, Chinese people carry some garlic with them while on a long journey, just in case they have to drink water from mountains or rivers. To prevent bad effects, they chew a garlic clove like chewing gum and spit it out before drinking water.

Many people don't want to eat garlic for fear of getting bad breath. According to some people, "garlic" breath can be eliminated by eating a few red dates or a persimmon. When garlic cloves are steamed (over boiling water), the strong smell will be gone before eating the garlic.

In daily cooking, a few garlic slices may be added to eliminate the strong smell of meats or fish. It is believed that a small quantity of garlic can counteract cancer, but an excessive quantity of garlic can cause cancer (based on the Chinese theory that excessive garlic is bad for the stomach and liver).

Chinese people eat large quantities of garlic only under special circumstances, such as severe malnutrition or edema.

In recent years, garlic has emerged as an important ingredient in Chinese medicine, mostly due to its powerful effects in treating dysentery and destroying germs. In fact, many modern medicines contain garlic as an important ingredient. For dysentery at its early stage, chew a garlic clove five or six times a day every four hours.

Contraindications of garlic include eye diseases and sore throat.

## PREPARATION

- Boil 70g horse beans and 70g wax gourd peels in water. Drink as tea to cure edema.
- Crush fresh horse beans into a cream. Apply externally to the affected region to relieve tinea capitis; or use dried horse beans, if necessary.
- Dry fresh horse beans in the sun to grind into powder. Take 2 teaspoonfuls of the powder dissolved in warm water each time, 3 times a day, to cure diarrhea and discharge of stools containing blood.
- Boil horse bean powder with sugar in water. Drink as tea to relieve poor appetite and diarrhea in children (white sugar should be used in the absence of discharge of blood but brown sugar in the presence of blood from the anus). The older the powder is, the better its effects will be.

## Hyacinth Bean Flowers

*Strengthen the spleen, balance the stomach, counteract summer heat, remove dampness; good for dysentery and diarrhea.*

## Hyacinth Beans

*Good for diarrhea and vomiting in summer, vaginal discharge, malnutrition in children.*

### DESCRIPTION

- Neutral; sweet; used as a spleen tonic; reduces water retention; affects the spleen and stomach.

### PREPARATION

- Grind hyacinth beans into powder. Take 15g of the powder dissolved in warm water each time, 3 times a day, to cure acute gastroenteritis, vomiting and diarrhea; or boil 50g hyacinth beans and drink as soup, 3 times a day. The same remedy may also be used to cure difficulty when urinating.
- Grind hyacinth beans into powder. Take 15g of the powder dissolved in rice soup each time, 3 times a day, to relieve quickening in women due to taking drugs; or, drink concentrated juice of hyacinth bean, twice a day.
- Cook a bowl of hyacinth beans with sugar and eat it at meals to cure chronic diarrhea.

## Japanese Cassia Bark

*Warms the middle region, strengthens the stomach and warms the loins and knees; particularly good for cold abdominal pain and swelling.*

### PREPARATION

- To relieve abdominal pain in women after childbirth, boil 50g of Japanese cassia bark with 15g of brown sugar; drink warm.
- To relieve swelling and pain in the lower abdomen before menstruation, boil 7g of Japanese cassia bark, 10g of hawthorn fruits, 40g of brown sugar. Drink before the onset of menstruation.
- To cure cold stomachaches, grind 4g of Japanese cassia bark and take once a day.

*Notes*

Japanese cassia bark tastes pungent and sweet with a slightly hot energy.

Japanese cassia bark can nurture the spirits and improve the complexion. One will feel light in the body after a prolonged consumption and live a long life, with complexion so shiny that one will always remain youthful.

## Job's Tears Roots

*Reduce internal heat, remove water in the body and strengthen the spleen; good for jaundice, edema and hernias.*

## Longan

*Good for insomnia, forgetfulness, palpitations, nervousness.*

### DESCRIPTION

- Warm; sweet; used as a spleen tonic, heart tonic, blood tonic and energy tonic; affects the heart and spleen.

### PREPARATION

- Steam 15g longans with 30g lean pork, 2 fresh ginger slices and an adequate amount of rice wine. Eat once a day to relieve dizziness and underweight.
- Mix 500g longans with 500g sugar; steam them to make longan jelly.
- Take 1 spoonful longan jelly with warm water to relieve dizziness and edema after childbirth; or boil 15g longans with 5 red dates, 30g brown sugar and 6g fresh ginger. Drink it as soup once a day.

## Lotus Fruit, Lotus Seed and Lotus Root

*Good for dreaminess, seminal emission, chronic diarrhea, vaginal bleeding and discharge.*

### DESCRIPTION

- Neutral; sweet; obstructive; used as a spleen tonic, heart tonic and kidney tonic; lotus root is also used as calmative; affects the heart, spleen and kidneys.

### PREPARATION

- Boil 30g dried lotus fruits and 30g brown sugar in 30g rice wine; add 1 chicken egg as in egg-drop soup. Drink the soup every evening for 1 month to improve physical conditions after childbirth or excessive fatigue due to old age.
- Steam lotus fruits until cooked. Leave them in the sun to dry; grind into powder. Take 15g of the powder each time, 3 times a day, to cure chronic diarrhea.
- Steam 250g dried lotus fruits with 6g rice wine and 6g lard. Take the entire dosage 3 times a day for 1 month to cure ulcers or during the recovery stage after stomach bleeding.
- Mix 180g lotus seeds and 30g licorice and grind into powder. Take 3 to 6g powder each time with warm water, 3 times a day, to relieve discharge of a short stream of red urine.
- Crush a few fresh lotus roots; squeeze out the juice. Drink a glass of the juice each time to stop bleeding of various kinds, including nosebleed, vaginal bleeding, discharge of blood from anus and vomiting of blood.

## Mullet (Black or Striped)

*Increases appetite and improves the conditions of internal organs; good for putting on weight.*

### Notes

It is interesting to note that lotus was referred to in Greek legend as yielding a fruit which induced a state of dreamy and contented forgetfulness in those who ate it. But in Chinese herbal remedies, it is believed that lotus fruit may be eaten to relieve dreaminess.

## Pearl Sago
*Good for indigestion and a weak stomach.*

## Perch
*Tones the liver and kidneys and strengthens the stomach and spleen; good for rheumatism and edema.*

## Pheasant
*Tones the internal region and strengthens body energy; good for diarrhea, frequent urination and diabetes.*

## Pineapples
*Good for edema, indigestion, diarrhea, vomiting, abdominal swelling.*

### DESCRIPTION
- Neutral; sweet and sour; promotes urination and digestion; quenches thirst; heals swelling.

### PREPARATION
- Fry 250g fresh pineapple, sliced, with 60g chicken in oil, seasoned with pepper and salt. Eat every day, or every other day, to relieve dizziness due to low blood pressure.
- Eat 4 slices fresh pineapple or drink a glass of fresh pineapple juice each time, twice a day, to relieve indigestion, abdominal swelling, vomiting, or diarrhea.
- Drink a glass of fresh pineapple juice seasoned with a little salt each time, twice a day, to relieve thirst from fever.

**Notes**

It is advisable to eat pineapple with a little salt to eliminate a slight itching at the tip of tongue.

Bromelain in pineapple has been used to heal various types of inflammation, edema and thrombus.

Pineapple is not recommended for people with eczema or carbuncle.

## Polished (White) Rice
*Good for diarrhea, morning sickness, difficult urination.*

### DESCRIPTION
- Neutral; sweet; used as an energy tonic and a spleen tonic; affects the spleen and stomach.

### PREPARATION
- Fry 1 bowlful polished rice with fresh ginger juice until the rice becomes yellowish. Chew 20 to 30 grains before getting up in the morning to relieve morning sickness.
- Boil rice in water as you would normally, but cook it a little longer than usual to allow a thick crust of charred rice to form on the bottom of the pan; rice is neutral and bitter and sweet.
- Boil 150g browned crust of rice with an equal amount of lotus fruits and sugar in an adequate amount of water. Drink 2 teaspoonfuls each time, 3 times a day, to cure diarrhea, particularly in children.

**Notes**

Rice sprouts are sweet and warm; they can promote digestion and also make the stomach stronger. Therefore, rice sprouts can be used to treat the digestive disorders effectively.

When fresh sprouts are to be used as a stomach tonic, they should be fried until yellowish but not burned.

Rice sprouts contain starch, protein, fat, amylase and vitamin B₁.

Unlike maltose, which is mostly used as a digestive aid, rice sprouts can strengthen the spleen and increase body energy.

## Rice Sprouts
*Beneficial for the spleen and stomach; good for hiccups and indigestion.*

## *Royal Jelly*

*Good for those suffering from underdevelopment, loss of weight, poor appetite, hepatitis, neurasthenia, nodular phlebitis, malnutrition, rheumatoid arthritis, anemia, gastric ulcers.*

### DESCRIPTION

- Royal jelly, a modern product not recorded in traditional Chinese diet classics, is now widely used to promote growth, slow down the aging process and prevent loss of hair; it is produced from a secretion of the worker bees' salivary glands and fermented with honey pollen and other ingredients and specially used as food for the queen bees. This explains why virtually all queen bees are able to live up to 5 years whereas worker bees can live only 2 to 4 months. On top of that, at the height of the laying season, a single queen bee can lay 2,500 to 3,000 ovules that weigh more than the queen bee's own body.

## *Sheep's or Goat's Blood*

*Treats nosebleeds, vomiting of blood, blood coagulations due to external injuries, bleeding from the anus as in hemorrhoids and heart pain.*

## *String Bean (Green Bean)*

*Good for diarrhea, vomiting, diabetes, seminal emission, whitish vaginal discharge, frequent urination.*

### DESCRIPTION

- Neutral; sweet; used as a kidney tonic and a spleen tonic; affects the spleen and kidneys.

### PREPARATION

- Boil 50g dried string beans (with the shells) in water. Drink as soup once a day to relieve diabetes, thirst and frequent urination.

## *Sweet (Glutinous) Rice*

*Good for excessive urination, excessive perspiration, diarrhea.*

### DESCRIPTION

- Warm; sweet; used as an energy tonic; affects the spleen, stomach and lungs.

### PREPARATION

- Fry sweet rice with wheat bran and grind into powder. Take 10g powder in warm water each time, 3 times a day, to stop excessive perspiration.
- Cook 50g sweet rice with 60g Job's tears and 8 red dates. Eat at meals to relieve pulmonary tuberculosis, neurasthenia, anemia and various kinds of chronic diseases.
- Boil sweet rice sprouts in water with malt. Drink the soup to relieve indigestion and to promote appetite.

## *Whitefish*

*Improves appetite, strengthens the spleen and promotes digestion and urination.*

Notes

Royal jelly is available in tablet form.

Notes

Sheep's or goat's blood contains 16.4 percent protein, primarily hemoglobin, with some hemocyania and serum globulin and a small amount of fibrin. Sheep's or goat's blood is salted and neutral. It can tone and cool the blood, which is why it is particularly good for women with blood deficiency, stroke and exhaustion after childbirth.

## Yam

*Good for chronic diarrhea, coughs, diabetes, seminal emission, vaginal discharge, frequent urination.*

### DESCRIPTION

- Neutral; sweet, spleen tonic, lung tonic and kidney tonic; affects the lungs, spleen and kidneys.

### PREPARATION

- Prepare 80g raw yam and grind into powder. Wash an equal amount of glutinous (sweet) rice and drain it; put rice in the sun to dry. Toast the rice in a pan, shaking or stirring, until yellowish and grind into powder. Mix the yam and rice. Take 4 spoonfuls of the powder, some sugar and black pepper dissolved in warm water each morning to treat chronic diarrhea and poor appetite.
- Boil yam with ginseng for 30 minutes and drink it as tea. Or make a soup with yam and beef or pork.

*T*he regulating foods for excess diseases caused by toxic heat are either cool or cold in nature.

# Foods for Eliminating Toxic Heat

## Adzuki Bean Flowers

*Reduce internal heat, quench thirst, relieve alcoholism and detoxicate; good
for malaria, dysentery, diabetes, headaches due to intoxication, bleeding in
hemorrhoids and erysipelas.*

## Adzuki Beans

*Good for edema, beriberi, jaundice, diarrhea, discharge of blood from anus,
carbuncle swelling, mumps, cirrhotic ascites.*

### DESCRIPTION

- Neutral; sweet and sour; facilitates urination; heals swelling; detoxicates; affects the heart and small intestine.

### PREPARATION

- Boil 100g adzuki beans in water with 300g wax gourd. Drink as soup
at meals once a day to relieve nephritis, beriberi and trophedema.
- Grind adzuki beans into powder and mix with honey. Apply to a carbuncle to heal the swelling.
- Boil 100g adzuki beans in water. Eat at meals to promote milk secretion
after childbirth.
- Fry 300g adzuki beans until charred. Add 6 bowlfuls of water and boil
until water is reduced to 3 bowlfuls. Add some brown sugar as seasoning. Drink 1 bowl of soup each time, 3 times a day, to relieve abdominal pain due to blood coagulations after childbirth.

### CLINICAL REPORT

- For a treatment of cirrhotic ascites: Boil 1 pound of adzuki beans with
a common carp (more than 1 pound) in 2 to 3 L water until the beans
break. Eat the beans and fish and drink the soup separately, daily or every
other day until cured. Results of 2 cases treated showed increased urination and reduced abdominal size, with good spirits and no side effects.
- A report on the treatment of mumps: Grind 50 to 70 adzuki beans into
powder; mix it with warm water and egg white or honey to make a cream
to apply to the affected region; cover it with a bandage. In general, swelling
disappears with one treatment; all 7 cases treated showed good results.

## Aloe Vera

*Reduces internal heat, promotes bowel movements, destroys worms; good for
constipation, suppression of menstruation, convulsions in children, atrophic
rhinitis and scrofula.*

## Bamboo Shoots

*Good for measles, mucous discharge.*

### DESCRIPTION

- Cold; sweet; glossy.

## Banana Rhizomes

*Reduce heat, cool the blood and detoxicate; good for asthma, blood in urine
and skin diseases.*

### Notes

There are many kinds of ordinary red
beans that should be distinguished
from adzuki beans under discussion. Ordinary red beans are round
in shape whereas adzuki beans are
long. Ordinary red beans have a neutral energy, bitter flavor, are normally
used to promote energy circulation
and menstrual flow and are considered good for hernia, abdominal pain
and the suppression of menstruation.

### Notes

Bamboo shoot is a valuable ingredient in cooking meats because it
has a cold energy. When it is cooked
with meat, the bamboo shoot neu-
tralizes the effects of the warm or
hot energy in meat and, therefore,
strikes a balance between the 2 ingredients. Like mushroom, bamboo
shoot is widely used in the Chinese
meat cookery.

Many centuries ago, a celebrated Chinese poet was so fond of the combination, he wrote a poem emphasiz-
ing that meats and bamboo shoots

## Bananas

*Good for constipation, hemorrhoids, hypertension, alcoholism.*

### DESCRIPTION

- Cold; sweet; lubricates the intestines; detoxicates.

### PREPARATION

- Eat 1 to 2 very soft bananas twice a day before bedtime and first thing in the morning on an empty stomach to relieve constipation.
- Eat 1 to 2 fresh bananas, three times a day, to relieve thirst in a hot disease.
- Steam 2 half-ripe bananas with their peels until very soft. Eat twice a day, the first thing in the morning on an empty stomach and before bedtime, to cure hemorrhoids and discharge of blood from anus after bowel movements.
- Boil 1 banana peel or stem in water and drink it as tea, a cupful each time, 3 times a day, to treat and prevent hypertension.
- Place 500g banana and 15g black sesame in a blender and mix them. Eat in one day to treat hypertension with constipation.
- Steam 2 very soft bananas with their peels. Eat the banana and peel twice a day, first thing in the morning on an empty stomach and before bedtime, to cure asthma and cough due to hot lungs.
- Boil 60g banana peel in water and drink the liquid for relief of alcoholism and hangover.

### EXPERIMENT

- An experiment on animals shows unripe banana is effective in the treatment and prevention of gastric ulcers.

## Bean Curd (Tofu)

*Good for pink eye, diabetes, periodic diarrhea, sulfur poisoning.*

### DESCRIPTION

- Cool; sweet; used as an energy tonic; produces fluids; lubricates dryness; detoxicates; affects the spleen, stomach and large intestine.

### PREPARATION

- Prepare 1 bowl bean curd, 70g maltose and half a cup of fresh radish juice; combine the 3 ingredients in a pan, add half a cup of water and bring to a boil once. Divide the soup into 2 dosages and drink twice a day to treat asthma with mucous discharge, including acute bronchial asthma.
- Crush a number of bean curds and apply the mash to the legs to heal erysipelas on the legs; change the dressing as soon as the mash dries.

## Bear's Gallbladder

*Reduces internal heat, relieves spasms, sharpens vision; often used to treat diarrhea, film in the eyes, convulsions and malnutrition in children and pain in the eyes.*

### PREPARATION

- To cure acute conjunctivitis and pink eye with swelling, mix a small bear's gallbladder with milk (human or cow's) for use as eye drops.
- Bear's gallbladder is also used as a stomach and heart tonic and to detoxicate and reduce inflammation. This has a great deal to do with its extreme cold and bitter nature.

are the 2 most appreciated ingredients at his dinner table.

As Western people consume a large quantity of meat every day, it is wise to use bamboo shoots when cooking.

Some people suffer from a skin disease that seems hidden beneath the skin, so to speak, because it won't go away nor will it erupt to the surface. When this happens, bamboo shoot can speed up the eruption, so that one can get it over with. This is also why bamboo shoot is good for measles before eruption of the rash.

Bamboo leaves have a cold energy and light-sweet flavor. The leaves produce fluids, promote urination, are good for difficult urination with discharge of short streams of red urine.

*Notes*

All gallbladders are extremely bitter and cold; they can act on the liver and gallbladder to reduce excessive heat in them.

Malnutrition in children often leads to film in the eyes, which often involve the liver, gallbladder and spleen, with excessive heat in those organs, for which bear's gallbladder can be an effective remedy.

## Bitter Endive

*Reduces internal heat, cools the blood and detoxicates; good for dysentery, jaundice, blood in urine and hemorrhoids.*

## Bitter Gourd (Wild Cucumber)

*Good for sunstroke, dysentery, pink eyes and pain in eyes.*

### DESCRIPTION

- Cold; bitter; detoxicates; sharpens the vision; affects the heart, spleen and stomach.

### PREPARATION

- Fry bitter gourd seeds and grind into powder. Take 10g of the powder dissolved in wine each time, twice a day, to cure impotence.
- Regular consumption of bitter gourd improves eyesight.

## Brake (Fern)

*Reduces internal heat, settles the intestines, removes phlegm.*

## Burdock

*Reduces internal heat and swelling, dissipates gas, detoxicates; good for coughs, sore throats and measles that fail to erupt.*

## Camphor Mint

*Promotes energy circulation, stops bleeding, reduces inflammation; good for common colds, vomiting of blood, nosebleeds, blood in stools.*

## Cattail

*Lubricates dryness, cools the blood; good for diminished urination and mastitis.*

## Celery Seeds

*Good for spasms and twitching muscles.*

## Chicken Egg White

*Good for sore throats, pink eyes, cough, diarrhea, burns.*

### DESCRIPTION

- Cool; sweet; detoxicates; lubricates the lungs; cools hot sensations; considered beneficial to the throat.

### PREPARATION

- Boil a chicken egg and remove it from the water as soon as it starts to boil; make a hole in the shell and slowly suck the white through the hole to lubricate the throat, once a day, for 3 or 4 months to relieve sore throat, hoarseness and loss of voice and to protect the throat in professional singers.
- Mix egg white with rice wine and use the mixture to wash the affected

**Notes**

Bitter gourd is regarded as the king of bitter foods. It is bad for people with a weak stomach because it could cause vomiting. But it is good for those with a hot physical constitution as it can cool down the internal region and relieve hot constipation.

According to Chinese medical theory, bitter foods can improve the conditions of the liver (which is why bitter gourd is good for liver disease).

region to heal burns and skin ulcers.
- Mix egg white with 3 teaspoonfuls rice vinegar. Drink it to resume menstruation after childbirth.

## CLINICAL REPORT

- For a treatment of burns, place a chicken egg in 75 percent alcohol and sterilize for 15 minutes; open 2 holes on 2 ends of the egg using a sterile instrument and let the egg white flow into a sterilized container. After debridement (cut off blisters, if any), use a sterilized cotton ball to apply egg white to the burned areas for 2 to 3 times on the first day. In general, a yellowish crust will form on the wound within 6 to 15 hours; by this time, the pain will decrease and the secretion of fluids either ceases or decreases. If the crust forms incompletely, with cracks, apply egg white again until it forms properly and completely. If, however, suppuration occurs under the crust (mostly seen in third degree burns), cut the crust open and incise the pus thoroughly and then apply egg white again. When burns involve a large area, a lamp may be used to maintain the desired temperature (25 and 31 degrees C). Among the 100 plus patients treated, the majority of patients with first degree and second degree burns (involving areas less than 10 percent) recovered within 10 days; the remaining patients recovered within 12 to 31 days. The majority of patients with first and second degree burns (involving areas between 10 to 20 percent) recovered within 7 to 20 days while the minority recovered within 37 to 60 days. It takes longer for patients to recover in cases of severe second and third degree burns with areas over 30 percent and complications.
- A report on treatment of infections on the body surface shows that egg white relieves pain, heals inflammation and prevents suppuration by external applications; and in case of suppurated regions, egg white is found to control inflammation and localize it. Among the 36 cases treated, the patients with smaller areas infected recovered within a single application; the patients with larger areas recovered within 3 to 4 applications. The method of application is similar to the one used in burns.
- A clinical report on the treatment of cervical erosion indicates the method of applications is similar to burns. Use a cotton ball to apply egg white to the erosive areas and then push the cotton ball filled with egg white into the cervix to be removed next day. Each treatment program lasts 3 to 5 days; a second program continues if no results are obtained and treatment stops during the menstruation period. Among the 32 cases treated, 18 cases recovered and 7 cases improved with 7 cases interrupted. It is indicated that those with bleeding show best results; in addition, the 7 cases treated for cervicitis and vaginitis (developed after childbirth) recovered completely.
- A clinical report on the treatment of otitis media purulenta shows that a mixture of equal quantities of egg white and sesame oil produce satisfactory results when used as ear drops.

## Chicken Gallbladder
*Cures blurred vision and boils on the skin.*

## PREPARATION

- To cure whooping cough, mix chicken gallbladder with white sugar: Give one Gallbladder every 3 days to children under one year old; one gallbladder every 2 days to those under 2 years old; one gallbladder every day to those over 2 years old. Divide into two dosages in each case to

be taken with warm water. Alternatively, bake the gallbladder and grind
it into powder. Take one gallbladder every day for those over 2 years old.
- To cure quartan malaria, swallow a chicken gallbladder 2 hours before
onset; repeat once every other day for 3 days.

## Chinese Endive
*Reduces heat and detoxicates; good for acute bacillary dysentery and acute
pharyngitis.*

## Chinese Rose
*Promotes blood circulation, regulates menstruation, reduces swelling and
detoxicates; good for period pain, injuries, swelling and pain caused by blood
coagulation carbuncle.*

## Chinese Toon
*Expels phlegm, removes water from the body, stops bleeding and relieves pain.*

## Chinese Toon Leaves
*Heal inflammation and detoxicate; good for enteritis and skin eruptions.*

## Chrysanthemums
*Reduce internal heat, sharpen vision and detoxicate; good for headaches,
dizziness, pink eye, skin eruptions.*

## Clam
*Saltwater clams good for edema, mucous discharge, goiter, vaginal discharge,
hemorrhoids; freshwater clams good for vaginal bleeding and discharge, pink
eyes, eczema and hemorrhoids; saltwater clamshell powder good for diabetes,
edema, goiter and hemorrhoids; freshwater clam saliva good for diabetes,
pink eyes and burns; freshwater clamshell powder good for cough with
mucous discharge, stomachache, hiccupping, vomiting, whitish vaginal discharge, eczema, swelling.*

### DESCRIPTION

- Sea (saltwater) clam—cold, salty, acts on the stomach, promotes water
passage, eliminates mucus and softens hardness; freshwater clam—cold,
sweet and salty, detoxicates, sharpens the vision, acts on the liver and
kidneys. Sea clamshell powder-cold, salty, promotes water passage, softens hardness, eliminates mucus, acts on the lungs and kidneys; river clam
saliva—sharpens vision; freshwater clamshell powder—cold, salty, eliminates mucus and dries dampness, acts on the lungs, liver and stomach.

### PREPARATION

- Sea clamshell may be baked and ground into very fine powder to make
sea clamshell powder. Freshwater clamshell may be washed clean (with
the black skin removed) and ground into powder or baked and ground
into powder to make freshwater clamshell powder. Apply saltwater
clam's saliva externally to the affected region to relieve itching and pain
and swelling of the vaginal orifice.

- Crush a few garlics to mix with clamshell powder and make into tablets of a normal size. Take 10 tablets with warm water each time, once a day, to relieve edema in weak persons.
- Mix clamshell powder with lard for external application to the affected region to relieve burns.
- Mix fine clamshell powder with an equal amount of raw licorice powder, take 7g each time with warm water, twice a day, to cure gastric ulcer and excessive gastric acid.
- Regular consumption of clam meat at meals relieves lymphadenitis scrofula in the neck and goiter.
- Cook clam with chive. Eat at meals to relieve pulmonary tuberculosis and night sweat.
- Boil 30g fine clamshell powder with 4g outer layer of peanuts and 6 red dates to make concentrated soup. Drink the soup once a day to relieve nosebleed, bleeding from gums and purpura hemorrhagica.
- Roast a whole freshwater clam until its outer part is charred and the inner part becomes yellow-brown with its original shape remaining intact; grind into fine powder and mix with sesame oil for external application to relieve eczema in infants.

## CLINICAL REPORT

- For treatment of gastric and duodenal ulcers, fry freshwater clamshell powder in a bronze fry pan (or any earthenware fry pan) until it becomes yellow-brown with the fishy smell gone; strain it before using. Take 1 to 2g each time mixed with warm water, once every hour during the daytime, 12 to 14 times a day, for 4 to 8 weeks. Among the 41 cases treated from 14 to 79 days, 28 cases showed disappearance of pain in the upper abdomen and 7 cases a decrease, 23 cases showed disappearance of pressure pain in the upper abdomen (pain that occurs on pressure by hand) and 6 cases a decrease; 21 cases had a follow-up X-ray examination, which indicated disappearance of the niche in 9 cases, disappearance of deformity in 1 case and a reduction in the size of the niche in 6 cases.

## Cow's Gallbladder

*Reduces heat in the internal region, quenches thirst; frequently used to treat diarrhea, dry and hot sensations in the mouth, blurred vision and carbuncle with swelling.*

## PREPARATION

- To treat blurred vision, soak black soybeans in bile for 100 days. Eat 14 beans every evening.
- To cure whooping cough, mix a cow's gallbladder with 100g of white sugar. Warm it over low heat until the sugar dissolves into the gallbladder completely. Take one teaspoon with warm water three times daily.
- To cure chronic tracheitis, coughs and asthma, take 3g of bile powder three times daily.

## Crabs

*Good for fractures and dislocations, tinea, skin eruption caused by lacquer.*

## DESCRIPTION

- Cold; salty; relieves blood coagulations; cools hot sensations; facilitates recovery of dislocations; affects the liver and stomach.

## PREPARATION

- Crush a fresh crab to mix with hot broth. Drink it frequently and apply remaining crab to the affected region to restore dislocations; or mix ash of burned crab with liquor for oral consumption to restore dislocations and heal fractures.
- Crush a fresh crab and apply it to the affected region to relieve lacquer-induced skin eruptions and tinea.
- Bake a crab until charred and grind into powder and mix with rice wine. Take 10g of the powder and wine each time, twice a day, to relieve jaundice.
- Roast a few crabs until charred and grind into powder. Take 10g powder with rice wine each time, twice a day, to relieve hypogastric pain after childbirth.
- Bake 1 male crab and 1 female crab and grind into powder; take the powder with wine all at once to facilitate the healing of breast cancer.
- Wrap a fresh crab in a clean cloth, crush it to squeeze out the juice; apply the juice to the affected region for relief of lacquer-induced skin eruptions, or drink the juice all at once to stop or suppress coughing.

## Eggplant

*Good for discharge of blood from anus, dysentery with discharge of blood, discharge of urine containing blood.*

### DESCRIPTION

- Cool; sweet; affects the spleen, stomach and large intestine.

### PREPARATION

- Boil in water white eggplants and drink the soup with honey to relieve cough.
- Bake some peel from a fresh eggplant until it appears black as charcoal on the outside but inside intact; mix with honey. Put it in the mouth like chewing gum to cure stomatitis.

### CLINICAL REPORT

- Eggplant contains vitamin P, which can prevent hardening of blood vessels and is useful in the treatment of arteriosclerosis, a report from China indicates. According to the statistics, the elderly Chinese are much less susceptible to apoplexy caused by cerebrovascular accident than their Western counterparts, attributed to the Chinese habit of eating eggplant. The same report points out two reasons for the elderly Chinese to consume more eggplants: Eggplants are much less expensive than other vegetables or meats; and eggplants can be cooked softer than other vegetables or meats, therefore easier for the elderly Chinese to eat (as most of them have lost most of their teeth). In addition, the Chinese people in general are fond of eggplants because of the taste.

## Figs

*Good for enteritis, dysentery, constipation, hemorrhoids, sore throat, diarrhea.*

### DESCRIPTION

- Neutral; sweet; detoxicates; used as stomachic tonic; affects the spleen and large intestine.

*Notes*

A male crab has a long navel while a female crab has a round navel.

Normally freshwater crabs are used in Chinese diet.

Crab claw is fairly strong in dissolving blood coagulations and is not recommended for pregnant women (it can cause miscarriage).

Crab shell powder may also be used for a variety of therapeutic purposes. To make the powder, bake crab shell and grind into powder. Take 10g powder with rice wine each time, twice a day, to relieve hypogastric pain after childbirth and acute mastitis.

*Notes*

Eggplant is considered obstructive to some extent, which explains why it can heal various kinds of bleeding. stops bleeding. Fresh eggplant can also relieve mushroom poisoning.

*Notes*

Fig leaf is neutral in energy and tastes sweet and slightly pungent; it can heal hemorrhoids and heart pain and swelling.

## PREPARATION

- Eat 1 to 2 fresh figs each time, in the morning and evening, to wake up appetite and correct indigestion.
- Eat 1 to 2 fresh figs at bedtime to relieve constipation, particularly in the elderly.
- Steam until very soft 1 to 2 fresh figs and 2 honey dates (processed in honey). Eat 1 to 2 figs each day to relieve dry cough and sore throat.
- Boil 1kg dry figs in water at low heat until they are soft as jelly. Add 750g sugar and heat until sugar dissolves. Then mix all the ingredients; take 1 teaspoonful fig jelly each time, in the morning and evening, to correct weakness after illness. Fig jelly is also used as adjuvant therapy for pulmonary tuberculosis and hepatitis.
- Boil until very soft 1 to 3 fresh figs or 30g dry figs with 60g lean pork and 2 red dates; eat once a day to increase milk secretion in women after childbirth.
- Boil 60g fresh figs with 60g pork or with 1 chicken egg and 15g rice wine. Eat once a day to relieve pain in muscles and bones and numbness from rheumatism.
- Fry 30g dry figs until aromatic; separately, fry 9g dry ginger until it looks like charcoal. Boil together the figs and ginger. Eat 3 times a day, to cure chronic diarrhea.
- Eat 2 unripe fresh figs in the morning and evening to alleviate pain and bleeding in hemorrhoids.

## Goose's Gallbladder

*Good for external applications for hemorrhoids.*

## Grapefruit

*Good for indigestion, bad breath due to intoxication, poor appetite in pregnant women.*

### DESCRIPTION

- Cold; sweet and sour.

### PREPARATION

- Steam 90g peeled grapefruit with half a cup rice wine and 1 cup honey. Drink it all in 1 day to relieve cough with mucous discharge.
- Eat 1 medium grapefruit each time, 3 times a day, to relieve indigestion, belching and mouth watering in pregnant women.
- Slowly eat 1 small grapefruit to relieve intoxication.

## Grape Leaves

*Good for edema, urination difficulty, pink eye, carbuncle swelling.*

## Hair Vegetable

*Reduces internal heat, eliminates congestion, softens hard spots, removes phlegm and purges intestines; used for hypertension, malnutrition, anemia, chronic tracheitis, goiter, tumors and cancer.*

*Notes*

Hair vegetable is a wild vegetable that grows like tangled hair on the ground; it is also called "dragon's mustache vegetable."

## Honey

*Good for dry coughs, constipation, stomachaches, sinusitis, mouth cankers, burns, neurasthenia, hypertension, pulmonary tuberculosis, heart disease, liver disease.*

### DESCRIPTION

- Neutral; sweet; detoxicates; lubricates dryness; relieves pain; affects the lungs, spleen and large intestine.

### PREPARATION

- Steam about half a cup honey. Eat it all at once on an empty stomach, 3 times a day, for 2 to 3 weeks on end, to relieve gastric and duodenal ulcers.
- Mix half a cup honey with warm water and drink once a day to treat hypertension, constipation, stomachache, neurasthenia, heart disease and coronary sclerosis.
- Drink a cup honey water at bedtime to cure insomnia due to neurasthenia. Externally apply honey to the affected region to relieve burns.
- Mix 3 large spoonfuls honey in boiling water. Drink it in the morning and in the evening to relieve insomnia, headache and anemia; or eat honey at meals with other foods.
- Using a sterilized cotton ball, externally apply honey to the anus to heal cracked skin in hemorrhoids; or externally apply to the ear to relieve swelling of the ear.
- Mix 2 teaspoonfuls honey with warm water. Drink it first thing in the morning on an empty stomach to relieve chronic constipation.
- Mix 1 teaspoonful honey with warm water and drink it 3 hours after meals, 3 times a day, for 5 consecutive days, to relieve hoarseness caused by excessive fatigue but unrelated to common cold, with sufficient rest to produce best results.

### CLINICAL REPORT

- For treatment of gastric and duodenal ulcers; among 20 cases treated, the niche disappeared in 15 cases, showed progress in 3 cases (32 days on the average), pain completely disappeared in 18 and pain decreased in 2; pain was gone as quickly as 6 days and within 22 days on the average. The method of treatment: each day, eat a third cup fresh honey before meals, 3 times a day; after the tenth day, increase the quantity of honey to half a cup each day.
- Clinical reports on treatment of other diseases showed good results: For treatment of acute bacillary dysentery, take 150g honey each day for adults (divide into 4 reduced dosages for children); for treatment of chronic and or temporary constipation in the elderly and in pregnant women, take honey first thing in the morning; for treatment of hypochromic anemia, take 80 to 100g honey each day, divided into 3 dosages; the results show an obvious increase in blood cells and hemoglobin.

## Honeysuckle

*Reduces internal heat and detoxicates; good for carbuncle, swelling of the skin, scrofula and hemorrhoids.*

## Honeysuckle Stem Leaf

*Good for enteritis, contagious hepatitis and arthritis.*

## Leaf Beets (Spinach Beets, Swiss Chard)

*Reduce internal heat, detoxicate, dissolve blood coagulations and arrest bleeding; good for measles that fail to erupt, dysentery and carbuncle.*

## Licorice

*Good for abdominal pain, poor appetites, fatigue, fever, coughs, palpitations, convulsions, sore throats, digestive ulcers, drug poisoning, food poisoning.*

### DESCRIPTION

- Neutral; sweet; slows down acute diseases, lubricates lungs, counteracts toxic effects, coordinates the effects of other herbs; affects the spleen, stomach and lungs.

### PREPARATION

- Prepare 150g processed licorice and 80g dry ginger; boil in only enough water to cover the 2 ingredients; boil until the water is reduced by half; strain and drink 1 cup of the warm soup each time, twice a day, to cure abscessed lungs, suppurative pneumonia and bronchitis without cough.
- Boil 10g licorice with 20g whole wheat kernels and 5 Chinese red dates. Drink as soup to treat hysteria in women, anxiety and stress. This is a time-honored herbal formula in Chinese medicine.

## Lily Flower

*Good for insomnia, cough, nervousness.*

### DESCRIPTION

- Cool; sweet; lubricates the lungs; relieves nervousness; affects the lungs.

### PREPARATION

- Boil 40g lily flowers for half an hour and sweeten with sugar. Drink the juice at bedtime to cure insomnia.

## Lotus Rhizomes

*Cooked lotus rhizomes can strengthen the spleen, improve appetite, nourish the blood, build muscles and stop diarrhea. Fresh lotus rhizomes can stop bleeding and relieve intoxication.*

### PREPARATION

- In case of stomach bleeding, crush a half pound of fresh lotus rhizomes and mix with an equal quantity of fresh radish juice. Drink a glass of juice two times daily. This remedy can also be used to stop bleeding in other parts of the body, such as nosebleeds and bleeding of hemorrhoids.
- Here is another way of using fresh lotus rhizomes to stop bleeding: Cut up five fresh lotus rhizomes and boil in water over low heat with brown sugar. Drink a glass of soup two or three times daily, for vomiting of blood, blood in stools, nosebleeds and bleeding from the uterus.
- To treat hemophilia, crush 900g of fresh lotus rhizomes, a fresh pear, 450g of fresh water chestnuts, 450g of fresh sugar canes. Drink a small cup of the juice three to four times daily.

**Notes**

Licorice is a very important herb in Chinese medicine. There are 2 kinds: raw licorice and licorice processed with honey. Raw licorice is slightly cool and tastes sweet, which can relieve hot symptoms and counteract toxic effects. Processed licorice is slightly warm and tastes sweet, which can tone up the spleen and increase energy.

**Notes**

Lily flower is referred to by the Chinese people as the "sorrow-forgetting flower" because it can relieve nervousness and let you forget your sorrow.

## Lotus Stems

*Reduce internal heat and relieve summer heat, detoxicate; good for sunstroke, diarrhea, congested chest and urination difficulty.*

## Mallow Roots

*Reduce internal heat, detoxicate, promote urination; good for diabetes, pain with diminished urination, shortage of milk secretion in breastfeeding mothers and vaginal discharge.*

## Mother Chrysanthemums

*Reduce internal heat and detoxicate; good for carbuncle, pink eye, scrofula and eczema.*

## Mung Bean Powder

*Reduces internal heat and detoxicates; good for carbuncle, skin diseases and alcoholism.*

## Mung Bean Sprouts

*Good for alcoholism.*

## Mung Beans

*Good for edema, diarrhea, drug poisoning, erysipelas.*

### DESCRIPTION

- Cool; sweet; detoxicates; reduces hot sensations of the body; promotes urination; affects the heart and stomach.

### PREPARATION

- Boil 200g mung beans in water; add a little honey or sugar as a seasoning. Drink as soup at meals, once a day, to cure red skin eruptions and urination difficulty due to fever; or grind mung beans into powder and take 15g powder dissolved in warm water each time, twice a day.

### CLINICAL REPORT

- A treatment of pesticide poisoning: Crush 500g mung beans and mix with 60g salt in about 2L cold water for a few minutes; strain and drink as much as possible, but no more than 3 to 5L each day. The 15 cases treated all recovered within 24 hours. No side effects were observed with the exception of occasional vomiting.
- A report on the treatment of lead poisoning: Boil 15g mung beans with 16g licorice to eat twice daily with 300mg vitamin C added each time. Each treatment program lasts 10 to 15 days. A total of 9 cases of light poisoning and 28 cases of lead absorption were treated and all the cases showed basic recovery.

## Orchid Leaves

*Reduce internal heat, cool the blood, regulate energy and promote water flow; good for coughs, pulmonary tuberculosis, vomiting of blood, discharge of blood from the mouth and vaginal discharge.*

*Notes*

Mung bean sprouts have a cold energy and sweet flavor and are used to counteract alcoholism and heat in the body.

Mung bean powder may be used for the same purpose as mung bean. Its particular uses are for burns, alcoholism and food poisoning.

## *Pear Peels*

*Reduce heat in the heart, lubricate the lungs and produce fluids; good for summer heat, coughs, vomiting of blood and boils on the skin.*

## *Pearl*

*Calms the spirits, nourishes yin energy in the body, reduces internal heat and sharpens vision; good for palpitations, nervousness and sore throats.*

## *Pepperment*

*Good for common colds, headaches, sore throats, indigestion, cankers, toothaches, skin eruptions.*

### DESCRIPTION

- Cool; pungent; affects the lungs and liver.

### PREPARATION

- Boil 5g peppermint in 1 cup water for a short while. Drink it as tea to treat discharge of stools containing blood (as in dysentery).
- Squeeze fresh peppermint juice for use as ear drops to relieve earache. (To squeeze the juice, use a pestle to pound the peppermint lightly, then wrap in a clean cloth and squeeze out the juice; or wrap peppermint, pound it and squeeze.)
- Boil 5g fresh peppermint in 1 cup water and add a little salt. Drink it like tea to relieve all kinds of pain involving the head and neck, such as headache, sore throat, pain in the mouth, pain in the tongue, toothache and also nosebleed, preferably at the early stage.
- Cook 70g fresh peppermint with 150g pork liver; eat it at meals to relieve pain in the eye, blurred vision and watering of the eyes.
- Boil fresh peppermint with bean curd and fresh ginger in water. Drink the soup and eat the bean curd to heal nasal congestion and nasal discharge, frequent sneezing and common cold.

### EXPERIMENT

- Local applications of menthol (a type of peppermint oil) are effective for headache, neuralgia and itching. When menthol is used, the skin feels cool sensations followed by light burning sensations. The cool sensations induced by menthol are not caused by a lowering of skin temperature but rather by the cold receptor of the nerve endings.

## *Pork Brain*

*Effective for dizziness, ringing in the brain and frostbite; produces bone marrow, reduces weakness and fatigue, treats neurasthenia and relieves migraine headaches.*

### PREPARATION

- To cure dizziness and ringing in the brain, wash pork brain and boil for 30 minutes. Eat warm, once a day, for 7 days.
- To cure a sore throat, steam a pork brain, season with ginger and vinegar and eat it at meals.

*Notes*

If skin itchiness is due to cold skin, menthol will make it worse; normally, when skin itchiness occurs in winter or on exposure to cold weather, it means that the person has a cold skin.

Peppermint can cure trigeminal neuralgia and I have a personal experience in this respect. About 10 years ago, I had developed trigeminal neuralgia, which was very painful and I had used peppermint for instant relief of pain. It was more effective than any pain killer. But treatment of trigeminal neuralgia must be based upon each person's physical constitution.

## Pork Gallbladder

*Heals swelling, relieves pain, counteracts toxic effects, removes dampness
from the body, clears the heart, cools the liver, sharpens vision and induces
bowel movements.*

### PREPARATION

- To cure hepatitis and diarrhea, squeeze bile from a pork gallbladder
  and then boil or steam it with 40g of honey.
- To cure jaundice, squeeze bile from a pork gallbladder and drink with
  warm water.
- To treat whooping cough, take 0.3g of pork gallbladder powder two to
  three times daily. To make pork gallbladder powder, bake bile and grind
  into powder; then mix 220g of bile powder with an equal amount of
  starch and 500g of white sugar.
- To cure hypertension, mix 130g of bile with 65g of mung bean powder
  and grind into powder. Take 6g of powder two times daily. Or, squeeze
  black soybeans into a pork gallbladder until it is full. Steam it until
  cooked and dry it in the sun. Take 20 to 30 beans two times daily.
- To relieve stomachaches, boil one pork gallbladder with 35g of rice
  vinegar over low heat until it becomes as concentrated as cream. Take
  one teaspoon two times daily.

## Potatoes (Irish Potatoes)

*Good for lack of energy, mumps, burns.*

### DESCRIPTION

- Neutral; sweet; heals inflammations; used as an energy tonic and a
  spleen tonic.

### PREPARATION

- Crush a potato and squeeze out the juice; mix it with vinegar. Apply
  the juice to the affected region to relieve mumps.
- Apply potato juice externally to burns.
- Prepare 5 potatoes (the size of eggs), 1 onion and an adequate amount
  of garlic and carrots. Wash and thoroughly clean the potatoes but do
  not peel them. Cut up the potatoes and onion; put all ingredients in
  about a few cups water; simmer over low heat until the water is reduced
  to half and add some salt. Drink 2 cups of the soup at each meal; or
  adjust the quantity and frequency according to individual needs. This
  soup is good for hypertension, malnutrition in infants, diarrhea, bronchial
  asthma, allergic skin, kidney disease and also for obesity.
- To relieve gastric and duodenal ulcers, eat a cupful of cooked potato
  liquid with a spoon once a day. To make the potato remedy, wash 30
  fresh unpeeled potatoes and grate them to squeeze out the juice. Simmer the juice in an earthenware pot (not a metal one) over low heat
  without a cover until the water evaporates completely to form a thick
  layer at the bottom of the pot. This substance is called potato glue and
  is full of protein. By taking this sticky liquid you can relieve pain and
  heal a sensitive stomach. It is reported that gastric and duodenal ulcers
  may recover within 20 to 30 days by taking this glue.

## Preserved Duck Eggs

*Sedate internal heat, counteract intoxication, eliminate fire in the large intes-
tines, cure diarrhea.*

*Notes*

Preserved duck eggs are readily
available in Chinese grocery stores.
They are usually preserved with
lime and salt.

## PREPARATION

- To cure hypertension, ringing in the ear and dizziness, cook a preserved duck egg with mussel powder and eat at meals on a regular basis.

## Pricking Amaranth (Amranth, Pigweed)
*Reduces internal heat, removes dampness, detoxicates and reduces swelling; good for dysentery, blood in stools, edema, gallstones, hemorrhoids, sore throats and snake bites.*

## Purslane
*Reduces internal heat, removes toxins from the body, promotes water flow and removes it from the body, heals swelling, stops bleeding; used to treat acute enteritis, dysentery, lung disease, pain in the nipples, bleeding from the uterus after childbirth, bleeding hemorrhoids and nephritis with edema.*

## PREPARATION

- To cure bacillary dysentery, squeeze juice from fresh purslane, add an equal amount of honey and drink with warm water. Or, crush 60 to 120g of fresh purslane and one garlic clove. Take the mixture with water three times daily. This recipe is also good for pulmonary tuberculosis.
- To cure urethritis, boil 60g of purslane with 6g of licorice over low heat. Strain it and drink the soup once a day.
- To cure jaundice and gingivitis, boil 70 to 140g of fresh purslane in water and eat at meals.
- To cure renal tuberculosis, crush one kilogram of fresh purslane and soak it in 800g of rice wine for 3 days. Strain and drink 10g of juice before meals.

## Rambutan
*Good for acute diarrhea and cold sensations in the abdomen.*

## Romaine Lettuce
*Detoxicates and quenches thirst.*

## Russian Olives (Oleaster)
*Good for diarrhea, stomachache and coughs.*

## Safflower Fruits
*Promote blood circulation and detoxicate; good for abdominal pain in women due to blood coagulation and for measles that fail to erupt.*

## Salt
*Good for constipation, bleeding from the gums, sore throat, toothache, carbuncle, cataract.*

*Notes*

Rarributan seeds contain 36.26 percent oil; bark contains 11.02 percent tannin; fruit peel contains 23.65 percent tannin.

*Notes*

Russian olives contain 43 to 59 percent sugar, of which 20 percent is fructose. They can be used as a tonic and sedative.

## DESCRIPTION

- Cold; salty, detoxicates; affects the stomach, kidneys, small and large intestines.

## PREPARATION

- Brush your teeth with fine table salt in the morning and evening to stop bleeding from gums.
- Mix salt with vinegar and drink it to relieve abdominal pain below the navel.
- Massage the surrounding regions of carbuncle and skin eruptions with salt to relieve itching.
- Drink a cup of salt water first thing in the morning on an empty stomach to relieve constipation.
- Gargle with salt water to prevent and relieve sore throat.
- Lick a little salt with the tip of the tongue before smoking to prevent forming a habit or to quit smoking within 1 month.
- Fry salt until brown; mix it with warm water. Drink the salt water to relieve fish and meat poisoning and abdominal pain due to eating the wrong foods.
- Mix salt with 2 glasses water and wash the affected region to relieve localized dermatitis, skin swelling and itching and contact skin poison.
- Lick a little salt and let it dissolve in the mouth and slowly swallow it to relieve hiccupping due to improper eating.

### Sheep's or Goat's Gallbladder

*Reduces fire in the internal region, cures pink eye, glaucoma, film in the eyes, vomiting of blood, sore throats, jaundice, constipation, carbuncle, esophagus disease, asthma.*

## PREPARATION

- To cure asthma, mix 100g of bile with 250g of honey and steam for 2 hours. Take one teaspoon twice a day. Or, bake the gallbladder and grind it into powder. Take one gram of powder three times a day. This recipe is equally good for pulmonary tuberculosis.

### Soybean Paste

*Reduces internal heart, counteracts food poisonings, relieves snake bites and bee stings.*

## PREPARATION

- To cure vaginal bleeding during pregnancy, drain 300g of soybean paste. Bake the beans and grind into powder. Take it with wine, three times daily.
- To relieve pain caused by snake bites and bee stings, apply soybean paste externally to the affected region.

### Squash

*Good for pulmonary abscessed, bronchiectasis, roundworms, opium addiction.*

## DESCRIPTION

- Warm; sweet; heals inflammation; relieves pain; affects the spleen and stomach.

*Notes*

According to one source, salt can counteract the toxic effects of vegetable alkaloid (this explains why salt can be used to relieve vegetable and herb poisoning).

According to the Yellow Emperor's Classic of Internal Medicine, "Salt travels to the blood and a person suffering from blood disease should avoid eating excessive salted foods; the kidneys are fond of salted foods." As salty flavor travels to the kidneys first, in taking a kidney tonic, it is customary to add a little salt to reinforce the effects; but salt is bad for edema associated with nephritis.

*Notes*

The major use of sheep's or goat's gallbladder is to sharpen vision. The eyes are outlets of the liver; a reduction in bile will cause blurred vision. The eyes are the external symbols of the liver. It is the essence of the gallbladder, which is why the gallbladder of various animals is beneficial to the eyes.

*Notes*

In the Chinese language, soybean paste is called "a general," meaning that it controls all food poisonings the same way that a general controls his soldiers.

*Notes*

Squash is not recommended for people suffering from chest congestion or water retention.

## PREPARATION

- Drink fresh squash juice frequently to relieve opium addiction.
- Cook 400g squash with 200g beef without salt or oil. Eat it to cure pulmonary abscess and bronchiectasis.
- Apply fresh squash juice to burns.

## CLINICAL REPORT

- Consumption of 400g fresh squash (reduced by half in children) followed by taking a purgative 2 hours later, once a day for 2 consecutive days, was found to expel roundworms (from 2 to over 100) in 6 out of 10 cases.
- Squash seeds have been found to expel tape worms, roundworms and blood flukes.
- Prepare 20g squash seeds and remove the shells; wrap the seeds in a cloth and crush them. Mix it with water or with a little soy sauce or sugar. Drink it in the morning and evening for 3 to 5 days. This has been found to promote milk secretion after childbirth; but fully cooked seeds have not been found effective.
- Squash leaves are effective for dysentery. Boil 10 leaves with a little salt. Drink it as tea twice a day to relieve dysentery.
- Squash flowers may be boiled to drink as tea to cure jaundice and cough.

## Star Fruit (Carambola)

*Good for coughs and fevers from a common cold, toothache, kidney and bladder stones, hemorrhoids, mouth canker, indigestion, hangover.*

## DESCRIPTION

- Cold; sweet and sour; reduces fever; produces fluids; promotes urination; detoxicates.

## PREPARATION

- Eat a fresh star fruit each time, twice a day, to relieve fever and cough in common cold.
- Boil 3 fresh star fruits with 2 teaspoonfuls honey. Eat the fruits and drink the juice once a day to relieve kidney and bladder stones and difficult urination.
- Crush 3 fresh star fruits to make juice. Drink it twice a day to relieve pharyngolaryngitis, mouth canker and toothache.
- Crush 3 fresh star fruits and mix the juice with cold water. Drink it 3 times a day to relieve painful urination and discharge of red urine.
- Eat 2 fresh star fruits each time, twice a day, first thing in the morning on an empty stomach and in the evening, to relieve hemorrhoids.

## Strawberries

*Good for dry coughs, thirst, sore throats, hoarseness, indigestion, difficulty when urinating, hangover.*

## DESCRIPTION

- Cool; sweet and sour; lubricates the lungs, produces fluids, strengthens spleen, relieves intoxication.

## PREPARATION

- Steam 60g fresh strawberries with 30g rock sugar. Eat 3 times a day to treat dry cough which drags on and on.

- Drink a glass of fresh strawberry juice in the morning and evening, to relieve thirst in fever, sore throat and hoarseness.
- Eat 60g fresh strawberries before meals, 3 times a day, to relieve indigestion and abdominal pain and swelling and to improve appetite.
- Crush 60g fresh strawberries and mix with cold water. Drink a glass of the juice each time, 3 times a day, to relieve difficult and painful urination and discharge of red urine.
- Eat 8 to 10 fresh strawberries all at once to relieve hangover.
- Mix fresh strawberry juice with an equal amount of rice wine. Drink it to correct malnutrition and for weakness after illness.

## Strawberry Plant
*Relieves coughs, reduces internal heat, detoxicates; good for whooping cough and stomatitis.*

## Sweet Basil
*Good for headaches in common cold, diarrhea, indigestion, stomachache, irregular menstruation.*

### DESCRIPTION
- Warm; pungent; promotes energy, blood circulation and digestion; affects the lungs, spleen, stomach and large intestine.

### PREPARATION
- Use sweet basil leaves as a seasoning to substitute for parsley or green onion for relief of headache in common cold.
- There are 2 ways sweet basil may be used to relieve menstrual pain: Cook a few leaves with chicken egg and consume it as a soup with some rice wine (good for women with premenstrual pain); another way is to cook a few sweet basil leaves with ginger, green onion and some meats or fish (good for menstrual pain due to coldness).
- Sweet basil, fresh ginger and licorice may be boiled in water; drink it like tea to cure acute gastroenteritis, abdominal swelling and pain.

## Tangerine Orange Peel
*Removes dampness, warms the internal region, disperses energy congestion, regulates energy flow.*

### PREPARATION
- To treat a cold stomach with vomiting, boil 120g of dried orange peel, 40g of fresh ginger and 7g of prickly ash in 4 cups of water until the water is reduced by half. Strain it and drink the soup.

## Tea Melon
*Promotes urination and detoxicates; good for thirst, diminished urination and alcoholism.*

## Tea Oil
*Reduces internal heat, removes dampness, destroys worms, detoxicates; good for abdominal pain, acute intestinal obstructions with roundworms, tinea and burns.*

### Notes

Tangerine orange peel has two layers: the red outer layer and white inner layer, which also has inner ribs. The peel may be used together or separately with different functions.

The red outer layer is pungent and can travel fast and disperse energy congestion and push it downwards. To remove phlegm from the body, it is necessary to regulate energy in the body.

On the other hand, the white inner layer can harmonize the stomach and eliminate grease from the body. The medicinal value of the white inner layer is far less than that of the red outer layer.

Another layer of peel deeper than the white inner layer is called the inner ribs, which contain vitamin P. It has a sweet and bitter flavor and a neutral energy. It can remove phlegm, regulate energy in the body and eliminate congestion. Inner ribs may be dried and used to make tea for tuberculosis of the lungs, coughs, phlegm, coughing blood and damp heat in the body.

*E*xcess diseases associated with both dampness and heat are treated with these regulating foods.

# Foods for Eliminating Damp Heat

## Alfalfa Roots

*Reduce internal heat, remove dampness, promote urination; good for jaundice, urinary stones and night blindness.*

## Brake Roots

*Reduce dampness and heat in the internal region, good for jaundice, vaginal discharge, diarrhea, abdominal pain and eczema.*

## Buckwheat

*Moves energy downwards, enlarges the intestines, checks sluggishness, eliminates internal heat, relieves swelling and pain, heals vaginal discharge, stops diarrhea.*

### PREPARATION

- To cure pain in the intestines with diarrhea: Fry 6g of wheat without oil, add one teaspoon of brown sugar and one cup of water. Drink it warm. To cure abdominal pain with diarrhea: Eat buckwheat or buckwheat noodles for three to four days.
- To cure skin erysipelas and furuncle in children, mix buckwheat powder with vinegar for external application to the affected region. Change the dressing twice a day.
- Buckwheat stems and leaves contain large amounts of rutin, which can prevent cerebral hemorrhage caused by hypertension. Externally, buckwheat stems and leaves can be crushed for application to wounds to stop bleeding.
- Purpura and bleeding from the eyes can be treated with a simple recipe: Boil 60g of buckwheat stems and leaves and drink like tea.

## Cantaloupe Calyx-Receptacle

*Induces vomiting, reduces jaundice, treats acute jaundice-type hepatitis.*

### PREPARATION

- Since cantaloupe calyx receptacle can induce vomiting, it is used for food poisoning. To treat food poisoning, grind one gram of cantaloupe calyx receptacle and 3g of adzuki beans into powder. Take the powder with water all at once.
- To treat jaundice-type hepatitis, bake and grind it into powder. Take 0.1g of powder with water once every 7 to 10 days. At the same time, inhale the same amount of powder into the nose after breakfast once every 40 minutes for a few times. This may cause a discharge of yellowish water from the nose, which should go away.

## Celery Roots

*To relieve vomiting, boil 10g of fresh celery roots with 15g of licorice. Crack a chicken egg into the soup when boiling and drink like soup.*

## Chinese Cabbage

*Good for constipation; thirst due to intoxication; ulcers.*

*Notes*

In one experiment, cantaloupe receptacle solution was injected into 103 cases of patients suffering from acute jaundice-type hepatitis. The results showed complete recovery within 10 days in 46.6 percent and complete recovery within 15 days in 92.2 percent.

## DESCRIPTION

- Neutral; sweet; glossy; promotes urination; beneficial to the kidneys and brain after prolonged consumption; affects the stomach and large intestine.

## PREPARATION

- Squeeze 1 to 2 fresh Chinese cabbages to obtain the juice; warm it. Drink the juice twice a day for 10 days to treat gastric and duodenal ulcers.

## Citron Leaves

*Good for jaundice.*

## Coconut Shells

*Good for pain in the bones.*

## Common Carp

*Promotes urination, reduces swelling, secures the fetus, promotes milk secretion in breastfeeding mothers, removes internal heat and detoxicates, suppresses coughs, relieves hiccups.*

## PREPARATION

- To cure edema, cook a large common carp with vinegar or with adzuki beans and eat at meals.
- To promote milk secretion in breastfeeding mothers, bake a common carp and grind it into powder. Take 4g of powder with a half glass of wine once a day.
- To promote urination and reduce swelling, prepare 450g of common carp. Wash it clean and place it in a pan with an equal amount of adzuki beans. Add water to boil until the carp becomes very soft. Cut off the head; remove scales, bones and internal organs. Eat the fish and beans and drink the soup without salt. This recipe is equally good for portal cirrhosis ascites.

## Corn Silk

*Promotes urination, reduces internal heat, calms the liver, benefits the gallbladder; good for nephritis, edema, beriberi, jaundice-type hepatitis, hypertension, gallstones, diabetes, vomiting of blood and nosebleeds.*

## Cucumber Vine (Stem)

*Good for epilepsy and hypertension.*

## Day Lilies

*Reduce internal heat, promote urination, nourish the blood, regulate the liver, promote milk secretion in breastfeeding mothers.*

*In Fukien province in China, fresh roots of day lily are used to treat arthritis with good results; In Jiangsu and Anwei provinces, the same roots are used to prevent schistosomiasis also with good results.*

**Notes**

It is reported that Chinese cabbage contains vitamin U, which is effective for the treatment of ulcers, reportedly better than artificial vitamin U.

Although Chinese cabbage is listed among foods with neutral energy, it is commonly regarded as a cold food, useful for hot symptoms, such as inflammation or ailments of various kinds. These include eye infections, sore throat, chest pain, cough with yellowish mucous discharge, difficult urination, abdominal swelling and constipation. The symptoms must be hot symptoms, if they are to be treated by Chinese cabbage.

It is reported that fresh Chinese cabbage juice can also relieve gas poisoning.

## PREPARATION

- To stop bleeding hemorrhoids, boil 30g of fresh day lilies in water. Strain them, add a teaspoon of brown sugar and drink one hour before breakfast for 5 days.
- To treat mumps with the roots of day lilies, boil 60g of roots with 10g of rock sugar. Strain it and drink soup at meals daily for one week.

## Dried Black Soybean Sprouts

*Good for edema, diminished urination and pain in the bones.*

## Eggplant Calyx

*Good for discharge of blood from the anus, mouth cankers and toothaches.*

## Fig Leaves

*Good for hemorrhoids, heart pain, painful swelling.*

## Glutinous Rice Stalks

*Good for hepatitis.*

## Hawthorn Fruit

*Good for meat indigestion, abdominal swelling, mucous discharge, discharge of blood from anus, lumbago, hernia, neck pain after childbirth.*

### DESCRIPTION

- Slightly warm; sweet and sour; promotes digestion; corrects blood coagulations; expels tapeworm; affects the spleen, stomach and liver.

### PREPARATION

- Soak hawthorn fruit in boiling water for less than 1 minute; slice the fruits and lay them in the sun to dry. (Hawthorn fruit slices are available in most Chinese herb shops.)
- Fry hawthorn slices until they look like charcoal to make hawthorn fruit charcoal.
- Mix together the following ingredients and marinate for 10 days to prepare hawthorn fruit wine: 250g hawthorn slices, 250g fresh longans, 30g red dates, 30g brown sugar and 4.5 cups rice wine.
- Drink 30 to 60g hawthorn fruit wine at every bedtime to relieve pain caused by excessive fatigue, muscular pain and arthritis pain, flying spots in front of the eyes, lumbago and pain in thigh in the elderly.
- Boil in water 60g hawthorn fruit slices with an equal amount fresh or dried chestnuts until very soft; add 30g sugar and stir thoroughly. Drink the juice once a day, first thing in the morning on an empty stomach, to cure scurvy.
- Boil 31g hawthorn slices with water; stir in 1.5g fennel powder. Drink the juice in the morning and evening to relieve hernia of the small intestine.
- Boil 15g hawthorn fruit slices in water and drink as tea on a long-term basis, to relieve hypertension, high level of blood fat and coronary heart disease.
- Grind 6 to 9g hawthorn fruit charcoal into powder. Take the powder with warm water, once a day, to relieve abdominal pain caused by acute

*Notes*

Hawthorn fruits are not recommended for people suffering from constipation due to internal heat or those who have excessive gastric acid.

Hawthorn fruits can effectively digest fat and prevent it from entering into the blood vessels by removing it through the bowel movements. Indeed, the fruits are so effective in softening hard substances, the Chinese people use it to cook stubborn and tough old chickens! When hawthorn fruits are used in the cooking water, the tough chickens become soft and tender—an indication of the tenderizing power of this fruit. Another example, when hawthorn fruits are used to cook fish, even the fish bones will become tender.

and chronic gastritis, enteritis and dysentery.

- Boil 3g hawthorn charcoal with 6g hawthorn fruit slices; drink the juice to relieve diarrhea in children; or crush 5 hawthorn fruits and squeeze out the juice to mix with a pinch of hawthorn fruit charcoal for oral administration to stop diarrhea in children.
- Crush 2 to 3 fresh hawthorn fruits and squeeze out the juice to drink; or boil 2 to 3 hawthorn fruits with 6g dry orange peels; drink the juice to correct indigestion, abdominal swelling and abdominal pain.

### EXPERIMENT

- An experiment on rabbits shows the effects of hawthorn fruit in lowering blood pressure.
- An experiment on toads shows the effects of hawthorn fruit in expanding blood vessels.
- Hawthorn fruits are reported to have the effects of contracting the uterus and reducing antibiosis.

## Olives

*Good for sore throats, coughing up blood, alcoholism, diarrhea.*

### DESCRIPTION

- Neutral; sweet and sour; obstructive; affects the lungs and stomach.

### PREPARATION

- Dry fresh olives in the shade for 1 to 2 days. Put olives in a large earthenware container, add salt and store for 2 weeks to make preserved olives.
- Remove the seed from a fresh or preserved olive and keep the olive in your mouth to relieve sore throat. Repeat with 1 olive each time, a few times a day.
- Boil 5 fresh pitted olives and a piece of crystallized ginger in water. Drink the juice 3 times a day, to cure dysentery and enteritis.
- Boil 5 fresh pitted olives in water; add 100g fresh lotus root and lean pork and a little salt. Drink the juice only, once a day, to stop bleeding from hemorrhoids and bleeding from the stomach.
- Mix 5 fresh pitted olives and some rock sugar; steam them for half an hour. Eat the olives to relieve chronic cough.
- Crush 5 to 10 fresh pitted olives; add 35g sugar and 4 cups water; boil for 10 minutes. Drink the juice, once a day, to relieve alcoholism.

### CLINICAL REPORT

- For treatment of acute bacillary dysentery: Use 100g fresh olives with seeds and boil in a cup of water over very low heat for 2 to 3 hours until reduced to a half cup; strain. Adults drink a half to 1 tablespoonful each time. Repeat 3 to 4 times until bowel movements return to normal. Treatment stops as soon as the patients have 1 to 2 bowel movements daily. In general, each treatment program continues for 5 days.

## Plantains

*Promote water flow, reduce internal heat, sharpen vision, remove phlegm; good for urination difficulty, blood in urine, edema, jaundice, diarrhea, nosebleeds, pink eye, sore throats and coughs.*

## Pumpkin Roots

*Reduce dampness and heat; good for jaundice.*

## River Snails

*Reduce internal heat, promote urination, counteract alcoholism, relieve pain
in the eyes.*

## Shells

*Reduce internal heat, promote urination; good for edema, pain on urination,
blood in urine, urination difficulty and film in the eyes.*

## Soybean Oil

*Good for gastric ulcers, duodenal ulcers, intestinal obstruction.*

### DESCRIPTION

- Hot; pungent and sweet; lubricates the intestines.

### PREPARATION

- Prepare 1 teaspoonful of soybean oil and add a few drops of lemon juice.
  Drink it on an empty stomach first thing in the morning; gradually
  increase the dosage to 5 or 6 teaspoonfuls each time to cure gastric
  ulcer, duodenal ulcer and intestinal obstruction.

## Squash Flowers

*Reduce heat and dampness, heal swelling; good for jaundice, dysentery,
coughs, carbuncle and swelling.*

## Squash Roots

*Reduce heat and dampness, promote milk secretion in breastfeeding mothers;
good for urination difficulty, swelling, jaundice and dysentery.*

## Star Fruit (Carambola)

*Good for coughs and fevers from a common cold, toothache, kidney and
bladder stones, hemorrhoids, mouth canker, indigestion, hangover.*

### DESCRIPTION

- Cold; sweet and sour; reduces fever; produces fluids; promotes urination; detoxicates.

### PREPARATION

- Eat a fresh star fruit each time, twice a day, to relieve fever and cough
  in common cold.
- Boil 3 fresh star fruits with 2 teaspoonfuls honey. Eat the fruits and
  drink the juice once a day to relieve kidney and bladder stones and
  difficult urination.
- Crush 3 fresh star fruits to make juice. Drink it twice a day to relieve
  pharyngolaryngitis, mouth canker and toothache.

### Notes

Cooked river snails can promote
bowel movements, remove accumulated heat in the abdomen, treat yellowish eyes, relieve beriberi and reduce edema in the hands and feet.
Juice squeezed from a fresh river
snail can relieve diabetes; its meat
can be crushed for external applications to heal carbuncle of heat.

### Notes

Soy sauce (a product of soybeans)
can promote digestion and it can also
be used as an external remedy to
heal burns. But an excessive consumption of soy sauce will cause a
cough and thirst and also is not recommended for people with jaundice.

- Crush 3 fresh star fruits and mix the juice with cold water. Drink it 3 times a day to relieve painful urination and discharge of red urine.
- Eat 2 fresh star fruits each time, twice a day, first thing in the morning on an empty stomach and in the evening, to relieve hemorrhoids.

## Sunflower Disc or Receptacle
*Good for hypertension, headaches, arthritis, blurred vision and toothaches.*

## Wheat Seedling
*Good for jaundice and alcoholism.*

## Yellow Soybean
*Good for malnutrition in children, diarrhea, abdominal swelling, underweight, gestosis.*

### DESCRIPTION
- Neutral, sweet; used as a spleen tonic; lubricates dryness; eliminates tissue fluids; affects the spleen and large intestine.

### PREPARATION
- Fry yellow soybeans until aromatic to eat at meals to promote milk secretion after childbirth.
- Fry yellow soybeans and then boil them in water to eat at meals to correct underweight.

### CLINICAL REPORT
- A treatment of acute gestosis: 92 cases of potential eclampsia and eclampsia are treated by soybean juice (soybean and water ratio 1 to 8) cooked with 120g sugar, divided into 6 dosages. Eat while drinking additional water. In general, treatment lasts 2 to 4 days and then, changes to a salt-free diet. On the second day of treatment, fruits or lotus root powder may be administered to relieve hunger. In the control group, 41 cases are given only a salt-free diet with other factors identical in both groups, including avoidance of sound and light stimuli and administration of sedatives and antispasmodic drugs. The results indicate that the experimental group shows a faster disappearance of edema and faster normalization of the blood pressure than the control group; the death rate in the experimental group is zero while in the control group it is more than 2 percent. The result is attributed to the fact that yellow soybean juice is low in calcium and sodium, higher in vitamin B-1 and niacin with more water intake, which contributes to the lowering of blood pressure and increased urination.

*Notes*

Yellow soybean sprouts are cool and sweet. They are used to relieve a cough with discharge of yellow mucus and to promote urination.

The presence of sputum in the body is responsible for many excess diseases. Sputum can be eliminated by eating the following regulating foods.

# Foods for Eliminating Sputum

## Adzuki Bean Sprouts

*Good for blood in stools, bleeding during pregnancy.*

## Almonds

*Lubricate the lung, suppress coughs, remove phlegm, balance energy.*

## Apple Peels

*Good for upset stomachs and phlegm.*

## Asafoetida

*Eliminates indigestion and destroys worms; good for cold abdominal pain, malaria and dysentery.*

## Asparagus

*Good for coughs, mucous discharge, swelling, various kinds of skin eruptions, shortage of milk secretion after childbirth.*

### DESCRIPTION

- Slightly warm; bitter and slightly pungent; promotes urination.

### EXPERIMENT

- An animal experiment shows the effects of asparagus in promoting urination, lowering blood pressure, expanding terminal blood vessels and reducing heartbeats.

## Azalea Flowers

*Regulate menstruation and relieve rheumatism.*

## Bamboo Liquid Oil

*Reduces internal heat, removes phlegm, calms spirits; good for epilepsy, thirst and excessive perspiration.*

## Bean Curd (Tofu)

*Good for pink eye, diabetes, periodic diarrhea, sulfur poisoning.*

### DESCRIPTION

- Cool; sweet; used as an energy tonic; produces fluids; lubricates dryness; detoxicates; affects the spleen, stomach and large intestine.

### PREPARATION

- Prepare 1 bowl bean curd, 70g maltose and half a cup of fresh radish juice; combine the 3 ingredients in a pan, add half a cup of water and bring to a boil once. Divide the soup into 2 dosages and drink twice a day to treat asthma with mucous discharge, including acute bronchial asthma.
- Crush a number of bean curds and apply the mash to the legs to heal erysipelas on the legs; change the dressing as soon as the mash dries.

## Bean Drink

*Increases body energy, reduces heat in the body, removes phlegm, promotes urination, relieves food poisoning.*

### PREPARATION

- To relieve whitish vaginal discharge in women, crush 10 ginkgo kernels and put into a glass of bean drink. Steam it and drink like tea.
- To relieve vaginal bleeding, mix a glass of bean drink with a half glass of chive juice. Drink it on an empty stomach.
- To relieve acute toxemia of pregnancy, mix 2,000 millilitres of bean drink with 120g of sugar. Divide into six dosages in one day for two to four days. Change to a no-salt diet on the fifth day; on the sixth day, eat some fruit and lotus root powder to check hunger. This food cure can also reduce edema and lower blood pressure.
- To cure peptic ulcers, mix one glass of bean drink with 20g of maltose. Bring to a boil and drink it first thing in the morning on an empty stomach.

## Bitter Apricot Seeds

*Remove phlegm from the body, suppress coughs, lubricate intestines; used to treat asthma and constipation.*

### PREPARATION

- To treat tracheitis, bore a hole into a pear, put 9g of crushed apricot seeds (bitter or sweet) into it and seal it. Boil in water, then drink the soup and eat the contents. Alternatively, crush bitter apricot seeds and mix with an equal amount of rock sugar to make apricot candy. Eat 9g of apricot candy two times daily, in the morning and evening, for 10 days.
- To treat stomachaches, crush five apricot seeds, seven black peppers and seven red dates. Make them into tablets and take with rice wine.

## Black and White Pepper

*Good for cold abdominal pain, upset stomach, vomiting of clear water, diarrhea, food poisoning.*

### DESCRIPTION

- Hot; pungent; pushes downwards; warms the internal regions; affects the stomach and large intestine.

### PREPARATION

- Boil 30g sliced fresh ginger with 1g ground black pepper in 3 cups water until water reduced to 1 cup. Drink this amount 3 times a day for 1 day to stop vomiting due to upset stomach.
- Grind 10 black peppercorns into powder and bring to the boil in 8 cups water; use the liquid to wash the affected region twice a day to cure eczema of the scrotum.

### EXPERIMENT

- Twenty-four normal adults were given 1g black pepper to put in their mouths without swallowing it to determine the effects of black pepper on blood pressure and pulse rates. It was found that black pepper can elevate blood pressure: On the average, systolic pressure rises 13.1mm of mercury; diastolic pressure rises 18.1mm of mercury; both pressures return to normal in 10 to 15 minutes; no effects were found on pulse rates. During the experiment, the majority of subjects felt hot sensations

### Notes

Bitter apricot seeds taste sour with a hot energy and slightly toxic. An excessive consumption is harmful to the tendons and bones. The seeds contain hydrocyanic acid, which is poisonous; consumption of 10 to 20 seeds in children and 40 to 60 seeds in adults will cause poisoning, dizziness, headaches, nausea, fatigue, vomiting, abdominal pain and diarrhea.

For this reason, sweet apricot seeds have been made into many forms of foods without danger, including cookies, tea and juice. Sweet apricot seeds, like bitter ones, are also toxic. They are larger than bitter ones with different actions, because they can lubricate the lungs, suppress cough and smooth the intestines.

### Notes

Traditionally, black and white peppers are considered useful in warming the body and eliminating the strong smell of meats and fish. But an excessive consumption of these spices is considered harmful and not recommended for people with eye diseases and sore throat.

in their entire bodies or in their heads in addition to the pungent and hot sensations at the tip of their tongues. The effects of black pepper were found to be similar to those of red pepper, only to a lesser degree.

## CLINICAL REPORT

- A report on simple indigestive diarrhea: grind 1g white pepper into powder and mix with 9g glucose powder in water; children less than a year old take .3 to .5g each time; children less than 3 years take .5 to 1.5 g, normally not exceeding 2 g, 3 times a day for 1 to 3 days as a treatment program; in case of dehydration, fluid retention therapy should be applied. Among the 20 cases of simple indigestive diarrhea treated, 18 cases recovered and 2 cases showed improvements.
- A report on nephritis: Make a hole in a chicken egg and squeeze 7 white peppercorns into the egg; seal the hole with flour. Wrap the egg with a wet sheet of paper; steam the egg until cooked. Peel the egg and eat it with the peppercorns. As a treatment program, adults eat 2 eggs a day and children eat 1 egg a day for 10 days. The second program begins 3 days after completing the first program. Generally, 3 treatment programs are administered. Among the 6 cases of nephritis treated, all recovered except a case of chronic nephritis with a ten-year history.

## Black Sesame Seed
*Good for constipation, dry skin, grey hair, shortage of milk secretion.*

### DESCRIPTION

- Neutral; sweet; used as a liver tonic and a kidney tonic; affects the liver and kidneys.

### PREPARATION

- Fry 15g black sesame seeds; add some salt. Eat it to increase milk secretion.
- Soak 1 cup rice for a few hours; drain and crush the rice; boil it with 1 cup black sesame seeds in water to make soup. Drink the soup at meals to correct constipation.

## Bottle Gourd (Autumn Bottle Gourd)
*Promotes urination and relieves pain; good for jaundice and edema.*

## Celery
*Good for hypertension, dizziness and headaches, discharge of urine containing blood.*

### DESCRIPTION

- Neutral; sweet; bitter; glossy; affects the stomach and liver.

### PREPARATION

- Sometimes an infant may feel hot sensations and is unable to sleep and cries day and night. If there are signs of hot symptoms (like mouth canker or redness in the region surrounding the anus or frequent urination with discharge of scanty and yellowish-red urine), then it is useful to cut a few pieces of celery, immerse them in boiling water for a few seconds and squeeze out the juice. This juice can reduce heat in the bladder, a useful remedy for urethritis.

There is a Chinese recipe to improve the conditions of liver and kidneys: Fry celery and pork kidneys. The celery can calm you down and prevent liver disorder while the pork kidneys can tone up the kidneys.

Celery is aromatic, the reason why the Chinese people call it "aromatic celery." Celery may be cooked with vinegar to lower blood pressure and relieve headache due to high blood pressure.

Fresh celery juice may be mixed with honey to relieve dizziness and headache and shoulder pain associated with hypertension.

In cases of hypertension of pregnancy and climacteric hypertension, drink fresh celery juice every day to relieve the symptoms.

## EXPERIMENT

Celery lowers blood pressure in rats.

## CLINICAL REPORT

A report on the effect of lowering blood pressure and the level of cholesterol: Wash fresh celery (with roots removed) in cold water. Squeeze out the juice and mix the juice with an equal quantity of honey or syrup. Drink 40 ml warm juice each time, 3 times a day. Among the 16 cases treated, 14 cases were effective and 2 cases had no effects. The results indicated effectiveness for primary hypertension, hypertension in pregnancy and climacteric hypertension. In general, blood pressure begins to drop after 1 day of treatment with subjective sensations, improved sleeping conditions and increased urination.

A clinical report on the effects of celery roots: As a treatment program, 10 celery roots are washed, crushed and boiled in water with 10 red dates for oral consumption twice a day for 15 to 20 days. Among the 21 cases treated for hypertension and coronary sclerosis heart disease with the cholesterol level over 200mg percent, it was found that the level of cholesterol was reduced between 8 and 75mg percent in 14 cases. It was also observed that fresh roots produce better results than dry ones and that dosages are flexible.

## REMARKS

According to Chinese theory, celery is effective for hypertension because it acts upon the liver; one type of hypertension is associated with the liver.

A physician wrote to me about the fact that celery contains sodium, which is considered bad for hypertension. Nevertheless, I would think that the quantity of sodium contained in celery (25mg in 1 stalk) is too small to cause any harm.

A classic Chinese food belief: Celery can reduce internal heat in children and also internal heat in adults due to intoxication.

## Citrons

*Strengthen the stomach, cure indigestion, relieve chest congestion, remove phlegm from the body, stop vomiting; used to cure chronic gastritis and nervous stomachaches.*

## PREPARATION

To cure coughs with phlegm, soak citrons in wine and drink on a regular basis. To treat chronic bronchitis, cut up one to two citrons, place them in a bowl, add an equal amount of maltose and steam for 2 hours, or until citrons are very soft. Take one teaspoon two times daily to remove phlegm, suppress cough and stop panting.

To cure stomachaches, chest congestion and indigestion, bake one or

## Notes

A citron is like an orange; its peel is aromatic. The most distinct feature of citron consists in its aroma, which is why the Chinese call it "aromatic orange," because its peel contains plenty of essential oil.

Although a citron is aromatic, it tastes extremely sour when eaten fresh; for this reason, the Chinese often preserve it with honey and sugar. When eaten, it can regulate energy flow in the body and disperse congestion.

more citrons (about 35g) and grind into powder. Add prickly ash and
fennel, 12g each and then grind the three ingredients into powder again
and mix thoroughly. Take 4g with water two times daily.

- To cure pain in the liver and stomachaches (including chronic gastritis),
  boil 12 to 15g of fresh citron (or 6g of dried citron) and drink like tea.

## *Clam*

*Saltwater clams good for edema, mucous discharge, goiter, vaginal discharge,
hemorrhoids; freshwater clams good for vaginal bleeding and discharge, pink
eyes, eczema and hemorrhoids; saltwater clamshell powder good for diabetes,
edema, goiter and hemorrhoids; freshwater clam saliva good for diabetes,
pink eyes and burns; freshwater clamshell powder good for cough with
mucous discharge, stomachache, hiccupping, vomiting, whitish vaginal discharge, eczema, swelling.*

### DESCRIPTION

- Sea (saltwater) clam—cold, salty, acts on the stomach, promotes water
  passage, eliminates mucus and softens hardness; freshwater clam—cold,
  sweet and salty, detoxicates, sharpens the vision, acts on the liver and
  kidneys. Sea clamshell powder-cold, salty, promotes water passage, softens
  hardness, eliminates mucus, acts on the lungs and kidneys; river clam
  saliva—sharpens vision; freshwater clamshell powder—cold, salty, eliminates mucus and dries dampness, acts on the lungs, liver and stomach.

### PREPARATION

- Sea clamshell may be baked and ground into very fine powder to make
  sea clamshell powder. Freshwater clamshell may be washed clean (with
  the black skin removed) and ground into powder or baked and ground
  into powder to make freshwater clamshell powder. Apply saltwater clam's
  saliva externally to the affected region to relieve itching and pain and
  swelling of the vaginal orifice.
- Crush a few garlics to mix with clamshell powder and make into tablets
  of a normal size. Take 10 tablets with warm water each time, once a day,
  to relieve edema in weak persons.
- Mix clamshell powder with lard for external application to the affected
  region to relieve burns.
- Mix fine clamshell powder with an equal amount of raw licorice powder, take 7g each time with warm water, twice a day, to cure gastric ulcer
  and excessive gastric acid.
- Regular consumption of clam meat at meals relieves lymphadenitis
  scrofula in the neck and goiter.
- Cook clam with chive. Eat at meals to relieve pulmonary tuberculosis
  and night sweat.
- Boil 30g fine clamshell powder with 4g outer layer of peanuts and 6 red
  dates to make concentrated soup. Drink the soup once a day to relieve
  nosebleed, bleeding from gums and purpura hemorrhagica.
- Roast a whole freshwater clam until its outer part is charred and the
  inner part becomes yellow-brown with its original shape remaining
  intact; grind into fine powder and mix with sesame oil for external
  application to relieve eczema in infants.

### CLINICAL REPORT

- For treatment of gastric and duodenal ulcers, fry freshwater clamshell
  powder in a bronze fry pan (or any earthenware fry pan) until it becomes
  yellow-brown with the fishy smell gone; strain it before using. Take 1 to

2g each time mixed with warm water, once every hour during the day-time, 12 to 14 times a day, for 4 to 8 weeks. Among the 41 cases treated from 14 to 79 days, 28 cases showed disappearance of pain in the upper abdomen and 7 cases a decrease, 23 cases showed disappearance of pressure pain in the upper abdomen (pain that occurs on pressure by hand) and 6 cases a decrease; 21 cases had a follow-up X-ray examination, which indicated disappearance of the niche in 9 cases, disappearance of deformity in 1 case and a reduction in the size of the niche in 6 cases.

## Common Button Mushrooms

*Regulate body energy and remove phlegm from the body; good for the stomach and intestines, measles, contagious hepatitis, coughs and hiccups.*

## Date

*Good for weak stomachs, palpitations, nervousness, hysteria in women, allergic purpura.*

### DESCRIPTION

- Warm; sweet; used as a spleen tonic, energy tonic and blood tonic; produces fluids; detoxicates; affects the spleen and stomach.

### PREPARATION

- Boil 30g red dates with 1 whole chicken egg, 4 fresh ginger slices and 30g brown sugar in water. Eat at meals to relieve weakness after childbirth.
- Prolonged consumption of 30g red dates in the evening every day improves physical conditions, such as skinniness and weakness.
- Boil 30g red dates with 5 green onion white heads. Eat it at bedtime to relieve insomnia.
- Eat 30 to 60g red dates each time, 3 times a day for 15 consecutive days, to cure allergic purpura.
- Boil 30g red dates and 30g yam with 2 fresh ginger slices until soft. Eat it once a day for 10 consecutive days to treat cold stomachache, abdominal pain and diarrhea due to digestive weakness.
- Boil 30g dried red dates with 15g yam, 15g whole wheat and 15g processed licorice. Drink the juice in the morning and evening to treat hysteria in women and jumpiness in women during menopause.
- Boil 15g black dates with 9g longans and 30g brown sugar. Eat the stewed fruit at meals on a long-term basis to treat anemia.
- To prepare date jelly, boil 1,500g fresh dates, seeded, or 500g red dates, seeded, until they look like jelly; add 500g sugar and stir until dissolved.
- Take a teaspoonful of date jelly with warm water on a long-term basis to relieve hepatitis, pulmonary tuberculosis and weakness after illness.

## Eggplant Roots

*Good for chronic diarrhea with blood in stools, beriberi, toothaches, frost-bite, rheumatic pain and hemorrhoids.*

### PREPARATION

- To cure chronic diarrhea, bake eggplant roots and pomegranate peels and grind into powder. Mix the two ingredients in equal amount and take one teaspoon of powder with white sugar in water two times daily.

## Epiphyllum

*Reduces heat in the lungs, stops coughs, removes phlegm; good for stomachaches, heart pain and vomiting of blood, particularly in pulmonary tuberculosis.*

## Figs

*Good for enteritis, dysentery, constipation, hemorrhoids, sore throat, diarrhea.*

### DESCRIPTION

- Neutral; sweet; detoxicates; used as stomachic tonic; affects the spleen and large intestine.

### PREPARATION

- Eat 1 to 2 fresh figs each time, in the morning and evening, to wake up appetite and correct indigestion.
- Eat 1 to 2 fresh figs at bedtime to relieve constipation, particularly in the elderly.
- Steam until very soft 1 to 2 fresh figs and 2 honey dates (processed in honey). Eat 1 to 2 figs each day to relieve dry cough and sore throat.
- Boil 1kg dry figs in water at low heat until they are soft as jelly. Add 750g sugar and heat until sugar dissolves. Then mix all the ingredients; take 1 teaspoonful fig jelly each time, in the morning and evening, to correct weakness after illness. Fig jelly is also used as adjuvant therapy for pulmonary tuberculosis and hepatitis.
- Boil until very soft 1 to 3 fresh figs or 30g dry figs with 60g lean pork and 2 red dates; eat once a day to increase milk secretion in women after childbirth.
- Boil 60g fresh figs with 60g pork or with 1 chicken egg and 15g rice wine. Eat once a day to relieve pain in muscles and bones and numbness from rheumatism.
- Fry 30g dry figs until aromatic; separately, fry 9g dry ginger until it looks like charcoal. Boil together the figs and ginger. Eat 3 times a day, to cure chronic diarrhea.
- Eat 2 unripe fresh figs in the morning and evening to alleviate pain and bleeding in hemorrhoids.

## Fingered Citrons (Buddha's Hand)

*Good for stomachaches, vomiting and alcoholism.*

## Fresh Ginkgo

*Removes phlegm and heals skin eruptions.*

## Garlic

*Good for cold abdominal pain, edema, diarrhea, dysentery, whooping cough.*

### DESCRIPTION

- Warm; pungent; promotes energy circulation, warms the stomach and spleen, destroys worms; affects the spleen, stomach and lungs.

### PREPARATION

- Boil 3 garlic cloves in water and eat with soy sauce at meals to relieve cough and abdominal pain and also to promote blood circulation and urination.

**Notes**

Fig leaf is neutral in energy and tastes sweet and slightly pungent, it can heal hemorrhoids and heart pain and swelling.

- For women, to relieve itch in the genital region, boil a few garlic cloves and use the liquid to wash the genital region.
- Crush a few garlic cloves to mix with mustard (powder or paste) and eat it with rice wine. Or, boil a few garlic cloves in water and drink it as tea to correct chronic cold sensations, particularly in women. If wine is desired, make garlic wine: Simply cut up a garlic clove in large pieces, drop into a small bottle of wine; put away for 1 month and it is ready to drink as a wine tonic.
- Eat 1 to 3 fresh garlic cloves daily by dividing them into 3 dosages; continue treatment for 5 to 10 consecutive days to heal amebic dysentery.
- Take 2 teaspoonfuls 10 to 20 percent garlic solution every 2 hours (mixed with some syrup or orange tincture to make it more appetizing) to relieve whooping cough in children.
- Eat garlic cloves regularly to prevent bacillary dysentery when it is widespread.
- Cut up a garlic clove and use the juicy slice to rub the skin to relieve pain caused by insect bite (such as bee sting) as an emergency measure.
- Garlic may be cooked with soybeans: Soak the soybeans overnight; cook soybeans with 5 to 10 garlic cloves. Eat as a tonic and also to promote urination, relieve edema and chronic nephritis.
- Another way to use garlic: Fry garlic cloves in vegetable oil with black pepper, sliced fresh ginger and salt; add dry shrimps, then sprinkle with sugar, vinegar and green onion. Add some tomato ketchup and flour to thicken, if desired. This recipe contains almost all the needed flavors— sweet, sour, pungent and salty.

### CLINICAL REPORT

- For treatment of lobar pneumonia; 1 tablespoon garlic syrup every 4 hours (in general 10 percent, but sometimes 100 percent). Among the 9 people treated, 6 cases show complete recovery, 3 show no satisfactory results.

## Grapefruit

*Good for indigestion, bad breath due to intoxication, poor appetite in pregnant women.*

### DESCRIPTION

- Cold; sweet and sour.

### PREPARATION

- Steam 90g peeled grapefruit with half a cup rice wine and 1 cup honey. Drink it all in 1 day to relieve cough with mucous discharge.
- Eat 1 medium grapefruit each time, 3 times a day, to relieve indigestion, belching and mouth watering in pregnant women.
- Slowly eat 1 small grapefruit to relieve intoxication.

## Grapefruit Peel

*Good for congestion in chest, mucous discharge, cough, intoxication.*

### DESCRIPTION

- Warm; pungent, sweet and bitter; pushes downwards; affects the spleen, kidneys and bladder.

### PREPARATION

- Collect grapefruit peels; cut off only the outer rind. Put rinds in the sun

---

### Notes

There have been fewer cases of pulmonary tuberculosis in Sandong, a province of China where people consume more garlic than in any other province. As a result of these findings, garlic has been made into tablets and used with good results.

In the northern provinces of China, Chinese people carry some garlic with them while on a long journey, just in case they have to drink water from mountains or rivers. To prevent bad effects, they chew a garlic clove like chewing gum and spit it out before drinking water.

Many people don't want to eat garlic for fear of getting bad breath. According to some people, "garlic" breath can be eliminated by eating a few red dates or a persimmon. When garlic cloves are steamed (over boiling water), the strong smell will be gone before eating the garlic.

In daily cooking, a few garlic slices may be added to eliminate the strong smell of meats or fish. It is believed that a small quantity of garlic can counteract cancer, but an excessive quantity of garlic can cause cancer (based on the Chinese theory that excessive garlic is bad for the stomach and liver).

Chinese people eat large quantities of garlic only under special circumstances, such as severe malnutrition or edema.

In recent years, garlic has emerged as an important ingredient in Chinese medicine, mostly due to its powerful effects in treating dysentery and destroying germs. In fact, many modern medicines contain garlic as an important ingredient. For dysentery at its early stage, chew a garlic clove five or six times a day every four hours.

Contraindications of garlic include eye diseases and sore throat.

to dry to make dry grapefruit peels. Or, instead of drying the peels in the sun, boil the peels in water for a while. Drain and put the peels in the sun to half-dry them; then add sugar to make candied grapefruit peels.

- Chew 30 to 60g candied grapefruit peels slowly, like chewing gum, to relieve motion sickness and vomiting.
- Boil 15g candied grapefruit peels or 3g dry grapefruit peels in water and drink like soup, 3 times a day, to alleviate abdominal swelling and pain and diarrhea caused by indigestion in children.

## Honey

*Good for dry coughs, constipation, stomachaches, sinusitis, mouth cankers, burns, neurasthenia, hypertension, pulmonary tuberculosis, heart disease, liver disease.*

### DESCRIPTION

- Neutral; sweet; detoxicates; lubricates dryness; relieves pain; affects the lungs, spleen and large intestine.

### PREPARATION

- Steam about half a cup honey. Eat it all at once on an empty stomach, 3 times a day, for 2 to 3 weeks on end, to relieve gastric and duodenal ulcers.
- Mix half a cup honey with warm water and drink once a day to treat hypertension, constipation, stomachache, neurasthenia, heart disease and coronary sclerosis.
- Drink a cup honey water at bedtime to cure insomnia due to neurasthenia. Externally apply honey to the affected region to relieve burns.
- Mix 3 large spoonfuls honey in boiling water. Drink it in the morning and in the evening to relieve insomnia, headache and anemia; or eat honey at meals with other foods.
- Using a sterilized cotton ball, externally apply honey to the anus to heal cracked skin in hemorrhoids; or externally apply to the ear to relieve swelling of the ear.
- Mix 2 teaspoonfuls honey with warm water. Drink it first thing in the morning on an empty stomach to relieve chronic constipation.
- Mix 1 teaspoonful honey with warm water and drink it 3 hours after meals, 3 times a day, for 5 consecutive days, to relieve hoarseness caused by excessive fatigue but unrelated to common cold, with sufficient rest to produce best results.

### CLINICAL REPORT

- For treatment of gastric and duodenal ulcers; among 20 cases treated, the niche disappeared in 15 cases, showed progress in 3 cases (32 days on the average), pain completely disappeared in 18 and pain decreased in 2; pain was gone as quickly as 6 days and within 22 days on the average. The method of treatment: each day, eat a third cup fresh honey before meals, 3 times a day; after the tenth day, increase the quantity of honey to half a cup each day.
- Clinical reports on treatment of other diseases showed good results: For treatment of acute bacillary dysentery, take 150g honey each day for adults (divide into 4 reduced dosages for children); for treatment of chronic and or temporary constipation in the elderly and in pregnant women, take honey first thing in the morning; for treatment of hypochromic anemia, take 80 to 100g honey each day, divided into 3 dosages; the results show an obvious increase in blood cells and hemoglobin.

中医疗法

## Jellyfish

*Reduces internal heat, lowers blood pressure, removes phlegm, eliminates internal congestion, lubricates the intestines, secures the fetus; good for asthma, chest pain, abdominal swelling, constipation, vaginal discharge, malnutrition and jaundice.*

### PREPARATION

- To treat chronic tracheitis, bake 40g of jellyfish, 6g of oyster shell and 6g of clam shell; then grind them into powder. Add 3g of honey and mix the powder and make into tablets. Divide into three dosages to take after meals in one day for 10 days.
- To treat pulmonary abscess, bronchiectasis and coughs with phlegm, prepare 150g of jellyfish and wash off the salt with boiling water. Cut up an equal amount of water chestnuts or carrots; then boil them in 3 cups of water and drink as soup at meals.
- To treat hypertension, prepare 150g of jellyfish and wash off the salt with boiling water. Cut up 400g of unpeeled water chestnuts and boil them in water until the water is reduced by half. Drink it warm on an empty stomach.
- To cure ulcers, boil jellyfish, red dates and brown sugar together over low heat until it becomes a thick soup. Take 1 teaspoon of soup two times daily.

## Jellyfish Skin

*Removes phlegm, eliminates internal congestion, removes dampness from the body, counteracts rheumatism. Frequently used for headaches, vaginal discharge, skin eruptions.*

### PREPARATION

- To treat internal congestion with hard spots, soak jellyfish skin and water chestnuts in wine. Eat at meals or boil for soup.
- Jellyfish skin can be boiled or soaked in wine or seasoned with ginger and vinegar.

## Kohlrabi Leaves

*Good for indigestion; remove phlegm.*

## Kumquat

*Good for chest congestion, thirst, indigestion, cough, whooping cough, stomachache, hernial pain, poor appetite.*

### DESCRIPTION

- Warm; pungent, sweet and sour; relieves cough; eliminates mucus, promotes energy circulation.

### PREPARATION

- Steam 5 to 10 fresh kumquats with 30g of rock sugar for half an hour and eat a few each time, twice a day, to stop senile cough and asthma.
- Eat a few fresh kumquats to relieve indigestion.
- To make dried kumquats, place fresh kumquats in the sun to dry.
- Boil 10 dried kumquats in 6 cups water until water is reduced to 3 cups; drink 1 cup of the juice each time, 3 times a day, to treat stomachache.
- Crush 10 dried kumquats and boil in a mixture of half water and half rice

### Notes

Jellyfish consists of two parts: the umbrellalike body, which is called jellyfish skin and the mouth or neck, which is called jellyfish head. After a jellyfish is caught, it is soaked in lime and alum solution; then its water is squeezed out, after which it is washed clean and preserved with salt. Before cooking jellyfish, its lime, alum and salt should be washed off with clean water.

wine. Drink a cup of the juice each time, twice a day, to relieve hernial pain.
- To make sugar kumquats, place fresh kumquats in the sun until half dry. Soak kumquats in syrup.
- Chew 30g sugar kumquats slowly, like chewing gum, to stimulate poor appetite due to common cold or motion sickness.

## Kumquat Cake
*Good for blood in stools.*

## Laver
*Removes phlegm from the body, softens up hard swelling in the body, reduces internal heat, promotes urination, strengthens the kidneys, nourishes the heart.*

**Notes**

There are many kinds of laver, but they all have similar effects. A report indicated that laver can lower cholesterol levels in the blood.

When one suffers from goiter and beriberi, it is wise to eat laver. When one has a sore throat, drink laver soup to cure it. Laver has also been found to be effective for curing hypertension.

## Leaf Mustard
*Good for mucous discharge, cough, chest congestion.*

### DESCRIPTION
- Warm; pungent; affects the lungs.

### PREPARATION
- Cook preserved leaf mustard and eat 30g a day to cure pulmonary abscess and bronchiectasis and laryngitis. Boil 5g fried leaf mustard seeds with 10g fried radish seeds, 5g dried orange peel and 5g licorice. Drink it as tea to cure chronic bronchitis and cough with mucous discharge.

**Notes**

A prolonged consumption of leaf mustard can warm up the internal region. It is not recommended for people suffering from eye diseases, hemorrhoids, or discharge of stools containing blood, which are normally regarded as hot symptoms.

Leaf mustard can relieve congestion because it has a warm energy and tastes pungent, which are the two important components of foods that are used to promote energy circulation and relieve congestion of various kinds.

## Lemon Leaves
*Remove phlegm, regulate body energy, improve appetite; good for coughs, asthma, abdominal swelling and diarrhea.*

## Lemon Peels
*Disperse congestion, strengthen the stomach, relieve pain; good for abdominal pain and poor appetite.*

## Licorice
*Good for abdominal pain, poor appetites, fatigue, fever, coughs, palpitations, convulsions, sore throats, digestive ulcers, drug poisoning, food poisoning.*

### DESCRIPTION
- Neutral; sweet; slows down acute diseases, lubricates lungs, counteracts toxic effects, coordinates the effects of other herbs; affects the spleen, stomach and lungs.

### PREPARATION
- Prepare 150g processed licorice and 80g dry ginger; boil in only enough water to cover the 2 ingredients; boil until the water is reduced by half; strain and drink 1 cup of the warm soup each time, twice a day, to cure abscessed lungs, suppurative pneumonia and bronchitis without cough.
- Boil 10g licorice with 20g whole wheat kernels and 5 Chinese red dates.

**Notes**

Licorice is a very important herb in Chinese medicine. There are 2 kinds: raw licorice and licorice processed with honey. Raw licorice is slightly cool and tastes sweet, which can relieve hot symptoms and counteract toxic effects. Processed licorice is slightly warm and tastes sweet, which can tone up the spleen and increase energy.

Drink as soup to treat hysteria in women, anxiety and stress. This is a time-honored herbal formula in Chinese medicine.

## Lobster (Sea Prawn)

*Tones the kidneys, increases sexual potency in men, improves appetite, removes phlegm; good for hemiplegia, pain in bones and impotence.*

## Longevity Fruits (Momordica Fruits)

*Suppress coughs, relieve asthma, reduce heat in the body, lubricate the intestines.*

### PREPARATION

- To suppress coughs with phlegm and constipation, boil longevity fruits with pork in water and eat at meals. To cure pharyngolaryngitis, cut up a longevity fruit in thin slices and make tea. To cure whooping cough, boil a longevity fruit with 15g of persimmon cake in water and drink as soup.

## Loquat Flowers

*Good for common colds, coughs and blood in phlegm.*

## Loquat Leaves

*Reduce heat in the lungs, settle the stomach, remove phlegm; good for coughs with discharge of phlegm, discharge of blood from the mouth and nosebleeds.*

## Loquat Seeds

*Reduce phlegm, relieve coughs, relax the liver, regulate body energy; good for hernia, edema and scrofula.*

## Mustard Seeds

*Warm the internal region, disperse cold, remove phlegm; good for vomiting, abdominal pain, coughs and sore throats.*

## Old Dried Radish Roots

*Expand the lungs, remove phlegm, promote digestion, remove water; good for cough with phlegm, chest congestion and abdominal pain.*

## Olives

*Good for sore throats, coughing up blood, alcoholism, diarrhea.*

### DESCRIPTION

- Neutral; sweet and sour; obstructive; affects the lungs and stomach.

### PREPARATION

- Dry fresh olives in the shade for 1 to 2 days. Put olives in a large earthenware container, add salt and store for 2 weeks to make preserved olives.

### Notes

Longevity fruits taste 300 times sweeter than sugar and are considered good for diabetics. In recent years, many reports indicate that this fruit contains an anticancerous agent.

When a singer is experiencing a throat problem, a Chinese physician will recommend longevity fruits as a remedy. In fact, longevity fruits can be consumed to treat many diseases, including common colds, coughs with mucous discharge, constipation, chronic pharyngitis and chronic tracheitis.

- Remove the seed from a fresh or preserved olive and keep the olive in your mouth to relieve sore throat. Repeat with 1 olive each time, a few times a day.
- Boil 5 fresh pitted olives and a piece of crystallized ginger in water. Drink the juice 3 times a day, to cure dysentery and enteritis.
- Boil 5 fresh pitted olives in water; add 100g fresh lotus root and lean pork and a little salt. Drink the juice only, once a day, to stop bleeding from hemorrhoids and bleeding from the stomach.
- Mix 5 fresh pitted olives and some rock sugar; steam them for half an hour. Eat the olives to relieve chronic cough.
- Crush 5 to 10 fresh pitted olives; add 35g sugar and 4 cups water; boil for 10 minutes. Drink the juice, once a day, to relieve alcoholism.

### CLINICAL REPORTS

- For treatment of acute bacillary dysentery: Use 100g fresh olives with seeds and boil in a cup of water over very low heat for 2 to 3 hours until reduced to a half cup; strain. Adults drink a half to 1 tablespoonful each time. Repeat 3 to 4 times until bowel movements return to normal. Treatment stops as soon as the patients have 1 to 2 bowel movements daily. In general, each treatment program continues for 5 days.

## Onions

*Increase urination and expel phlegm; good for urination difficulty and coughs in common colds.*

## Orange Cake

*Balances energy, expands the chest, removes phlegm, suppresses coughs, improves appetite, stops diarrhea.*

### PREPARATION

- To cure bronchitis, crush 30g of orange cake and 15g of garlic. Boil them in water for consumption as soup.
- To cure diarrhea, boil 30g of orange cake, 15 longan nuts and 15g of rock sugar in 2 cups of water until the water is reduced to one cup. Drink it warm.

## Orange Leaves

*Relax the liver, promote energy circulation, remove phlegm, heal swelling; good for pain in the ribs, mastitis, coughs and hernias.*

## Orange Peels (Sweet Old Orange Peels)

*Regulate energy, remove phlegm and congestion, strengthen the spleen; good for common colds, coughs, poor appetite, abdominal pain and swelling, diarrhea and mastitis.*

## Oregano (Wild Marjoram)

*Induces perspiration, regulates energy, removes dampness; good for common colds, fevers, vomiting, chest congestion, diarrhea, jaundice and malnutrition in children.*

**Notes**

Onions have healing properties for wounds, ulcers, constipation and trichomonas vaginitis. According to a report, a normal healthy adult can inhibit an elevation of cholesterol level due to consumption of fatty foods by eating 60 grams of onion that is fried in oil.

Experiments with laboratory animals showed that onions can elevate gastric secretion, which indicates that they can be used to treat weakness of the intestines and nonbacterial enteritis.

The Chinese people cook onion and season it with soy sauce and vinegar as a remedy for urination difficulty.

A report indicated that the onion is the only known vegetable containing prostaglandins, which act on the cardiovascular system, smooth muscle and induce contraction of the uterus. In contemporary China, the onion is regarded as an important food cure for hypertension.

**Notes**

Orange cake is orange preserved with honey.

## Oyster Shells

*Check perspiration, control semen, remove phlegm and soften up hard spots; good for dizziness, seminal emission, scrofula, vaginal discharge and bleeding and goiter.*

## Peach Blossoms

*Treat edema with puffiness, ascites, beriberi, swelling of feet, constipation with dry stools, urination difficulty.*

### PREPARATION

- Bake peach blossom and grind into powder. Take one to 3g of powder with honey water one to two times daily.

## Peanuts

*Tone the spleen, balance the stomach, lubricate the lungs, remove phlegm from the body, nourish body energy.*

### PREPARATION

- To cure hypertension, soak peanuts in vinegar for 7 days. Eat 10 peanuts two times daily, in the morning and evening.
- To promote milk secretion in breastfeeding mothers, boil peanuts for regular consumption.
- To cure stomachaches, excessive gastric acids and peptic ulcers, take 2 to 4 teaspoons of peanut oil first thing in the morning for one week.
- To cure edema as in nephritis, boil peanuts (with the outer layers unremoved) and red dates in equal amounts and drink like tea.
- There is a Chinese remedy made of peanuts' outer layer to arrest bleeding in the digestive system, discharge of blood in pulmonary tuberculosis and tracheitis.

### Notes

Peanuts contain large amounts of protein (about 27 percent), including all eight essential amino acids. Over 80 percent of the fats contained in peanuts are unsaturated fatty acids that can lower the cholesterol level in the blood.

## Pear

*Good for cough with mucus, constipation, difficulty when swallowing, alcoholism, difficult urination, indigestion.*

### DESCRIPTION

- Cool; sweet and slightly sour; produces fluids; lubricates dryness; eliminates mucus; affects the lungs and stomach.

### PREPARATION

- Drink a glass of fresh pear juice in the morning and evening to relieve cough and thirst from fever.
- Soak fresh unpeeled pears in vinegar to make vinegar pears.
- Peel 2 vinegar pears and eat them to relieve indigestion and alcoholism.
- Crush 2 vinegar pears to squeeze out the juice. Drink the juice slowly in the morning and evening to cure sore throat and difficulty when swallowing.
- Boil 60g dried pear peels in water. Drink the juice to relieve difficult urination and pain when urinating.

## Peppermint

*Good for common colds, headaches, sore throats, indigestion, cankers, toothaches, skin eruptions.*

## DESCRIPTION

- Cool; pungent; affects the lungs and liver.

## PREPARATION

- Boil 5g peppermint in 1 cup water for a short while. Drink it as tea to treat discharge of stools containing blood (as in dysentery).
- Squeeze fresh peppermint juice for use as ear drops to relieve earache. (To squeeze the juice, use a pestle to pound the peppermint lightly, then wrap in a clean cloth and squeeze out the juice; or wrap peppermint, pound it and squeeze.)
- Boil 5g fresh peppermint in 1 cup water and add a little salt. Drink it like tea to relieve all kinds of pain involving the head and neck, such as headache, sore throat, pain in the mouth, pain in the tongue, toothache and also nosebleed, preferably at the early stage.
- Cook 70g fresh peppermint with 150g pork liver; eat it at meals to relieve pain in the eye, blurred vision and watering of the eyes.
- Boil fresh peppermint with bean curd and fresh ginger in water. Drink the soup and eat the bean curd to heal nasal congestion and nasal discharge, frequent sneezing and common cold.

## EXPERIMENT

- Local applications of menthol (a type of peppermint oil) are effective for headache, neuralgia and itching. When menthol is used, the skin feels cool sensations followed by light burning sensations. The cool sensations induced by menthol are not caused by a lowering of skin temperature but rather by the cold receptor of the nerve endings.

## *Persimmons*

*Good for coughing, vomiting of blood, mouth canker, stomachache, diarrhea, hemorrhoids, hypertension, endemic goiter, discharge of urine containing blood, hiccupping.*

## DESCRIPTION

- Cold; sweet; obstructive; quenches thirst; lubricates the lungs; strengthens the spleen; affects the heart, lungs and large intestine.

## PREPARATION

- Eat a fresh persimmon, peeled, each time, twice a day, to relieve stomachache that gets worse on exposure to heat.
- Crush a partially ripe persimmon and squeeze out the juice. Drink the juice with warm water once a day to treat hypertension and endemic goiter.
- Pick persimmons when the outer layers just begin to turn yellow; peel persimmons and leave them in the sun on hot days and frequently apply pressure to flatten them until the surface appears coated with white powder. In the Chinese language, the powder is called white frost of persimmon. Persimmons dried in this manner are called persimmon cakes.
- Steam 2 persimmon cakes with 30g honey. Eat in the morning and evening to treat senile asthma and cough with mucus.
- Cook 2 persimmon cakes in water with 60g glutinous (sweet) rice and 2 slices dried orange peel. Eat with meals, once a day for 3 consecutive days, to cure chronic enteritis and diarrhea.
- Mix a persimmon cake with a little long-grain rice and water and crush them to make a paste. Use to feed children 3 times a day for 2 to 3 consecutive days to relieve diarrhea.
- Boil 2 persimmon cakes until very soft. Eat 2 persimmon cakes each

*Notes*

If skin itchiness is due to cold skin, menthol will make it worse; normally, when skin itchiness occurs in winter or on exposure to cold weather, it means that the person has a cold skin.

Peppermint can cure trigeminal neuralgia and I have a personal experience in this respect. About 10 years ago, I had developed trigeminal neuralgia, which was very painful and I had used peppermint for instant relief of pain. It was more effective than any pain killer. But treatment of trigeminal neuralgia must be based upon each person's physical constitution.

time, twice a day, to cure hemorrhoids.

- Cook rice soup and add 2 persimmon cakes to the soup. Eat once a day for 5 consecutive days to relieve discharge of urine containing blood with no pain on urination.
- Crush 3 to 9g white frost of persimmon; boil in water and drink it slowly, a few times each day, to cure mouth canker, sore throat and dry cough.
- Gather the calyx and receptacle of a persimmon and leave in the sun to dry. The dried calyx and receptacle, important in Chinese herbal remedies, have a neutral energy, obstructive power and have the effect of pushing downwards.
- Boil 3 persimmon cakes in water with the calyxes and receptacles until soft. Drink the juice in the morning and evening to treat cough and chest pain in lung disease.
- Boil 9g calyxes and receptacles in water with 3g fresh ginger. Drink like tea to relieve hiccupping; or fry 3g persimmon calyxes and receptacles until aromatic and grind into powder. Dissolve in rice wine and drink once a day to relieve hiccupping.

## Plantain Seeds
*Promote urination, reduce internal heat, sharpen vision, remove phlegm; good for blocked urination, blood in urine and coughs.*

## Plum Blossoms
*Promote appetite, produce fluids, quench thirst; good for prevention of chicken pox and globus hystericus.*

## Radish
*Good for abdominal swelling due to indigestion, laryngitis due to continual cough with mucous discharge, vomiting of blood, nosebleed, dysentery, headache.*

### DESCRIPTION

- Cool; pungent and sweet; affects the lungs and stomach; detoxicates; downwards movements; promotes digestion and eliminates hot mucous discharge.

### PREPARATION

- Drink fresh radish juice mixed with ginger juice to cure laryngitis.
- Drink fresh radish juice to relieve intoxication.
- Regular consumption of fresh radishes prevents common cold, flu and respiratory infections.

## Radish Seeds
*Good for coughs, asthma and indigestion.*

## Salt
*Good for constipation, bleeding from the gums, sore throat, toothache, carbuncle, cataract.*

### DESCRIPTION

- Cold; salty, detoxicates; affects the stomach, kidneys, small and large intestines.

### PREPARATION

- Brush your teeth with fine table salt in the morning and evening to stop bleeding from gums.
- Mix salt with vinegar and drink it to relieve abdominal pain below the navel.
- Massage the surrounding regions of carbuncle and skin eruptions with salt to relieve itching.
- Drink a cup of salt water first thing in the morning on an empty stomach to relieve constipation.
- Gargle with salt water to prevent and relieve sore throat.
- Lick a little salt with the tip of the tongue before smoking to prevent forming a habit or to quit smoking within 1 month.
- Fry salt until brown; mix it with warm water. Drink the salt water to relieve fish and meat poisoning and abdominal pain due to eating the wrong foods.
- Mix salt with 2 glasses water and wash the affected region to relieve localized dermatitis, skin swelling and itching and contact skin poison.
- Lick a little salt and let it dissolve in the mouth and slowly swallow it to relieve hiccupping due to improper eating.

## Sea Grass

*Good for tuberculosis of the lymph node, goiter, edema, beriberi, pain in the testes.*

### DESCRIPTION

- Cold; bitter and salty; softens hardness, eliminates mucus; promotes water passage; reduces hot sensations.

### PREPARATION

- Boil 20g sea grass at low heat in 4 cups water until water is reduced to 2 cups. Drink 1 cup each time, twice a day, to relieve tuberculosis of the lymph node and goiter and to prevent hypertension and arteriosclerosis.
- Boil 50g sea grass with 20g fried orange seeds and 15g fried caraway seeds in water. Drink the soup once a day to relieve swollen testes.

### EXPERIMENT

- One experiment shows that sea grass extract can be used as an anticoagulant; another experiment on rats indicates various kinds of sea grass can lower cholesterol in the serum and internal organs; another experiment on dogs and rats shows that when large dosages (.75g per kilogram) are used, sea grass can lower blood pressure for a prolonged period of time; but smaller dosages will temporarily elevate blood pressure.

## Seaweed

*Good for goiters, edema, beriberi.*

### DESCRIPTION

- Cold; salty; softens hardness; eliminates mucus; promotes water passage.

## PREPARATION

- Prepare 40g seaweed and wash off the salt; boil it in 2 or 3 glasses water over low heat until the water is reduced by half. Drink to cure simple goiter.
- Boil 20g seaweed and sea grass each with 5g caraway seeds in an adequate amount of water over low heat until the water is reduced by half. Drink it to relieve swollen testes.
- Wash seaweed and cut about 1 inch in length; soak seaweed in boiling water 3 times, about 30 seconds each time; strain and eat the seaweed with sugar at meals for 1 month to relieve senile chronic bronchitis.

## *Shiitake Mushrooms*
*Good for prevention of rickets, anemia, measles.*

### DESCRIPTION

- Neutral; sweet; affects the stomach.

### PREPARATION

- Boil some shiitake mushrooms in water until the soup becomes yellowish. Drink only the liquid (without eating the mushrooms) to relieve vomiting caused by careless eating; another alternative is to place shiitake mushrooms in boiling water and steep until the soup becomes yellowish. Drink it as tea.
- Dissolve some sugar or honey in the shiitake mushroom soup to treat coughing.
- Drink shiitake mushroom soup, or dissolve shiitake mushroom powder in hot water and drink it as tea to relieve fish poisoning. A prolonged consumption by this method is believed to prevent arteriosclerosis.
- In case of difficult urination or discharge of urine containing blood, bake some shiitake mushroom until it appears burned on the surface. Eat 10g each time, twice a day, or eat fresh shiitake mushrooms.

### EXPERIMENT

- Studies with rats show shiitake mushroom lowers blood fat levels.

### CLINICAL REPORT

- Shiitake mushroom counteracts cholesterol, a recent report indicates.

## *Sour Orange Peels*
*Remove phlegm, stop vomiting, promote digestion.*

## *Squash Calyx*
*Good for boils on the skin, burns and mouth cankers.*

### PREPARATION

- To cure boils on the skin, apply squash calyx powder with sesame oil externally to the affected region.
- To heal burns, apply squash calyx powder with tea oil externally to the affected region; or apply to mouth cankers and ulcers externally to heal them.

### Notes

Shiitake mushroom is believed to counteract stomach and cervical cancers. (When I visited Japan in October 1985, I learned that a new pro-duct containing the extract from shiitake mushroom had been approved by the Japanese government as an anti-cancerous agent.) The Chinese people are very fond of mushrooms, including shiitake mushrooms, which are produced primarily in Japan. Shiitake mushroom may be cooked by itself and it may also be cooked with other vegetables. In either case, avoid excessive amounts of soy sauce and salt because they are quickly absorbed by the mushroom and spoil its good taste.

### Notes

Squash calyx can be baked or dried in the sun and ground into powder for food cures either externally or internally.

An experiment indicated that among 34 cases of late-stage ascites with a light degree of schistosomiasis treated with squash calyx powder, 0.5 grams three times daily for 2 to 3 weeks increased urine production, reduced symptoms in four cases, improved 23 cases and had no effects in eight cases.

## *Sweet Green Orange Peels*

*Disperse liver energy and clear phlegm; good for stomachaches, hernias, indigestion and swollen breasts.*

## *Tangerine Orange Seeds*

*Regulate energy flow in the body and relieve pain; used to treat hernias, swollen testes, with pain, pain in the nipples, lumbago and pain in the bladder.*

### PREPARATION

- To cure hernia of the small intestine and swollen testes, fry 20g of orange seeds without oil, boil them in wine, strain and drink the soup. Or, boil orange seeds, litchi nut seeds and longan seeds in water, strain and drink the soup.
- To cure brandy nose, fry orange seeds without oil and grind into powder; then grind a walnut into powder and mix with some warm wine. Make ointment for external application to the affected region.

## *Tea*

*Good for headaches, blurred vision, sleepiness, thirst, indigestion, enteritis, bacillary dysentery, edema in heart disease, herpes zoster.*

### DESCRIPTION

- Bitter; sweet; slightly cold; quenches thirst; wakes up the spirits; promotes digestion and urination; affects the heart, lungs and stomach.

### PREPARATION

- Grind into powder 10g tea leaves and 10g dried ginger. Take one teaspoonful powder with warm water each time, 2 to 3 times daily, to cure acute gastroenteritis.
- Grind tea leaves into powder; dissolve the powder in strong tea and apply externally to the affected region 2 to 3 times daily to cure herpes zoster.

### CLINICAL REPORT

- It is reported that among 168 cases of bacillary dysentery treated by drinking 2 ml strong tea 3 to 4 times daily, 40.6 percent recovered within a few days to a few weeks.
- Strong tea was also used to treat 87 cases of acute enteritis and more than 90 percent of patients recovered within 2 days; the same method was used to treat 12 cases of chronic enteritis. Ten cases completely recovered within 4 to 21 days with stools returning to normal; 2 cases improved to a very significant degree. The method of treatment: Drink 2 to 5 ml of very strong tea 3 to 4 times a day. (Tea leaves are boiled over low heat to make very strong tea, which is different from the normal way of making tea by pouring hot water over tea leaves.)

## *Thyme*

*Good for whooping cough, acute bronchitis, laryngitis.*

### DESCRIPTION

- Suppresses cough; also used as an aromatic calmative.

## EXPERIMENT

- Thyme can be used as an antibacterial agent and an anthelmintic. Thyme leaf may be used as an expectorant, according to experiments.

## *Turnip Seeds*

*Sharpen vision, reduce internal heat, remove dampness from the body; good for jaundice, dysentery and diminished urination.*

## *Walnut*

*Good for coughs, lumbago, impotence, seminal emission, frequent urination, kidney and bladder stones, constipation.*

### DESCRIPTION

- Warm; sweet; used as kidney tonic and to lubricate intestines and check seminal emission; affects the kidneys and lungs.

### PREPARATION

- Steam 30g walnuts with 15g rock sugar and 6g radish seeds for half an hour. Eat the mixture twice a day to cure chronic asthma and cough.
- Chew 90g of walnuts slowly each day to relieve sore throat, hoarseness, constipation and gastric and duodenal ulcers.
- Boil 15g walnut with 15g crushed fresh ginger. Drink it twice a day to relieve headache and fever and fear of cold due to common cold and also to induce perspiration in common cold.
- Steam 250g walnuts and persimmon cakes each for 1 hour. Divide into 3 portions and eat 1 portion each time, 3 times a day, for 1 month to relieve cough and underweight due to pulmonary tuberculosis.
- Prepare 30g walnuts, 2 pork kidneys, sliced and a little lard; fry them together. Eat it hot every day at bedtime for 3 days to cure seminal emission with sudden urination.
- Fry 120g walnuts in vegetable oil until crunchy. Mix walnuts with some sugar and water to make syrup. Eat it within 2 days to relieve stones in urinary tract.

### CLINICAL REPORT

- For the treatment of kidney and bladder stones: Fry 120g walnuts in vegetable oil until crunchy. Add sugar and grind into an emulsion or cream. Eat the walnuts within 1 to 2 days. (Reduce the dosage for children.) Treatment continues until stones are passed or the symptoms disappear. In general, stones are passed once or several times within a few days. They also appear smaller and softer than earlier stones or they are dissolved in urine to look like cream. Thus, walnut is considered effective for dissolving the stones.

## *Water Chestnut*

*Good for diabetes, jaundice, urinary strains, pink eyes, sore throat, hypertension.*

### DESCRIPTION

- Cold; sweet; relieves fever and indigestion; promotes urination; affects the lungs and stomach.

## PREPARATION

- Boil 5 water chestnuts in water with 1 fresh mandarin orange peel. Drink as tea, 3 times a day, to relieve hypertension.
- Peel 100g water chestnuts and chew them slowly in the morning and evening; or drink water chestnut juice to cure sore throat, hemorrhoids and mouth canker.
- Prepare 500g water chestnuts; wash in water and dry thoroughly; put them in half a bottle of rice wine; seal it and set aside for a few days. Slowly chew 2 water chestnuts each time and wash down with the rice wine in the bottle, twice a day, to cure diarrhea with discharge of whitish or reddish substances.
- Warm a glass of water chestnut juice and mix with 2 teaspoonfuls rice wine. Drink it to relieve discharge of blood from anus (as in hemorrhoids).

## White or Yellow Mustard

*Warms the internal regions and disperse cold; good for coughs, cold stomachaches and abdominal pain.*

## White Sugar

*Good for dry coughs, thirst, stomachaches.*

### DESCRIPTION

- Neutral; sweet; lubricates the lungs; produces fluids; affects the spleen.

### PREPARATION

- Boil 3 spoonfuls sugar in 1 glass rice wine over low heat. Drink it to relieve a tight sensation in the abdomen.
- Mix sugar with red dates and chew 2 dates after meals like chewing gum to relieve a dry cough.
- Boil sugar in water to make concentrated syrups to treat stomachache, abdominal discomfort caused by eating fish and crabs and bad breath caused by eating garlic and onion.

### Notes

Sugar may be boiled and made into the shape of a rock; this is called rock sugar (rock candy) with a neutral energy and sweet flavor. Rock sugar is regarded as the best quality of sugar and is frequently used in combination with other foods in Chinese remedies.

## Yellow Soybeans

*Heal swelling and relieve pain, remove water from the body, reduce internal heat, dissolve blood coagulations, regulate the functions of internal organs, cure kidney disease, promote urination and blood circulation.*

### PREPARATION

- Use this simple recipe to prevent common cold: Boil 50g of yellow soybeans, 3g of dry coriander (or three green onion heads), three slices of radish. Drink the soup at meals.

### Notes

Yellow soybeans are regarded as the king of beans; they contain about 40 percent protein, which is comparable to animal protein. For this reason, yellow soybeans are sometimes called "vegetable meat" or "green beef." Yellow soybeans contain 18 to 20 percent fat, which is better than animal fat in quality, because the former has no cholesterol in it.

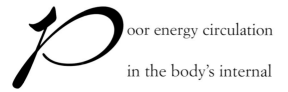

*P*oor energy circulation in the body's internal environments can affect various vital organs and cause pain. These regulating foods are good for promoting energy circulation.

# Foods for Promoting Energy Circulation

## Beef

*Good for those who are underweight and for diabetes, edema.*

### DESCRIPTION

- Neutral; sweet; used as a spleen, stomach, energy and blood tonic; affects the spleen and stomach.

### PREPARATION

- Eat regularly concentrated beef soup to relieve chronic diarrhea and prolapse of anus caused by chronic diarrhea.
- Mix together 1,000g beef, 10g ground black pepper, 5g dried orange peel powder; add 1 cup fresh ginger juice and an adequate amount of salt; marinate for 2 hours; cook the beef. Eat at meals to improve the conditions of stomach and stimulate the appetite. To make ginger juice, grate fresh ginger and boil it in water.

## Cantaloupe Seeds

*Remove phlegm from the body, relieve abdominal swelling and blood coagulations in the abdomen; good for gastrointestinal disorders.*

### PREPARATION

- Here's a simple way of treating bad breath: grind cantaloupe seeds into powder and mix with honey. Make into tablets as big as a date; take a tablet after brushing teeth in the morning.

## Caraway Seeds

*Good for stomachaches, abdominal pain, hernias, lumbago.*

### DESCRIPTION

- Warm; slightly pungent; promotes energy circulation; good for the stomach; affects the kidneys and stomach.

### PREPARATION

- Boil 10g caraway seed with 5g cinnamon and 5g dried ginger; drink it as soup to treat vomiting and hiccupping.
- Boil 10g fennel seed in 3 cups water over low heat until water is reduced to 1 cup. Drink a cupful each time, twice a day, to relieve cough.

### EXPERIMENT

- Caraway has been found to relieve asthma in rats.

## Carrot

*Good for chronic diarrhea; coughs; indigestion; difficulty when urinating.*

### DESCRIPTION

- Neutral; sweet; pushes downwards; used as a diuretic and digestive; affects the lungs and spleen.

### PREPARATION

- Regular consumption of fresh or cooked carrot prevents night blindness.
- Boil carrot and red dates in water to make soup to treat whooping cough in children.

### Notes

Beef kidney is used as kidney tonic to improve sexual capacity and to cure temporary and permanent impotence in men; cut a kidney into small pieces to boil with one bowl of rice and when the kidney is cooked, add five green onion white heads.

Beef liver is neutral and sweet, is used as a liver tonic and to sharpen the vision and relieve glaucoma and night blindness.

### Notes

Cantaloupe seeds can soften up hard spots, produce body fluids and lubricate dryness in the body. They contain about 27 percent fat and 5.78 percent glutelin, which is a simple protein soluble in alkalies and diluted acids.

An experiment showed that the ratio of 1:10 cantaloupe seed solution was able to destroy roundworms and tapeworms within 10 to 90 minutes, but when the skin was removed from the seeds, the action slowed and some worms were still not destroyed after 1.5 to 3 hours.

### Notes

Basically, the actions of caraway are similar to fennel.

- Carrot may be cooked with parsley and water chestnut for facilitating eruption in measles.
- Fresh carrot juice may be used for external application to heal burns.
- Boil 5g carrot seeds in 2 glasses water over low heat until water is reduced to 1 glass. Drink the soup to promote urination for treatment of edema.
- Bake the peels of carrots until they appear burned. Eat the peels while hot to relieve frequent urination at night. Divide 1 carrot into 3 dosages and eat them 3 times a day.
- To use carrot as a blood tonic, cook it with spinach and lotus roots in soup; or, cook carrot with tomatoes, onion and beef; or, cook carrot with pork liver.
- For sharpening the vision, cook carrot with chicken liver or duck liver.

## EXPERIMENT

- Shows the effect of lowering blood sugar in animals.

## Cherry Roots

*Good for roundworm disease.*

## Chicken Eggs

*Good for dry cough, hoarseness, pink eyes, sore throat, quickening, diarrhea, burns.*

### DESCRIPTION

- Neutral; sweet; used as a blood tonic; lubricates dryness.

### PREPARATION

- Egg may be eaten fresh or mixed with hot water; or use a mixture of egg white and yolk for external applications.
- Break an egg into a cup and mix with a few teaspoonfuls rice wine. Drink it to relieve heart pain in pregnant women.
- Boil 20 chicken eggs in their shells until fully cooked. Crush the eggs, including the shell; boil the eggs again in water with 500g black soybeans for 2 or 3 hours until the eggs and beans are thoroughly mixed and become black; remove and discard the black soybeans. Store the eggs in a container until needed. Peel the eggs and eat 2 to 3 warm eggs each time, once a day, for as long as necessary, to sharpen vision and correct blurred vision.

### CLINICAL REPORT

- For treatment of neurodermatitis and psoriasis, sterilize 2 chicken eggs with alcohol and place in a jar slightly larger than the eggs; add vinegar to cover the eggs and seal; set aside for 7 days. Break the eggs and pour the egg white and egg yolk into another sterilized jar and seal the jar. Use a cotton ball to rub the egg on the affected region for 1 to 2 minutes each time, several times a day; the treatment should continue without interruption. In general, scales begin to fall off after a number of treatments; severe itching either improves or stops completely. If treatment continues, then the focus of the skin ailment will gradually be reduced in size; but if treatment is interrupted at this point, symptoms will recur. The longer the history of symptoms, the longer the treatment needed. Among the 12 cases of neurodermatitis treated, 9 cases recovered completely and 3 cases improved; among the 5 cases of psoriasis treated, 2 cases recovered completely and 3 cases improved.

*Notes*

I remember one day my friend told me that his 3-year-old son had wet the bed the previous night. I asked him casually if his son ate any carrot before going to bed. Quite unexpectedly, this friend was taken by surprise. "How did you know?" he asked. I told him that carrot can promote urination. In fact, carrot is also good to promote the outbreak of rash in measles and for inflammation of the bladder and the kidneys not only because carrot is a diuretic, but also because it is an effective food for healing inflammations.

## Chives

*Good for chest pain; difficulty when swallowing; upset stomach; vomiting blood; nosebleed; discharge of urine containing blood; prolapse of anus; injuries from a fall, causing internal blood coagulations.*

### DESCRIPTION

- Warm; pungent; promotes energy circulation; counteracts blood coagulations; affects the liver, stomach and kidneys.
- Contraindications: eye diseases and skin eruptions.

### PREPARATION

- Squeeze the juice from fresh chive (leaves or roots). Drink 1 teaspoonful of the warm juice each time with milk to treat difficulty when swallowing. The same juice, cold without milk, is effective to treat sunstroke and also to wash skin eruptions caused by lacquer poisoning.
- Cook chive with pork or lamb liver to cure excessive perspiration and stimulate the appetite.
- Crush chive leaves or roots and externally apply the juice to the wound to relieve bruises, swelling and pain.
- Cut chive leaves and roots into small pieces; boil with wine. Drink it hot to relieve injuries resulting from twisting the waist.
- Cook chive with egg to relieve diarrhea, night sweat and nocturia.

## Clam

*Saltwater clams good for edema, mucous discharge, goiter, vaginal discharge, hemorrhoids; freshwater clams good for vaginal bleeding and discharge, pink eyes, eczema and hemorrhoids; saltwater clamshell powder good for diabetes, edema, goiter and hemorrhoids; freshwater clam saliva good for diabetes, pink eyes and burns; freshwater clamshell powder good for cough with mucous discharge, stomachache, hiccupping, vomiting, whitish vaginal discharge, eczema, swelling.*

### DESCRIPTION

- Sea (saltwater) clam—cold, salty, acts on the stomach, promotes water passage, eliminates mucus and softens hardness; freshwater clam—cold, sweet and salty, detoxicates, sharpens the vision, acts on the liver and kidneys. Sea clamshell powder-cold, salty, promotes water passage, softens hardness, eliminates mucus, acts on the lungs and kidneys; river clam saliva—sharpens vision; freshwater clamshell powder—cold, salty, eliminates mucus and dries dampness, acts on the lungs, liver and stomach.

### PREPARATION

- Sea clamshell may be baked and ground into very fine powder to make sea clamshell powder. Freshwater clamshell may be washed clean (with the black skin removed) and ground into powder or baked and ground into powder to make freshwater clamshell powder. Apply saltwater clam's saliva externally to the affected region to relieve itching and pain and swelling of the vaginal orifice.
- Crush a few garlics to mix with clamshell powder and make into tablets of a normal size. Take 10 tablets with warm water each time, once a day, to relieve edema in weak persons.
- Mix clamshell powder with lard for external application to the affected region to relieve burns.
- Mix fine clamshell powder with an equal amount of raw licorice powder, take 7g each time with warm water, twice a day, to cure gastric ulcer

### Notes

Chive is an important food for external injuries because it can counteract blood coagulations. When a person gets hurt (like in an automobile accident) he or she may feel pain long after the accident caused by internal blood coagulations not diagnosed by X-ray examination. The blood coagulation that is causing pain may be so light that it cannot be seen on the X-ray. One useful way to determine whether blood coagulation occurred or not, however, is to determine if the pain recurs in the same body region or if it shifts around; if the patient always feels pain in the same region, it is very likely that blood coagulation has occurred, which may be relieved by eating chive. The Chinese people believe that pain may be caused either by blood coagulations or energy congestion. (When blood fails to circulate, it coagulates; when energy fails to circulate, it gets congested.) When pain is caused by blood coagulations, it will recur in the same region; when caused by energy congestion, the pain will shift around.

Here's a convenient way to use chive to relieve pain caused by blood coagulations: Cut chive into small pieces; boil it in water with wine and then drink the whole thing as soup. For example, in the past, Chinese authorities used to severely beat prisoners to force a confession from them but the severe beating caused internal bleeding and subsequently, internal blood coagulations. To prevent blood coagulations, it had become a routine practice to give prisoners chive at meals after the beating.

Chive is warm in energy and acts upon the stomach. Therefore, chive is often used to relieve stomachache of a cold nature. As a matter of fact, the Chinese people always make a point of regularly eating chive, which is also effective for enteritis, if they have weak digestive functions. Fresh chive juice may also be drunk to relieve nosebleed (but its awful taste often makes the juice difficult to administer).

and excessive gastric acid.

- Regular consumption of clam meat at meals relieves lymphadenitis scrofula in the neck and goiter.
- Cook clam with chive. Eat at meals to relieve pulmonary tuberculosis and night sweat.
- Boil 30g fine clamshell powder with 4g outer layer of peanuts and 6 red dates to make concentrated soup. Drink the soup once a day to relieve nosebleed, bleeding from gums and purpura hemorrhagica.
- Roast a whole freshwater clam until its outer part is charred and the inner part becomes yellow-brown with its original shape remaining intact; grind into fine powder and mix with sesame oil for external application to relieve eczema in infants.

### CLINICAL REPORT

- For treatment of gastric and duodenal ulcers, fry freshwater clamshell powder in a bronze fry pan (or any earthenware fry pan) until it becomes yellow-brown with the fishy smell gone; strain it before using. Take 1 to 2g each time mixed with warm water, once every hour during the daytime, 12 to 14 times a day, for 4 to 8 weeks. Among the 41 cases treated from 14 to 79 days, 28 cases showed disappearance of pain in the upper abdomen and 7 cases a decrease, 23 cases showed disappearance of pressure pain in the upper abdomen (pain that occurs on pressure by hand) and 6 cases a decrease; 21 cases had a follow-up X-ray examination, which indicated disappearance of the niche in 9 cases, disappearance of deformity in 1 case and a reduction in the size of the niche in 6 cases.

## Dillseed

*Good for abdominal pain, poor appetite, shortage of milk secretion after childbirth.*

### DESCRIPTION

- Warm; pungent; warms the body, promotes energy circulation and counteracts fish and meat poisoning; affects the spleen and kidneys.

### PREPARATION

- Fry dillseeds until aromatic and grind into powder; dissolve 5g of the powder in warm rice wine and drink each time to cure lumbago due to twisted muscles.

## Fennel Seed

*Good for hernias, cold pain in lower abdomen, lumbago, stomachache, vomiting, dry and wet beriberi.*

### DESCRIPTION

- Warm; pungent; warms the internal region and promotes energy circulation; affects the kidneys, the bladder and stomach.

### PREPARATION

- Prepare 40g apricot seeds; crush 20g fresh green onion white heads with roots and bake until dry; prepare 40g fennel seed; grind all the ingredients into a powder. Drink 10g of the powder dissolved in rice wine each time, twice a day, to relieve pain in hernia of small intestine.
- Fry equal amounts of fennel and litchi seeds and grind into powder; dissolve 10g of the powder in rice wine and drink each time, twice a

*Notes*

Dill leaf is warm, pungent and oppressive. According to 1 experiment, dill leaf is found to have the effect of lowering blood pressure and expanding blood vessels in animals.

day, to relieve pain in hernia of the small intestine.

- Measure equal amounts fennel and black pepper and grind them into powder; dissolve 10g of the powder in rice wine each time, twice a day, to relieve pain in small intestine.
- For lumbago, when unable to turn sideways and extreme fatigue, cook slices of pork kidneys with fried fennel and eat at meals.
- To heal cold stomachache and abdominal pain, use fennel and ginger as seasonings when preparing meals.

## CLINICAL REPORT

- For treatment of incarcerated hernia of small intestine, use 10 to 20g fennel (less for children) to make tea; drink it hot; if no effects are shown within 15 to 30 minutes, repeat once more. Or, use hot water to make fennel soup (4 to 8g fennel seed for adults and 2g for children) and drink the soup; 10 minutes later, repeat and drink once more, then lie down on your back with your legs together and knees half bent for 40 minutes. In general, the incarcerated hernia should restore itself within half an hour and the pain should disappear or improve, otherwise, surgery is indicated, according to this clinical report. Among the 26 cases treated from 2 hours to 3 days, 22 cases have recovered and 4 cases have shown no effects (3 cases of incarcerated omenturn majus and 1 case of parietal necrosis). The report also indicates that the treatment results are better in cases with a shorter history of the disease; if the symptoms have a long history, necrosis and perforation may have already occurred and they should not be treated by this method. In case of incarcerated momentum majus, surgery should be considered, according to this report.
- For treatment of hydrocele of tunica vaginalis and elephantiasis scroti: Fry 16g fennel and 5g salt until black; grind them into powder to make cakes with 2 raw duck eggs; eat the cakes while drinking warm rice wine at bedtime. Each treatment program continues for 4 days; the second treatment program begins 2 to 5 days after completing the first program. Treatment may continue, if necessary. Among the 64 cases of hydrocele of tunica vaginalis treated for 1 to 6 programs, 59 cases recovered, 1 case has shown progress, 4 cases have shown no results. The majority of patients suffering from elephantiasis scroti have shown results only after 4 treatment programs; the results are rather satisfactory with no side effects (except the cases in which the scrotum was as hard as stone).

## Fig Roots
*Good for pain in muscles and bone, hemorrhoids, tuberculosis of lymph node.*

## PREPARATION

- Boil fresh or dried fig or fig roots in water with pork or eggs for pain in muscles and bones.
- Crush fig roots (with rough surfaces removed); boil in water to make tea to remedy itching in the throat.
- Boil 30g fig and fig roots to relieve tuberculosis of lymph node.

## Fingered Citron Roots
*Good for pain and weakness in limbs.*

### Notes

Chinese herbalists believe that fennel travels very fast in the body and it can quickly warm up the internal region. Therefore, fennel can treat cold pain in the body; but since it is warm in nature, fennel should not be used to treat any hot disease, such as hot diarrhea or pain that occurs on exposure to hot surroundings (sunburn, burn, or warm temperatures). Fennel is not recommended for men with excessively strong erection and premature ejaculation. Fennel should be of the best quality, fresh and aromatic; it is considered an aromatic digestive and carminative, good for regulation of intestines, expelling intestinal gas, warming up internal region and exciting the nervous system. Fennel root is warm and tastes pungent and sweet, it can warm the kidneys and promote energy circulation to relieve pain; good for cold pain in hernia, cold vomiting, abdominal pain and arthritis.

## Garlic

*Good for cold abdominal pain, edema, diarrhea, dysentery, whooping cough.*

### DESCRIPTION

- Warm; pungent; promotes energy circulation, warms the stomach and spleen, destroys worms; affects the spleen, stomach and lungs.

### PREPARATION

- Boil 3 garlic cloves in water and eat with soy sauce at meals to relieve cough and abdominal pain and also to promote blood circulation and urination.
- For women, to relieve itch in the genital region, boil a few garlic cloves and use the liquid to wash the genital region.
- Crush a few garlic cloves to mix with mustard (powder or paste) and eat it with rice wine. Or, boil a few garlic cloves in water and drink it as tea to correct chronic cold sensations, particularly in women. If wine is desired, make garlic wine: Simply cut up a garlic clove in large pieces, drop into a small bottle of wine; put away for 1 month and it is ready to drink as a wine tonic.
- Eat 1 to 3 fresh garlic cloves daily by dividing them into 3 dosages; continue treatment for 5 to 10 consecutive days to heal amebic dysentery.
- Take 2 teaspoonfuls 10 to 20 percent garlic solution every 2 hours (mixed with some syrup or orange tincture to make it more appetizing) to relieve whooping cough in children.
- Eat garlic cloves regularly to prevent bacillary dysentery when it is widespread.
- Cut up a garlic clove and use the juicy slice to rub the skin to relieve pain caused by insect bite (such as bee sting) as an emergency measure.
- Garlic may be cooked with soybeans: Soak the soybeans overnight; cook soybeans with 5 to 10 garlic cloves. Eat as a tonic and also to promote urination, relieve edema and chronic nephritis.
- Another way to use garlic: Fry garlic cloves in vegetable oil with black pepper, sliced fresh ginger and salt; add dry shrimps, then sprinkle with sugar, vinegar and green onion. Add some tomato ketchup and flour to thicken, if desired. This recipe contains almost all the needed flavors—sweet, sour, pungent and salty.

### CLINICAL REPORT

- For treatment of lobar pneumonia; 1 tablespoon garlic syrup every 4 hours (in general 10 percent, but sometimes 100 percent). Among the 9 people treated, 6 cases show complete recovery, 3 show no satisfactory results.

## Grapefruit

*Good for indigestion, bad breath due to intoxication, poor appetite in pregnant women.*

### DESCRIPTION

- Cold; sweet and sour.

### PREPARATION

- Steam 90g peeled grapefruit with half a cup rice wine and 1 cup honey. Drink it all in 1 day to relieve cough with mucous discharge.
- Eat 1 medium grapefruit each time, 3 times a day, to relieve indigestion, belching and mouth watering in pregnant women.
- Slowly eat 1 small grapefruit to relieve intoxication.

*Notes*

There have been fewer cases of pulmonary tuberculosis in Sandong, a province of China where people consume more garlic than in any other province. As a result of these findings, garlic has been made into tablets and used with good results.

In the northern provinces of China, Chinese people carry some garlic with them while on a long journey, just in case they have to drink water from mountains or rivers. To prevent bad effects, they chew a garlic clove like chewing gum and spit it out before drinking water.

Many people don't want to eat garlic for fear of getting bad breath. According to some people, "garlic" breath can be eliminated by eating a few red dates or a persimmon. When garlic cloves are steamed (over boiling water), the strong smell will be gone before eating the garlic.

In daily cooking, a few garlic slices may be added to eliminate the strong smell of meats or fish. It is believed that a small quantity of garlic can counteract cancer, but an excessive quantity of garlic can cause cancer (based on the Chinese theory that excessive garlic is bad for the stomach and liver).

Chinese people eat large quantities of garlic only under special circumstances, such as severe malnutrition or edema.

In recent years, garlic has emerged as an important ingredient in Chinese medicine, mostly due to its powerful effects in treating dysentery and destroying germs. In fact, many modern medicines contain garlic as an important ingredient. For dysentery at its early stage, chew a garlic clove five or six times a day every four hours.

Contra-indications of garlic include eye diseases and sore throat.

## Grapefruit Roots

*Regulate body energy, relieve pain, counteract wind and cold; good for stomachaches, hernia pain and coughs in common colds.*

## Grapefruit Flowers

*Promote energy circulation, remove phlegm from the body, relieve pain; often used to relieve stomachaches and chest pain.*

## Green Onion Roots

*Good for headaches and sore throats.*

## Green Onion White Heads

*Stimulate sweat glands to perspire, inhibit or destroy the growth of bacteria for diphtheria, dysentery, tuberculosis.*

### PREPARATION

- For common colds, boil 30g of green onion white heads with 9g of fresh ginger in water. Add 30g of brown sugar when the water is boiling. Drink it hot to induce perspiration three times a day.
- For acute mastitis, crush a half pound of green onion white heads and boil in water. Strain quickly and use the soup to wash the affected region two to three times a day.

## Hawthorn Fruit

*Good for meat indigestion, abdominal swelling, mucous discharge, discharge of blood from anus, lumbago, hernia, neck pain after childbirth.*

### DESCRIPTION

- Slightly warm; sweet and sour; promotes digestion; corrects blood coagulations; expels tapeworm; affects the spleen, stomach and liver.

### PREPARATION

- Soak hawthorn fruit in boiling water for less than 1 minute; slice the fruits and lay them in the sun to dry. (Hawthorn fruit slices are available in most Chinese herb shops.)
- Fry hawthorn slices until they look like charcoal to make hawthorn fruit charcoal.
- Mix together the following ingredients and marinate for 10 days to prepare hawthorn fruit wine: 250g hawthorn slices, 250g fresh longans, 30g red dates, 30g brown sugar and 4.5 cups rice wine.
- Drink 30 to 60g hawthorn fruit wine at every bedtime to relieve pain caused by excessive fatigue, muscular pain and arthritis pain, flying spots in front of the eyes, lumbago and pain in thigh in the elderly.
- Boil in water 60g hawthorn fruit slices with an equal amount fresh or dried chestnuts until very soft; add 30g sugar and stir thoroughly. Drink the juice once a day, first thing in the morning on an empty stomach, to cure scurvy.
- Boil 31g hawthorn slices with water; stir in 1.5g fennel powder. Drink the juice in the morning and evening to relieve hernia of the small intestine.

- Boil 15g hawthorn fruit slices in water and drink as tea on a long-term basis, to relieve hypertension, high level of blood fat and coronary heart disease.
- Grind 6 to 9g hawthorn fruit charcoal into powder. Take the powder with warm water, once a day, to relieve abdominal pain caused by acute and chronic gastritis, enteritis and dysentery.
- Boil 3g hawthorn charcoal with 6g hawthorn fruit slices; drink the juice to relieve diarrhea in children; or crush 5 hawthorn fruits and squeeze out the juice to mix with a pinch of hawthorn fruit charcoal for oral administration to stop diarrhea in children.
- Crush 2 to 3 fresh hawthorn fruits and squeeze out the juice to drink; or boil 2 to 3 hawthorn fruits with 6g dry orange peels; drink the juice to correct indigestion, abdominal swelling and abdominal pain.

## EXPERIMENT

- An experiment on rabbits shows the effects of hawthorn fruit in lowering blood pressure.
- An experiment on toads shows the effects of hawthorn fruit in expanding blood vessels.
- Hawthorn fruits are reported to have the effects of contracting the uterus and reducing antibiosis.

## Jasmine Flowers

*Regulate energy in the body and balance the internal region; good for abdominal pain, diarrhea and conjunctivitis.*

## Kumquat

*Good for chest congestion, thirst, indigestion, cough, whooping cough, stomachache, hernial pain, poor appetite.*

### DESCRIPTION

- Warm; pungent, sweet and sour; relieves cough; eliminates mucus, promotes energy circulation.

### PREPARATION

- Steam 5 to 10 fresh kumquats with 30g of rock sugar for half an hour and eat a few each time, twice a day, to stop senile cough and asthma.
- Eat a few fresh kumquats to relieve indigestion.
- To make dried kumquats, place fresh kumquats in the sun to dry.
- Boil 10 dried kumquats in 6 cups water until water is reduced to 3 cups; drink 1 cup of the juice each time, 3 times a day, to treat stomachache.
- Crush 10 dried kumquats and boil in a mixture of half water and half rice wine. Drink a cup of the juice each time, twice a day, to relieve hernial pain.
- To make sugar kumquats, place fresh kumquats in the sun until half dry. Soak kumquats in syrup.
- Chew 30g sugar kumquats slowly, like chewing gum, to stimulate poor appetite due to common cold or motion sickness.

## Kumquat Roots

*Good for stomachaches, vomiting, hernias, abdominal pain in women after childbirth and prolapse of the uterus.*

## Ladle Gourd

*Promotes urination, reduces swelling, disperses congestion.*

### PREPARATION

- To heal ascites and edema all over the body, boil 30 to 60g of ladle gourd with 30g of winter gourd peel and 30g of watermelon peel. Drink like tea.
- To relieve urination difficulty, reduce jaundice and lower blood pressure, squeeze fresh juice from a ladle gourd and add honey. Drink a cup of juice two times daily.

## Leaf Mustard

*Good for mucous discharge, cough, chest congestion.*

### DESCRIPTION

- Warm; pungent; affects the lungs.

### PREPARATION

- Cook preserved leaf mustard and eat 30g a day to cure pulmonary abscess and bronchiectasis and laryngitis. Boil 5g fried leaf mustard seeds with 10g fried radish seeds, 5g dried orange peel and 5g licorice. Drink it as tea to cure chronic bronchitis and cough with mucous discharge.

## Litchi (Lychee)

*Good for hiccupping, stomachache, diarrhea, asthma, hernial pain.*

### DESCRIPTION

- Warm; sweet and sour; produces fluids; stimulates energy; relieves pain; affects the spleen and liver.

### PREPARATION

- Eat 60 to 150g fresh litchis to improve physical conditions after prolonged illness.
- Fresh litchis may be left in the sun to dry. Dried litchis are widely used in the Chinese diet.
- Boil 30 to 60g dried litchis and 5 dried red dates with adequate water. Drink the soup twice a day to cure chronic diarrhea.
- Steam 120g dried litchis and eat once a day to cure asthma.
- Collect litchi seeds and leave them in the sun to dry to use in remedies.
- Crush 30g dried litchi seeds; boil in water with 6g fresh ginger or dried orange peels. Drink it once a day to relieve stomachache and abdominal pain.
- Crush 60g dried litchi seeds and 15g caraway seeds; boil them in an adequate amount of water. Drink the soup once a day to relieve hernial pain, elephantiasis, hydrocele of tunica vaginalis and swelling and pain in the testes.

## Limes (Young Trifoliate Oranges)

*Remove phlegm; good for chest pain and congestion, edema, constipation, gastroptosis, falling of the uterus and falling of the anus.*

### Notes

A prolonged consumption of leaf mustard can warm up the internal region. It is not recommended for people suffering from eye diseases, hemorrhoids, or discharge of stools containing blood, which are normally regarded as hot symptoms.

Leaf mustard can relieve congestion because it has a warm energy and tastes pungent, which are the two important components of foods that are used to promote energy circulation and relieve congestion of various kinds.

## Longan Seeds

*Arrest bleeding, relieve pain, regulate energy, remove dampness; good for injuries, hernias, scrofula and eczema.*

## Malt

*Good for indigestion, abdominal swelling, poor appetite, vomiting, diarrhea, swelling of breasts.*

### DESCRIPTION

- Slightly warm; sweet; promotes digestion; pushes downwards; affects the spleen and stomach.

### PREPARATION

- Boil 50g malt in water and drink as soup to cure indigestion, abdominal swelling and swelling of breast with pain.
- Boil 50g malt with 10g orange peel in water. Drink as tea to relieve the aftereffects of acute and chronic hepatitis.
- Fry malt and grind into powder. Take 2 teaspoonfuls with wine each time, twice a day, to cure abdominal swelling and tightness after childbirth; or take 2 teaspoonfuls with warm water each time, twice a day, to relieve fever after childbirth or shortage of milk after childbirth, or swelling of breasts after childbirth.
- Boil 40g each of fresh malt and fried malt. Drink as soup once a day for three consecutive days to cure swelling of breasts at weaning; if swelling and hardness and pain are observed, double the quantities of fresh malt and fried malt.
- Boil 10g hawthorn fruits and 10g fried malt (to be reduced in case of children) and drink as tea, 3 times a day, to relieve indigestion.

### CLINICAL REPORT

- For treatment of acute and chronic hepatitis: Prepare tender roots of malt sprouts. (To make malt sprouts, wash barley, then immerse in water for 12 hours; drain, then wrap tightly in a wet cloth and splash water on them a few times daily until they sprout; dry the sprouts in the sun.) Dry and grind into powder and mix with syrup for a remedy. Take 10ml (containing 15g malt powder) each time, 3 times a day, after meals; in addition, an adequate amount of yeast and vitamin B-complex tablets should be administered. In general, one treatment program consists of 30 days and one additional treatment program should be administered after recovery. Among the 161 cases treated, 108 cases showed effects and 53 cases showed no effects, which means the effective rate is 67.1 percent. Among the subjects treated, of the 56 cases of acute hepatitis, 48 cases showed effects of the treatment; of the 105 cases of chronic hepatitis, 60 cases showed effects. After treatments, there are decreases of various degrees in symptoms, such as pain in liver, anorexia, fatigue and low temperature, particularly the symptom of anorexia. Among the cases that showed effects, there are various degrees of decreases in the size of a swollen liver and in transaminase. A few patients showed some side effects, including dry sensations in the mouth, bitter taste in the mouth, anxiety and diarrhea. The long-term effects of this treatment should be determined by further research.

## Mango Leaves

*Promote energy flow and eliminate congestion; good for abdominal pain and swelling due to energy congestion.*

## Mussel

*Good for night sweats, lumbago, impotence, vomiting of blood, vaginal discharge, goiter.*

### DESCRIPTION

- Warm; salty; increases the energy of kidneys and liver; cures simple goiter; affects the liver and kidneys.

### PREPARATION

- Bake 100g mussels and grind into powder. Grind into powder 10g dried orange peel. Mix the two powders with honey. Dissolve 3 teaspoonfuls in water each time, 3 times daily, to cure insomnia and dizziness.
- Use rice wine to wash mussels and cook with chive. Eat to cure lumbago and to counteract cold sensations in the lower abdomen in women.
- Boil 10g mussels with 30g celery. Eat at meals to lower blood pressure.

## Green Onion White Head

*Good for headaches, abdominal pain, constipation, suppression of urination, dysentery.*

### DESCRIPTION

- Warm; pungent; induces perspiration; affects the lungs and stomach.

### PREPARATION

- For relief of nasal congestion and nasal discharge in infants associated with common colds, steam a green onion white head and a mushroom with 30 to 50 ml mother's milk. Feed infants the soup without the mushroom or white head.
- Crush 4 to 6 white heads; warm it up with wine. Drink the soup to remedy a common cold.

## Radish Leaves

*Good for chest congestion, hiccupping, indigestion, diarrhea, sore throat, swelling of breast in women, shortage of milk secretion.*

### DESCRIPTION

- Neutral; pungent and bitter; promotes digestion and energy circulation; affects the spleen and stomach.

### PREPARATION

- Cut up dry radish leaves, boil them in water and add some salt. Use the warm liquid to wash the genital areas in women to relieve itching, or pour the liquid into the bathtub and sit in it to relieve cold sensations in the genital region.

## Rapeseed

*Good for abdominal pain in women after childbirth and blood in stools.*

## Red Beans

*Regulate energy in the body and facilitate menstruation.*

## Roses

*Good for discharge of blood from the mouth, irregular menstruation, dysentery and mastitis.*

## Saffron

*Good for congested chest, vomiting of blood, suppression of menstruation, abdominal pain after childbirth due to blood coagulations, injuries from falls.*

### DESCRIPTION

- Neutral; sweet; promotes energy and blood circulation, eliminates blood coagulations; affects the heart and liver.

### EXPERIMENT

- On animals, an experiment shows that saffron can induce tensions and contractions of the uterus with signs of excitation. Another experiment on cats shows the effect of saffron in lowering blood pressure. A third experiment on rats shows the effect of saffron in prolonging their estrous cycle from 1 or 2 to 3 or 4 days.

**Notes**

Saffron styles, stigmas and flowers are used by Chinese people for therapies.

## Scallion Bulbs

*Good for chest congestion and dry vomiting.*

## Shiitake Mushrooms

*Good for prevention of rickets, anemia, measles.*

### DESCRIPTION

- Neutral; sweet; affects the stomach.

### PREPARATION

- Boil some shiitake mushrooms in water until the soup becomes yellowish. Drink only the liquid (without eating the mushrooms) to relieve vomiting caused by careless eating; another alternative is to place shiitake mushrooms in boiling water and steep until the soup becomes yellowish. Drink it as tea.
- Dissolve some sugar or honey in the shiitake mushroom soup to treat coughing.
- Drink shiitake mushroom soup, or dissolve shiitake mushroom powder in hot water and drink it as tea to relieve fish poisoning. A prolonged consumption by this method is believed to prevent arteriosclerosis.
- In case of difficult urination or discharge of urine containing blood, bake some shiitake mushroom until it appears burned on the surface. Eat 10g each time, twice a day, or eat fresh shiitake mushrooms.

### EXPERIMENT

- Studies with rats show shiitake mushroom lowers blood fat levels.

**Notes**

Shiitake mushroom is believed to counteract stomach and cervical cancers. (When I visited Japan in October 1985, I learned that a new product containing the extract from shiitake mushroom had been approved by the Japanese government as an anti-cancerous agent.) The Chinese people are very fond of mushrooms, including shiitake mushrooms, which are produced primarily in Japan. Shiitake mushroom may be cooked by itself and it may also be cooked with other vegetables. In either case, avoid excessive amounts of soy sauce and salt because they are quickly absorbed by the mushroom and spoil its good taste.

## CLINICAL REPORT

- Shiitake mushroom counteracts cholesterol, a recent report indicates.

### *Spearmint*

*Regulates energy and relieves pain; good for common colds, coughs, headaches, period pain and abdominal pain.*

### *Star Anise*

*Good for hernias, abdominal pain, lumbago, beriberi, vomiting.*

#### DESCRIPTION

- Warm; pungent and sweet; warms up yang energy (energy that travels in the skin and muscles as opposed to yin energy that travels through internal organs) and promotes energy circulation; affects the spleen, kidneys and liver.

#### PREPARATION

- Crush 7 star anises and 7 fresh onion white heads and boil them in 3 cups water over low heat until liquid is reduced to 1 cup. Drink it like tea, twice a day, to cure constipation, urination difficulty and abdominal swelling.
- Bake 40g star anise and grind into powder; drink 5g of the powder dissolved in warm rice wine each time, twice a day, to relieve hernia of the small intestine.
- Fry star anise and grind into powder; dissolve 7g of the powder with a little salt in warm water before meals, twice a day, to cure lumbago.

### *String Bean (Green Bean)*

*Good for diarrhea, vomiting, diabetes, seminal emission, whitish vaginal discharge, frequent urination.*

#### DESCRIPTION

- Neutral; sweet; used as a kidney tonic and a spleen tonic; affects the spleen and kidneys.

#### PREPARATION

- Boil 50g dried string beans (with the shells) in water. Drink as soup once a day to relieve diabetes, thirst and frequent urination.

### *Sweet Basil*

*Good for headaches in common cold, diarrhea, indigestion, stomachache, irregular menstruation.*

#### DESCRIPTION

- Warm; pungent; promotes energy, blood circulation and digestion; affects the lungs, spleen, stomach and large intestine.

#### PREPARATION

- Use sweet basil leaves as a seasoning to substitute for parsley or green onion for relief of headache in common cold.
- There are 2 ways sweet basil may be used to relieve menstrual pain: Cook a few leaves with chicken egg and consume it as a soup with

### Notes

According to traditional Chinese theory, star anise heals all sorts of cold symptoms, as well as hernia, swollen scrotum, lumbago and beriberi. It is wise to take star anise with a little salt, rice wine and cinnamon for better results. If you have an eye or skin disease, you should avoid star anise.

some rice wine (good for women with premenstrual pain); another way
is to cook a few sweet basil leaves with ginger, green onion and some
meats or fish (good for menstrual pain due to coldness).
- Sweet basil, fresh ginger and licorice may be boiled in water; drink it
  like tea to cure acute gastroenteritis, abdominal swelling and pain.

## Sword Bean Roots

*Good for headaches, rheumatism, hernias, diarrhea and suppression of menses.*

## Tangerine Oranges

*Good for chest congestion, vomiting, hiccupping.*

### DESCRIPTION

- Cool; sweet and sour; promotes energy circulation; strengthens the
  spleen; relieves coughing; affects the lungs, stomach and kidneys.

### PREPARATION

- Eat a half-ripe tangerine to relieve indigestion and help your digestion.
- Drink fresh tangerine juice to relieve thirst from fever and dry throat
  and to relieve a hangover.
- Steam 2 unpeeled tangerines with 30g rock sugar; eat the tangerines at
  bedtime to relieve cough with yellowish mucous discharge.

## Tea Seeds

*Camellin contained in tea seeds is an anticancerous agent; good for abdominal pain and diarrhea.*

## Turmeric

*Promotes energy circulation, facilitates menstruation, relieves pain; good for
pain in the abdomen and upper arms and suppression of menses.*

## Vinegar

*Increases appetite, promotes digestion, disperses blood coagulation, detoxicates, kills bacteria.*

### PREPARATION

- To prevent flu, cholecystitis and meningitis, mix vinegar with water and
  boil over low heat; inhale before bedtime.
- To cure biliary ascariasis, drink 30g of rice vinegar with warm water,
  three to four times daily. Or, mix 30g of rice vinegar with 30g of water.
  Drink it when pain occurs and take anthel-mintics after the pain is gone.
- To treat hypertension, soak peanuts in vinegar and eat at meals.
- To cure hepatitis, soak peeled pears in vinegar and eat regularly.

## Notes

Dried tangerine peels can be made
by putting tangerine peels in the
sun to dry. Dried tangerine peels
have a warm energy and pungent-
bitter flavor.

Boil 6g dried tangerine peels with
3g fresh ginger in water; drink a cup
of the juice each time, twice a day,
to relieve vomiting.

Spread fresh tangerines in the sun
until half dry. Press to flatten them;
soak the flat tangerines in syrup to
make tangerine cakes.

Chew 1 small tangerine cake slowly,
like chewing gum, to relieve vomiting
and diarrhea; repeat 4 hours later.

Tangerine seeds have a neutral
energy and bitter flavor.

To relieve pain and swelling in mastitis, boil 15g tangerine seeds in a
mixture of half water and half wine.
Drink a cup of the juice each time,
3 times a day.

Fry until yellowish 30g tangerine
seeds and grind them; mix the powder with a quarter cup rice wine.
Drink the juice twice a day to relieve
hernial pain, swelling and pain in
testes and lumbago.

Fresh tangerine is not recommended for people with a cough from
common cold and edema. Tangerine peel is not recommended for
anyone with a dry cough or who is
vomiting blood.

Poor blood circulation in the internal environments can lead to various painful conditions due to blood coagulation. These regulating foods promote blood circulation.

# Foods for Promoting Blood Circulation

## Arrowhead

*Good for swelling and inflammation.*

### PREPARATION

- To heal local inflammatory, symptoms, such as swelling, burning, or pain on the skin, crush 60g of fresh arrowhead; then add a little fresh ginger juice. Mix thoroughly and apply it to the affected region on the skin. Change the dressing twice daily.

## Bayberry Roots

*Regulate energy in the body, arrest bleeding, dissolve blood coagulations; good for stomachaches, vomiting, hernias, vomiting of blood, vaginal bleeding and bleeding due to external injuries.*

## Bean Curd (Tofu)

*Good for pink eye, diabetes, periodic diarrhea, sulfur poisoning.*

### DESCRIPTION

- Cool; sweet; used as an energy tonic; produces fluids; lubricates dryness; detoxicates; affects the spleen, stomach and large intestine.

### PREPARATION

- Prepare 1 bowl bean curd, 70g maltose and half a cup of fresh radish juice; combine the 3 ingredients in a pan, add half a cup of water and bring to a boil once. Divide the soup into 2 dosages and drink twice a day to treat asthma with mucous discharge, including acute bronchial asthma.
- Crush a number of bean curds and apply the mash to the legs to heal erysipelas on the legs; change the dressing as soon as the mash dries.

## Black Soybeans

*Good for edema, beriberi, jaundice, rheumatism, muscular cramps, lockjaw, drug poisoning.*

### DESCRIPTION

- Neutral; sweet; promotes blood circulation and water passage; counteracts rheumatism; detoxicates; affects the spleen and kidneys.

### PREPARATION

- Boil 5g fresh black soybeans in water as 1 dosage, 3 times a day; or boil until soft, then add sugar and salt as seasonings. Eat at meals; or fry and grind into powder. Take 1 large teaspoonful of the powder each time, dissolved in water, twice a day to relieve cough, kidney disease and peritonitis.
- Regular consumption of black soybeans at meals promotes urination, relieves muscular cramps and rheumatism and pain in the knees.

### EXPERIMENT

- An experiment on rats indicates that black soybeans produce effects that resemble a female sex hormone and the effects of an antispasmodic on the small intestine equal to 37 percent of those produced by papaverine hydrochloride.

### Notes

Arrowhead is an excellent source of potassium; 100g of arrowhead contain 1003mg of potassium.

## *Brown Sugar*

*Good for abdominal pain, dysentery, lochiastasis.*

### DESCRIPTION

- Warm; sweet; used as an energy tonic; promotes blood circulation; counteracts or eliminates blood coagulations; affects the liver, spleen and stomach.

### PREPARATION

- Mix brown sugar with rice wine. Drink it to relieve lochiostasis and faintness after childbirth due to excessive loss of blood.
- Boil brown sugar with 2 plums and drink as tea to relieve dysentery.

## *Camellia*

*Cools the blood, arrests bleeding, disperses blood coagulations, eliminates swelling; good for vomiting of blood, nosebleeds and vaginal bleeding.*

## *Castor Bean*

*Good for carbuncles, swelling, tuberculosis of the lymph node, sore throats, edema, constipation.*

### DESCRIPTION

- Neutral; sweet and pungent; heals swelling with its detoxicating effects; induces bowel movements; affects the large intestine and lungs.

### PREPARATION

- Grind 20 uncooked castor beans (shells removed) and add a little salt to apply to cure swelling of a carbuncle.
- Fry castor beans in vegetable oil until fully cooked; peel the beans. Chew 3 beans at bedtime and gradually increase to 10 or more beans each time, to relieve tuberculosis of the lymph node.

### CLINICAL REPORT

- For treatment of facial paralysis: Grind castor beans (shells removed) to make into a cream. Apply externally to the affected side of the mandibular joint and angle of mouth (the layer of cream should be 3mm or about ⅛" thick) and covered with a bandage; change dressing once every day. Among the 3 cases treated, all recovered within 3 days.
- A report on castor bean poisoning and treatment: The toxic substances in castor beans are destroyed by heat. Most cases of castor bean poisoning are due to consumption of fresh castor beans. A report indicates that 3 children who ate 2 to 7 fresh castor beans vomited continually, with abdominal pain; one child suffered from unclear consciousness with dehydration, cold limbs, enlargement of the pupils and poor reactions to light. All cases recovered after treatment by standard procedures of treating poisoning.

## *Cattail Pollen*

*Cools the blood, stops bleeding, promotes blood circulation, dissolves blood coagulations; good for injuries, blood in urine and nosebleeds.*

## Celery

*Good for hypertension, dizziness and headaches, discharge of urine containing blood.*

### DESCRIPTION

- Neutral; sweet; bitter; glossy; affects the stomach and liver.

### PREPARATION

- Sometimes an infant may feel hot sensations and is unable to sleep and cries day and night. If there are signs of hot symptoms (like mouth canker or redness in the region surrounding the anus or frequent urination with discharge of scanty and yellowish-red urine), then it is useful to cut a few pieces of celery, immerse them in boiling water for a few seconds and squeeze out the juice. This juice can reduce heat in the bladder, a useful remedy for urethritis.
- There is a Chinese recipe to improve the conditions of liver and kidneys: Fry celery and pork kidneys. The celery can calm you down and prevent liver disorder while the pork kidneys can tone up the kidneys.
- Celery is aromatic, the reason why the Chinese people call it "aromatic celery." Celery may be cooked with vinegar to lower blood pressure and relieve headache due to high blood pressure.
- Fresh celery juice may be mixed with honey to relieve dizziness and headache and shoulder pain associated with hypertension.
- In cases of hypertension of pregnancy and climacteric hypertension, drink fresh celery juice every day to relieve the symptoms.

### EXPERIMENT

- Celery lowers blood pressure in rats.

### CLINICAL REPORT

- A report on the effect of lowering blood pressure and the level of cholesterol: Wash fresh celery (with roots removed) in cold water. Squeeze out the juice and mix the juice with an equal quantity of honey or syrup. Drink 40 ml warm juice each time, 3 times a day. Among the 16 cases treated, 14 cases were effective and 2 cases had no effects. The results indicated effectiveness for primary hypertension, hypertension in pregnancy and climacteric hypertension. In general, blood pressure begins to drop after 1 day of treatment with subjective sensations, improved sleeping conditions and increased urination.
- A clinical report on the effects of celery roots: As a treatment program, 10 celery roots are washed, crushed and boiled in water with 10 red dates for oral consumption twice a day for 15 to 20 days. Among the 21 cases treated for hypertension and coronary sclerosis heart disease with the cholesterol level over 200mg percent, it was found that the level of cholesterol was reduced between 8 and 75mg percent in 14 cases. It was also observed that fresh roots produce better results than dry ones and that dosages are flexible.

### REMARKS

- According to Chinese theory, celery is effective for hypertension because it acts upon the liver; one type of hypertension is associated with the liver.
- A physician wrote to me about the fact that celery contains sodium, which is considered bad for hypertension. Nevertheless, I would think that the quantity of sodium contained in celery (25mg in 1 stalk) is too small to cause any harm.
- A classic Chinese food belief: Celery can reduce internal heat in children and also internal heat in adults due to intoxication.

## Chicken

*Good for those who are underweight, have poor appetite, diarrhea, edema, frequent urination, vaginal bleeding and discharge, shortage of milk secretion after childbirth, weakness after childbirth.*

### DESCRIPTION

- Warm; sweet; used as an energy tonic; warms up the internal region; affects the spleen and stomach.

### PREPARATION

- Cut up a chicken and remove the skin; pat dry with a paper towel; heat and lightly oil a fry pan; drop chicken cubes into the pan, stirring constantly; add a little vegetable oil and 5 slices fresh ginger and continue to stir-fry for a while. Add 1 cup water and 1 cup rice wine; continue to cook for about 20 minutes; add more rice wine, if desired. Eat at meals to alleviate fatigue and increase milk secretion of lactating mothers.
- Cut up a chicken and remove the skin; wash chicken cubes with rice wine and place the cubes in a fry pan; stir-fry until dried. Steam the chicken cubes with 20g longans for 3 hours until reduced to half a cup of pure chicken and longan soup. Drink the strained soup (without eating the chicken or longans) to relieve neurasthenia and forgetfulness. This is an expensive recipe; dried longans are available in most Chinese foods shops.

## Chicken Blood

*Promotes blood circulation and counteracts rheumatism. The blood of a three-year-old rooster is considered the best for food cures.*

## Chili Leaves

*Good for rheumatism and blood coagulation.*

## Chili Peppers (Cayenne Pepper)

*Aid in digestion, improve appetite, stimulate the secretion of salivary glands and gastric juices; normally used as a stomachic and carminative to expel gas from the intestines; externally, used as a local skin stimulant to promote blood circulation. Good for frostbite, rheumatism and lumbago.*

## Chili Rhizomes

*Reduce cold and dampness, dissolve blood coagulations; good for arthritis, rheumatism and frostbite.*

## Chinese Rose Leaves

*Promote blood circulation and reduce swelling; good for scrofula and pain and swelling caused by injuries.*

## Chives

*Good for chest pain; difficulty when swallowing; upset stomach; vomiting blood; nosebleed; discharge of urine containing blood; prolapse of anus; injuries from a fall, causing internal blood coagulations.*

### Notes

Chicken liver is slightly warm and tastes sweet; it acts on the liver and kidneys, is used as a liver and kidney tonic and also for such symptoms as blurred vision, malnutrition in children and habitual miscarriage.

### Notes

People with hot constitutions should avoid chili peppers. The Chinese have a popular saying to the effect that chili peppers are so good that nobody can eat a full meal without them. There are different kinds of chili peppers, notably, sweet chili peppers, half pungent and hot chili peppers and pungent and hot chili peppers. Large-size chili peppers are not hot but sweet. They are normally consumed like other vegetables, but they contain large amounts of vitamin C, as much as 198 milligrams per 100 grams.

## DESCRIPTION

- Warm; pungent; promotes energy circulation; counteracts blood coagulations; affects the liver, stomach and kidneys.
- Contraindications: eye diseases and skin eruptions.

## PREPARATION

- Squeeze the juice from fresh chive (leaves or roots). Drink 1 teaspoonful of the warm juice each time with milk to treat difficulty when swallowing. The same juice, cold without milk, is effective to treat sunstroke and also to wash skin eruptions caused by lacquer poisoning.
- Cook chive with pork or lamb liver to cure excessive perspiration and stimulate the appetite.
- Crush chive leaves or roots and externally apply the juice to the wound to relieve bruises, swelling and pain.
- Cut chive leaves and roots into small pieces; boil with wine. Drink it hot to relieve injuries resulting from twisting the waist.
- Cook chive with egg to relieve diarrhea, night sweat and nocturia.

## Clam

*Saltwater clams good for edema, mucous discharge, goiter, vaginal discharge, hemorrhoids; freshwater clams good for vaginal bleeding and discharge, pink eyes, eczema and hemorrhoids; saltwater clamshell powder good for diabetes, edema, goiter and hemorrhoids; freshwater clam saliva good for diabetes, pink eyes and burns; freshwater clamshell powder good for cough with mucous discharge, stomachache, hiccupping, vomiting, whitish vaginal discharge, eczema, swelling.*

## DESCRIPTION

- Sea (saltwater) clam—cold, salty, acts on the stomach, promotes water passage, eliminates mucus and softens hardness; freshwater clam—cold, sweet and salty, detoxicates, sharpens the vision, acts on the liver and kidneys. Sea clamshell powder-cold, salty, promotes water passage, softens hardness, eliminates mucus, acts on the lungs and kidneys; river clam saliva—sharpens vision; freshwater clamshell powder—cold, salty, eliminates mucus and dries dampness, acts on the lungs, liver and stomach.

## PREPARATION

- Sea clamshell may be baked and ground into very fine powder to make sea clamshell powder. Freshwater clamshell may be washed clean (with the black skin removed) and ground into powder or baked and ground into powder to make freshwater clamshell powder. Apply saltwater clam's saliva externally to the affected region to relieve itching and pain and swelling of the vaginal orifice.
- Crush a few garlics to mix with clamshell powder and make into tablets of a normal size. Take 10 tablets with warm water each time, once a day, to relieve edema in weak persons.
- Mix clamshell powder with lard for external application to the affected region to relieve burns.
- Mix fine clamshell powder with an equal amount of raw licorice powder, take 7g each time with warm water, twice a day, to cure gastric ulcer and excessive gastric acid.
- Regular consumption of clam meat at meals relieves lymphadenitis scrofula in the neck and goiter.
- Cook clam with chive. Eat at meals to relieve pulmonary tuberculosis and night sweat.

*Notes*

Chive is an important food for external injuries because it can counteract blood coagulations. When a person gets hurt (like in an automobile accident) he or she may feel pain long after the accident caused by internal blood coagulations not diagnosed by X-ray examination. The blood coagulation that is causing pain may be so light that it cannot be seen on the X-ray. One useful way to determine whether blood coagulation occurred or not, however, is to determine if the pain recurs in the same body region or if it shifts around; if the patient always feels pain in the same region, it is very likely that blood coagulation has occurred, which may be relieved by eating chive. The Chinese people believe that pain may be caused either by blood coagulations or energy congestion. (When blood fails to circulate, it coagulates; when energy fails to circulate, it gets congested.) When pain is caused by blood coagulations, it will recur in the same region; when caused by energy congestion, the pain will shift around.

Here's a convenient way to use chive to relieve pain caused by blood coagulations: Cut chive into small pieces; boil it in water with wine and then drink the whole thing as soup. For example, in the past, Chinese authorities used to severely beat prisoners to force a confession from them but the severe beating caused internal bleeding and subsequently, internal blood coagulations. To prevent blood coagulations, it had become a routine practice to give prisoners chive at meals after the beating.

Chive is warm in energy and acts upon the stomach. Therefore, chive is often used to relieve stomachache of a cold nature. As a matter of fact, the Chinese people always make a point of regularly eating chive, which is also effective for enteritis, if they have weak digestive functions. Fresh chive juice may also be drunk to relieve nosebleed (but its awful taste often makes the juice difficult to administer).

- Boil 30g fine clamshell powder with 4g outer layer of peanuts and 6 red dates to make concentrated soup. Drink the soup once a day to relieve nosebleed, bleeding from gums and purpura hemorrhagica.
- Roast a whole freshwater clam until its outer part is charred and the inner part becomes yellow-brown with its original shape remaining intact; grind into fine powder and mix with sesame oil for external application to relieve eczema in infants.

## CLINICAL REPORT

- For treatment of gastric and duodenal ulcers, fry freshwater clamshell powder in a bronze fry pan (or any earthenware fry pan) until it becomes yellow-brown with the fishy smell gone; strain it before using. Take 1 to 2g each time mixed with warm water, once every hour during the daytime, 12 to 14 times a day, for 4 to 8 weeks. Among the 41 cases treated from 14 to 79 days, 28 cases showed disappearance of pain in the upper abdomen and 7 cases a decrease, 23 cases showed disappearance of pressure pain in the upper abdomen (pain that occurs on pressure by hand) and 6 cases a decrease; 21 cases had a follow-up X-ray examination, which indicated disappearance of the niche in 9 cases, disappearance of deformity in 1 case and a reduction in the size of the niche in 6 cases.

## Coriander (Chinese Parsley)

*Induces perspiration, promotes digestion, suppresses hiccups, strengthens the stomach.*

### PREPARATION

- When a child develops measles that don't erupt, coriander can be a good remedy. Boil a bunch of coriander and drink as soup at meals.
- Coriander is good for indigestion, particularly coriander seeds, which can be boiled with orange peels and fresh ginger. Drink the juice only. All the ingredients in this recipe are warm, which means that it is good for indigestion due to a cold stomach.

## Corn Roots

*Promote urination and remove blood coagulations; good for stones and vomiting of blood.*

## Crab Claws

*Break up blood coagulation and cause miscarriage; good for abdominal pain in women after difficult labor and childbirth.*

## Crab Shells

*Break up blood coagulation, eliminate internal congestion; good for pain in the ribs and abdomen, mastitis, breast cancer and frostbite.*

### PREPARATION

- To treat breast cancer, bake crab shells and grind into powder. Take 7g of powder with white wine two times daily for a prolonged period of time (not for pregnant women). The same recipe is also good for twisting injuries to the loins and suppression of menses after childbirth.

*Notes*

Coriander has a pungent flavor and warm energy. It is connected with the heart and the spleen internally; externally, it reaches the four limbs.

Coriander can remove all undesirable elements in the body, disperse stomach gas and cold, reduce fever and relieve headache, promote digestion and reduce abdominal swelling, regulate urination and bowel movements, promote hair growth.

*Notes*

About three-quarters of crab shell is calcium carbonate, with the remaining one-quarter containing chitin and protein in equal amounts.

- To treat mastitis at its early stage, bake five crab shells and grind into powder. Take 9g of powder with warm water or wine each time. Or, crush a live crab, strain it and drink with white wine.
- To relieve swelling with hard spots in breast cancer, bake a dozen crab shells and grind into powder. Take 6g of powder with wine three times daily. Avoid spicy foods.

## Deer Horns (Antlers)

*Calm the liver, reduce internal heat, relieve convulsions, detoxicate; good for delirium, headaches and dizziness.*

## Distillers' Grains

*Warm the internal region, promote digestion, relieve pain, disperse blood coagulation; good for frostbite and rheumatism.*

## Eel Blood

*Increases yang energy in the body and promotes blood circulation; good for dry mouth and eyes, pain in the ears, nosebleeds and impotence.*

## Eggplant

*Good for discharge of blood from anus, dysentery with discharge of blood, discharge of urine containing blood.*

### DESCRIPTION

- Cool; sweet; affects the spleen, stomach and large intestine.

### PREPARATION

- Boil in water white eggplants and drink the soup with honey to relieve cough.
- Bake some peel from a fresh eggplant until it appears black as charcoal on the outside but inside intact; mix with honey. Put it in the mouth like chewing gum to cure stomatitis.

### CLINICAL REPORT

- Eggplant contains vitamin P, which can prevent hardening of blood vessels and is useful in the treatment of arteriosclerosis, a report from China indicates. According to the statistics, the elderly Chinese are much less susceptible to apoplexy caused by cerebrovascular accident than their Western counterparts, attributed to the Chinese habit of eating eggplant. The same report points out two reasons for the elderly Chinese to consume more eggplants: Eggplants are much less expensive than other vegetables or meats; and eggplants can be cooked softer than other vegetables or meats, therefore easier for the elderly Chinese to eat (as most of them have lost most of their teeth). In addition, the Chinese people in general are fond of eggplants because of the taste.

## Eggplant Leaves

*Good for blood in urine, discharge of blood from the anus, carbuncle and frostbite.*

**Notes**

Eggplant is considered obstructive to some extent, which explains why it can heal various kinds of bleeding. Further, it has a cool energy that stops bleeding. Fresh eggplant can also relieve mushroom poisoning.

## Fish Air Bladder

*Tones the kidneys, increases semen, nourishes tendons, arrests bleeding, disperses blood coagulations, reduces swelling; good for vomiting of blood, vaginal bleeding and bleeding due to external injuries.*

## Ginger Leaves

*Good for blood coagulation and indigestion.*

## Green Onion Juice

*Disperses blood coagulation, detoxicates, expels worms; good for headaches, nosebleeds, blood in urine, parasites, swelling and injuries.*

### Notes

Green onion white head is an important herb in Chinese medicine. It can induce perspiration and warm the body. It is most frequently used to relieve common cold at its early stages.

## Fresh Ham

*Good for diarrhea, nervousness, poor appetite.*

### DESCRIPTION

- Warm; salty; used as a spleen tonic; stimulates the appetite; produces fluids; pushes downwards.

### PREPARATION

- Boil ham in water with red pepper to make soup; skim off and discard the floating fat. Drink the hot soup to relieve hiccupping and abdominal pain that has lasted for 3 to 4 days.
- Boil 200g ham in water over low heat for a full day until extremely tender; discard the fat from the surface. Drink as soup to relieve chronic diarrhea.

## Hawthorn Fruit

*Good for meat indigestion, abdominal swelling, mucous discharge, discharge of blood from anus, lumbago, hernia, neck pain after childbirth.*

### DESCRIPTION

- Slightly warm; sweet and sour; promotes digestion; corrects blood coagulations; expels tapeworm; affects the spleen, stomach and liver.

### PREPARATION

- Soak hawthorn fruit in boiling water for less than 1 minute; slice the fruits and lay them in the sun to dry. (Hawthorn fruit slices are available in most Chinese herb shops.)
- Fry hawthorn slices until they look like charcoal to make hawthorn fruit charcoal.
- Mix together the following ingredients and marinate for 10 days to prepare hawthorn fruit wine: 250g hawthorn slices, 250g fresh longans, 30g red dates, 30g brown sugar and 4.5 cups rice wine.
- Drink 30 to 60g hawthorn fruit wine at every bedtime to relieve pain caused by excessive fatigue, muscular pain and arthritis pain, flying spots in front of the eyes, lumbago and pain in thigh in the elderly.
- Boil in water 60g hawthorn fruit slices with an equal amount fresh or dried chestnuts until very soft; add 30g sugar and stir thoroughly. Drink the juice once a day, first thing in the morning on an empty stomach, to cure scurvy.

### Notes

Hawthorn fruits are not recommended for people suffering from constipation due to internal heat or those who have excessive gastric acid.

Hawthorn fruits can effectively digest fat and prevent it from entering into the blood vessels by removing it through the bowel movements. Indeed, the fruits are so effective in softening hard substances, the Chinese people use it to cook stubborn and tough old chickens! When hawthorn fruits are used in the cooking water, the tough chickens become soft and tender—an indication of the tenderizing power of this fruit. Another example, when hawthorn fruits are used to cook fish, even the fish bones will become tender.

- Boil 31g hawthorn slices with water; stir in 1.5g fennel powder. Drink the juice in the morning and evening to relieve hernia of the small intestine.
- Boil 15g hawthorn fruit slices in water and drink as tea on a long-term basis, to relieve hypertension, high level of blood fat and coronary heart disease.
- Grind 6 to 9g hawthorn fruit charcoal into powder. Take the powder with warm water, once a day, to relieve abdominal pain caused by acute and chronic gastritis, enteritis and dysentery.
- Boil 3g hawthorn charcoal with 6g hawthorn fruit slices; drink the juice to relieve diarrhea in children; or crush 5 hawthorn fruits and squeeze out the juice to mix with a pinch of hawthorn fruit charcoal for oral administration to stop diarrhea in children.
- Crush 2 to 3 fresh hawthorn fruits and squeeze out the juice to drink; or boil 2 to 3 hawthorn fruits with 6g dry orange peels; drink the juice to correct indigestion, abdominal swelling and abdominal pain.

## EXPERIMENT

- An experiment on rabbits shows the effects of hawthorn fruit in lowering blood pressure.
- An experiment on toads shows the effects of hawthorn fruit in expanding blood vessels.
- Hawthorn fruits are reported to have the effects of contracting the uterus and reducing antibiosis.

## Hemp

*Lubricates dryness, settles intestines, promotes urination, increases blood circulation; good for constipation, diabetes, rheumatism and irregular menstruation.*

## Kiwifruit Roots (Chinese Gooseberry Roots)

*Reduce internal heat, promote urination, activate the blood, reduce swelling; good for hepatitis, edema, injuries, rheumatic pain and vaginal discharge.*

## Leaf Mustard

*Good for mucous discharge, cough, chest congestion.*

## DESCRIPTION

- Warm; pungent; affects the lungs.

## PREPARATION

- Cook preserved leaf mustard and eat 30g a day to cure pulmonary abscess and bronchiectasis and laryngitis. Boil 5g fried leaf mustard seeds with 10g fried radish seeds, 5g dried orange peel and 5g licorice. Drink it as tea to cure chronic bronchitis and cough with mucous discharge.

## Lemon Roots

*Relieve pain and remove blood coagulation; good for injuries and animal bites.*

## Lotus Flowers

*Promote blood circulation, arrest bleeding, remove dampness; good for vomiting of blood.*

### Notes

A prolonged consumption of leaf mustard can warm up the internal region. It is not recommended for people suffering from eye diseases, hemorrhoids, or discharge of stools containing blood, which are normally regarded as hot symptoms.

Leaf mustard can relieve congestion because it has a warm energy and tastes pungent, which are the two important components of foods that are used to promote energy circulation and relieve congestion of various kinds.

## *Lotus Sprouts*

*Good for vomiting of blood.*

## *Green Onion White Head*

*Good for headaches, abdominal pain, constipation, suppression of urination, dysentery.*

### DESCRIPTION

- Warm; pungent; induces perspiration; affects the lungs and stomach.

### PREPARATION

- For relief of nasal congestion and nasal discharge in infants associated with common colds, steam a green onion white head and a mushroom with 30 to 50ml mother's milk. Feed infants the soup without the mushroom or white head.
- Crush 4 to 6 white heads; warm it up with wine. Drink the soup to remedy a common cold.

## *Peaches*

*Good for coughs, hernial pain, excessive perspiration.*

### DESCRIPTION

- Warm; sweet and sour; obstructive; promotes blood circulation; lubricates the intestines; produces fluids; checks perspiration.

### PREPARATION

- Peel 3 fresh peaches and steam the peaches with 30g rock sugar. Eat once a day to treat asthma and cough.
- Fresh unripe peaches may be left in the sun to dry to make dried peaches.
- Boil 30g dried peaches and a mango in water. Eat twice a day to relieve hernial pain.
- Fry 30g dried peaches until the surface is brown and yellowish. Add water immediately and then add 30g red dates; boil for a few minutes. Eat at bedtime to relieve seminal emission, excessive perspiration and night sweat.
- Eat 1 to 2 peaches each time, twice a day, or boil 30g dried peaches in water and drink like tea to treat hypertension.
- Break peach seeds to obtain the kernels; leave them in the sun to dry. Peach kernels are important and widely used in Chinese herbal remedies. The kernels have a neutral energy and bittersweet flavor. They are considered slightly toxic and capable of promoting blood circulation and lubricating the intestines.
- Crush 15g peach kernels and boil with 30g honey. Drink it to cure constipation.
- Boil 15g each of peach kernels, fresh ginger and red dates with 30g rice wine and an adequate amount of water. Drink as tea in the morning and evening to relieve abdominal pain after childbirth and suppression of menstruation.

## *Peach Kernels*

*Break up blood coagulation, which is essential in the treatment of many illnesses, including hypertension with headache, injuries, suppression of menstruation, whiplash.*

## Peach Roots

*Good for jaundice, vomiting of blood, nosebleeds, suppression of menses.*

## Peony Flowers

*Good for irregular menstruation and period pain.*

## Peony Root Bark

*Reduces internal heat, cools the blood, dissolves blood coagulation; good for hypertension and rhinitis.*

## Plum Kernels

*Disperse blood coagulation, promote water flow, lubricate the intestines; good for pain caused by injuries, coughs with phlegm, edema and constipation.*

## Pumpkin Pedicels

*Promote blood circulation and remove blood coagulation.*

## Radish

*Good for abdominal swelling due to indigestion, laryngitis due to continual cough with mucous discharge, vomiting of blood, nosebleed, dysentery, headache.*

### DESCRIPTION

- Cool; pungent and sweet; affects the lungs and stomach; detoxicates; downwards movements; promotes digestion and eliminates hot mucous discharge.

### PREPARATION

- Drink fresh radish juice mixed with ginger juice to cure laryngitis.
- Drink fresh radish juice to relieve intoxication.
- Regular consumption of fresh radishes prevents common cold, flu and respiratory infections.

## Rape

*Breaks up blood coagulations, strengthens the loins and legs, heals rheumatism. Rape oil can be applied externally to the head to promote hair growth.*

### PREPARATION

- To cure lochiostasis in women after childbirth with pricking pain, fry rapeseeds and cinnamon in equal amounts without oil and grind into powder. Make into tablets as big as olive seeds. Take one to two tablets three times daily with warm rice wine.
- To cure acute pain in nipples and swelling on skin of unknown cause, boil rape in water or crush it to make juice. Drink a small glass of warm juice three times daily. Alternatively, apply crushed rape externally to the affected region. Change dressings three times daily.
- To correct intestinal intussusception (the slipping of one part of the intestine into another part just below it), drink 120g of rape oil, or drink 6g of cooked rape oil four times a day.

## Saffron

*Good for congested chest, vomiting of blood, suppression of menstruation, abdominal pain after childbirth due to blood coagulations, injuries from falls.*

### DESCRIPTION

- Neutral; sweet; promotes energy and blood circulation, eliminates blood coagulations; affects the heart and liver.

### EXPERIMENT

- On animals, an experiment shows that saffron can induce tensions and contractions of the uterus with signs of excitation. Another experiment on cats shows the effect of saffron in lowering blood pressure. A third experiment on rats shows the effect of saffron in prolonging their estrous cycle from 1 or 2 to 3 or 4 days.

**Notes**

Saffron styles, stigmas and flowers are used by Chinese people for therapies.

## Sea Grass

*Good for tuberculosis of the lymph node, goiter, edema, beriberi, pain in the testes.*

### DESCRIPTION

- Cold; bitter and salty; softens hardness, eliminates mucus; promotes water passage; reduces hot sensations.

### PREPARATION

- Boil 20g sea grass at low heat in 4 cups water until water is reduced to 2 cups. Drink 1 cup each time, twice a day, to relieve tuberculosis of the lymph node and goiter and to prevent hypertension and arteriosclerosis.
- Boil 50g sea grass with 20g fried orange seeds and 15g fried caraway seeds in water. Drink the soup once a day to relieve swollen testes.

### EXPERIMENT

- One experiment shows that sea grass extract can be used as an anti-coagulant; another experiment on rats indicates various kinds of sea grass can lower cholesterol in the serum and internal organs; another experiment on dogs and rats shows that when large dosages (.75g per kilogram) are used, sea grass can lower blood pressure for a prolonged period of time; but smaller dosages will temporarily elevate blood pressure.

**Notes**

One source indicates that sea grass can inhibit appetite and cause weight loss. See Kelp for effects on the thyroid gland.

## Shark

*Reduces swelling, removes blood coagulation, strengthens internal organs.*

## Sweet Basil

*Good for headaches in common cold, diarrhea, indigestion, stomachache, irregular menstruation.*

### DESCRIPTION

- Warm; pungent; promotes energy, blood circulation and digestion; affects the lungs, spleen, stomach and large intestine.

### PREPARATION

- Use sweet basil leaves as a seasoning to substitute for parsley or green onion for relief of headache in common cold.

**Notes**

In ancient China, shark was called "the healthy son of water," because of its body strength.

The shark has a very strong immune system. A shark will not develop cancer after cancerous cells are injected into its body. Shark's fin is a precious food considered beneficial to the blood, body energy, kidneys and lungs; it is an ideal food for chronic deficiency.

- There are 2 ways sweet basil may be used to relieve menstrual pain: Cook a few leaves with chicken egg and consume it as a soup with some rice wine (good for women with premenstrual pain); another way is to cook a few sweet basil leaves with ginger, green onion and some meats or fish (good for menstrual pain due to coldness).
- Sweet basil, fresh ginger and licorice may be boiled in water; drink it like tea to cure acute gastroenteritis, abdominal swelling and pain.

## Sweet (Glutinous) Rice

*Good for excessive urination, excessive perspiration, diarrhea.*

### DESCRIPTION

- Warm; sweet; used as an energy tonic; affects the spleen, stomach and lungs.

### PREPARATION

- Fry sweet rice with wheat bran and grind into powder. Take 10g powder in warm water each time, 3 times a day, to stop excessive perspiration.
- Cook 50g sweet rice with 60g Job's tears and 8 red dates. Eat at meals to relieve pulmonary tuberculosis, neurasthenia, anemia and various kinds of chronic diseases.
- Boil sweet rice sprouts in water with malt. Drink the soup to relieve indigestion and to promote appetite.

## Sword Bean Shells

*Balance the internal region, disperse blood coagulation, promote blood circulation; good for lumbago, diarrhea and hiccups.*

## Vinegar

*Good for jaundice, vomiting of blood, nosebleeds, discharge of blood from anus, itching in the genital region, fish, meat and vegetable poisoning.*

### DESCRIPTION

- Warm; sour and bitter; disperses coagulations; detoxicates; arrests bleeding; affects the liver and stomach.

### PREPARATION

- Crush a small piece fresh ginger and mix it with 1 or 2 cups rice vinegar; drink it to correct indigestion caused by an excessive consumption of fish, salads and fruits.
- Add some vinegar to meats when cooking to promote digestion and stimulate the appetite.
- Cook celery with vinegar as a seasoning to treat hypertension with headache.
- In Chinese folk medicine, when a child suffers from convulsions and faints, with body temperature decreasing rapidly, vinegar is boiled at high heat with the doors closed so that the patient will inhale the vinegar vapor to regain consciousness. The same method may be used to arouse women who faint following childbirth.
- Drink a cup of hot vinegar to relieve pain caused by binary ascariasis and intestinal ascariasis.
- Combine half a bowl of vinegar, 70g brown sugar and 35g sliced fresh ginger; bring to a boil twice and strain it. Drink 1 small cup of the liquid each time with warm water, 3 times a day, to relieve itchiness and

*Notes*

Vinegar is called bitter wine in the Chinese language and vinegar and wine are considered the 2 friends of Chinese herbs. Why? Vinegar and wine are very frequently used to process Chinese herbs, not only to inhibit the side effects of herbs but also to increase their effects.

Drink between 30 to 50ml vinegar or more, according to your age, to alleviate the pain caused by biliary ascariasis. This treatment may be repeated until pain is gone. After pain is significantly reduced, apply anthelmintic as usual. Among the 15 cases of biliary ascariasis observed, with a total of 300 to 500ml vinegar administered in each case, pain stopped completely in 12 cases within 2 days and pain stopped within 3 to 4 days in 3 cases.

skin eruptions from allergic reactions after eating fish and crab.

- Soak overnight 10 peanuts in a small cup of vinegar. Drink the vinegar and eat the peanuts the next morning to treat hypertension; repeat for 10 to 15 days as a treatment program.

## CLINICAL REPORT

- A child was suffering from epidemic encephalitis and the Chinese doctor told the patient's father that it was necessary to use lactic acid sterilization; but lactic acid was not readily available. So the father used vinegar as a substitute and obtained good results.
- Once a Chinese food factory reported an epidemic of influenza. All workers in the factory were stricken except the workers in the vinegar division; none of them became ill.
- According to a report from a Chinese food-processing plant, an average 8 percent of the factory workers are sick with respiratory infections yearly; but only 1 percent of the workers in the vinegar division have suffered from respiratory infections each year. Moreover, when the workers in the vinegar division do suffer from respiratory infections, the attack is lighter, too.
- Boil 500g pork bones and 100g white sugar in 4 cups vinegar for 30 minutes; strain it. Adults take 30 to 40ml and children take 10 to 15ml each time after meals, 3 times a day for 1 month as a treatment program. Chronic patients undergo 2 to 3 treatment programs (except patients with high fever who should not be treated by this method). Among the 3 cases of acute and chronic contagious hepatitis treated, all recovered within 40 to 60 days.
- In Hu Bei Yeecang People's Hospital in China, 51 cases of acute contagious jaundice-type hepatitis were treated with 10ml rice vinegar and 2 vitamin B-1 tablets. All patients recovered from the illness within an average of 4 days and their poor appetites were significantly improved.

## EXPERIMENT

- In an experiment conducted by the Research Institute of Epidemic Diseases at the Chinese Academy of Medical Science, 200 bacteria colonies were cultured, consisting of 5 bacteria most frequently causing respiratory infections, such as pneumonia, catarrh and influenza. It was found that all but a few isolated bacteria colonies were exterminated within 30 minutes by vinegar vaporized at 100 degrees C; the same experiment also indicated that vinegar has no obvious bacteria-exterminating power when vaporized below 100 degrees C.

## White or Yellow Mustard
*Warms the internal region; good for coughs, stomachaches and abdominal pain.*

## Yellow Soybean
*Good for malnutrition in children, diarrhea, abdominal swelling, underweight, gestosis.*

## DESCRIPTION

- Neutral, sweet; used as a spleen tonic; lubricates dryness; eliminates tissue fluids; affects the spleen and large intestine.

*Notes*

Yellow soybean sprouts are cool and sweet. They are used to relieve a cough with discharge of yellow mucus and to promote urination.

## PREPARATION

- Fry yellow soybeans until aromatic to eat at meals to promote milk secretion after childbirth.
- Fry yellow soybeans and then boil them in water to eat at meals to correct underweight.

## CLINICAL REPORT

- A treatment of acute gestosis: 92 cases of potential eclampsia and eclampsia are treated by soybean juice (soybean and water ratio 1 to 8) cooked with 120g sugar, divided into 6 dosages. Eat while drinking additional water. In general, treatment lasts 2 to 4 days and then, changes to a salt-free diet. On the second day of treatment, fruits or lotus root powder may be administered to relieve hunger. In the control group, 41 cases are given only a salt-free diet with other factors identical in both groups, including avoidance of sound and light stimuli and administration of sedatives and antispasmodic drugs. The results indicate that the experimental group shows a faster disappearance of edema and faster normalization of the blood pressure than the control group; the death rate in the experimental group is zero while in the control group it is more than 2 percent. The result is attributed to the fact that yellow soybean juice is low in calcium and sodium, higher in vitamin B-1 and niacin with more water intake, which contributes to the lowering of blood pressure and increased urination.

# Miscellaneous Useful Foods

中医疗法

## Apricot and Apricot Seed

*Apricot is good for thirst and asthma; bitter apricot seed for cough, sore throat, constipation, asthma; sweet apricot seed for cough, constipation and sore throat.*

### DESCRIPTION

- Apricot is neutral, sweet and sour. Apricot lubricates the lungs and produces fluids. Bitter apricot seed is warm, pungent and bitter and toxic. It is used to suppress cough, relieve asthma and lubricate intestines. Sweet apricot seed is warm, pungent and sweet. It is used to lubricate the intestines and suppress a cough and also as an energy tonic.

### PREPARATION

- Eat 2 to 3 fresh or dry apricots in the morning and evening to relieve a dry throat and to quench thirst.
- Chew 5 to 10 sweet apricot seeds once a day to cure chronic cough and shivering with cold.
- Combine 15g sweet apricot seeds, 30g each of rice and sugar; add water and crush them to make a cream. Eat it in the morning and evening to correct constipation in the elderly and in pregnant women.
- Prepare 2 pears and remove the seeds. Crush 6g bitter apricot seeds and grind into powder; stuff the powder into the pears and steam for half an hour. Eat once a day to cure dry cough.
- Boil 9g bitter apricot seeds in water with 6g fresh ginger and 2 red dates. Drink as tea twice a day to cure a cough with watery mucus.

## Barley

*Good for indigestion, diarrhea, pain when urinating, edema, burns.*

### DESCRIPTION

- Cool; sweet and salty; regulates the stomach; expands the intestines; promotes urination; affects the spleen and stomach.

### PREPARATION

- Fry barley until aromatic and slightly brown. Use it to make tea to relieve summer heat, indigestion, fatigue and excessive perspiration in summer.
- Fry 1 cup barley until aromatic and slightly brown to make tea with a few slices of fresh ginger. Drink it as a substitute for regular tea or juice, which is good for people who feel thirsty in hot weather but cannot drink tea or juice for one reason or another.
- Boil 100g barley in water and mix with fresh ginger juice to drink before meals to cure difficult urination and pain when urinating.
- Fry barley until charred; grind into powder and mix in vegetable oil for external application to relieve burns.
- Regular consumption of barley cures uremia and indigestion.
- Boil 5g tender barley leaves and stalks. Drink as tea to promote urination.

## Beetroot

*Good for congested chests, poor energy circulation.*

### DESCRIPTION

- Neutral; sweet; promotes menstruation; promotes downwards movements.

### Notes

Fresh apricots are not recommended for frequent or excessive consumption or for people with diarrhea. Bitter apricot seeds are toxic and should not be consumed in fresh or raw form.

## Carp

*Common carp good for edema, beriberi, jaundice, cough and shortage of milk secretion; grass carp good for headache and rheumatism; gold carp for weak stomach, poor appetite, dysentery, discharge of blood from anus, edema, urinary strains and ulcers.*

### DESCRIPTION

- Common carp—neutral, sweet, pushes downwards, facilitates water passage, promotes milk secretion and heals swelling, acts on the spleen and kidneys; grass carp—warm and sweet, acts on the spleen and stomach; gold carp—neutral and sweet, used as a spleen tonic, facilitates water passage, acts on the spleen, stomach and large intestine.

## Cherry Seed

*Good for measles, sty in the eyelid, scar.*

### DESCRIPTION

- Neutral; bitter and pungent; helps promote outbreak of rash in measles; counteracts toxic effects.

### PREPARATION

- Grind cherry seeds into powder and mix with water for external application to the affected region to cure a sty.
- Boil cherry seeds in water; use the liquid to wash the affected skin to eliminate a scar.
- Boil 9g cherry seeds in 1 cup water and drink the liquid to promote outbreak of rash in measles. In addition, boil 150g cherry seeds in 4 cups water; wash the body with the liquid.
- Crush 90 to 150g cherry seeds with a pestle or hammer and boil in water. Wash the affected skin with the liquid to heal a carbuncle.

## Chestnut

*Good for upset stomachs, diarrhea, weak legs, vomiting of blood, nosebleed, discharge of stools containing blood.*

### DESCRIPTION

- Warm; sweet; used as a stomach tonic, spleen tonic and kidney tonic; promotes blood circulation and arrests bleeding; affects the spleen, stomach and kidneys.

### PREPARATION

- Slowly chew 30 to 60g fresh raw chestnuts (with shells removed) as chewing gum to cure chronic pharyngolaryngitis.
- Boil 30 to 60g fresh or dried chestnuts in water with some brown sugar. Eat chestnuts at bedtime to relieve weakness and numbness of limbs.
- Bake 30g dried chestnuts. Eat them in the morning and evening to cure frequent urination and weak legs due to kidney weakness.
- Boil 60g fresh chestnuts with 4 red dates and some lean pork. Eat it all at once to cure asthma and cough.
- Crush 15g chestnuts and mix with a persimmon cake to make jelly and then cook it. Eat it to cure diarrhea in children.
- Chestnut shells may be left to dry in the sun to use for remedies.
- Bake dried chestnut shells until they look like charcoal; grind them into powder. Take 6g of the powder with 30g honey to relieve hemorrhoids.

## Chicken Egg Yolk

*Good for insomnia, muscular twitching, vomiting of blood, hiccupping, diarrhea, miscarriage, burns, hepatitis, malnutrition in children, eczema.*

### DESCRIPTION

- Neutral; sweet; used as a blood tonic; and to lubricate dryness; affects the heart and kidneys.

### PREPARATION

- Swallow a few egg yolks to relieve acute vomiting.
- Mix fresh egg yolk with milk and let children drink it to stop convulsions.

### CLINICAL REPORT

- For treatment of burns use egg-yolk oil after filtration and high-pressure sterilization. Apply the oil to the areas of burns after debridement; exposure is preferred. In more than 100 cases treated for first and second degree burns with small and medium areas, all of them showed good results and no secondary infections occurred. After application of egg-yolk oil, the patients feel cool with decreased pain and effusion of fluids and quicker crusting (which falls by itself) with either no scars or only obscure scars.
- To make egg-yolk oil, boil about 5 to 10 eggs until hard-cooked. Remove the yolks and mash them thoroughly. Fry the yolks in a pan over high heat, stirring constantly, until they gradually turn very dark and close to black, as if the oil is about to flow out; use a clean cloth to wrap the yolks and squeeze out the oil. Apply the oil to burns.
- A report on the treatment of varicose ulcer (stasis ulcer): use the same method as in burns to extract the egg-yolk oil; clean up the affected areas and then apply flat cotton bandage soaked in the oil to the affected region; change the dressing every other day or once every 3 days until recovery.

## Chicken Eggshell

*Good for stomachache, gastritis, rickets in children, various types of bleeding, ceruminosis (excessive buildup of earwax).*

### DESCRIPTION

- Checks gastric acid; arrests bleeding.

### PREPARATION

- Crush an eggshell into powder; dissolve 7g of the powder in rice wine. Drink this amount each time, twice a day, to relieve upset stomach.
- Bake eggshell until dried and crush into powder (the finer, the better). Take 4g each time with warm water before meals, 3 times a day, to reduce excessive gastric acid and gastric and duodenal ulcers.
- Break 12 large chicken eggs and mix thoroughly; add 500g rock sugar and 500g rice wine; boil until charred and yellowish. Eat a large spoonful each time before meals, 3 times a day, to relieve gastric spasms.

### CLINICAL REPORT

- A clinical report on the treatment of malnutrition in children (56 cases) and rickets (139 cases) and twitching of hands and feet (10 cases) shows that all except 9 cases of chronic indigestion recovered completely within 20 days to 3 months. The treatment: Wash an eggshell and dry it thoroughly; grind it into powder and sieve it (the finer, the better); administer .5g each time to a 1-year-old child, 1g for children up to 2 years old, twice a day.

Notes

One source indicates that boiled egg yolk may be used to quit smoking.

A clinical report on the treatment of various kinds of bleeding: Simply apply the powder (as made above) to the affected areas with standard precautions of sterilization; the 600 cases treated for traumatic bleeding by this method did not develop suppuration. For the treatment of coughing up blood, vomiting blood, nosebleed and discharge of blood from anus, apply 6g of the fine powder with some salt and vitamin C. Administer orally 3 times a day for 2 to 7 days. It is also reported that taking the powder dissolved in water (2g each time, 3 times a day) relieves allergic skin rash, urticaria, bronchial asthma, excessive stomach acid and bad breath.

## Chive Seed

*Good for impotence, seminal emission with erotic dreams, frequent urination, uncontrolled or involuntary urination, diarrhea, vaginal discharge.*

### DESCRIPTION

Warm; pungent and salty; affects the liver and kidneys.

### PREPARATION

For men having a strong erection with stinging pain in the penis, take 10g chive seed ground into powder, with warm water each time, 3 times day.

For impotence and sexual weakness, boil over low heat 15g chive seeds in 2 glasses water until reduced to 1 glass. Drink it as soup, 3 times a day; alternatively take about 20 chive seeds with salt water first thing in the morning (which should produce the same results).

**Notes**

Chive seed is an important herb in Chinese herbal remedies and it is normally used as a yang tonic.

## Chive Root

*Good for chest pain; vomiting of blood; vaginal discharge; nosebleeds; internal blood coagulations caused by injuries from a fall.*

### DESCRIPTION

Warm; pungent; warms up the internal region; promotes energy circulation; counteracts blood coagulations.

### PREPARATION

Chive root may be applied the same as chive stem, except that the root is normally not used in cookery.

## Chicory

*Good for icterohepatitis.*

### DESCRIPTION

Affects the liver and gall bladder.

### EXPERIMENT

The entire plant was found to excite the central nervous system and increase heart actions in animals. The roots were found to increase appetite and improve digestive functions.

## Corn Silk (Corn Stule and Stigma)

*Good for edema in nephritis, beriberi; icterohepatitis, hypertension, gallstones, diabetes; vomiting of blood; nosebleed; cholecystitis; sinusitis; mastitis.*

## DESCRIPTION

- Neutral; sweet; promotes urination; affects the liver and gall bladder.

## PREPARATION

- Boil 40g corn silk and 40g banana peel in water. Drink the juice cold to relieve hypertension, nosebleed and vomiting of blood.
- Boil corn silk with watermelon peel and small red beans in water. Drink it as soup for relief of chronic nephritis with edema and ascites.

## CLINICAL REPORT

- A report on the treatment of chronic nephritis: Place 50g dry corn silk in 600ml warm water; boil it over low heat for 20 to 30 minutes until reduced to about 300 to 400ml soup; strain and drink the soup once a day; or divide it and drink it a few times a day. This remedy was used to treat 9 cases of chronic glomerular nephritis under observation for 10 months. The results indicate that among the 9 cases treated, 3 cases show complete recovery, 2 improvements and 4 significant results. Corn silk promotes urination, improves kidney functions, heals or reduces edema and eliminates or reduces urinary albumin, according to the report.

## EXPERIMENTS

- Corn silk promotes urination, lowers blood sugar, is beneficial to the gall bladder and arrests bleeding, according to experiments on animals.

## PREPARATION

- Boil 40g corn silk and 40g banana peel in water. Drink the juice cold to relieve hypertension, nosebleed and vomiting of blood.
- Boil corn silk with watermelon peel and small red beans in water. Drink it as soup for relief of chronic nephritis with edema and ascites.

## Cinnamon Twig (Stick)

*Good for pain in the back and shoulder, chest pain, menopause.*

## DESCRIPTION

- Warm; pungent and sweet; induces perspiration, warms the upper region of the body; affects the bladder, heart, lungs.

## PREPARATION

- Boil 20g cinnamon twigs with 30g fresh ginger in enough water to cover the spices; boil until the water is reduced by half. Drink a cupful each time, 3 times a day, to cure arthritis.
- Cook 10g cinnamon twig with 100g lean pork in water as a soup; drink it to relieve menopause and excessive gas in the intestine. (Drink the soup as slowly as if consuming liquor.) There is no need to induce perspiration because cinnamon twig is capable of inducing perspiration by itself.
- Boil 3g cinnamon twigs in water over low heat. Drink it like tea just before bedtime to cure numbness of the skin, fingers and muscles.

## Cottonseed

*Good for impotence, falling of testes, enuresis, hemorrhoids, prolapse of anus, vaginal bleeding and discharge, night sweat.*

*Notes*

Cinnamon twigs are branches from the cinnamon tree. For that reason, the twigs are most effective for arthritis involving the joints of the 4 limbs, because tree branches are comparable to a person's 4 limbs. Many Chinese herbalists describe the functions of cinnamon twigs like streets of a city branching out, with the effects reaching every part of the body. Cinnamon twigs are particularly effective for the symptoms of the limbs and fingers, because fingertips are considered the most remote areas in the human body, beyond the reach of many other herbs.

Cinnamon twig is basically a warm herb. It can induce perspiration, eliminate cold, promote blood circulation, facilitate menstrual flow and promote urination. Obviously, this herb is good for rheumatic pain that worsens on exposure to cold and for cold abdominal pain. But on the other hand, this herb is bad for hot symptoms and ailments, including dry lips, thirst, sore throat, vomiting of blood, fever, ulcers and alcoholism.

## DESCRIPTION

- Hot; pungent; warms up kidneys; arrests bleeding; used as a tonic.

## PREPARATION

- Prepare 300g cottonseeds and fry with a few teaspoonfuls rice wine; separately fry 100g chive seeds; grind into powder. Take 10g with wine on an empty stomach once a day to cure impotence.
- Boil 10g cottonseeds in 1 glass water over low heat until water is reduced by half. Drink as tea on an empty stomach once a day to cure night sweat.

## Crab Apple

*Good for diarrhea, diabetes, seminal emission.*

## DESCRIPTION

- Neutral; sweet and sour; quenches thirst; obstructive; affects the heart, liver and lungs.

## PREPARATION

- Boil 10 partially ripe fresh crab apples in an adequate amount of water until the water is reduced by half. Drink the soup and eat the crab apples first thing in the morning to cure watery diarrhea.
- Crush 60g partially ripe fresh crab apples; boil crab apples in water. Drink a cup of the juice each time, 3 times a day, to relieve abdominal pain and diarrhea in enteritis and dysentery.
- Crush 15 to 30g fresh crab apples; squeeze out the juice. Drink 3 times a day to cure diarrhea in children.
- Fry 30g dried crab apples until yellowish; boil crab apples in water. Eat them at bedtime to cure seminal emission and premature ejaculation.

## Cucumber

*Good for sore throat, pink eyes, inflammation, burns.*

## DESCRIPTION

- Cool; sweet, detoxicates; promotes urination and quenches thirst; affects the spleen, stomach and large intestine.

## PREPARATION

- Squeeze the juice from the cucumber or the leaf. Apply externally to the affected region to relieve burns.
- When cucumber becomes old, it appears yellowish. Cucumber may then be boiled as soup to alleviate dry cough in autumn (when people are more likely to develop cough due to a dry climate). The Chinese people believe that the lungs are most susceptible to the external energy of dryness in autumn.

## Black Fungus

*Good for discharge of blood from anus, dysentery with discharge of blood, vaginal bleeding, hemorrhoids.*

## DESCRIPTION

- Neutral; sweet; arrests bleeding; cools the blood; affects the stomach and the large intestine.

### Notes

Cottonseed oil is hot and pungent. It may be used externally to relieve boils, tinea and frostbites. An experiment on chicks shows it can elevate the level of blood fat more than corn or sunflower oil.

### Notes

It is not wise to consume crab apples in large quantities because they have an obstructive nature. Crab apples are not recommended for people with constipation.

### Notes

Cucumber is effective to relieve common acne, because common acne is due to excessive heat in the lungs and stomach. Since cucumber has a cool energy and acts upon the stomach, fresh cucumber may be eaten to cure acne.

The Chinese people preserve cucumber and eat it as a vegetable to cleanse the blood, clear up internal heat to cure hot diarrhea or hot skin conditions. Cut a cucumber lengthwise, remove and discard the seed portion and put the cucumber in the sun to dry.

### Notes

It is reported that black fungus has been used as a contraceptive with results: Boil 450g black fungus in water until very soft; mash it with brown sugar to make a syrup. Take the syrup with yellow rice wine, twice a day, for 3 to 7 days after childbirth.

## APPLICATION

- Drink black fungus cooked with wine to relieve or prevent blood coagulations after external injuries or after childbirth.
- Cook black fungus as soup to relieve hemorrhoids.
- Boil black fungus in water and add brown sugar. Drink to relieve vaginal bleeding.

## *Fresh Ginger*

*Good for common cold, vomiting, cough, asthma, diarrhea.*

### DESCRIPTION

- Warm; pungent; induces perspiration, disperses cold and relieves vomiting; affects the lungs, stomach and spleen.

### PREPARATION

- Grate fresh old ginger (see Remarks below) and boil in water for 10 minutes; drink it like tea to cure edema or vomiting or cough and also to warm up the body.
- Crush 100g fresh old ginger and boil it; use the hot liquid to wash the body and stimulate the skin to induce perspiration for relief of fever in common cold.
- Grate fresh old ginger and squeeze the juice; mix the juice with sugar or honey in 1 to 2 cups boiling water; drink a cupful each time, 3 times a day, to relieve cough.
- Eat a few pieces of tender, fresh ginger to relieve indigestion.
- Squeeze fresh ginger juice and drink it as orange juice to heal motion sickness, hiccup, or vomiting; it is also effective to counteract food poisoning.
- Boil 2g dried ginger or 7g fresh ginger with some brown sugar and drink it hot to relieve discomfort of cold and fever with cold abdominal pain due to common cold.
- Boil 4g fresh ginger with 8g dried orange peel and drink it like tea to heal vomiting and cough due to common cold.
- Western doctors normally use ginger as a digestive and carminative.

### CLINICAL REPORT

- Injection of 5 to 10 percent fresh ginger juice into the affected areas is effective to relieve rheumatic pain.
- Mix 50g fresh ginger with 30g brown sugar; to treat acute bacillary dysentery, eat 3 times a day, for 7 days as a treatment program. Among the 50 cases treated, 70 percent recover from the disease and 30 percent show improvements. After eating the ginger mixture, abdominal pain and tenesmus disappear within an average of 1 and 5 days respectively. Stools and bowel movements return to normal within an average of 4 and 5 days respectively.

## *Dried Ginger*

*Good for cold abdominal pain, vomiting and diarrhea, cold limbs, rheumatism.*

### DESCRIPTION

- Hot; pungent; warms the internal region; affects the spleen, stomach and lungs.

### Notes

In everyday cooking, fresh tender ginger is used; but when used for therapeutic purposes, fresh old ginger gives better effects. (Fresh ginger, also called "baby" ginger, is available in Chinese shops seasonally, usually in June and July and can be used to make ginger pickle; old ginger, known as "mother" ginger, is difficult to chew and usually available in Chinese markets.)

Like garlic, ginger is widely used in cooking; a few slices added to cooking will counteract the strong smell of meats, fish, or shellfish and it can also counteract toxic effects.

### Notes

Dried ginger, available in herb shops, is normally used as herb; when fresh old ginger is peeled and put under the sun to dry, it becomes dried ginger with a hot energy instead of a warm energy.

## PREPARATION

- Dissolve 7g dried ground ginger in warm water and drink each time, once a day, to relieve diarrhea with discharge of very watery stools.

## *Guava*

*Good for diarrhea, diabetes, hemorrhoids.*

### DESCRIPTION

- Warm; sweet; obstructive and constrictive; stops diarrhea and bleeding.

### PREPARATION

- Crush 250g fresh guavas and bring to a boil. Drink it all each time, 3 times a day, to relieve diarrhea in acute gastroenteritis and dysentery.
- Fry 30g dry guavas; boil guavas in water and divide into 3 dosages to drink in 1 day to relieve diarrhea in children.
- Crush 90g fresh guavas; squeeze out the juice to drink before meals, 3 times a day, to alleviate the symptoms associated with diabetes.
- Boil 90g dry guavas and drink as tea, to relieve acute and chronic pharyngolaryngitis and hoarseness.
- Boil 500g fresh guavas or 250g dry guavas until the liquid becomes very concentrated; use the guava liquid to wash the affected region, 2 to 3 times a day, to remedy hemorrhoids, bleeding, eczema, itching and heat rash.

## *Guava Leaf*

*Good for diarrhea, chronic dysentery, eczema, bleeding due to injuries.*

### DESCRIPTION

- Neutral; sweet; obstructive.

### PREPARATION

- Boil about 50g fresh guava leaves in water; drink the juice to cure or prevent enteritis, dysentery and diarrhea.
- Apply fresh guava leaf juice to injuries to stop bleeding.

## *Hops*

*Good for indigestion, abdominal swelling, edema, cystitis, pulmonary tuberculosis, insomnia.*

### DESCRIPTION

- Slightly cool; bitter; used as a stomach tonic, digestive and diuretic.

### PREPARATION

- Boil 15g hops in 2 glasses water over low heat until water is reduced by half. Drink once a day to relieve the early stage of pulmonary tuberculosis and low fever in the afternoon.
- Use 4g hops to make tea every day to relieve neurasthenia, insomnia and decreased appetite.

### CLINICAL REPORT

- On treatment of leprosy, pulmonary tuberculosis, silicosis, silicotuberculosis, tuberculosis of the lymph node and acute bacillary dysentery, all indicate positive results.

*Notes*

One report reveals that Chinese women picking hops in the field normally start to have menstrual flow on the second or third day after they start picking and they do not experience menstrual pain. The actions of hops and those of a female sex hormone are similar.

## Kelp

*Good for tuberculosis of the lymph node, goiter, hiccupping, difficulty when swallowing, edema, swelling and pain of the testes, vaginal discharge.*

### DESCRIPTION

- Cold; salty; softens hardness; facilitates water passage; affects the stomach.

### PREPARATION

- Regular consumption of kelp at meals relieves goitre; or eat kelp powder with honey.

### EXPERIMENT

- One experiment shows kelp is effective for hypothyroidism due to iodine deficiency, kelp also temporarily inhibits the basal metabolic rate in hyperthyroidism and improves the symptoms for a short duration.
- Another experiment indicates that kelp reduces blood pressure, asthma attacks and coughing.

## Kohlrabi

*Good for indigestion, jaundice, diabetes, alcoholism, nosebleed.*

### DESCRIPTION

- Neutral; bitter, sweet and pungent; detoxicates.

### PREPARATION

- Drink fresh kohlrabi juice to stop nosebleed.
- Crush fresh kohlrabi seeds into powder. Take 10g powder each time, twice a day, to relieve difficult urination after childbirth and improve the eyesight.
- Crush 10g kohlrabi seeds into powder. Mix with a glass of boiling water. Strain through cheesecloth over a bowl and squeeze out all the liquid. Drink the liquid as tea first thing in the morning to induce bowel movements and urination.

## Lamb or Mutton

*Good for general weakness, underweight, abdominal pain, lumbago.*

### DESCRIPTION

- Warm; sweet; used as an energy tonic and to warm up the internal region; affects the spleen and kidneys.

### PREPARATION

- Cook lamb or mutton with garlic and eat at meals to strengthen erection of the penis and also to relieve upset stomach in men and women.
- Boil 500g mutton with 1 bowl rice and 1 glass papaya juice; season with sugar and salt. Drink to cure lumbago and beriberi.

## Leek

*Good for diarrhea in enteritis of large intestine, bleeding, dysphagia, upset stomach.*

### DESCRIPTION

- Warm; pungent; obstructive; affects the liver and lungs.

*Notes*

Kelp is cold and can cool hot symptoms; and it is salty and can soften hardness.

Prolonged consumption of kelp will cause weight loss. Kelp is not recommended for pregnant women and people with weak digestion.

To make kelp powder, roast the kelp; dry and grind into powder.

*Notes*

Mutton can warm the internal region and for that reason, it is not recommended for people with a hot physical constitution; moreover, mutton is very fatty, not recommended for people with a high level of blood fat.

Mutton is beneficial for weak and underweight people. Since it may not be easily digested, the quantity eaten each time should be limited.

Sheep's milk is warm and sweet, is used to lubricate dryness and to relieve fatigue, underweight, diabetes and vomiting of acid.

Sheep's liver is cool, sweet and bitter, is used as a liver tonic and to sharpen vision and to relieve glaucoma and night blindness.

Sheep's kidney is warm and sweet, is used as a kidney tonic and to strengthen sexual capacity and erection of the penis.

## Lettuce

*Good for diminished urination, discharge of bloody urine, shortage of milk secretion.*

### DESCRIPTION

- Cool; bitter and sweet; promotes urination and milk secretion; affects the stomach and large intestine.

## Lettuce Seed

*Good for swollen scrotum, hemorrhoids, shortage of milk secretion after childbirth.*

### DESCRIPTION

- Cold; bitter; promotes milk secretion and urination.

### PREPARATION

- Grind 30 seeds into powder and dissolve in wine. Drink it for shortage of milk secretion after childbirth; or cook equal amounts of lettuce seeds and sweet rice and add a little licorice to eat at meals.

## Dried Manadarin Orange Peel

*Good for chest congestion, abdominal swelling, lack of appetite, vomiting, hiccupping, coughing with mucous discharge, fish and crab poisoning.*

### DESCRIPTION

- Warm; pungent and bitter; pushes downwards; stimulates energy; relieves water retention; eliminates mucus; affects the spleen and lungs.

### PREPARATION

- Dried mandarin orange peel is an important Chinese herb. It is widely used in remedies.
- Dissolve 1.5g dry mandarin orange peel powder in warm water. Drink each time, 3 times a day, to relieve chest congestion and abdominal swelling and pain due to indigestion.
- Mix 40g dry mandarin orange peel powder with 100g cuttlefish bone powder. Take 3g dissolved in warm water each time, 3 times a day, to treat stomachache, swelling of stomach, belching and excessive gastric acid.

### CLINICAL REPORT

- For treatment of acute mastitis: Mix 40g dried mandarin orange peels and 7g licorice in water. Bring to a boil and then boil it again for a second time. Divide into 2 dosages to take in 1 day. Double the dosage in severe cases. Clinical observations show that early treatment (within 1 to 2 days of onset) produces good results with a 70 percent success rate in 2 to 3 days. This treatment is less effective when acute mastitis has a longer duration. No results are obtained after suppuration has occurred.

## Marjoram

*Good for common colds, fever, vomiting, diarrhea, jaundice, malnutrition in children, skin rash.*

*Notes*

It is believed that excessive consumption of lettuce will cause dizziness and pain in the eyes.

*Notes*

In Chinese folk medicine, marjoram is believed to regulate body temperature and prevent hot diseases; it is widely used in summer as substitute for tea.

## DESCRIPTION

- Cool; pungent; induces perspiration; promotes energy circulation; relieves water retention.

## PREPARATION

- Boil marjoram in water and drink it like tea to induce perspiration.
- Boil marjoram in water and use the liquid to wash the mouth to counteract bad breath.
- To relieve itch, boil 150g fresh marjoram and use the liquid to wash the affected region.

## EXPERIMENT

- Marjoram promotes urination, induces perspiration, increases the appetite and also relieves mucous discharge, experiments show.

## Button Mushroom

*Good for diarrhea, mucous discharge, vomiting.*

## DESCRIPTION

- Cool; sweet; affects the stomach, lungs and intestines.

## PREPARATION

- Cook common button mushroom to relieve leukocytopenia and contagious hepatitis and to prevent metastasis after a cancer operation.

## EXPERIMENT

- Common button mushroom has the effects of antibiosis and lowers blood fat, according to an experiment.

## Muskmelon

*Good for coughs, difficult urination, constipation, liver disease.*

## DESCRIPTION

- Cold; sweet; reduces fever; quenches thirst; promotes urination; affects the heart and stomach.

## PREPARATION

- Eat 250 to 500g muskmelon each time, twice a day, to relieve thirst in fever, pain on urination and constipation.
- Steam 250g fresh muskmelon with an adequate amount of rock sugar. Eat twice a day to relieve cough in pulmonary tuberculosis.
- To make dried calyx and receptacle of muskmelon, cut off calyx and receptacle of a muskmelon and leave them in the shade to dry. This is an important Chinese herb whose extracts are reported to have been made into tablets for hepatitis.

## Nutmeg

*Good for abdominal swelling and pain, diarrhea, vomiting, indigestion.*

## DESCRIPTION

- Warm; pungent; pushes downwards; warms the internal region; promotes digestion; affects the spleen and large intestine.

### Notes

Muskmelon and seeds are not recommended for people with diarrhea and edema. Dried calyx and receptacle of muskmelon are not recommended for people with heart disease.

### Notes

Nutmeg is bad for hemorrhoids, hot diarrhea and toothache. Mace, the spice ground from the layer between the nutmeg shell and its outer husk, is used as a carminative, stomach tonic and stimulant.

## Onion

*Good for external applications on ulcers and trichomonas vaginitis.*

### DESCRIPTION

- In folk medicine, onion is used as a diuretic and expectorant.

### PREPARATION

- Boil 10g onion over low heat. Eat it to lower blood pressure.
- Eat onion regularly to increase muscular strength.

### EXPERIMENT

- Sauté 60g onion with vegetable oil. Healthy males who eat onion inhibit a rise in cholesterol caused by a high level of fat intake. Onion also acts to reduce fibrinolysis activity and is considered beneficial in the treatment of arteriosclerosis.
- An experiment on animals indicates that onion increases intestinal tension and secretion and is considered beneficial to weak intestines and nondysenteric enteritis.

## Green Onion Leaf

*Good for headaches and nasal congestion associated with common cold.*

### DESCRIPTION

- Warm; pungent; induces perspiration.

## Papaya

*Good for stomachaches, dysentery, difficulty in bowel movements, rheumatism.*

### DESCRIPTION

- Neutral; sweet; promotes digestion; destroys intestinal worms.

### PREPARATION

- Boil 500g partially ripe papayas with 2 pork forelegs until very soft. Eat papayas and pork once each day for 3 consecutive days to stimulate lactation after childbirth.
- Steam 250 to 500g fresh papayas. Eat papayas once a day to relieve thirst from fever and chronic cough.
- Prepare a few unripe papayas: peel and remove seeds; soak papayas in vinegar to make sour papayas (save the soaking vinegar).
- Eat 30g sour papaya or 60g fresh papaya twice a day to relieve indigestion and abdominal pain and swelling.
- At bedtime, eat 250g sour papayas and drink 60g of the vinegar in which papayas have been soaked, for 3 consecutive days, to destroy tapeworms, roundworms and whipworms and other worms of the intestinal tract.

### REMARKS

- Papaya is reported to be antitumorigenic because it contains carpaine.
- It is reported that papaya has a paralytic effect on the central nervous system, which may explain why papaya can relieve rheumatic pain.

## Chinese Parsley (Coriander)

*Good for indigestion, measles prior to the rash.*

## DESCRIPTION

- Warm; pungent; induces perspiration, promotes digestion, speeds the outbreak of measles rash; affects the lungs and spleen.

## PREPARATION

- Boil Chinese parsley with water chestnut and carrot to make soup to facilitate eruptions in measles; or, cut up a few whole parsleys (including leaves and roots) and cook in water; wash the measles patient while the liquid is warm to facilitate measles eruptions.
- Regular consumption of Chinese parsley will reduce the bad smell of urine due to internal heat.
- Cook whole Chinese parsley (including leaves and roots) with fish, pork, or beef to remove offensive smells (including vaginal odors and bad breath).
- Use Chinese parsley as a seasoning in cooking to relieve excessive gastric acid and cold stomachache.

## *Peanut*

*Good for dry coughs, upset stomachs, beriberi, shortage of milk secretion after childbirth.*

## DESCRIPTION

- Neutral; sweet; lubricates the lungs; considered good for stomachache; affects the spleen and lungs.

## PREPARATION

- Fry 3 cups roasted peanuts until aromatic; soak 1 cup rice (any kind except sweet [glutinous]) in water for at least 2 hours; drain and add the peanuts and boil together in water until they become soft to make peanut-rice congee soup. Drink the soup once a day to relieve beriberi and to promote milk secretion.
- Roast peanuts and eat them to stimulate the appetite, lubricate the intestines and relieve a dry cough.
- Consume fresh peanuts to relieve a cough with mucous discharge.
- Boil 100g fresh peanuts with an equal amount of small red beans and red dates. Drink as soup at meals to relieve beriberi.
- Boil 100g peanuts with 1 pork foreleg. Eat at meals to promote milk secretion after childbirth.
- Boil 1 glass peanuts with 3 glasses water over low heat for 3 hours; add a little rock sugar and drink it on an empty stomach to relieve beriberi.
- Consume fresh peanuts on a regular basis to relieve deafness.

## EXPERIMENT

- Initial experiments indicate peanuts arrest bleeding in hemophilia patients. Subsequent experiments show peanuts can arrest various kinds except severe bleeding. It is also found that fried or roasted peanuts are 20 times less effective than raw peanuts and the effects of the outer brown skins of the peanut are 50 times stronger than the peanut itself.

## CLINICAL REPORT

- For the treatment of chronic tracheitis: Boil 70g of the outer layers of peanuts in water for about 10 hours. Strain it to obtain 100ml of the liquid; add sugar. Drink 50ml each time, twice a day, for 10 days as a treatment program. Among the 407 cases of chronic tracheitis treated, 74 cases show significant results, 230 cases show improvements, 95 cases show no effects.

*Notes*

Chinese people use Chinese parsley as a seasoning when cooking shrimps, crabs, oysters, clams and other fish for 3 purposes: To make the food look better, to increase the aromatic fragrance and to increase the warm energy.

When Chinese parsley is used to facilitate eruptions in measles, a number of things should be kept in mind: Chinese parsley is not intended for prolonged consumption; when there are signs of eruptions on the second or third day of fever in measles, it is the best time to administer Chinese parsley. But if eruptions have already occurred, Chinese parsley should not be used, because it may increase the internal heat.

People with constant thirst or cracked lips or constipation should not eat Chinese parsley.

*Notes*

The outer layers of peanuts should not be removed if possible when peanuts are used in a Chinese remedy, unless otherwise specified.

Eating large quantities of peanuts is considered harmful to the digestive functions and to the skin.

Peanut oil is neutral and sweet and is used to lubricate the intestines. Use a cotton ball to apply peanut oil to the scrotum region to relieve itching and wet sensations, 5 or 6 times a day, without washing with hot water.

## *Red or Green Pepper*

*Good for abdominal pain, vomiting, diarrhea.*

### DESCRIPTION

- Hot; pungent; warms the internal region, increases appetite, promotes digestion; affects the heart and spleen.

### PREPARATION

- Red pepper may be used in cooking to excite the spirits, induce perspiration, promote urination, increase appetite and soften up blood vessels. Some people believe that red pepper can prevent heart disease.
- Cook red pepper leaves with chicken egg and fresh ginger as a soup to warm up the stomach.
- Use red pepper as a seasoning in cooking to promote blood circulation and also to soften up blood vessels (good for relief of arteriosclerosis and for prevention of hypertension).

## *Plum*

*Good for liver disease, diabetes, ascites*

### DESCRIPTION

- Neutral; sweet and sour; produces fluids; promotes urination and digestion; affects the liver and kidneys.

### PREPARATION

- Eat 2 fresh plums every day in the morning and evening to promote digestion and to arrest bleeding from gums.
- To cure cirrhosis and diminished urination, crush 2 sweet plums with seeds and mix with hot water. Drink like tea, 1 cup each time, twice a day.
- Soak fresh plums in vinegar to make vinegar plums.
- Crush 2 vinegar plums with their seeds, mix with boiling water and a little salt; let it cool down. Wash your mouth and throat with the juice a few times a day to cure chronic pharyngolaryngitis, tonsillitis, periodontitis, mouth canker and tongue ulcer.
- Crush 30g plum seeds and boil with water. Drink a cupful each time, twice a day, to relieve constipation.

## *Sour Plum*

*Good for diarrhea, dry cough, thirst.*

### DESCRIPTION

- Neutral; extremely sour; constrictive and obstructive; produces fluids and destroys worms; affects the liver.

### PREPARATION

- Eat 2 fresh sour plums, or crush a fresh sour plum and mix with sugar and a little salt to make tea. Drink the tea to relieve thirst from fever and shortage of gastric acid and poor appetite.
- To make preserved sour plums (good for checking diarrhea), put ripe fresh sour plums in a large earthenware container; add salt and marinate until the plums become so soft that juice begins to flow out.

*Notes*

Consumption of red pepper in excessive quantities will cause abdominal pain and constipation: Red pepper is not recommended for people with eye disease, cough, gastritis, or nephritis.

In addition to the color of peppers (which may be red or green), there are also different degrees of intensity: Peppers with a round shape are not as hot as peppers that are long and pointed.

It is said that there are 4 stages in the psychology of eating red or green pepper: At the beginning, before one starts eating it, one is afraid of its hot nature; gradually, one can tolerate its hot nature; and then, one is used to it and no longer afraid of its hot nature; and finally, one starts complaining that it is not hot enough any more.

*Notes*

Plum is not recommended for people with weak stomachs, ulcers and acute or chronic gastroenteritis.

*Notes*

A friend who is now practicing acupuncture in Montreal told me that once he joined a group of people on an extreme diet and was told to eat a very large quantity of preserved plums every day. After a few days of consuming plums, he became so jumpy that while he was working at a store, he felt a strong urge to chase customers out and tell them to go to hell. The plums can act upon the liver and thus, eating too many of them may disturb the liver and cause an emotional outbreak.

## Pumpkin

*Good for bronchial asthma, cough, edema.*

### DESCRIPTION

- Neutral; sweet and slightly bitter.

### CLINICAL REPORT

- More than 30 sufferers of bronchial asthma were given each day about a pound of steamed pumpkin mixed with honey and sugar. The majority of patients were able to control the symptoms with either an absence of asthma attacks or significant improvements. Some patients did not have recurring attacks during the observation periods, ranging from 6 months to 2 years. Preliminary observations indicated that the patients of simple bronchial asthma have the best results and patients of complicated bronchial asthma also show some improvements.

## Rice Bran

*Good for difficulty when swallowing, beriberi.*

### DESCRIPTION

- Neutral; sweet and pungent; pushes downwards; affects the stomach and large intestine.

## Rosemary

*Good for headaches.*

### DESCRIPTION

- Warm; pungent; induces perspiration; used as a stomachic.

## Sesame Oil

*Good for constipation due to dryness, ulcers, cracked skin, scabies and tinea.*

### DESCRIPTION

- Cool; sweet; detoxicates; lubricates dryness; promotes bowel movements; produces muscles.

### PREPARATION

- Add a few drops of sesame oil in cooking to relieve constipation.
- Apply sesame oil externally to the affected region and massage it repeatedly to relieve rheumatic pain and fatigue.

### CLINICAL REPORT

- For the treatment of chronic simple rhinitis: Cook sesame oil over low heat until boiling. Use as nose drops; apply 2 to 3 drops on each side each time, gradually increasing to 5 to 6 drops, 3 times a day. Among the 63 cases treated, 52 cases showed significant improvements, 3 cases showed progress or improvements, 8 cases showed no effects. Treatment duration ranges from 10 days to 3 months.

*Notes*

Mix rice bran with honey and shape into tablets. Keep 1 tablet at a time in the mouth just as a cough drop. This remedy relieves difficulty when swallowing.

Fry 250g rice bran until yellowish but not burned. Store in a jar for application. Take 10g of the yellowish rice bran with water each time, twice a day, to relieve beriberi.

*Notes*

One source indicates that rosemary preparation can be used as an emmenagogue to speed up menstrual flow in menopause syndrome. Another source indicates that rosemary oil and hollylock root mixtures can promote growth of hair on head. Still another source indicates that infusions of rosemary and borax can prevent baldness.

## *Spearmint*

*Good for common cold, coughs, headaches, abdominal pain, menstrual pain.*

### DESCRIPTION

- Warm; pungent and sweet; promotes energy circulation, relieves pain.

### PREPARATION

- Cook tender, fresh peppermint leaves in water with chicken egg and eat as soup to treat headache.
- Spearmint calms down the spirits and relieves common cold at the same time. It has been used in Chinese folk medicine to treat headache and dizziness. It is reported that a woman was suffering from chronic headache for a decade, particularly when she was under stress, with headache attacks, sometimes many times a day. Her malady was diagnosed by Western doctors as a case of cerebral anemia and by traditional Chinese doctors as something else, but no relief was offered. She eventually healed herself by drinking spearmint soup for less than 1 month.
- It is believed that Vietnamese women regard spearmint as an important herb for relief of headache; they just drink it as tea.

## *Sunflower Seed*

*Good for constipation, diarrhea with discharge of blood.*

### DESCRIPTION

- Warm and neutral; sweet and light flavor; stops diarrhea; facilitates eruption of rash in measles.

### PREPARATION

- Crush 30g sunflower seeds (with shells removed); add 1 cup boiling water and an adequate amount of honey and stir. Drink in the morning and evening to cure constipation.
- Crush 30 9 sunflower seeds; add 30g rock sugar and some water; boil over low heat for 1 hour. Drink 1 cup each time, 3 times a day, to cure diarrhea with discharge of blood.
- Crush 5g sunflower seeds and make tea. Drink twice a day, to promote eruptions in measles.
- Crush 30g sunflower seeds with shells, add 30g rock sugar and boil over low heat for half an hour; drink twice a day to cure ringing in the ears.

### EXPERIMENT

- A normal person consuming unrefined sunflower oil on an empty stomach will temporarily increase the level of their cholesterol; and young women using sunflower oil for cooking for 7 days will slightly lower their levels of cholesterol.

## *Taro*

*Good for tuberculosis of the lymph nodes, scrofula, external application to relieve inflammation, swelling and pain.*

### DESCRIPTION

- Neutral; sweet and pungent; glossy; affects the stomach and large intestine.

### PREPARATION

- Peel about 30 fresh taros (roots); cut into pieces and fry in vegetable

*Notes*

Spearmint could be effective for relief of headache because it can act upon the liver and in Chinese medicine the liver is responsible for headache due to stress.

oil. Dry taro in the sun; grind into powder. Take 15g of the powder dissolved in warm water each time, twice a day, to cure scrofula.

## Taro Flower

*Good for stomachache, vomiting of blood, prolapse of uterus, hemorrhoids, prolapse of anus.*

### DESCRIPTION

- Neutral; numbing taste.

## Taro Leaf

*Good for diarrhea, excessive perspiration, night sweat.*

### DESCRIPTION

- Cool; pungent; checks perspiration and diarrhea; heals swelling.

## Tobacco

*Good for indigestion, abdominal swelling, headache, numbness and pain in arthritis.*

### DESCRIPTION

- Warm; pungent; toxic; promotes energy circulation, relieves pain; counteracts cold and damp symptoms.

### PREPARATION

- Boil or squeeze tobacco juice or smoke cigarettes to cure blood coagulations, rheumatic pain and to warm the body and the womb in women. (Using cigarettes as a form of therapy is a far cry from habitual smoking, which is a form of addiction.)

### EXPERIMENT

- Heavy smokers can develop chronic pharyngitis and other respiratory symptoms; heavy smokers (over 20 cigarettes a day) are 4 to 7 times more susceptible to an attack of bronchitis than nonsmokers.
- Smoking may also be related to lung cancer: Among lung cancer patients over 45 years old, there are approximately 50 times as many smoking more than 25 cigarettes a day as nonsmokers.
- Smokers are also more susceptible to gastroenteric disorders (such as indigestion, nervous stomach diseases, ulcers and constipation).
- Heavy smokers may develop headache and insomnia.
- The primary ingredient of tobacco is nicotine, which is very easily absorbed by mucous membranes. When 2 drops are placed on the tongue surface of dogs, they die within 1 to 2 minutes. Nicotine may also be absorbed by the skin surface and cause death.

## Wax Gourd
## (Winter Gourd or Winter Melon)

*Good for edema, beriberi, sunstroke, hemorrhoids, alcoholism.*

### Notes

Boil fresh taro flower in small quantities.

### Notes

The Chinese people believe that lung cancer may be attributed to excessive heat in the lungs. This may explain why smoking contributes to lung cancer, because tobacco is considered capable of generating the heat that dries the lungs. Thus the lungs become easy targets of cancer when they are hot and dry. For this reason, when a person displays the symptoms of cough and vomiting of blood, smoking could prove fatal.

Many people gain weight after they quit smoking, which may be due to 2 possible reasons: First, many physicians attribute it to overeating, because when a person quits smoking, he or she needs something else to compensate for smoking and eating is the easiest candidate; second, according to Chinese medicine, smoking can make the body dry; many overweight persons have a wet physical constitution and smoking may help them stay slim; when they quit smoking, their body begins to retain water and they gain weight.

My personal speculation is that if a person has a damp physical constitution (which often means overweight), he or she is less likely to be harmed by smoking; on the other hand, a person with a dry and hot physical constitution is very easily harmed by smoking and it is wise and urgent for such a person to quit smoking.

## DESCRIPTION

- Cool; sweet and light tastes; detoxicates; promotes urination; eliminates mucus; affects the lungs, bladder and small and large intestines.

## PREPARATION

- Drink fresh wax gourd juice to relieve sunstroke and thirst.
- Cook 100g dry wax gourd peel until it becomes syrup. Drink it in large quantities each day to relieve all kinds of edema associated with diminished urination, including kidney disease, heart disease, beriberi and cirrhotic ascites.
- Boil 100g wax gourd over low heat. Drink it as soup. Or bake a wax gourd until its skin appears charred. Take 30g each time, twice a day. Or eat cooked wax gourd on a regular basis to promote urination and bowel movements, cure edema, beriberi and hemorrhoids.

*Notes*

Chinese wax gourd peel is commonly used in Chinese medicine. It may be used as wax gourd but with greater effects.

## *Wheat Bran*

*Good for stomatitis, oral herpes, rheumatism, beriberi, discharge of urine containing blood.*

## DESCRIPTION

- Cool; sweet; affects the stomach.

## CLINICAL REPORT

- A treatment of diabetes: steam 60 percent wheat bran and 40 percent all-purpose flour; add an adequate amount of vegetable oil, eggs and vegetables. Eat at meals to relieve diabetes. The proportion of wheat bran decreases as conditions improve. No drugs or nutritional supplements are given in this treatment. Among the 13 diabetes cases treated, blood sugar dropped to below 140mg percent in 3 cases and to 180mg percent in 7 cases; after treatment (which lasts from 4 days to 98 days), sugar in the urine changed from + + + + or + + + to negative in 10 cases; but in general, sugar in the urine changed to negative within 1 month along with the disappearance of neuritis associated with diabetes.

*Notes*

The grains that float on the water are used as an important Chinese remedy for the above symptoms.

## *Whole Wheat*

*Good for hysteria in women, diarrhea, burns.*

## DESCRIPTION

- Cool; sweet; used as a heart tonic and a kidney tonic; affects the heart, spleen and kidneys.

## PREPARATION

- Boil 30g whole wheat kernels with 10g licorice and 5 red dates in water. Eat once a day to cure hysteria in women. This is a time-honored recipe frequently used in Chinese medicine for hysteria in women.
- Fry wheat until charred and grind into powder to mix with oil for external applications to relieve burns.

## *Wine*

*Good for rheumatism, muscular spasms, chest pain, cold abdominal pain.*

## DESCRIPTION

- Warm; sweet, bitter and pungent; promotes blood circulation; expels cold energy; speeds up the effects of herbs; affects the heart, liver, lungs and stomach.

## PREPARATION

- Drink a glass of wine to relieve diarrhea due to cold and with the discharge of a clear and long stream of urine, which indicates a cold symptom.
- Mix honey with rice wine and drink it to treat itching all over the body in women.
- Fry 500g black soybeans until they appear over-fried and begin to crack. Place in an earthenware pot and pour 2 to 4 glasses rice wine into the pot; let it cool and strain it. Drink a cupful each time, twice a day, to heal numbness and pain in the joints, rheumatic pain, neuralgia and anemia.
- Drink 1 glass hot rice wine or grape wine to relieve pain caused by external injuries.

## CLINICAL REPORT

- For treatment of simple diarrhea after childbirth, bring 3 glasses rice wine to a boil; add 150g brown sugar and continue boiling for 2 to 3 minutes; let it cool and drink it all, or divide it into 2 parts to drink 3 to 4 hours apart. Among the 14 cases treated, 10 cases completely recovered. One case recovered naturally after stopping the treatment, 2 cases showed improvements and 1 case no significant results. Some cases recovered completely within 3 days. Only 1 case complained about light headache during the treatment. No side effects were shown in all other cases.

*Notes*

There are basically 2 kinds of wine used in Chinese herbal therapy—rice wine (also called yellow wine) and hot wine (also called white wine or fire wine). Yellow wine contains only 10 to 20 percent alcohol; white wine contains a much higher alcohol level. White wine is usually used to manufacture medicated herbal wine. Yellow wine is suitable for drinking with Chinese meals.

Wine is sometimes considered more harmful than beneficial, because many people have a tendency to become intoxicated when drinking wine.

# Appendices

*Bibliography*

*These publications were all published in China in the Chinese language

Chinese Medical Journal (monthly). Peking, 1959-1984.

Chinese Scientific Nutritional Research Institute. Nutritional Chart of Chinese Foods, Peking: People's Health Press, 1963.

Dai Yin-Fong and Liu Cheng-Jun. Medicinal Uses of Fruits. Peking: Guang-Xi People's Press, 1982.

Jiangsu New Medical College. A Complete Dictionary of Chinese Herbs. Shanghai: Shanghai Technical Press, 1977.

Journal of New Chinese Medicine (monthly). Canton, 1956-1985.

Li Shih-Chen. An Outline of Materia Medica, 1578.

Li Yan. Self Healing of Cancers and Tumors by Herbs and Diet. Peking: People's Health Press, 1983.

Luo He-Sheng. Common Herbs for Prevention and Cure of Cancers and Tumors. Canton: Canton Technical Press, 1981.

Sun Shu Mao. One Thousand Ounces of Gold Classic, seventh century. AD

Yeh Ju-Quan. Chinese Diet and Herbal Formulas. Hong Kong: Shang-Wu Press, 1978.

Yellow Emperor's Classic of Internal Medicine, third century BC

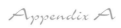

## Conversion Guides & Approximate Equivalents

| CUSTOMARY TERMS | | METRIC SYMBOLS | |
|---|---|---|---|
| t. | teaspoon | ml or mL | millilitre |
| T. | tablespoon | L | litre |
| c. | cup | mg | milligram |
| pkg. | package | g | gram |
| pt. | pint | kg | kilogram |
| qt. | quart | mm | millimeter |
| oz. | ounce | cm | centimeter |
| lb. | pound | ºC | degrees Celsius |
| ºF | degrees Fahrenheit | | |
| in. | inch | | |

## Guide to Approximate Equivalents

| CUSTOMARY | | | | METRIC | |
|---|---|---|---|---|---|
| Ounces Pounds | Cups | Tblespoons | Teaspoons | Milliliters Liters | Grams Kilograms |
| | | | 1/2 t. | 1 ml | 1 g |
| | | | 1/2 t. | 2 ml | |
| | | | 1 t. | 5 ml | |
| | | | 2 t. | 10 ml | |
| 1/2 oz. | | 1 T. | 3 t. | 15 ml | 15 g |
| 1 oz. | | 2 T. | 6 t. | 30 ml | 28 g |
| 2 oz. | 1/2 c. | 4 T. | 12 t. | 60 ml | 60 g |
| 4 oz. | 1/2 c. | 8 T. | 24 t. | 125 ml | 120 g |
| 8 oz. | 1 c. | 16 T. | 48 t. | 250 ml | 225 g |
| 1 lb. | | | | | 450 g |
| | 4 c. | | | 1 L | |
| 2.2 lb. | | | | | 1 kg |

Keep in mind that this is not an exact conversion, but generally may be used for food measurement.

*Appendix B*

| Foods | Tonic Food | | | | | |
|---|---|---|---|---|---|---|
| | COMMON TONICS | | | | ORGANIC | |
| | ENERGY | BLOOD | YIN | YANG | LUNG | LIVER |
| ABALONE | | | ♠ | | | |
| ADZUKI BEAN FLOWERS | | | | | | |
| ADZUKI BEAN SPROUTS | | | | | | |
| ADZUKI BEANS | | | | | | |
| ALFALFA ROOTS | | | | | | |
| ALMONDS | | | | | | |
| ALOE VERA | | | | | | |
| AMBERGRIS | | | | | | |
| APPLE CUCUMBERS | | | | | | |
| APPLE PEELS | | | | | | |
| APPLES | | | ♠ | | | |
| ARECA NUTS MALE FLOWERS | | | | | | |
| ARROWHEAD | | | | | | |
| ASAFOETIDA | | | | | | |
| ASPARAGUS | | | | | | |
| AZALEA FLOWERS | | | | | | |
| AZALEA ROOTS | | | | | | |
| BAMBOO OIL | | | | | | |
| BAMBOO SHOOTS | | | | | | |
| BANANA RHIZOMES | | | | | | |
| BANANAS | | | | | | |
| BAYBERRY ROOTS | | | | | | |
| BEAN DRINK | | | | | | |
| BEAR GALL BLADDER | | | | | | |
| BEEF | ♠ | ♠ | | | | |
| BEEF KIDNEYS | | | | ♠ | | |
| BEEF LIVER | ♠ | | | | | ♠ |
| BEER | | | | | | |
| BIRD'S NEST | ♠ | | ♠ | | | |
| BITTER APRICOT SEEDS | | | | | | |
| BITTER ENDIVE | | | | | | |
| BITTER GOURD (BALSAM PEAR) | | | ♠ | | | |
| BITTER GOURD SEEDS | ♠ | | | | | |
| BLACK PEPPER | | | | | | |
| BLACK SESAME SEEDS | | | | | | ♠ |
| BLACK SOYBEAN SKINS | | ♠ | | | | |
| BLACK SOYBEANS | | | | | | |
| BLOOD CLAM | | ♠ | | | | |
| BOTTLE GOURD | | | | | | |
| BRAKE | | | | | | |
| BRAKE ROOTS | | | | | | |
| BROOMCORN | | ♠ | | | | |
| BROWN SUGAR | | | ♠ | | | |
| BUCKWHEAT | | | | | | |
| BURDOCK | | | | | | |

中医疗法

## *Regulating Foods*

| TONICS | | | | | | | | |
|--------|--------|--------|------------|-----------|--------|----------------------|---------------------|
| HEART | STOMACH | SPLEEN | TONIC HEAT | DAMP HEAT | SPUTUM | ENERGY CIRCULATION | BLOOD CIRCULATION |
| | | | ♠ | | | | |
| | | | | ♠ | | | |
| | | | | ♠ | | | |
| | | | ♠ | | | | |
| ♠ | | | | | | ♠ | ♠ |
| | | ♠ | | | | | |
| | ♠ | | | | ♠ | | |
| | | | | | | | ♠ |
| | | | | | ♠ | | |
| | | | | | ♠ | | |
| | | | | | ♠ | | |
| | ♠ | | | | ♠ | | |
| | | | ♠ | | | | |
| | | | ♠ | | | | |
| | | | | | ♠ | | ♠ |
| | | | | | ♠ | | |
| | ♠ | ♠ | | | | ♠ | |
| ♠ | | | | | | | |
| | | | ♠ | | | | |
| | | | ♠ | | ♠ | | |
| | | | ♠ | | | | |
| | | | | | ♠ | | |
| | | | | | ♠ | | |
| | | | | | | | ♠ |
| | ♠ | | | | ♠ | | |
| | | | ♠ | | ♠ | | |
| | | ♠ | | ♠ | | | ♠ |
| | | | ♠ | | | | |

Foods

## Tonic Food

| | COMMON TONICS | | | | ORGANIC | |
| Foods | ENERGY | BLOOD | YIN | YANG | LUNG | LIVER |
|---|---|---|---|---|---|---|
| CAMELLIA | | | | | | |
| CAMPHOR MINT | | | | | | |
| CANTALOUPE (MUSKMELON) | | | ♠ | | | |
| CANTALOUPE CALYX & RECEPTACLE | | | | | | |
| CANTALOUPE SEEDS | | | | | | |
| CARAWAY SEEDS | | | | | | |
| CARDAMOM SEEDS | | | | | | |
| CARROTS | | | | | | |
| CASTOR BEAN ROOTS | | | | | | |
| CATTAILS | | | | | | |
| CATTAIL POLLEN | | | | | | |
| CELERY | | | | | | |
| CELERY ROOTS | | | | | | |
| CELERY SEEDS | | | | | | |
| CHEESE | | | ♠ | | ♠ | |
| CHERRIES | ♠ | | | | | |
| CHERRY LEAVES | | | | | | |
| CHERRY ROOTS | | | | | | |
| CHESTNUTS | | | | ♠ | | |
| CHICKEN | ♠ | | | | | |
| CHICKEN BLOOD | | | | | | |
| CHICKEN EGG WHITES | | | | | | |
| CHICKEN EGGS | | ♠ | ♠ | | | |
| CHICKEN GALLBLADDER | | | | | | |
| CHICKEN LIVER | | | | | | ♠ |
| CHICORY | | | | | | |
| CHILI LEAVES | | | | | | |
| CHILI PEPPER | | | | | | |
| CHILI RHIZOMES | | | | | | |
| CHINESE CABBAGES | | | | | | |
| CHINESE ENDIVE | | | | | | |
| CHINESE MAGNOLIA VINE FRUITS | | | | | | |
| CHINESE ROSES | | | | | | |
| CHINESE ROSE LEAVES | | | | | | |
| CHINESE TOON | | | | | | |
| CHINESE TOON LEAVES | | | | | | |
| CHINESE ROOTS & BULBS | | | | | | |
| CHIVE SEEDS | | | | ♠ | | ♠ |
| CHIVES | | | | | | |
| CHRYSANTHEMUM | | | | | | |
| CINNAMON BARK | | | | ♠ | | |
| CITRON LEAVES | | | | | | |
| CITRONS | | | | | | |
| CLAMS | | | | | | |
| CLOVE OIL | | | | ♠ | | |

中医疗法

## Regulating Foods

| TONICS | | | | | | | |
|---|---|---|---|---|---|---|---|
| HEART | STOMACH | SPLEEN | TONIC HEAT | DAMP HEAT | SPUTUM | ENERGY CIRCULATION | BLOOD CIRCULATION |

*Foods*                                                                    *Tonic Food*

| | COMMON TONICS | | | | | ORGANIC |
| | ENERGY | BLOOD | YIN | YANG | LUNG | LIVER |
|---|---|---|---|---|---|---|
| CLOVES | | | | ♠ | | |
| COCONUT MILK | | | ♠ | | | |
| COCONUT MEAT | ♠ | | | | | |
| COCONUT SHELL | | | | | | |
| COFFEE | | | | | | |
| COMMON BUTTON MUSHROOMS | | | | | | |
| COMMON CARP | | | | | | |
| COOKED GINKGO | ♠ | | | | ♠ | |
| CORIANDER | | | | | | |
| CORN ROOTS | | | | | | |
| CORN SILK | | | | | | |
| CORNCOBS | | | | | | |
| COW GALL BLADDER | | | | | | |
| COW MILK | | | ♠ | | ♠ | |
| CRAB CLAWS | | | | | | |
| CRAB SHELLS | | | | | | |
| CRABS | | | ♠ | | | |
| CRANE MEAT | ♠ | | | | | |
| CROWN DAISIES | | | | | | |
| CUCUMBER VINES | | | | | | |
| CUTTLEFISH | | ♠ | ♠ | | | |
| DATES | ♠ | | ♠ | | | |
| DAY LILIES | | | | | | |
| DEER KIDNEYS | | | | ♠ | | |
| DEER HORNS (ANTLERS) | | | | | | |
| DILL SEEDS | | | | ♠ | | |
| DISTILLERS GRAINS | | | | | | |
| DOG'S BONE | | | | | | |
| DONGGUI | | ♠ | | | | |
| DRIED BLACK SOYBEAN SPROUTS | | | | | | |
| DUCK | | | ♠ | | | |
| DUCK EGGS | | | ♠ | | | |
| EEL | ♠ | | | | | |
| EEL BLOOD | | | | | | |
| EGGPLANT CALYX | | | | | | |
| EGGPLANT LEAVES | | | | | | |
| EGGPLANT ROOTS | | | | | | |
| EGGPLANTS (AUBERGINE) | | | | | | |
| EPIPHYLLUM | | | | | | |
| FENNEL ROOTS | | | | ♠ | | |
| FENNEL SEEDS | | | | ♠ | | |
| FENUGREEK SEEDS (ORIENTAL FENUGREEK) | | | | ♠ | | |
| FERMENTED GLUTINOUS RICE | ♠ | | | | | |
| FIG LEAVES | | | | | | |
| FIG ROOTS | | | | | | |

## Regulating Foods

| TONICS | | | Regulating Foods | | | | |
| --- | --- | --- | --- | --- | --- | --- | --- |
| HEART | STOMACH | SPLEEN | TONIC HEAT | DAMP HEAT | SPUTUM | ENERGY CIRCULATION | BLOOD CIRCULATION |

*Foods*      *Tonic Food*

| | COMMON TONICS | | | | ORGANIC | |
| --- | --- | --- | --- | --- | --- | --- |
| | ENERGY | BLOOD | YIN | YANG | LUNG | LIVER |
| FIGS | | | | | | |
| FINGERED CITRON | | | | | | |
| FINGERED CITRON ROOTS | | | | | | |
| FISH AIR BLADDER | | | | | | |
| FRESH GINKGO | | | ♠ | | | |
| FRESHWATER CLAMS | | | ♠ | | | |
| FROG | | | | | ♠ | |
| GARLIC | | | | | | |
| GINGER LEAVES | | | | | | |
| GINGKO LEAVES | ♠ | | | | | |
| GINSENG | ♠ | | | | ♠ | |
| GLUTINOUS RICE | | | | | | |
| GLUTINOUS RICE STALKS | | | | | | |
| GOOSE GALLBLADDER | ♠ | | | | | |
| GOOSE MEATS | | | | | | |
| GRAPEFRUIT FLOWERS | | | | | | |
| GRAPEFRUIT PEELS | | | | | | |
| GRAPEFRUIT ROOTS | | | | | | |
| GRAPEFRUITS | ♠ | ♠ | | | | |
| GRAPES | | | | | | |
| GRAPE LEAVES | | | | | | |
| GRASS CARP | | | | | | |
| GRASS CARP GALL | | | | | | |
| GREEN ONION FIBROUS ROOTS | | | | | | |
| GREEN ONION FRESH JUICE | | | | ♠ | | |
| GREEN ONION SEEDS | | | | | | |
| GREEN ONION WHITE HEADS | | | ♠ | | | |
| GREEN TURTLE | | | | | | |
| HAIR VEGETABLE | | | | | | |
| HAIRTAIL | | ♠ | | | | |
| HAM | | | | | | |
| HAWTHORN FRUITS | | | | | | |
| HEMP | ♠ | | | | | |
| HERRING | ♠ | | ♠ | | | |
| HONEY | | | | | | |
| HONEYSUCKLE STEMS & LEAVES | | | | | | |
| HONEYSUCKLE | | | | | | |
| HORSE BEANS | | ♠ | | | | |
| HUMAN MILK | | | | | | |
| HYACINTH BEAN FLOWERS | | | | | | |
| HYACINTH BEANS | ♠ | | | | | |
| JACKFRUITS | | | | | | |
| JAPANESE CASSIA BARK | | | | ♠ | | |
| JAPANESE CASSIA FRUITS | | | | | | |
| JASMINE FLOWERS | | | | | | |
| JELLYFISH | | | | | | |

中
医
疗
法

## *Regulating Foods*

### TONICS

| HEART | STOMACH | SPLEEN | TONIC HEAT | DAMP HEAT | SPUTUM | ENERGY CIRCULATION | BLOOD CIRCULATION |
|-------|---------|--------|------------|-----------|--------|--------------------|-------------------|

*Foods* — *Tonic Food*

| | COMMON TONICS | | | | ORGANIC | |
| --- | --- | --- | --- | --- | --- | --- |
| | ENERGY | BLOOD | YIN | YANG | LUNG | LIVER |
| JELLYFISH SKIN | | | | | | |
| JOB'S TEARS | | | | | | |
| JOB'S TEARS LEAVES | | | | | ⚓ | |
| JOB'S TEARS ROOTS | | | | | | |
| KIDNEY BEANS | | | ⚓ | | | |
| KIWIFRUIT ROOTS | | | | | | |
| KOHLRABI LEAVES | | | | | | |
| KUMQUATS | | | ⚓ | | | |
| KUMQUAT CAKE | | | | | | |
| KUMQUAT ROOTS | | | | | | |
| LADLE GOURD | | | | | | |
| LARD | | | ⚓ | | | |
| LAVER | | | | | | |
| LEAF BEETS | | | | | | |
| LEAF BROWN MUSTARD | | | | | | |
| LEMON LEAVES | | | | | | |
| LEMON PEELS | | | | | | |
| LEMON ROOTS | | | | | | |
| LEMONS | | | ⚓ | | | |
| LICORICE | ⚓ | | | | | |
| LILY FLOWERS | | | | | | |
| LIMES | | | | | | |
| LITCHI NUTS | | ⚓ | ⚓ | | | |
| LOBSTER | | | | | | |
| LONGAN SEEDS | | | | | | |
| LONGAN SHELLS | | | | | | |
| LONGANS | ⚓ | ⚓ | | | | |
| LONGEVITY FRUITS | | | | | | |
| LOQUATS | | | ⚓ | | | |
| LOQUAT FLOWERS | | | | | | |
| LOQUAT LEAVES | | | | | | |
| LOQUAT SEEDS | | | | | | |
| LOTUS FLOWERS | | | | | | |
| LOTUS FRUIT SEEDS | | | | | | |
| LOTUS RHIZOME POWDER | ⚓ | | | | | |
| LOTUS RHIZOMES | | | | | | |
| LOTUS SPROUTS | | | | | | |
| LOTUS STEMS | | | | | | |
| LUCID ASPARAGUS | | | ⚓ | | | |
| MACKEREL | ⚓ | | | | | |
| MALLOW ROOTS | | | | | | |
| MALT | | | | | | |
| MALTOSE | | | ⚓ | | | |
| MANDARIN FISH | ⚓ | ⚓ | | | | |
| MANDARIN ORANGES | | | ⚓ | | | |
| MANGOES | | | ⚓ | | | |

## Regulating Foods

| TONICS | | | | | | | |
|---|---|---|---|---|---|---|---|
| HEART | STOMACH | SPLEEN | TONIC HEAT | DAMP HEAT | SPUTUM | ENERGY CIRCULATION | BLOOD CIRCULATION |
| | | | | | | | ♠ |
| | ♠ | | | | | | |
| | | ♠ | | ♠ | | | |
| | | | | | | | ♠ |
| | | | | | ♠ | ♠ | |
| | | | | | ♠ | | |
| | | | | | ♠ | | |
| | | | | | | ♠ | |
| | | | | | | ♠ | |
| | | | | ♠ | | | |
| | | | ♠ | | ♠ | ♠ | ♠ |
| | | | | | ♠ | ♠ | ♠ |
| | | | | | ♠ | | ♠ |
| | | | ♠ | | ♠ | | |
| | | | ♠ | | | | |
| | | | | | | ♠ | |
| | | | | | ♠ | ♠ | |
| ♠ | | ♠ | | | ♠ | | |
| ♠ | | | | | ♠ | | |
| | | | | | ♠ | | |
| | | | | | ♠ | ♠ | ♠ |
| ♠ | | ♠ | | | | | |
| | | | ♠ | | | | ♠ |
| | | | ♠ | | | ♠ | ♠ |
| | | | ♠ | | | | |
| | | | ♠ | | | ♠ | |
| | ♠ | | | | | | |

## Foods

### Tonic Food

| | COMMON TONICS | | | | ORGANIC | |
| | ENERGY | BLOOD | YIN | YANG | LUNG | LIVER |
|---|---|---|---|---|---|---|
| MANGO LEAVES | | ♠ | | | | |
| MARE MILK | | | | | | ♠ |
| MATRIMONY VINE FRUITS | | | | | | |
| MOTHER CHRY-SANTHEMUMS | | | | | | ♠ |
| MULBERRY | | | | | | |
| MULLET | | | | | | |
| MUNG BEAN SPROUTS | | | | | | |
| MUNG BEANS | | | ♠ | | | ♠ |
| MUSSELS | | | | | | |
| MUSTARD SEEDS | ♠ | ♠ | | | | |
| OCTOPUS | | | | | | |
| OLD DRIED RADISH ROOTS | | | | | | |
| OLIVES | | | | | | |
| ONIONS | | | | | | |
| ORANGE CAKE | | | | | | |
| ORANGE LEAVES | | | | | | |
| ORANGE PEELS | | | | | | |
| ORCHID LEAVES | | | | | | |
| OREGANO (WILD MARJORAM) | | ♠ | | ♠ | | |
| OXTAIL | | | | | | |
| OYSTER SHELLS | | ♠ | ♠ | | | |
| OYSTERS | | ♠ | | | | |
| PALM SEEDS | | | | | | |
| PEACH BLOSSOMS | | | | | | |
| PEACH KERNELS | | | | | | |
| PEACH ROOTS | | | | | | |
| PEACHES | | | | | | |
| PEANUTS | | | | | | |
| PEAR PEELS | | | | | | |
| PEARL | | | | | | |
| PEARL SAGO | | | ♠ | | | |
| PEARS | | | ♠ | | | |
| PEAS | | | | | | |
| PEONY FLOWERS | | | | | | |
| PEONY ROOT BARK | | | | | | |
| PEPPERMINT | | | | | | ♠ |
| PERCH | | | | | | |
| PERSIMMONS | | | | | | |
| PHEASANT | ♠ | | | | | |
| PIGEON EGGS | ♠ | | | | | |
| PIGEON MEAT | | | ♠ | | | |
| PINEAPPLES | | | | ♠ | | |
| PISTACHIO NUTS | | | | | | |
| PLANTAINS | | | | | | |
| PLANTAIN SEEDS | | | | | | |
| PLUM BLOSSOM | | | | | | |

中医疗法

| TONICS | | | Regulating Foods | | | | |
| HEART | STOMACH | SPLEEN | TONIC HEAT | DAMP HEAT | SPUTUM | ENERGY CIRCULATION | BLOOD CIRCULATION |
| --- | --- | --- | --- | --- | --- | --- | --- |

*Foods* — *Tonic Food*

| | COMMON TONICS | | | | ORGANIC | |
| --- | --- | --- | --- | --- | --- | --- |
| | ENERGY | BLOOD | YIN | YANG | LUNG | LIVER |
| PLUM KERNELS | ♠ | | ♠ | | | |
| POLISHED RICE | | | ♠ | | | |
| POMEGRANATES (SWEET FRUITS) | | | | | | |
| PORK | | | | | | |
| PORK BRAIN | | | | | | ♠ |
| PORK GALLBLADDER | | ♠ | | | ♠ | |
| PORK LIVER | | | ♠ | | | |
| PORK LUNGS | | | | | ♠ | |
| PORK MARROW | | | | ♠ | | |
| PORK PANCREAS | | | | | | |
| PORK TESTES | | ♠ | | | | |
| PORK TROTTER | ♠ | | | | | |
| POTATOES | | | | | | |
| PRESERVED DUCK EGGS | | | | ♠ | | |
| PRICKING AMARANTH | | | | | | |
| PRICKLY ASH ROOTS | | | | | | |
| PUMPKIN PEDICEL | | | | | | |
| PUMPKIN ROOTS | | | ♠ | | | |
| PURSLANE | ♠ | | | | | ♠ |
| RABBIT | | | | | | |
| RABBIT LIVER | | | | | | |
| RADISH LEAVES | | | | | | |
| RADISH SEEDS | | | | | | |
| RADISHES | | | | | | |
| RAMBUTAN | | | | | | |
| RAPES | | | | ♠ | | ♠ |
| RAPESEEDS | | | ♠ | | | |
| RASPBERRIES | | | | | | |
| RED BAYBERRIES | | | | | | |
| RED BEANS | ♠ | | | | | |
| RED & BLACK DATES | | | | | | |
| RICE SPROUTS | | | | | | |
| RIVER SNAILS | | | | | | |
| ROCK SUGAR | | | | | | |
| ROMAINE LETTUCE | | | ♠ | | | ♠ |
| ROSES | | | | | | |
| ROYAL JELLY | | | | | | |
| RUSSIAN OLIVES (OLEASTER) | | | | | | |
| SAFFLOWER FRUITS | | | | | | |
| SAFFRON | | | ♠ | | | |
| SALT | | | | | | |
| SALTWATER CLAMS | | | | | | |
| SCALLION BULBS | | | | | | |
| SEA CUCUMBER | | | | | | |
| SEAGRASS | | | | | | |
| SEAWEED | | ♠ | | | | |

中
医
疗
法

## Regulating Foods

### TONICS

| HEART | STOMACH | SPLEEN | TONIC HEAT | DAMP HEAT | SPUTUM | ENERGY CIRCULATION | BLOOD CIRCULATION |
|---|---|---|---|---|---|---|---|

## Foods — *Tonic Food*

| Foods | COMMON TONICS | | | | ORGANIC | |
|---|---|---|---|---|---|---|
| | ENERGY | BLOOD | YIN | YANG | LUNG | LIVER |
| SHARK'S FIN | ● | | ● | ● | ● | |
| SHARK AIR BLADDER | | | | | | |
| SHARK MEAT | | | | | | |
| SHEEP OR GOAT BLOOD | | | | | | |
| SHEEP OR GOAT GALLBLADDER | | ● | | | | |
| SHEEP OR GOAT LIVER | | | | | | ● |
| SHELLS | ● | | | | | |
| SHIITAKE MUSHROOMS | | | ● | | | |
| SHRIMP | | | | | | |
| SOUR DATES | | | | | | ● |
| SOUR ORANGE PEELS | | | | | | |
| SOYBEAN OIL | | | | | | |
| SOYBEAN PASTE | | | | | | |
| SPEARMINT | | ● | | | | |
| SPINACH | ● | | | | | |
| SQUASH | | | | | | |
| SQUASH CALYX | | | | | | |
| SQUASH FLOWERS | | | | | | |
| SQUASH ROOTS | | | | ● | | |
| STAR ANISE | | | ● | | | |
| STAR FRUITS (CARAMBOLA) | | | | | | |
| STRAWBERRIES | | | | | | ● |
| STRAWBERRY WHOLE PLANTS | | | ● | | | |
| STRING BEANS | ● | | | | | |
| STURGEON | | | ● | | | |
| SUGAR CANE | | | | | | |
| SUNFLOWER DISC RECEPTACLE | | | ● | | | |
| SWEET APRICOT SEEDS | | | | | | |
| SWEET BASIL | | | | | | |
| SWEET GREEN ORANGE PEELS | ● | | | | | |
| SWEET POTATOES | | | | | | |
| SWEET BEAN ROOTS | | | | | | |
| SWORD BEAN SHELLS | | | | ● | | |
| SWORD BEANS (SABER BEANS) | | | | | | |
| TANGERINE PEELS | | | | | | |
| TANGERINE SEEDS | | | | | | |
| TANGERINE ORANGES | | | | | | |
| TEA | | | | | | |
| TEA GROWN IN YUNNAN | | | | | | |
| TEA MELONS | | | | | | |
| TEA OIL | | | | | | |
| TEA SEEDS | | | | | | |
| THYME | ● | | ● | | | |
| TOFU | | | ● | | | |
| TOMATOES | | | | | | |
| TRIFOLIATE ORANGES | | | | | | |

中医疗法

## Regulating Foods

### TONICS

| HEART | STOMACH | SPLEEN | TONIC HEAT | DAMP HEAT | SPUTUM | ENERGY CIRCULATION | BLOOD CIRCULATION |
|-------|---------|--------|------------|-----------|--------|--------------------|-------------------|

*Foods*　　　　　　　　　　　　　　　　　　　　　　　　　　*Tonic Food*

| | | COMMON TONICS | | | | | ORGANIC |
|---|---|---|---|---|---|---|---|
| | | ENERGY | BLOOD | YIN | YANG | LUNG | LIVER |
| TUMERIC | | | | | | | |
| TURNIP FLOWERS | | | | | | | ♠ |
| TURNIP SEEDS | | | | | | | |
| VINEGAR | | | | | | | |
| WALNUTS | | | | ♠ | | ♠ | |
| WATER CHESTNUTS | | | | | | | |
| WATERMELONS | | | | ♠ | | | |
| WESTERN GINSENG | | | | | | ♠ | |
| WHEAT | | | | | | | |
| WHEAT SEEDLINGS | | | | | | | |
| WHITE FUNGUS | | | | ♠ | | | |
| WHITE OR YELLOW MUSTARD | | | | | | | |
| WHITE PEPPER | | | | | | | |
| WHITE STRING BEANS | | ♠ | | | | | |
| WHITE SUGAR | | | | ♠ | | | |
| WHITE BAIT | | | | ♠ | | ♠ | |
| WHITEFISH | | | | | | | |
| YAMS | | | | ♠ | | ♠ | |
| YELLOW SOYBEANS | | | | | | | |
| | | | | | | | |
| TOTAL FOODS LISTED | 386 | 39 | 23 | 58 | 21 | 13 | 16 |
| TONIC FOODS | 253 | | | | | | |
| REGULATING FOODS | 336 | | | | | | |

## Regulating Foods

### TONICS

| HEART | STOMACH | SPLEEN | TONIC HEAT | DAMP HEAT | SPUTUM | ENERGY CIRCULATION | BLOOD CIRCULATION |
|---|---|---|---|---|---|---|---|
| | | | | | | ♠ | ♠ |
| | | | | ♠ | | | |
| | | | | | ♠ | ♠ | ♠ |
| | | | | | ♠ | | |
| ♠ | | | ♠ | | | | |
| ♠ | | | | ♠ | | | |
| | | | | | | | ♠ |
| | | | | | ♠ | | |
| | | ♠ | | | | | |
| | | | | | ♠ | | |
| | ♠ | | | | | | |
| | ♠ | ♠ | | | | | |
| | | ♠ | | | | | |
| | | | | ♠ | | | ♠ |
| 14 | 29 | 40 | 74 | 37 | 85 | 63 | 77 |

*Appendix C*

| Foods | Yang | | | | | | | | Y-Scores | Yin | | | | | | | |
|---|---|---|---|---|---|---|---|---|---|---|---|---|---|---|---|---|---|
| | OUTWARD | | | | UPWARDS | | | | NEUTRAL | DOWNWARDS | | | | INWARD | | | |
| | SUMMER | | | | SPRING | | | | | AUTUMN | | | | WINTER | | | |
| | +8 | +7 | +6 | +5 | +4 | +3 | +2 | +1 | 0 | -1 | -2 | -3 | -4 | -5 | -6 | -7 | -8 |
| ABALONE | | | | | | | | | | ♠ | | | | | | | |
| APPLE | | | | | | | | | | | ♠ | | | | | | |
| APRICOT | | | | | | | | | ♠ | | | | | | | | |
| APRICOT SEED (BITTER) | | | | | | | ♠ | | | | | | | | | | |
| APRICOT SEED (SWEET) | | | | | | | | ♠ | | | | | | | | | |
| ASPARAGUS | | | | | | | | ♠ | | | | | | | | | |
| BAMBOO SHOOT | | | | | | | | | | | ♠ | | | | | | |
| BANANA | | | | | | | | | | | ♠ | | | | | | |
| BARLEY | | | | | | | | | | | | ♠ | | | | | |
| BEAN CURD | | | | | | | | | ♠ | | | | | | | | |
| BEEF | | | | | | | ♠ | | | | | | | | | | |
| BEETROOT | | | | | | | ♠ | | | | | | | | | | |
| BITTER GOURD | | | | | | | | | | | | | | | | ♠ | |
| BLACK AND WHITE PEPPER | ♠ | | | | | | | | | | | | | | | | |
| BLACK FUNGUS | | | | | | | ♠ | | | | | | | | | | |
| BLACK SESAME SEED | | | | | | | ♠ | | | | | | | | | | |
| BROWN SUGAR | | | | | ♠ | | | | | | | | | | | | |
| BUTTER | | | | | ♠ | | | | | | | | | | | | |
| CABBAGE (CHINESE) | | | | | | | ♠ | | | | | | | | | | |
| CARAWAY | | | ♠ | | | | | | | | | | | | | | |
| CARP (COMMON) | | | | | | | ♠ | | | | | | | | | | |
| CARP (GOLD) | | | | | | | ♠ | | | | | | | | | | |
| CARP (GRASS) | | | | | ♠ | | | | | | | | | | | | |
| CARROT | | | | | | | ♠ | | | | | | | | | | |
| CASTOR BEAN | | | | | | | | | | ♠ | | | | | | | |
| CELERY | | | | | | | | | | | | | | | | | |
| CHERRY | | | | | ♠ | | | | | | | | | | | | |
| CHERRY SEED | | | | | | | | | ♠ | | | | | | | | |
| CHESTNUT | | | | | ♠ | | | | | | | | | | | | |
| CHICKEN | | | | | ♠ | | | | | | | | | | | | |
| CHICKEN EGG | | | | | | | ♠ | | | | | | | | | | |
| CHICKEN EGG WHITE | | | | | | | | | | | ♠ | | | | | | |
| CHICKEN EGG YOLK | | | | | | | ♠ | | | | | | | | | | |
| CHICORY | | | | | | | | | | | | | | | | | |
| CHINESE WAX GOURD | | | | | | | | | ♠ | | | | | | | | |
| CHIVE | | | ♠ | | | | | | | | | | | | | | |
| CHIVE ROOTS | | | ♠ | | | | | | | | | | | | | | |
| CHIVE SEEDS | | | | | | ♠ | | | | | | | | | | | |
| CINNAMON BARK | | ♠ | | | | | | | | | | | | | | | |
| CINNAMON TWIG | | | | ♠ | | | | | | | | | | | | | |
| CLAM (FRESHWATER) | | | | | | | | | | | | | | ♠ | | | |
| CLAM (SALTWATER) | | | | | | | | | | | | | | | | ♠ | |
| CLAMSHELL (RIVER) | | | | | | | | | | | | | | ♠ | | | |
| CLAMSHELL (SEA) | | | | | | | | | | | | | | | | ♠ | |
| CLOVE | | | ♠ | | | | | | | | | | | | | | |
| COCONUT LIQUID | | | | | ♠ | | | | | | | | | | | | |
| COCONUT MEAT | | | | | | | ♠ | | | | | | | | | | |

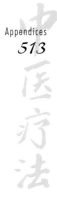

| Foods | Yang | | | | | | | | Y-Scores | Yin | | | | | | | |
|---|---|---|---|---|---|---|---|---|---|---|---|---|---|---|---|---|---|
| | OUTWARD | | | | UPWARDS | | | | NEUTRAL | DOWNWARDS | | | | INWARD | | | |
| | SUMMER | | | | SPRING | | | | | AUTUMN | | | | WINTER | | | |
| | +8 | +7 | +6 | +5 | +4 | +3 | +2 | +1 | 0 | -1 | -2 | -3 | -4 | -5 | -6 | -7 | -8 |
| COCONUT SHELL | | | | | | | | | ⚓ | | | | | | | | |
| COFFEE | | | | | | | | ⚓ | | | | | | | | | |
| COMMON BUTTON MUSHROOM | | | | | | | | | ⚓ | | | | | | | | |
| CORIANDER (CHINESE PARSLEY) | | | ⚓ | | | | | | | | | | | | | | |
| CORN | | | | | | | ⚓ | | | | | | | | | | |
| CORN SILK | | | | | | | ⚓ | | | | | | | | | | |
| COTTONSEED | ⚓ | | | | | | | | | | | | | | | | |
| CRAB | | | | | | | | | | | | | | | ⚓ | | |
| CRAB APPLE | | | | | | | | | ⚓ | | | | | | | | |
| CUCUMBER | | | | | | | | | ⚓ | | | | | | | | |
| CUTTLEBONE | | | | | | | | | | | ⚓ | | | | | | |
| CUTTLEFISH | | | | | | | | | | | | ⚓ | | | | | |
| DATE (RED AND BLACK) | | | | | ⚓ | | | | | | | | | | | | |
| DILLSEED | | | ⚓ | | | | | | | | | | | | | | |
| DRY MANDARIN ORANGE PEEL | | | | | | | ⚓ | | | | | | | | | | |
| DUCK | | | | | | | | | | ⚓ | | | | | | | |
| EEL | | | | | ⚓ | | | | | | | | | | | | |
| EEL BLOOD | | | | | | | | | | | | ⚓ | | | | | |
| EGG (DUCK) | | | | | | | | | ⚓ | | | | | | | | |
| EGGPLANT | | | | | | | | | ⚓ | | | | | | | | |
| FENNEL | | | ⚓ | | | | | | | | | | | | | | |
| FIG | | | | | | | ⚓ | | | | | | | | | | |
| FIG ROOT | | | | | | | | | | | | | | | | | |
| GARLIC | | | | | | | | | | | | | | | | | |
| GINGER (DRIED) | ⚓ | | | | | | | | | | | | | | | | |
| GINGER (FRESH) | | | ⚓ | | | | | | | | | | | | | | |
| GINSENG | | | | | | | | ⚓ | | | | | | | | | |
| GRAPE | | | | | | | | ⚓ | | | | | | | | | |
| GRAPEFRUIT | | | | | | | | | | | | | ⚓ | | | | |
| GRAPEFRUIT PEEL | | | | | | ⚓ | | | | | | | | | | | |
| GREEN ONION LEAF | | | ⚓ | | | | | | | | | | | | | | |
| GREEN ONION WHITE HEAD | | | ⚓ | | | | | | | | | | | | | | |
| GUAVA | | | | | ⚓ | | | | | | | | | | | | |
| GUAVA LEAF | | | | | | | ⚓ | | | | | | | | | | |
| HAM | | | | | | | | | | ⚓ | | | | | | | |
| HAWTHORN FRUIT | | | | | | | ⚓ | | | | | | | | | | |
| HONEY | | | | | | | ⚓ | | | | | | | | | | |
| HOPS | | | | | | | | | | | | | | ⚓ | | | |
| HORSE BEAN (BROAD BEAN) | | | | | | | ⚓ | | | | | | | | | | |
| HYACINTH BEAN | | | | | | | ⚓ | | | | | | | | | | |
| JOB'S TEARS | | | | | | | | | ⚓ | | | | | | | | |
| KELP | | | | | | | | | | | | | | | | ⚓ | |
| KIDNEY (BEEF) | | | | | | | ⚓ | | | | | | | | | | |
| KIDNEY (PORK) | | | | | | | | | | | | ⚓ | | | | | |
| KIDNEY BEAN | | | | | | | ⚓ | | | | | | | | | | |
| KIDNEY (SHEEP) | | | | | ⚓ | | | | | | | | | | | | |
| KOHLRABI | | | | | | | | ⚓ | | | | | | | | | |

| Foods | Yang | | | | | | | | Y-Scores | Yin | | | | | | | |
|---|---|---|---|---|---|---|---|---|---|---|---|---|---|---|---|---|---|
| | OUTWARD SUMMER | | | | UPWARDS SPRING | | | | NEUTRAL | DOWNWARDS AUTUMN | | | | INWARD WINTER | | | |
| | +8 | +7 | +6 | +5 | +4 | +3 | +2 | +1 | 0 | -1 | -2 | -3 | -4 | -5 | -6 | -7 | -8 |
| KUMQUAT | | | | | | | ♠ | | | | | | | | | | |
| LEAF MUSTARD | | | ♠ | | | | | | | | | | | | | | |
| LEEK | | | ♠ | | | | | | | | | | | | | | |
| LEMON | | | | | | | ♠ | | | | | | | | | | |
| LETTUCE | | | | | | | | | | | | ♠ | | | | | |
| LETTUCE (LEAF) | | | | | | | | | | | ♠ | | | | | | |
| LETTUCE (STALK) | | | | | | | | | | | | | | | | | |
| LICORICE | | | | | | | ♠ | | | | | | | | | | |
| LILY FLOWER | | | | | | | | | ♠ | | | | | | | | |
| LITCHI | | | | | | | ♠ | | | | | | | | | | |
| LIVER (BEEF) | | | | | | | ♠ | | | | | | | | | | |
| LIVER (CHICKEN) | | | | | ♠ | | | | | | | | | | | | |
| LIVER (PORK) | | | | | | | | ♠ | | | | | | | | | |
| LIVER (SHEEP) | | | | | | | | | | | | ♠ | | | | | |
| LONGAN | | | | | ♠ | | | | | | | | | | | | |
| LOQUAT | | | | | | | | | | | ♠ | | | | | | |
| LOTUS (FRUIT, SEED, ROOT) | | | | | | | ♠ | | | | | | | | | | |
| LOTUS PLUMULE | | | | | | | | | | | | | | | | | ♠ |
| MALT | | | | | ♠ | | | | | | | | | | | | |
| MALTOSE | | | | | ♠ | | | | | | | | | | | | |
| MANDARIN ORANGE | | | | | | | | | | | ♠ | | | | | | |
| MANGO | | | | | | | | | | | ♠ | | | | | | |
| MARJORAM | | | | | | | ♠ | | | | | | | | | | |
| MILK (COW'S) | | | | | | | ♠ | | | | | | | | | | |
| MILK (HUMAN) | | | | | | | | | | ♠ | | | | | | | |
| MILK (SHEEP'S) | | | | | ♠ | | | | | | | | | | | | |
| MUNG BEAN | | | | | | | | | ♠ | | | | | | | | |
| MUSKMELON | | | | | | | | | | | ♠ | | | | | | |
| MUSSEL | | | | | | | | | | ♠ | | | | | | | |
| MUTTON | | | | | ♠ | | | | | | | | | | | | |
| NUTMEG | | | ♠ | | | | | | | | | | | | | | |
| OLIVE | | | | | | | | | ♠ | | | | | | | | |
| ONION | | | | | | | | | | | | | | | | | |
| OYSTER | | | | | | | | | | ♠ | | | | | | | |
| OYSTER SHELL | | | | | | | | | | | | | | ♠ | | | |
| PAPAYA | | | | | | | ♠ | | | | | | | | | | |
| PEACH | | | | | | | ♠ | | | | | | | | | | |
| PEANUT | | | | | | | ♠ | | | | | | | | | | |
| PEAR | | | | | | | | | | | ♠ | | | | | | |
| PEPPERMINT | | | | | | | | | | | | | | | | | |
| PERSIMMON | | | | | | | | | | | ♠ | | | | | | |
| PINEAPPLE | | | | | | | | | ♠ | | | | | | | | |
| PLUM | | | | | | | | | ♠ | | | | | | | | |
| POLISHED RICE | | | | | | | ♠ | | | | | | | | | | |
| PORK | | | | | | | | | | ♠ | | | | | | | |
| POTATO | | | | | | | ♠ | | | | | | | | | | |
| PUMPKIN | | | | | | | | | ♠ | | | | | | | | |
| RADISH | | | | | | | ♠ | | | | | | | | | | ♠ |

中医疗法

| Foods | Yang | | | | | | | | Y-Scores | | | | Yin | | | | |
|---|---|---|---|---|---|---|---|---|---|---|---|---|---|---|---|---|---|
| | OUTWARD | | | | UPWARDS | | | | NEUTRAL | DOWNWARDS | | | | INWARD | | | |
| | SUMMER | | | | SPRING | | | | | AUTUMN | | | | WINTER | | | |
| | +8 | +7 | +6 | +5 | +4 | +3 | +2 | +1 | 0 | -1 | -2 | -3 | -4 | -5 | -6 | -7 | -8 |
| RADISH LEAF | | | | | | | | | ● | | | | | | | | |
| RASPBERRY | | | | | | | ● | | | | | | | | | | |
| RED OR GREEN PEPPER | ● | | | | | | | | | | | | | | | | |
| RED SMALL BEAN | | | | | | | | | ● | | | | | | | | |
| RICE BRAN | | | | | | ● | | | | | | | | | | | |
| ROSEMARY | | | ● | | | | | | | | | | | | | | |
| ROYAL JELLY | | | | | | | ● | | | | | | | | | | |
| SAFFRON | | | | | | | ● | | | | | | | | | | |
| SALT | | | | | | | | | | | | | | | | ● | |
| SEA GRASS | | | | | | | | | | | | | | | | | ● |
| SEAWEED | | | | | | | | | | | | | | | | ● | |
| SESAME OIL | | | | | | | | | ● | | | | | | | | |
| SHIITAKE MUSHROOM | | | | | | | ● | | | | | | | | | | |
| SHRIMP | | | | | ● | | | | | | | | | | | | |
| SOUR PLUM | | | | | | | | | | | | ● | | | | | |
| SOYBEAN (BLACK) | | | | | | | ● | | | | | | | | | | |
| SOYBEAN (YELLOW) | | | | | | | ● | | | | | | | | | | |
| SOYBEAN OIL | | ● | | | | | | | | | | | | | | | |
| SPEARMINT | | | | ● | | | | | | | | | | | | | |
| SPINACH | | | | | | | | | ● | | | | | | | | |
| SQUASH | | | | | ● | | | | | | | | | | | | |
| STAR ANISE | | | | ● | | | | | | | | | | | | | |
| STAR FRUIT (CARAMBOLA) | | | | | | | | | | | | | ● | | | | |
| STRAWBERRY | | | | | | | | | | | ● | | | | | | |
| STRING BEAN | | | | | | | ● | | | | | | | | | | |
| SUGAR CANE | | | | | | | | | | | ● | | | | | | |
| SUNFLOWER SEED | | | | | | ● | | | | | | | | | | | |
| SWEET BASIL | | | ● | | | | | | | | | | | | | | |
| SWEET POTATO | | | | | | | | | | | ● | | | | | | |
| SWEET RICE | | | | | ● | | | | | | | | | | | | |
| SWORD BEAN | | | | | ● | | | | | | | | | | | | |
| TANGERINE ORANGE | | | | | | | | | | | ● | | | | | | |
| TARO | | | | | | ● | | | | | | | | | | | |
| TARO FLOWER | | | | | | | | | ● | | | | | | | | |
| TARO LEAF | | | | | | | ● | | | | | | | | | | |
| THYME | | | | | | | | | | | | | | | | | |
| TOBACCO | | | ● | | | | | | | | | | | | | | |
| TOMATO | | | | | | | | | | | | | ● | | | | |
| VINEGAR | | | | | | | | | | ● | | | | | | | |
| WALNUT | | | | | ● | | | | | | | | | | | | |
| WATER CHESTNUT | | | | | | | | | | | ● | | | | | | |
| WATERMELON | | | | | | | | | | | ● | | | | | | |
| WHEAT | | | | | | | | | ● | | | | | | | | |
| WHEAT BRAN | | | | | | | | | ● | | | | | | | | |
| WHITE FUNGUS | | | | | | | ● | | | | | | | | | | |
| WHITE SUGAR | | | | | | | ● | | | | | | | | | | |
| WINE | | | | | | ● | | | | | | | | | | | |
| YAM | | | | | | | ● | | | | | | | | | | |

*Appendix D*

## Comprehensive Y-Scores

| | YANG | | | | | | | 0 | YIN | | | | | | | |
|---|---|---|---|---|---|---|---|---|---|---|---|---|---|---|---|---|
| | +8 | +7 | +6 | +5 | +4 | +3 | +2 | +1 | 0 | -1 | -2 | -3 | -4 | -5 | -6 | -7 | -8 |

| | | | | | | |
|---|---|---|---|---|---|---|
| ENERGIES OF FOODS | hot | warm | neutral | cool | | cold |
| Y-SCORES | +8 | +4 | 0 | -4 | | -8 |
| FLAVORS OF FOODS | pungent | sweet | light | sour | salty | bitter |
| Y-SCORES | +8 | +4 | 0 | -4 | -6 | -8 |
| MOVEMENTS OF FOODS | outward | upwards | neutral | downwards | | inward |
| Y-SCORES | +8 | +4 | 0 | -4 | | -8 |
| HOT-COLD | hot | warm | neutral | cool | | cold |
| Y-SCORES | +8 | +4 | 0 | -4 | | -8 |

| | | | | | |
|---|---|---|---|---|---|
| DRY-DAMP (INDIVIDUAL BODY TYPES) | dry (underweight) | | neutral | | damp (overweight) |
| Y-SCORES | +8 +7 +6 +5 | +4 +3 +2 +1 | 0 | -1 -2 -3 -4 | -5 -6 -7 -8 |
| EXCESSIVE—DEFICIENT | normally energetic | normally not tired | neutral | normally lazy | normally tired |
| Y-SCORES | +8 | +4 | 0 | -4 | -8 |
| DISPOSITIONS | restless or impatient | fairly active | neutral | fairly relaxed | easy-going or patient |
| Y-SCORES | +8 | +4 | 0 | -4 | -8 |
| SEX LIFE | very high sex drive | sex > foods | neutral | foods > sex | very low sex drive |
| Y-SCORES | +8 | +4 | 0 | -4 | -8 |
| MOODS | cheerfull or joyful | hopeful or comfortable | thinking or reasoning | depressed or sad | scary or fearful |
| Y-SCORES | +8 | +4 | 0 | -4 | -8 |
| FOUR SEASONS | summer | spring | summer—autumn | autumn | winter |
| Y-SCORES | +8 | +4 | 0 | -4 | -8 |

## Y-Scores of Foods

| | YANG | | | | | | | | | | YIN | | | | | |
|---|---|---|---|---|---|---|---|---|---|---|---|---|---|---|---|---|
| | +8 | +7 | +6 | +5 | +4 | +3 | +2 | +1 | 0 | -1 | -2 | -3 | -4 | -5 | -6 | -7 | -8 |
| ENERGIES OF FOODS | hot | | | | warm | | | | neutral | cool | | | | cold | | | |
| Y-SCORES | +8 | | | | +4 | | | | 0 | -4 | | | | -8 | | | |
| FLAVORS OF FOODS | pungent | | | | sweet | | | | light | sour | | | | salty | bitter | | |
| Y-SCORES | +8 | | | | +4 | | | | 0 | -4 | | | | -6 | -8 | | |

### Y-SCORES OF MOVEMENTS OF FOODS

| | | | | | | | | | | | | | | | | | |
|---|---|---|---|---|---|---|---|---|---|---|---|---|---|---|---|---|---|
| MOVEMENTS OF FOODS | outward | | | | upwards | | | | neutral | downwards | | | | inward | | | |
| Y-SCORES | +8 | | | | +4 | | | | 0 | -4 | | | | -8 | | | |

### YIN AND YANG BODY TYPES

| | | | | | | | | | | | | | | | | | |
|---|---|---|---|---|---|---|---|---|---|---|---|---|---|---|---|---|---|
| HOT-COLD | hot | | | | warm | | | | neutral | cool | | | | cold | | | |
| Y-SCORES | +8 | | | | +4 | | | | 0 | -4 | | | | -8 | | | |
| DRY-DAMP (INDIVIDUAL BODY TYPES) | dry (underweight) | | | | | | | | neutral | | | | | damp (overweight) | | | |
| Y-SCORES | +8 | +7 | +6 | +5 | +4 | +3 | +2 | +1 | 0 | -1 | -2 | -3 | -4 | -5 | -6 | -7 | -8 |
| EXCESSIVE—DEFICIENT | normally energetic | | | | normally not tired | | | | neutral | normally lazy | | | | normally tired | | | |
| Y-SCORES | +8 | | | | +4 | | | | 0 | -4 | | | | -8 | | | |
| DISPOSITIONS | restless or impatient | | | | fairly active | | | | neutral | fairly relaxed | | | | easy-going or patient | | | |
| Y-SCORES | +8 | | | | +4 | | | | 0 | -4 | | | | -8 | | | |
| SEX LIFE | very high sex drive | | | | sex > foods | | | | neutral | foods > sex | | | | very low sex drive | | | |
| Y-SCORES | +8 | | | | +4 | | | | 0 | -4 | | | | -8 | | | |

### Y-SCORES OF MOODS

| | | | | | | | | | | | | | | | | | |
|---|---|---|---|---|---|---|---|---|---|---|---|---|---|---|---|---|---|
| MOODS | cheerfull or joyful | | | | hopeful or comfortable | | | | thinking or reasoning | depressed or sad | | | | scary or fearful | | | |
| Y-SCORES | +8 | | | | +4 | | | | 0 | -4 | | | | -8 | | | |

### Y-SCORES OF FOUR SEASONS

| | | | | | | | | | | | | | | | | | |
|---|---|---|---|---|---|---|---|---|---|---|---|---|---|---|---|---|---|
| FOUR SEASONS | summer | | | | spring | | | | summer—autumn | autumn | | | | winter | | | |
| Y-SCORES | +8 | | | | +4 | | | | 0 | -4 | | | | -8 | | | |

*Appendix E*

| Foods | Flavors | | | | | Energies | | | |
|---|---|---|---|---|---|---|---|---|---|
| | PUNGENT | SWEET | SOUR | BITTER | SALTY | COLD | HOT | WARM | COOL |
| ABALONE | | ▲ | | | ▲ | | | | |
| APPLE | | ▲ | ▲ | | | | | | ▲ |
| APRICOT | | ▲ | ▲ | | | | | | |
| APRICOT SEED (BITTER) | ▲ | ▲ | | ▲ | | | | ▲ | |
| APRICOT SEED (SWEET) | | ▲ | | ▲ | | | | ▲ | |
| ASPARAGUS | -▲ | | | ▲ | | | | ▲ | |
| BAMBOO SHOOT | | ▲ | | | | ▲ | | | |
| BANANA | | ▲ | | | | ▲ | | | |
| BARLEY | | ▲ | | | ▲ | | | | ▲ |
| BEAN CURD | | ▲ | | | | | | | ▲ |
| BEEF | | ▲ | | | | | | | |
| BEETROOT | | ▲ | | | | | | | |
| BITTER GOURD | | | | ▲ | | ▲ | | | |
| BLACK AND WHITE PEPPER | ▲ | | | | | | ▲ | | |
| BLACK FUNGUS | | ▲ | | | | | | | |
| BLACK SESAME SEED | | ▲ | | | | | | | |
| BROWN SUGAR | | ▲ | | | | | | ▲ | |
| BUTTER | | ▲ | | | | | | ▲ | |
| CABBAGE (CHINESE) | | ▲ | | | | | | | |
| CARAWAY | ▲ | | | | | | | ▲ | |
| CARP (COMMON) | | ▲ | | | | | | | |
| CARP (GOLD) | | ▲ | | | | | | | |
| CARP (GRASS) | | ▲ | | | | | | ▲ | |
| CARROT | | ▲ | | | | | | | |
| CASTOR BEAN | ▲ | ▲ | | | | | | | |
| CELERY | | ▲ | | ▲ | | | | | |
| CHERRY | | ▲ | | | | | | ▲ | |
| CHERRY SEED | ▲ | | | ▲ | | | | | |
| CHESTNUT | | ▲ | | | | | | ▲ | |
| CHICKEN | | ▲ | | | | | | ▲ | |
| CHICKEN EGG | | ▲ | | | | | | | |
| CHICKEN EGG WHITE | | ▲ | | | | | | | |
| CHICKEN EGG YOLK | | ▲ | | | | ▲ | | | |
| CHICORY | | | | | | | | | |
| CHINESE WAX GOURD | | ▲ | | | | | | | ▲ |
| CHIVE | ▲ | | | | | | | ▲ | |
| CHIVE ROOTS | ▲ | | | | | | | ▲ | |
| CHIVE SEEDS | ▲ | | | | ▲ | | | ▲ | |
| CINNAMON BARK | ▲ | ▲ | | | | | ▲ | | |
| CINNAMON TWIG | ▲ | ▲ | | | | | | ▲ | |
| CLAM (FRESHWATER) | | ▲ | | | ▲ | ▲ | | | |
| CLAM (SALTWATER) | | | | | ▲ | ▲ | | | |
| CLAMSHELL (RIVER) | | ▲ | | | ▲ | ▲ | | | |
| CLAMSHELL (SEA) | | | | | ▲ | ▲ | | | |
| CLOVE | ▲ | | | | | | | | |
| COCONUT LIQUID | | ▲ | | | | | | | |
| COCONUT MEAT | | ▲ | | | | | | ▲ | |
| COCONUT SHELL | | | | | | | | | |

中医疗法

## Internal Organs

| NEUTRAL | LUNGS | LARGE INTESTINE | SMALL INTESTINE | GALL BLADDER | BLADDER | LIVER | KIDNEYS | SPLEEN | HEART | STOMACH | OTHERS |
|---|---|---|---|---|---|---|---|---|---|---|---|
| • | | | | | | | | | | | |
| • | | | | | | | | | | | |
| | | | | | | | | | | | toxic |
| | | | | | | | | | | | glossy |
| | | | | | | | | • | | • | |
| | | • | | | | | | • | | • | |
| • | | | | | | | | • | | • | |
| • | | | | | | | | • | • | • | |
| | | • | | | | | | | | • | |
| | | • | | | | | | | | • | |
| • | | | | | | • | • | | | | |
| • | | | | | | • | | • | | • | |
| • | | • | | | | | | | | • | glossy |
| | | | | | | | | | | • | |
| • | | • | | | | | • | | | • | |
| • | | | | | | | • | • | | • | |
| • | • | | | | | | | • | | | |
| • | • | • | | | | | | • | | | |
| • | | | | | | • | | • | | • | |
| • | | | | | | | • | • | | • | |
| | | | | | | | | • | | • | |
| • | | | | | | | | | | | |
| • | | | | | | | • | | • | | |
| | | | | • | | • | | | | | |
| | • | • | • | | • | | | | | | |
| | | | | | | • | • | | | • | |
| | | | | | | • | • | | | | |
| | • | | | | • | | | • | | | |
| | | | | | • | | | | • | | |
| | | | | | | • | | | | | |
| | | | | | | | | | | • | |
| | | | | | | • | • | | | | |
| | | | | | | | | | | • | |
| | | | | | | | • | • | | • | |
| | | | | | | | | | | | obstructive |

CHINESE NATURAL CURES
520

| Foods | Flavors | | | | | Energies | | | |
|---|---|---|---|---|---|---|---|---|---|
| | PUNGENT | SWEET | SOUR | BITTER | SALTY | COLD | HOT | WARM | COOL |
| COFFEE | | ♠ | | | ♠ | | | ♠ | |
| COMMON BUTTON MUSHROOM | | ♠ | | | | | | | ♠ |
| CORIANDER (CHINESE PARSLEY) | ♠ | ♠ | | | | | | ♠ | |
| CORN | | ♠ | | | | | | | |
| CORN SILK | | ♠ | | | | | | | |
| COTTONSEED | ♠ | | | | | | ♠ | | |
| CRAB | | | | | ♠ | ♠ | | | |
| CRAB APPLE | | ♠ | ♠ | | | | | | |
| CUCUMBER | | ♠ | | | | | | | ♠ |
| CUTTLEBONE | | | | | ♠ | | | ♠ | |
| CUTTLEFISH | | | | | ♠ | | | | |
| DATE (RED AND BLACK) | | ♠ | | | | | | ♠ | |
| DILLSEED | ♠ | | | | | | | ♠ | |
| DRY MANDARIN ORANGE PEEL | ♠ | | | ♠ | | | | ♠ | |
| DUCK | | | ♠ | | ♠ | | | | |
| EEL | | ♠ | | | | | | ♠ | |
| EEL BLOOD | | ♠ | | | | | | | |
| EGG (DUCK) | | ♠ | | | | | | | ♠ |
| EGGPLANT | | ♠ | | | | | | | ♠ |
| FENNEL | ♠ | | | | | | | ♠ | |
| FIG | | ♠ | | | | | | | |
| FIG ROOT | | | | | | | | | |
| GARLIC | ♠ | | | | | | | ♠ | |
| GINGER (DRIED) | ♠ | | | | | | ♠ | | |
| GINGER (FRESH) | ♠ | | | | | | | ♠ | |
| GINSENG | | ♠ | | ♠ | | | | ♠ | |
| GRAPE | | ♠ | ♠ | | | | | | |
| GRAPEFRUIT | | ♠ | ♠ | | | ♠ | | | |
| GRAPEFRUIT PEEL | ♠ | ♠ | | ♠ | | | | ♠ | |
| GREEN ONION LEAF | ♠ | | | | | | | ♠ | |
| GREEN ONION WHITE HEAD | ♠ | | | | | | | ♠ | |
| GUAVA | | ♠ | | | | | | | |
| GUAVA LEAF | | ♠ | | | | | | | |
| HAM | | | | | ♠ | | | ♠ | |
| HAWTHORN FRUIT | | ♠ | ♠ | | | | | ♠ | |
| HONEY | | ♠ | | | | | | | |
| HOPS | | | | ♠ | | | | | ♠ |
| HORSE BEAN (BROAD BEAN) | | ♠ | | | | | | | |
| HYACINTH BEAN | | ♠ | | | | | | | |
| JOB'S TEARS | | ♠ | | | | | | | ♠ |
| KELP | | | | | | ♠ | | | |
| KIDNEY (BEEF) | | | | | | | | ♠ | |
| KIDNEY (PORK) | | | | | | | | | |
| KIDNEY BEAN | | ♠ | | | | | | | |
| KIDNEY (SHEEP) | | ♠ | | | | | | ♠ | |
| KOHLRABI | ♠ | ♠ | | ♠ | | | | | |
| KUMQUAT | ♠ | ♠ | ♠ | | | | | ♠ | |
| LEAF MUSTARD | ♠ | | | | | | | ♠ | |

## Internal Organs

| NEUTRAL | LUNGS | LARGE INTESTINE | SMALL INTESTINE | GALL BLADDER | BLADDER | LIVER | KIDNEYS | SPLEEN | HEART | STOMACH | OTHERS |
|---|---|---|---|---|---|---|---|---|---|---|---|

obstructive
& constrictive

obstructive

| Foods | Flavors | | | | | Energies | | | |
|---|---|---|---|---|---|---|---|---|---|
| | PUNGENT | SWEET | SOUR | BITTER | SALTY | COLD | HOT | WARM | COOL |
| LEEK | | | | | | | | ♠ | |
| LEMON | | | ♠ | | | | | | |
| LETTUCE | | ♠ | | ♠ | | | | | ♠ |
| LETTUCE (LEAF) | | ♠ | | ♠ | | | | | ♠ |
| LETTUCE (STALK) | | | | | | | | | |
| LICORICE | | ♠ | | | | | | | |
| LILY FLOWER | | ♠ | | | | | | | ♠ |
| LITCHI | | ♠ | ♠ | | | | | ♠ | |
| LIVER (BEEF) | | ♠ | | | | | | ♠ | |
| LIVER (CHICKEN) | | ♠ | | | | | | ♠ | |
| LIVER (PORK) | | ♠ | | ♠ | | | | ♠ | |
| LIVER (SHEEP) | | ♠ | | ♠ | | | | | ♠ |
| LONGAN | | ♠ | | | | | | ♠ | |
| LOQUAT | | ♠ | ♠ | | | | | | ♠ |
| LOTUS (FRUIT, SEED, ROOT) | | ♠ | | | | | | | |
| LOTUS PLUMULE | | | | ♠ | | ♠ | | | |
| MALT | | ♠ | | | | | | ♠ | |
| MALTOSE | | ♠ | | | | | | ♠ | |
| MANDARIN ORANGE | | ♠ | ♠ | | | | | | ♠ |
| MANGO | | ♠ | ♠ | | | | | | ♠ |
| MARJORAM | ♠ | | | | | | | | ♠ |
| MILK (COW'S) | | ♠ | | | | | | | |
| MILK (HUMAN) | | ♠ | | | ♠ | | | | |
| MILK (SHEEP'S) | | ♠ | | | | | | ♠ | |
| MUNG BEAN | | ♠ | | | | | | | ♠ |
| MUSKMELON | | ♠ | | | | ♠ | | | |
| MUSSEL | | | | | ♠ | | | ♠ | |
| MUTTON | | ♠ | | | | | | ♠ | |
| NUTMEG | ♠ | | | | | | | ♠ | |
| OLIVE | | ♠ | ♠ | | | | | | |
| ONION | | | | | | | | | |
| OYSTER | | ♠ | | | ♠ | | | | |
| OYSTER SHELL | | | | | ♠ | | | | ♠ |
| PAPAYA | | ♠ | | | | | | | |
| PEACH | | ♠ | ♠ | | | | | ♠ | |
| PEANUT | | ♠ | | | | | | | |
| PEAR | | ♠ | ♠ | | | | | | ♠ |
| PEPPERMINT | ♠ | | | | | | | | ♠ |
| PERSIMMON | | ♠ | | | | ♠ | | | |
| PINEAPPLE | | ♠ | ♠ | | | | | | |
| PLUM | | ♠ | | | | | | | |
| POLISHED RICE | | ♠ | | | | | | | |
| PORK | | ♠ | | | ♠ | | | | |
| POTATO | | | | | | | | | |
| PUMPKIN | ♠ | | | ♠ | | | | | |
| RADISH | ♠ | ♠ | | | | | | | ♠ |
| RADISH LEAF | ♠ | | | ♠ | | | | | |
| RASPBERRY | | ♠ | ♠ | | | | | ♠ | |

中医疗法

| | Internal Organs | | | | | | | | | | |
|---|---|---|---|---|---|---|---|---|---|---|---|
| NEUTRAL | LUNGS | LARGE INTESTINE | SMALL INTESTINE | GALL BLADDER | BLADDER | LIVER | KIDNEYS | SPLEEN | HEART | STOMACH | OTHERS |
| | ▲ | | | | | ▲ | | | | | obstructive |
| | | ▲ | | | | | | | | ▲ | |
| | | ▲ | | | | | | | | ▲ | |
| ▲ | ▲ | | | | | | | ▲ | | ▲ | |
| | ▲ | | | | | | | | | | |
| | | | | | | ▲ | | | | | |
| ▲ | | | | | | ▲ | | | | | |
| | | | | | | ▲ | ▲ | | | | |
| | | | | | | ▲ | | | | | |
| | | | | | | ▲ | | | | | |
| | ▲ | | | | | ▲ | | ▲ | ▲ | | obstructive |
| ▲ | ▲ | | | | | ▲ | ▲ | ▲ | ▲ | | obstructive |
| | | | | | | | | ▲ | | ▲ | |
| | | | | | | | | ▲ | | ▲ | |
| ▲ | ▲ | | | | | | | | ▲ | ▲ | |
| ▲ | ▲ | | | | | | | | ▲ | ▲ | |
| | | | | | | ▲ | ▲ | ▲ | | | |
| | | | | | | | | ▲ | | | |
| | | ▲ | | | | | | ▲ | | | |
| ▲ | ▲ | | | | | | | | | ▲ | obstructive |
| ▲ | | | | | | | | | | | |
| | | | | | | ▲ | ▲ | | | | obstructive |
| ▲ | ▲ | | | | | | | ▲ | | | |
| | ▲ | | | | | ▲ | | | | | |
| | ▲ | | | | | | | | ▲ | | obstructive |
| ▲ | ▲ | | | | | ▲ | | ▲ | | ▲ | |
| ▲ | ▲ | | | | | | ▲ | ▲ | | ▲ | |
| ▲ | ▲ | | | | | | | | | | |
| | ▲ | | | | | ▲ | | | | ▲ | |
| ▲ | | | | | | | | ▲ | | ▲ | |

| Foods | Flavors | | | | | Energies | | | |
|---|---|---|---|---|---|---|---|---|---|
| | PUNGENT | SWEET | SOUR | BITTER | SALTY | COLD | HOT | WARM | COOL |
| RED OR GREEN PEPPER | ♠ | | | | | | ♠ | | |
| RED SMALL BEAN | | ♠ | ♠ | | | | | | |
| RICE BRAN | ♠ | ♠ | | | | | | | |
| ROSEMARY | ♠ | | | | | | | ♠ | |
| ROYAL JELLY | | ♠ | | | | | | | |
| SAFFRON | | ♠ | | | | | | | |
| SALT | | | | | ♠ | ♠ | | | |
| SEA GRASS | | | | ♠ | ♠ | ♠ | | | |
| SEAWEED | | | | | ♠ | ♠ | | | |
| SESAME OIL | | ♠ | | | | | | | ♠ |
| SHIITAKE MUSHROOM | | ♠ | | | | | | | |
| SHRIMP | | ♠ | | | | | | ♠ | |
| SOUR PLUM | | | ♠ | | | | | | |
| SOYBEAN (BLACK) | | ♠ | | | | | | | |
| SOYBEAN (YELLOW) | | ♠ | | | | | | | |
| SOYBEAN OIL | ♠ | ♠ | | | | | ♠ | | |
| SPEARMINT | ♠ | ♠ | | | | | | ♠ | |
| SPINACH | | ♠ | | | | | | | ♠ |
| SQUASH | | ♠ | | | | | | ♠ | |
| STAR ANISE | ♠ | ♠ | | | | | | ♠ | |
| STAR FRUIT (CARAMBOLA) | | ♠ | ♠ | | | ♠ | | | |
| STRAWBERRY | | ♠ | ♠ | | | | | | ♠ |
| STRING BEAN | | ♠ | | | | | | | |
| SUGAR CANE | | ♠ | | | | ♠ | | | |
| SUNFLOWER SEED | | ♠ | | | | | | ♠ | |
| SWEET BASIL | ♠ | | | | | | | ♠ | |
| SWEET POTATO | | ♠ | | | | | | | |
| SWEET RICE | | ♠ | | | | | | ♠ | |
| SWORD BEAN | | ♠ | | | | | | ♠ | |
| TANGERINE ORANGE | | ♠ | ♠ | | | | | | ♠ |
| TARO | ♠ | ♠ | | | | | | | |
| TARO FLOWER | | | | | | | | | |
| TARO LEAF | ♠ | | | | | | | | ♠ |
| THYME | | | | | | | | | |
| TOBACCO | ♠ | | | | | | | ♠ | |
| TOMATO | | ♠ | ♠ | | | ♠ | | | |
| VINEGAR | | | ♠ | ♠ | | | | | |
| WALNUT | | ♠ | | | | | | ♠ | |
| WATER CHESTNUT | | ♠ | | | | ♠ | | | |
| WATERMELON | | ♠ | | | | ♠ | | | |
| WHEAT | | ♠ | | | | | | | ♠ |
| WHEAT BRAN | | ♠ | | | | | | | ♠ |
| WHITE FUNGUS | | ♠ | | | | | | | |
| WHITE SUGAR | | ♠ | | | | | | | |
| WINE | ♠ | ♠ | | ♠ | | | | ♠ | |
| YAM | | ♠ | | | | | | | |

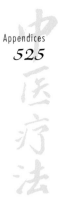

| | Internal Organs | | | | | | | | | | |
|---|---|---|---|---|---|---|---|---|---|---|---|
| NEUTRAL | LUNGS | LARGE INTESTINE | SMALL INTESTINE | GALL BLADDER | BLADDER | LIVER | KIDNEYS | SPLEEN | HEART | STOMACH | OTHERS |
| | | | | | | | | ✓ | ✓ | | |
| ✓ | | | ✓ | | | | | | ✓ | | |
| ✓ | | ✓ | | | | | | | | ✓ | |
| | | | | | | | | | | | |
| | | | | | | | | | | | |
| ✓ | | | | | | ✓ | | | ✓ | | |
| | | ✓ | ✓ | | | | ✓ | | | ✓ | |
| | | | | | | | | | | | |
| | | | | | | | | | | | |
| | | | | | | | | | | | |
| ✓ | | | | | | | | | | ✓ | |
| | | | | | | | | | | | |
| ✓ | | | | | | ✓ | | | | | obstructive & constrictive |
| ✓ | | | | | | | ✓ | ✓ | | | |
| ✓ | | ✓ | | | | | | ✓ | | | |
| | | | | | | | | | | | |
| | | | | | | | | | | | |
| | | ✓ | ✓ | | | | | | | | glossy |
| | | | | | | | | ✓ | | ✓ | |
| | | | | | | ✓ | ✓ | ✓ | | | |
| | | | | | | | | | | | |
| | | | | | | | | | | | |
| ✓ | | | | | | | ✓ | ✓ | | | |
| | ✓ | | | | | | | | | ✓ | |
| ✓ | | | | | | | | | | | |
| | | ✓ | | | | | | ✓ | | ✓ | |
| ✓ | | | | | | | | | | | |
| | ✓ | | | | | | | | | ✓ | |
| | | ✓ | | | | | | | | ✓ | |
| | | | | | | | ✓ | | | ✓ | |
| ✓ | | ✓ | | | | | | | | ✓ | glossy |
| ✓ | | | | | | | | | | | numbing taste |
| | | | | | | | | | | | |
| | | | | | | | | | | | |
| | | | | | | | | | | | |
| | | | | | | | | | | | |
| | | | | | | ✓ | | | | ✓ | |
| | ✓ | | | | | | ✓ | | | | |
| | ✓ | | | | | | | | | ✓ | |
| | | | | | ✓ | | | | ✓ | ✓ | |
| | | | | | | | ✓ | ✓ | ✓ | | |
| | | | | | | | | | | ✓ | |
| ✓ | | | | | | | | | | | glossy |
| ✓ | | | | | | | | ✓ | | | |
| | ✓ | | | | | ✓ | | | | ✓ | |
| ✓ | ✓ | | | | | | ✓ | ✓ | | | |

# *Index*

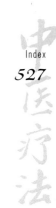